TECHNIQUES OF
VETERINARY RADIOGRAPHY

TECHNIQUES OF VETERINARY RADIOGRAPHY

FIFTH EDITION

Edited by

Joe P. Morgan, D.V.M., Vet med dr

Iowa State University Press / Ames

Joe P. Morgan is Diplomate of the American College of Veterinary Radiology and a Professor in the Department of Radiological Sciences, School of Veterinary Medicine, University of California, Davis.

First edition, 1974; second edition, 1977; originally published by Veterinary Radiology Associates, Davis, Calif. 95617-0222

Third edition, 1982; fourth edition, 1984 (second printing, 1985); copyright © J. P. Morgan and S. Silverman

Fourth edition, 1984 (third through sixth printings, 1987–1990); fifth edition, 1993; copyright © Iowa State University Press, Ames, Iowa 50014

♾ Printed on acid-free paper in the United States of America

Fifth edition, 1993
Second printing, 1993
Third printing, 1994
Fourth printing, 1996

Library of Congress Cataloging-in-Publication Data

Morgan, Joe P.
    Techniques of veterinary radiography/Joe P. Morgan.—5th ed.
         p.   cm.
    Includes bibliographical references and index.
    ISBN 0-8138-1727-7
      1. Veterinary radiography. 2. Veterinary radiography—Methodology. I. Title.
    SF757.8.M685   1993
    636.089′607572—dc20   92-41342

CONTRIBUTORS

Thomas Baker, Principle Radiologic Technologist, Ultrasound Service, Veterinary Medical Teaching Hospital, School of Veterinary Medicine, University of California, Davis.

Uri Bargai, A.B. (Zool.), V.M.D., D.V.Sc., Associate Professor of Radiology, Koret School of Veterinary Medicine, The Hebrew University of Jerusalem, Rehovot, Israel.

John Doval, Senior Artist, Department of Radiological Sciences, School of Veterinary Medicine, University of California, Davis.

John Neves, Staff Research Associate, Large Animal Radiology Service, Veterinary Medical Teaching Hospital, School of Veterinary Medicine, University of California, Davis.

Paul E. Fisher, Staff Research Associate, Department of Radiological Sciences, School of Veterinary Medicine, University of California, Davis.

John Pharr, D.V.M., M.S., Diplomate, American College of Veterinary Radiology, Professor of Radiology, Department of Veterinary Anesthesia, Radiology and Surgery, University of Saskatchewan—Western College of Veterinary Medicine, Saskatoon, Saskatchewan, Canada.

Sam Silverman, D.V.M., Ph.D., Diplomate, American College of Veterinary Radiology, Clinical Professor, Department of Radiological Sciences, School of Veterinary Medicine, University of California, Davis.

Robert Smith, Principle Radiologic Technologist, Small Animal Radiology Service, Veterinary Medical Teaching Hospital, School of Veterinary Medicine, University of California, Davis.

Candi Stafford, Senior Radiologic Technologist, Small Animal Radiology Service, Veterinary Medical Teaching Hospital, School of Veterinary Medicine, University of California, Davis.

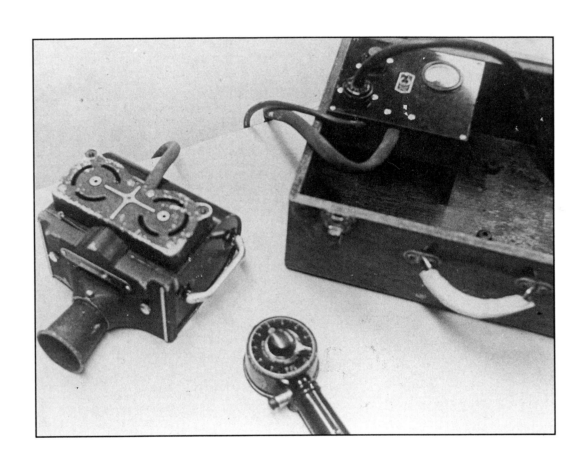

CONTENTS

PREFACE

The final diagnosis of a lesion on a radiograph of a clinic patient is the end product of a series of events comprising the "radiological process". This process consists of three distinct parts: 1) selecting the patient for an appropriate radiological examination, 2) conducting the examination, and 3) interpreting the resulting radiograph. The radiographic interpretation can be subdivided into: 1) the detection of findings, 2) the description of these findings, 3) how they may deviate from a normal pattern, and finally, 4) preparation of a list of diseases, a differential diagnosis, that might cause these particular radiographic findings. It is possible that each part of the process may be performed by a different individual, although, in an average small hospital or clinic, a single individual may be responsible for all three parts. The quality of a radiograph is equated with the visibility of the pertinent findings, since they constitute the raw material from which a diagnosis is made. The visibility of the lesion depends mainly upon the many physical factors chosen to conduct the radiographic examination and this manual is designed to investigate the effects of these physical parameters on the quality of the resultant radiograph. It will become obvious that you need to know about x-rays, their production and usage, if you are to be able to use this valuable diagnostic technique.

Little similarity remains between Veterinary Radiology today and the time of the first edition of this manual in 1974. Major changes have taken place in equipment production with solid state construction that requires only a few self-contained components, integrated circuit timers, digital read-out control panels, and silicon controlled rectifiers. Wet-tank processing was important at the time of the first edition, while table-top automatic processors are now economically feasible and used commonly. This means the concept of film artifacts has changed completely with the frequency of artifacts being less, however, the type of artifacts is entirely different. Increase in the speed of film-screen systems makes many radiographic studies possible that could not be considered earlier because of the problem of patient motion. The manual remains directed toward those who are studying about diagnostic radiology and those who are performing radiographic examinations in a clinical setting. This includes the student in Veterinary Medicine or a student in an Animal Health Technician Program, in addition to those performing diagnostic radiographic studies in a clinic or hospital.

The manual is written so that it can serve as the basic text for the student enrolled in a course in Radiography in a curriculum in Veterinary Medicine or in a curriculum training Animal Health Technicians. For those in practice, the format remains that of a "loose-leaf" manual that is most valuable when placed near the x-ray machine where it is readily available for referral during the radiographic examinations.

The advent of Ultrasound has created an entirely new diagnostic technique for evaluation of disease in animals that has in part replaced diagnostic radiology. Since it is a non-painful study, usually does not require anesthesia, and causes no injury to the patient, it has become a most attractive diagnostic procedure. We have, in this edition, introduced the basic aspects of ultrasound equipment and the method of its operation. For those beginning their training, this provides an introduction to this fascinating diagnostic procedure.

It is impossible to list all of the individuals who have contributed to the editions of this manual. Much of what was good in the first editions has been carried over into this edition, while much new information and many new figures have been included. In an effort to recognize the contributions of these people, authors have been listed for each of the separate chapters. I have played a role of coordinating these contributions and fitting them in place within the manual.

Davis, CA January 1993
Joe P. Morgan, DVM, Vet. med. dr.

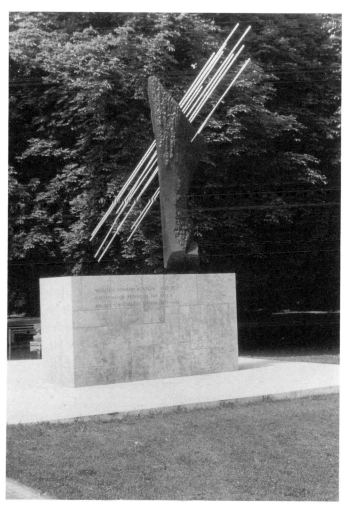

MONUMENT TO WILHELM CONRAD RONTGEN (1845-1923)
Professor of Experimental Physics at Wurzburg University. Discoverer of x-rays.

SECTION A

X-RAY TO
FINAL RADIOGRAPH

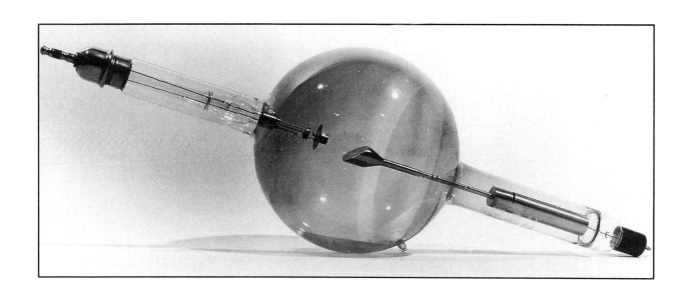

1. RADIATION PHYSICS

A. ATOMIC STRUCTURE

A discussion of the structure of matter will provide the reader with definitions and an understanding of matter that will make certain concepts easier to understand when discussed later in the book. Atomic structure consists of two major components, nuclear and orbital (Fig. 1-1). The nucleus consists of two types of particles. The positively charged particles, <u>protons</u>, have a positive charge and a large mass approximately 1900 times that of an electron. The number of protons in a nucleus defines the atom with the letter, Z, equalling the atomic number of the atom. In addition to the protons, the nucleus contains <u>neutrons</u> that have no charge and a large mass similar to that of the proton. The number of neutrons is indicated by the letter, N. The <u>mass number</u> (A) of the atom equals the number of protons (Z) and neutrons (N) (A=Z+N). Electrostatic repulsion and nuclear forces holds the nucleus together with an energy that increases as the Z of the element increases.

Orbital electrons have a negative charge and remain outside the nucleus because of their high velocity and small mass. The number of electrons equals the number of protons. Electron energy is important in the production of x-rays and it is necessary to understand the role electrons play within the atom (Fig 1-1). Specific numbers of electrons are positioned in shells or energy levels around the nucleus and are numbered K for the inner shell, L for the next shell, M for the next shell, up to the outermost shell or the Q shell. They have a high centripital force (electrostatic attractive force) exerted by the nucleus that keeps the electrons from escaping and this force must be overcome if the electron is to become free. The energy required to remove an electron from the atom is termed the <u>binding energy</u> for that electron and the energy level is unique for a particular shell electron in a particular atom (Table 1-1).

Table 1-1
K-SHELL ELECTRON BINDING ENERGIES OF ELEMENTS IMPORTANT IN DIAGNOSTIC RADIOLOGY

Atomic number	Atom	K-shell energy (keV)
6	Carbon	0.284
7	Nitrogen	0.400
8	Oxygen	0.532
13	Aluminum	1.560
20	Calcium	4.038
39	Yttrium	17.00
50	Tin	29.20
53	Iodine	33.17
56	Barium	37.44
57	Lanthanum	38.90
64	Gadolinium	50.20
74	Tungsten	69.53
82	Lead	88.00

Binding energies are greater for inner shell electrons and decrease with increasing distance from the nucleus. As the Z number of the atom increases, the binding energy of the electrons also increases because the nuclear charge increases. Binding energies are thought of as being negative because they represent amounts of energy which must be supplied to the atom to release the electron from its position. Binding energies are measured in electron volts (eV). Any vacancy existing within an electron shell is promptly filled by electrons cascading from lower energy levels at a greater distance from the nucleus. During the shifting of electrons, the difference in binding energies between the original and final energy level of the electron is released as a photon of energy. This excess in energy is considered an x-ray photon if its energy exceeds a level of 100 electron volts (eV). Remember that an electron volt is the amount of energy that an electron gains as it is accelerated by a potential difference of 1 volt. When these forms of energy are sufficient to cause release of electrons from the atoms with which they interact, they are referred to as <u>ionizing radiation.</u>

Later in the book we will find that the amount of energy possessed by an electron is important in production of x-rays and in determining the ability of the x-ray to penetrate tissue. This energy is described as an electron volt (eV) and is the amount of energy that an electron gains as it is accelerated by a potential difference of 1 volt. <u>Voltage</u> is a way of describing the potential energy that can be held by an electron and is similar to the energy held by a block of wood because of its location on a tabletop. When the block is pushed from the tabletop, it expresses its energy by hitting your foot which is on the floor. An electron can be given potential energy (eV) by expressing an electrical potential difference between two wires. When electrons are available that can move between the wires, this flow of electrons (electrical current) can be measured in <u>amperage</u> (numbers

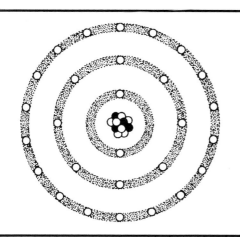

Fig. 1-1
SCHEMATIC REPRESENTATION OF AN ATOM
A model of an atom with the nucleus containing protons and neutrons as shown by the solid and hollow spheres in the center. The hollow spheres shown in the peripheral rings around the nucleus represent the electrons that rotate around the nucleus.

of electrons) and permits the potential energy difference to be expressed. A block of wood has potential energy (eV) as it rests on the tabletop but the block needs to move to express its potential. If it falls through gravity, similar to flow of electrons, it expresses its energy when it strikes your foot. Electrons can have potential energy but need to flow through a wire or "jump" across a gap in the wire to express their energy.

Electrons can flow through a wire (conductor) in one direction only and this flow is referred to as <u>direct current</u> (DC). It is also possible for the flow to alternate in the direction of flow and this flow is referred to as <u>alternating current</u> (AC). The flow of electrical energy in our homes and businesses is AC with the change in direction being 120 times per second in the United States. Later in the book we will see how x-rays are produced within the x-ray tube and how the character of flow of electrical energy influences how efficient this production is.

B. RADIATION

Radiation needs to be defined at this point in your reading, since you are studying about x-rays which are one form of radiation. A very general definition of radiation is <u>the propagation of energy through space and matter</u>. Two different types of radiation are recognized, one is <u>particulate,</u> or <u>corpuscular,</u> and the other is <u>electromagnetic.</u>

<u>Particulate radiation</u> is the transport of energy through space with the energy contained in moving particles of matter that are usually submolecular in nature. The level of energy contained by the particulate radiation is dependent on the mass and speed of the particle and the energy is disseminated through a "billiard ball" effect. The particles have a finite range that is dependent on their energy and the material through which they are traveling. Particulate radiation may include particles that are electrically charged or are neutral electrically. They include <u>alpha particles</u> (helium nuclei) that consist of 2 neutrons and 2 protons and are similar to the nucleus of a helium atom. Alpha particles have a positive charge and large mass and are emitted by radioactive decay of an atom in which the mass number (A) decreases by 4 and the atomic number (Z) decreases by 2 at the time of release of the alpha particle. <u>Beta particles</u> are another form of particulate radiation and are electrons that have a negative charge and a small mass. Beta particles form through the destruction of a neutron if they are spontaneously emitted by radioactive nuclei. The mass number (A) of the parent atom remains the same during formation of the beta particle while the atomic number (Z) increases by one as a proton is created by the radioactive decay. A second method of creating beta particles (electrons) is to create a beam of electrons (<u>cathode ray</u>) that have been freed from nuclear attraction of their parent atom through the heating of a wire filament. This beam of electrons can be accelerated and made to move across an x-ray tube. Other particulate energy that is not of importance in diagnostic radiology can be found in the form of protons or neutrons.

Because electrons (beta particles) are particulate and charged, they lose energy at a constant rate and their ability to penetrate tissue is limited (usually <<1 mm). In a similar fashion, alpha particles, being even heavier and charged, lose energy rapidly and are capable of penetrating only short distances in tissue (<1 μ). The depth to which an alpha particle or beta particle can penetrate tissue is entirely predictable and is a function of initial energy. The main danger to radiation workers from exposure to alpha particles and beta particles occurs with the ingestion or inhalation of isotopes emitting these radiations that places the isotope within your body at a location near radiosensitive cells.

An excess or lack of neutrons may make the atom radioactive with the release of particulate radiation being a randomly occuring event and is referred to as naturally occurring <u>radioactive decay</u>. It is also possible to produce atoms that undergo radioactive decay with the decay controlled through the manner of generation of the radioactive atom. These atoms are described as being an <u>isotope</u> of an element that possesses the same number of protons (atomic number), however, the number of neutrons (mass number) varies. While this atomic variation is important in the field of nuclear medicine, both diagnostic and therapeutic, it is not important in diagnostic radiology that depends on x-rays. Some particles with a high mass when made to achieve high speeds can be used for radiation therapy in the treatment of malignant tumors.

<u>Electromagnetic radiation</u> is the other major form of radiation and is the transport of energy through space without mass. <u>X-rays</u> are members of the electromagnetic spectrum (Fig. 1-2) and their properties and creation are described in greater detail below. <u>Gamma rays</u> are another form of electromagnetic radiation that are similar to x-rays except that they originate from unstable (radioactive) nucleus as they decay to become more stable. Production of gamma rays from radioactive nuclei is usually associated with emission of some type of particulate radiation as well. The energy spectrum of gamma ray(s) is characteristic for each individual radioisope. Gamma rays have a high energy that cannot be controlled since it is dependent on the radioisotope. They play an important role as a form of radiation therapy in the treatment of malignant tumors.

C. DEFINITION OF X-RAYS

<u>X-rays are a form of radiation that results from the transfer of kinetic energy held by electrons into a form of electromagnetic radiation</u>. Thus, x-rays are a method of propagating energy through space or matter. The energy x-rays carry is sufficient to cause the freeing of electrons from an atom, forming ions, and therefore x-rays are also referred to as <u>ionizing radiation</u>. X-rays, or <u>photons</u>, as members of the electromagnetic spectrum, have different wavelengths and energy levels (Fig. 1-2). The physical properties of x-rays are important in several aspects in the production of radiographs (Table 1-2). The wavelength of an individual photon can vary, and is a function of the energy level with shorter wavelengths possessing greater photon energy. The energy characteristics of a given photon beam can be altered as needed in diagnostic radiology. X-rays travel at a constant speed measured in a vacuum, which is 3×10^{10} cm/second, or the speed of visible light, travel in a straight line, possess

no electrical charge so are not affected by an electromagnetic field, and interact with matter in predictable ways. They penetrate matter dependent on the density of the tissue, atomic number, and the energy of the x-ray photon.

D. PRODUCTION OF X-RAYS

The production of x-rays occurs through the conversion of energy contained within particulate radiation (electrons) to energy within the electromagnetic spectrum (x-rays). A cloud of electrons made to form within the x-ray tube is forced to travel across the tube where the electrons interact with the target material. This electron cloud is referred to as particulate or corpuscular radiation and obeys the rules relative to the propagation of energy through space or matter in the form of moving particles of matter. The velocity of the electrons can be altered and their path is highly influenced by electrical charge. The electrons that travel across the x-ray tube have different energies (measured in keV). The energy of the electrons is determined by a setting on the x-ray machine that determines kilovoltage of the x-ray beam. Electrons of 100 keV (thousand electron volts) energy can produce x-rays with an energy of 100 kVp (kilovolts).

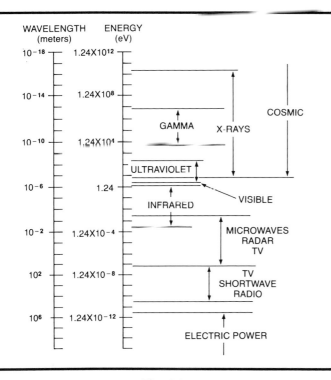

Fig. 1-2
ELECTROMAGNETIC SPECTRUM
Members of the electromagnetic spectrum with appropriate wavelength and energy levels. They are conveniently divided into: (1) short wavelength and high energy—cosmic rays, gamma rays, and x-rays, (2) medium wavelength and medium energy—visible light, ultraviolet light, and infrared rays, and (3) long wavelength and low energy—television waves and radio waves.

Table 1-2
PHYSICAL PROPERTIES OF X-RAY PHOTONS

1. Speed of the photons is constant, unchangeable, and equal to that of light in a vacuum (3×10^{10} cm/sec).
2. Wavelength of the photons is variable and inversely related to the energy of the photon.
3. Photons cannot be reflected or refracted in the manner of visible light.
4. Photons possess no electrical charge and are unaffected by magnetic or electrical fields.
5. Travel of the photons is in a straight line until there is interaction with matter after which, direction of the primary photons can be altered.
6. Photon interaction with matter is through absorption (photoelectric absorption) or scatter (Compton scatter).
7. Penetration of tissue by the photons is dependent on the energy of the photon and the density and atomic number of the tissue.
8. Average photon beam energy is increased after penetrating absorbers and the change in energy is referred to as attenuation or beam hardening.
9. Photons interact with certain substances causing fluorescence (emission of radiation within the visible spectrum).
10. Photons interact with photographic emulsion causing changes made visible through chemical processing of the film.
11. Photons interact causing ionization of gases resulting in ions that are electrically conductive.
12. Photon interact with living tissue causing both somatic and genetic damage.

When the electron beam interacts with the target on the other side of the x-ray tube, the energetic (high speed) electrons lose their energy, and x-rays are produced. There are two different methods by which this occurs. One method is the result of sudden deceleration of the electrons as they respond to the electrical field of the atomic nuclei in the target material. When a negatively charged electron passes near the nucleus of a tungsten atom in the target of the x-ray tube, the positive charge of the nucleus acts on the negative charge of the electron, causing a sudden change in direction of travel toward the nucleus and a marked deceleration of the electron. The kinetic energy lost through this process of radiative interaction is called <u>general radiation</u> or <u>Bremsstrahlung</u> (from the German "bremsen," to brake) (Fig. 1-3).

The energy of the resulting photon varies, being dependent on the energy of the incoming electron, but cannot exceed that energy. The maximum energy of the electron and, therefore, the maximum energy of a resulting photon are dependent on the kVp setting of the x-ray machine. To create a maximum energy photon, loss of <u>all</u> of the electron's energy is required through <u>one</u> interaction in the creation of <u>one</u> photon. However, in most interactions, the electron gives up only a part of its energy so that a continuous spectrum of energies is produced in the resulting photons. The resulting beam containing many different energy photons is referred to as <u>heterogenic</u>, <u>heterochromic</u>, or <u>polychromic</u>. The ability of an atomic nucleus within the target material to affect the path of an electron is related to the positive charge of the atom. The higher the atomic number (Z), of the target material, the greater the probability usable x-rays will be produced. Much of the energy carried by the incoming electron beam is unfortunately lost by conversion into heat and not into useful x-rays. Most of the photons produced when the electron beam interacts with the target are low-energy general radiation or Bremsstrahlung. The relative percentage is dependent on x-ray tube voltage (Table 1-3).

A second method of x-ray production, called <u>characteristic or line radiation</u>, follows the removal of one of the tightly held electrons and subsequent electron rearrangement within the atoms in the target material. A statistically determined probability exists that one of the incoming electrons will collide with an electron tightly bound in one electron shell of an atom of target material, creating the possibility of ejection of that electron. The resulting vacancy in the electron shell is filled immediately by: (1) an electron from an adjacent ring within the same atom, (2) an electron from a ring within another atom, or (3) by a free electron (Fig. 1-4). The energy of the resulting photon of energy exactly equals the difference in the binding energies between that of the electron ejected and that of the replacement electron. This "filling" process can take place in a single transition with one photon emitted or

Table 1-3
RELATIVE PERCENTAGES OF
X-RAY PHOTONS EMITTED

Tube Voltage (kVp)	Characteristic Radiation %	General Radiation %
80	10	90
100	19	81
120	24	76
150	28	72

*(Ter-Pogossian, M.M., 1967)

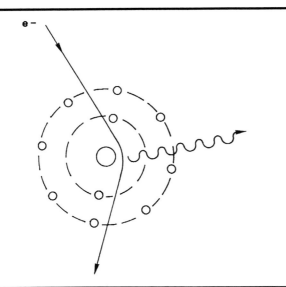

Fig. 1-3
GENERAL OR BREMSSTRAHLUNG RADIATION
An electron is made free by heating the filament or cathode of the x-ray tube and is accelerated toward the anode because of the difference in electrical charge. If the incident electron passes close to the nucleus of an atom in the target, it is attracted by the positively charged nucleus, and the direction of its path and its speed are both altered. This interaction results in the release of an x-ray photon of energy referred to as general or Bremsstrahlung radiation. Usually, the electron gives up only a portion of the energy it carries and continues to travel in a new direction after the interaction.

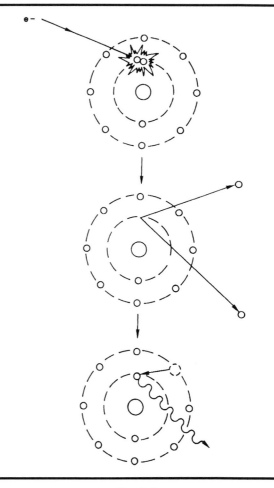

Fig. 1-4
CHARACTERISTIC RADIATION
An electron is made free by heating the filament or cathode of the x-ray tube and is accelerated toward the anode because of the difference in electrical charge. An incident electron with sufficient energy (in excess of 70 keV) may strike an inner shell electron within the tungsten target causing its ejection from an atom within the target and the impinging electron continues with a lower energy level. The vacancy in the inner electron shell of an atom of the tungsten target is quickly filled by an electron from one of the adjacent shells or by a free electron. The difference in the binding energies of the two electrons is emitted as a characteristic x-ray photon.

through multiple transitions with multiple lower energy photons emitted. Thus, for any given atom, there is a finite set of x-ray energies that can be produced, depending on which electron is ejected and which electron fills the void. Since electron binding energy increases with the size of the nucleus, materials with high Z are more likely to produce useable characteristic x-rays. It should be emphasized that the incident electron per se is not converted into a photon; rather it is the kinetic energy of the electron that is converted into photons and heat energy. After the electron gives up all of its energy through interaction with atoms within the target, the electron simply continues to flow within the electrical circuit of the x-ray tube where it receives a new energy potential. The relative percentage of characteristic radiation is dependent on x-ray tube voltage (Table 1-3).

The resulting spectrum of energies of the photons produced in these two ways can be drawn (Fig. 1-5). The shortest wave length photon produced is dependent on an interaction in which all of the energy carried by the electron within the cathode beam is lost through one Bremsstrahlung interaction. Following this maximum energy level is a curve showing production of other photons of progressively decreasing energy. Superimposed over this curve are spikes showing the production of characteristic radiation, the energy of which is determined by the energy levels of the electrons within the atoms of the target material. The different energies of the spikes reflect the differences in binding energy between the specific electron that was displaced and the energy of the replacing electron and are thus specific for the target material. Since electron binding energy increases with the size of the nucleus, high Z atoms are more likely to produce useable characteristic z-rays and this is one reason the anode of the x-ray tube is made of a high Z atom such as tungsten.

Because of the use of alternating current to supply the x-ray machine, the voltage varies rapidly between zero and the maximum voltage supplied by the high voltage power supply. This, plus the fact that the Bremsstrahlung photons vary in energy from zero to the maximum electron energy, means that many low energy x-ray photons are produced with few having the maximum energy that permits them to participate in the effective or useful x-ray beam. The resulting x-ray beam is described as being polychromatic, that is, as the beam leaves the target within the x-ray tube, it contains photons of varying energy levels. The number of photons within the beam is immediately reduced because many have a lesser energy and are not able to escape from the x-ray tube glass envelope. Since the x-rays travel in all directions at the time of production, the number of photons in the useful x-ray beam is further reduced because only a small percentage of the x-ray beam passes through the tube window to the outside. These features determine the longest wave length photon seen on the curve representing the spectrum of energies produced (Fig. 1-5). The heterochromatic primary x-ray beam as it leaves the tube has an average energy that is between one-half to one-third of the energy of the highest energy photon produced.

In later chapters you will learn how the pattern of energies found within the emerging x-ray beam can also be affected by changes made by controlling the energy of the electrons that flow across the x-ray tube. Also by increasing the number of electrons that flow across the x-ray tube the number of x-rays produced can be changed. Both the energy limits and the maximum number of x-rays produced are determined at the time of x-ray machine construction. In addition, we will learn that the energy level of the x-ray beam is influenced by filtration of the x-ray beam because the mean energy of the beam increases as it passes through any material which acts as an attenuator through the selective absorption of a higher percentage of the lower energy photons.

This implies that the number and energy of the x-ray photons is precisely determined through the machine settings. This is not always true and the reproducibility of an exposure made with similar machine settings may vary as much as 18 to 75 % in smaller portable units to as little as ± 5% in larger units.

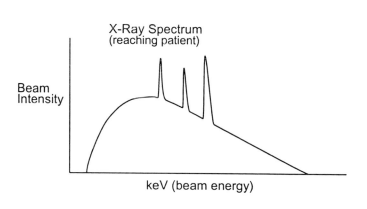

Fig. 1-5
SPECTRUM OF PHOTON PRODUCTION
A curve with spikes showing the intensity and energy level of photons produced in the x-ray tube through interaction of the cathode beam with the target. Energy of the characteristic radiation (spikes) is dependent on the target atom and the electron shell from which the replacement electron was derived. The shortest wavelength photon (most energetic) is dependent on the kVp setting and occurs with the transfer of total energy from an electron through Bremsstrahlung interaction. Notice how the energy of the beam within the x-ray tube is changed by absorption of the low energy portion by the tube housing.

2. X-RAY TUBE

The purpose of the x-ray tube is to produce in the shortest time possible a beam of x-ray photons in which the number and mean energy of the photons can be determined. The penetrating power (mean energy) and the number of x-rays produced must be controllable to permit selection of the photon beam to be used for a radiographic examination. The x-ray tube provides for: (1) a source of electrons, (2) a method of accelerating the electron beam, (3) a glass envelope to maintain an evacuated path in which the accelerated electrons can travel, (4) a target in which the electrons interact with the kinetic energy of the electrons changed into x-ray photons or heat, and (5) a method of heat dissipation. All of this is within a lead shield that offers protection from radiation exposure to the user. The tube is called a diode because of the two principle components, the cathode and the anode, and an x-ray tube is, therefore, a special type of diode tube (Figs. 2-1, 2-2).

A. CATHODE

The <u>cathode</u> is the electrically negative side of the x-ray tube and is made of a fine tungsten-rhenium wire filament placed within a metallic cup and is referred to as the <u>filament</u> because of its physical appearance (Figs. 2-1, 2-3). The purpose of the cathode is: (1) to serve as the source of electrons for x-ray production and (2) to direct the flow of the electrons toward the anode. By heating the filament to a temperature of about 2000° C, the electrons are held less tightly by the nucleus of the atom and if the energy level exceeds the binding energy of the electrons, a cloud of electrons forms around the filament. This phenomenon is called <u>thermionic emission</u>. The number of electrons that are "boiled off" is determined by the temperature of the filament, which is directly controlled by the milliamperage (mA) setting on the x-ray machine. Tungsten is used in construction of the cathode filament

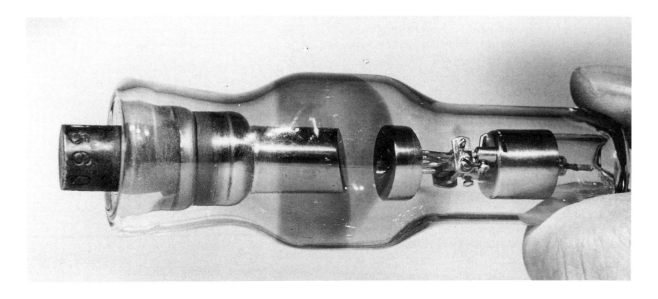

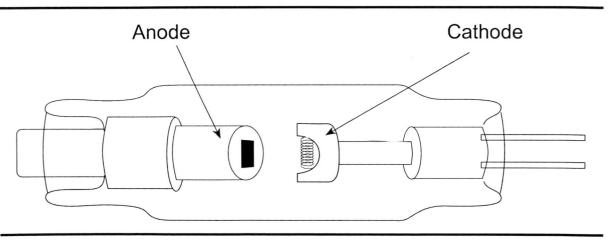

Fig. 2-1
STATIONARY ANODE X-RAY TUBE
A photograph and drawing of a stationary anode x-ray tube. Note the absence of any moving parts. The cathode with filament is on the right and the target is embedded within the non-moving anode on the left. The small size of the tube can be appreciated when comparing it with the size of the fingers holding the tube.

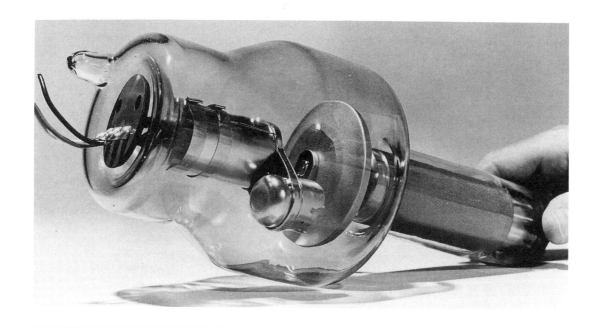

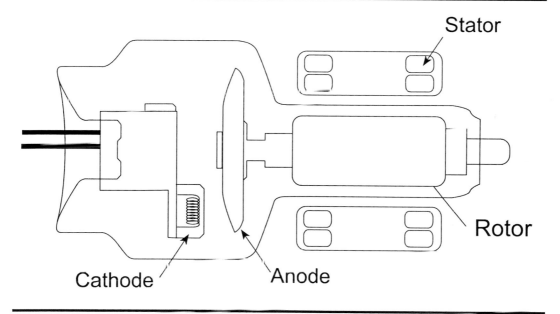

Fig. 2-2
ROTATING ANODE X-RAY TUBE
A photograph and drawing of a rotating anode x-ray tube. The cathode with filament is on the left displaced from the tube axis. The target is on the surface of the disc shaped anode on the right. The focal spot is seen to be on the edge of the disc.

because of its high melting point (3410° C) and a vapor pressure that prevents the wire from vaporizing at the high temperatures imposed. The wire forming the filament is small, only about 0.2 mm in diameter. It may help to think of the thin filament within an electrical lightbulb becoming "red-hot" when the lightbulb is turned on as being analogous to heating the filament within an x-ray tube at the time an exposure is made.

The filament sits within a cavity or <u>focusing cup</u> that is maintained at the same negative potential as the heated filament. The cup is made of molybdenum that has a high melting point and is a poor conductor of heat. Therefore, a repulsive charge from the focusing cup tends to direct the electrons toward a relatively small area on the target, preventing them from traveling in all directions and interacting with the wall of the x-ray tube. It is possible to place two wires of different sizes adjacent to each other. A selection is made of which wire is to be heated with the resulting electron beam being directed across the tube. More recent developements in cathode construction have the surfaces of the cathode head inclined inwards toward each other so that the electrons that originate from the two different sized filaments are directed toward the same area on the target. The level of heat supplied to the filament(s) is determined by the low-tension circuit of the x-ray machine.

B. ANODE

The <u>anode</u> is the electrically positive side of the x-ray tube (Figs. 2-1, 2-2, 2-3). The anode serves four functions and: (1) provides a structure for placement of the target, (2) receives electrons and provides for their interaction with the target producing x-ray photons, (3) further conducts electrons through the tube to the connecting cables and back to the high-voltage section of the x-ray machine, and (4) the copper construction accommodates the tremendous heat production. The <u>target</u> is defined as the area of the anode struck by the electron beam. Because more than 99% of the energy within the electron beam is converted to heat energy at the time of interaction of the electron beam with the target, the basic construction of the anode must deal with this massive heat accumulation. The amount of heat that the target can withstand and the rate of dissipation of the heat are of great importance in determining the maximum quantity and quality of the x-ray photons produced.

<u>Tungsten</u> is chosen as the material of choice for the target because of its: (1) high atomic number (74) that results in higher-efficiency x-ray production and higher-energy x-ray production, (2) thermal conductivity that is nearly equal to that of copper and thus is efficient in dissipating heat, and (3) high melting point (3410°C) that accepts the high tube current without pitting. Newer rotating anodes are built up from three separate layers with a substrate of molydenum, alloyed with titanium and zirconium that is covered with a layer of tungsten alloyed with rhenium. By compressing the layers in a single blow from a heavy press, discs are formed that are not subject to cracking from high temperatures.

There are two basic types of anode construction that strongly influence x-ray tube function;: (1) <u>stationary anode</u> and (2) <u>rotating anode</u>.

The <u>stationary anode</u> consists of a small plate of tungsten embedded in the end of a copper cylinder (Fig. 2-1). Despite the high melting point of the tungsten, a copper cylinder is still needed to rapidly dissipate the heat generated during an exposure. The tungsten block sits on the end of the copper cylinder with the surface of the tungsten plate at a predetermined angle of 15° to 22.5°. An advantage of this type of tube, which is found in small portable x-ray units, is that there are no moving parts. Therefore, it has a long lifetime and is difficult to damage if treated with care. The production and elimination of heat is the limiting factor in the size of an exposure that can be obtained through use of a stationary anode.

The <u>rotating anode</u> consists of a plate or disc on a slender molybdenum stem with the target material coated along a path around the edge of the disc (Figs. 2-2, 2-3).

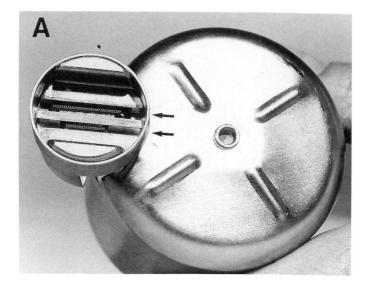

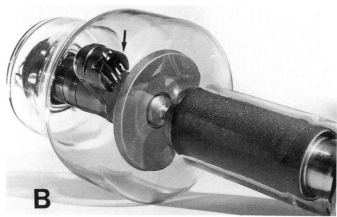

Fig. 2-3
X-RAY TUBE CATHODE
A photograph of the cathode assembly (A) with the filaments (arrows) within the focusing cup of the cathode from a rotating anode x-ray tube (B). The "en face" view shows the filaments sitting within the focusing cup. The filaments are of differing sizes and produce electrons beams of differing size partially determining the focal spot size of the tube.

Molybdenum is used in construction of the anode because of its high melting point and because the weight is only one-half of tungsten thus permitting higher speed rotation. Contrary to the construction of the stationary anode tube, the stem in the rotating anode tube must provide a barrier to heat transfer between the anode and the bearings of the anode assembly. Molybdenum was selected for the stem because it has a high melting point (2600° C) and is a poor conductor of heat. Diameter of anode discs are 3 to 5 inches (75 to 100 mm). Newer anode discs are constructed of a bimetal unit of tungsten and molybdenum that are sintered together and have 200 mm diameters. The angle of the target surface is much smaller than in the stationary anode tube, usually 10° to 17°, increasing radiographic detail because the x-ray beam originates from what is essentially a point source.

By rotating the disc during the exposure, the surface area of target material with which the electron beam can interact is greatly increased, up to several hundred times more area for election beam interaction than is found in a stationary anode tube (Fig. 2-4). This results in dissipation of the heat produced over a larger target area and permits the production of many more photons for a single exposure resulting in the use of much higher mA exposures within much shorter exposure times. The speed of rotation of the rotating anode varies with revolutions per minute of 3,000 and 3,600 being common. High speed rotating anodes achieve speeds of 8,000 to 10,500 rpm. The "whirring" noise made by the rotating anode can be heard easily prior to the exposure. Because of the moving parts, these tubes are much more expensive to produce than stationary anode tubes and are more subject to damage with improper use.

Rotation of the anode at high speeds was not accomplished without overcoming many difficulties. High speed anode rotation requires excellent bearing surfaces that must function satisfactorily over a wide range of temperatures. Another problem to overcome was discovery of a satisfactory method of lubrication of vacuum-enclosed bearing surfaces.

It is important to understand that the electron beam remains fixed in position within the tube and only the anode rotates. The rotating anode disc plus the anode stem is often referred to as a "rotor" and is actually a part of an electromagnetic induction motor that creates anode rotation. The other portion of the electromagnetic induction motor consists of the stationary windings positioned outside the glass envelope and is referred to as the "stator" or the stationary part of the anode. It is formed of a series of electromagnets equally spaced around the neck of the x-ray tube (Fig. 2-5).

The term <u>focal spot</u> defines the area on the target in either type of anode tube that is bombarded by the electron beam during the exposure and from which the x-ray beam originates. Size of the focal spot is determined by: (1) length of the filament coil used to generate the electron beam, (2) structure and function of the focusing cup, and (3) position of the filament within the focusing cup. The <u>actual focal spot size</u>, which determines the heat distribution and thus limits the rate of x-ray production, is determined by viewing the focal spot perpendicularly to its surface. By looking through the window of the x-ray tube at an angle to the target surface, a smaller <u>effective</u> or <u>projected focal spot</u> can be identified (Fig. 2-6). The effective focal spot size, or effective target area, is the area projected onto the x-ray

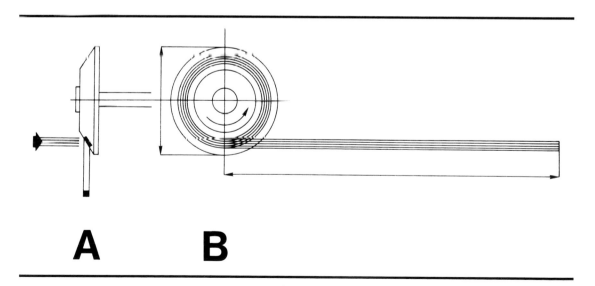

A   **B**

Fig. 2-4
FOCAL SPOT AS DRAWN FROM A ROTATING ANODE TUBE
A drawing of an edge-on projection of the rotating anode (A) shows the small size of the focal spot on the rotating disc being struck by the electron beam (arrow). The "en face" projection of the rotating anode (B) shows the total target area on the anode face displayed on the disc and also displayed in a linear manner. The total target area on the rotating anode tube through which heat can be dissipated is much larger than the target area in the stationary anode tube.

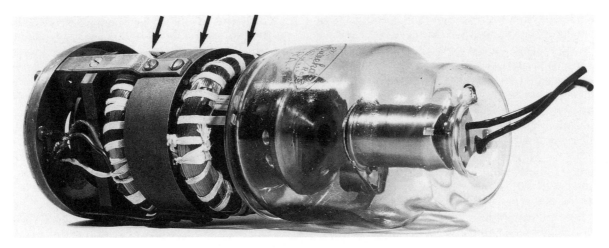

Fig. 2-5
ELECTROMAGNETIC INDUCTION MOTOR
The rotating anode disc plus the anode stem is often referred to as a "rotor" and is actually a part of an electromagnetic induction motor that creates anode rotation. The second portion of the electromagnetic induction motor consists of the stationary windings positioned outside the glass envelope and is referred to as the "stator". It is formed of a series of electromagnets equally spaced around the neck of the x-ray tube (arrows).

film and determines resolution characteristics of the x-ray beam and radiographic detail. The smaller the effective focal spot size, the greater is the detail or sharpness of the images created on the film. However, as the focal spot size decreases, the heating of the target is concentrated to the smaller area thus limiting the size of the electron beam that can be safely used. Focal spot size is more easily determined on examination of a stationary anode tube since it is possible to visualize the discolored square area on the target (Fig. 2-1). In a rotating anode tube, the location and size of the focal spot is much smaller and remains fixed in space while the anode rotates (Fig. 2-2).

The primary x-ray beam that takes origin from the anode is not of equal intensity throughout. It is more intense toward the cathode end of the tube and rather quickly diminishes toward the anode end of the tube (Fig. 2-7). This difference in beam intensity is due to: (1) most electron-target interactions occuring deep to the surface of the target so escape of the resulting photons is greater in the zone perpendicular to the surface where the target is not as thick, (2) the greater focal-film distance to the margin of the field than to the center of the field causing around a 7% decrease in beam intensity around the margin, and (3) the variation in the thickness of the filter through which the beam passes resulting in a greater thickness at the margin of the field causing around 4% decrease in beam intensity. This difference in beam intensity can be recognized only in the event that you are using the largest size film and a low kVp beam setting such as might be observed in radiography of birds. The difference is called the "heel" effect. In the past, it has been stated that the heaviest part of the patient should

be at the cathode end of the table to take advantage of the "heel" effect. With faster film-screen systems and the use of higher kVp techniques, it is uncommon to see the "heel" effect on a radiograph and positioning of the patient is therefore not as critical.

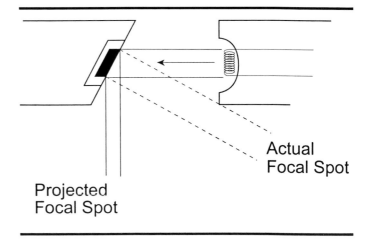

Fig. 2-6
FOCAL SPOT AS DRAWN FROM A STATIONARY ANODE TUBE
A drawing shows the electron beam (arrow) produced by the cathode striking the angled target surface. The size of the actual focal spot is determined by viewing the target perpendicular to its surface. The projected focal spot is determined by viewing the target at an angle through the window of the x-ray tube. Note the difference in size between the actual and projected focal spot.

Most diagnostic x-ray tubes have two focal spots or dual focal spots, one large and the other small, matching the two different sized filaments within the cathode (Fig. 2-3). The smaller filament in the cathode produces the smaller focal spot while the larger filament produces the larger focal spot. The small focal spot is used when finer detail images are required and the mA setting can be low. Use of the large focal spot results in a decrease in film detail but must be used when higher mA settings are required that produce more heat. The selection of the focal spot to be used in a given exposure is made with the mA station selector on the control console and is often indicated by the use of the letters "S" or "L" or the words "small" or "large". Small focal spots (projected) range in size from 0.3 to 1.0 mm while large focal spots usually range from 1.0 to 2.5 mm.

C. TUBE ENVELOPE

The technical properties of glass are remarkable and glass envelopes have been used for most tube construction up to the past few years. Glass serves simultaneously as a vacuum vessel and high-voltage insulator, and as the mechanical carrier of vibrating and incandescent electrodes (Fig. 2-1, 2-2, 2-3). A thin region in the tube envelope allows the primary x-ray beam to exit with a part of the low energy radiation filtered out. The envelope is able to expand and contract due to the heat produced during photon production. The vacuum prevents collision of electrons with air molecules and prevents oxidation of the hot filament. Partial loss of the vacuum results in a "gassy" tube with loss in emitted useful radiation.

It has been noted that high-output tubes last longer when the glass envelope is replaced by a metal envelope. This is because the electron current flowing across the tube "sprays" back from the anode, like a high-pressure water jet, and bombards the walls of the tube with electrons and ions. During the life of the tube, metal atoms from the incandescent filament and focal spot are also deposited on the walls of the glass envelope. In the course of time, these metal deposits inevitably affect the surface of the glass and its insulating properties. It was observed that metal shielding within the tube enabled heat conduction and electrical conduction to be better controlled. A window made of a material with minimal x-ray absorption such as beryllium can easily be incorporated into a metal tube envelope. This permits emission of low energy photons that would otherwise be absorbed by the glass envelope.

D. TUBE OR MACHINE HOUSING

The housing is the heavy metallic structure visible from the outside that covers the x-ray tube, or if it is a small portable type, it covers the entire x-ray machine (Fig. 2-8). The housing is lined internally with lead which prevents the escape of x-ray photons and is thus important in radiation protection. Within the lead shielding is an opening that coincides with the x-ray tube window, creating an exit port for the primary x-ray beam. This is the site of attachment for the externally located device that can be used to control the size of the x-ray beam. The housing also contains insulating oil to protect the operator from electrical hazards present because of the high kilovoltage potential within the electrical cables attached to the housing. Newer and more expensive x-ray units are planned that have a much smaller modified electrical transformer within the tube housing, thus eliminating the high tension cables that are so commonly seen leading to the tube housing.

Lightweight x-ray units are available that use a cooling gas instead of heavy oil to eliminate a great deal of the tubehead weight. These units have a very low error factor in beam reproducability but cost more than conventional portable x-ray units.

E. CAUSES OF X-RAY TUBE FAILURE

Causes of x-ray tube failure or malfunction are usually related to the thermal characteristics of the tube, and are important since the cost of replacement tubes is high. Stationary anode tubes are difficult to damage and breakage usually occurs as a result of dropping the machine with the enclosed tube. Damage to tubes with a rotating anode is much more common and almost 95% of the damaged x-ray tubes requiring replacement are the result of operator technical error (Thompson, 1983). Common operator errors cause increased heat accumulation within the tube and lead to: (1) filament evaporation, (2) broken filaments, (3) cracked

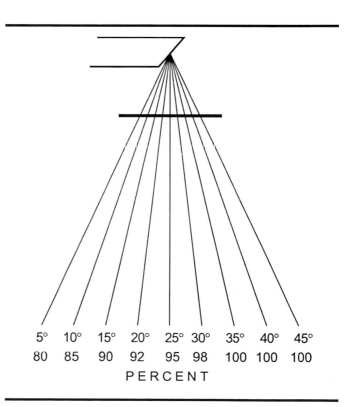

5°	10°	15°	20°	25°	30°	35°	40°	45°
80	85	90	92	95	98	100	100	100

PERCENT

Fig. 2-7
DISTRIBUTION OF X-RAY PHOTONS WITHIN THE PRIMARY BEAM
Differences in the numbers of the x-ray photons within the x-ray beam are plotted relative to an angle measured from the plane of the target on the anode face. This drawing is of a tube with approximately a 22° angle of the target face. This phenomonon of unequal beam intensity creates what is referred to as the "heel effect".

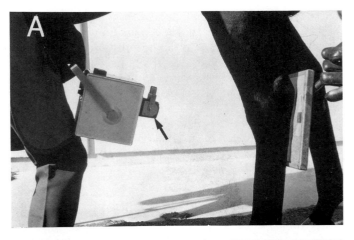

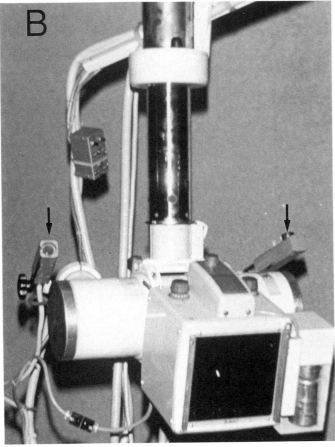

anodes, (3) anode melting or pitting, and (4) "burned-out" or "frozen" bearings. Most of these types of damage are controllable and their prevention would result in significantly extending the useful life of the x-ray tube.

Filament vaporization is probably the most common cause of tube failure, occuring in about 33% of all tube failure and results: (1) from high-mA operation for prolonged periods of time, or (2) from activating the switch, providing full heat to the filament for prolonged periods of time prior to making exposures. This is called the "boost and hold" method of exposure. Because of the high temperature of the filament, tungsten atoms are slowly vaporized and plate the inside of the glass envelope altering the electrical balance within the x-ray tube. The filament wire eventually becomes thin due to the tungsten vaporization and may break causing an nonfunctioning tube (Fig. 2-9).

The filament is built to last for approximately 500 minutes "on-time" when operated at a temperature required to produce an x-ray beam. By using the shortest time to bring the filament to maximum temperature, plus the exposure times, each exposure time probably consists of a total of 2 seconds. Under these conditions, 15,000

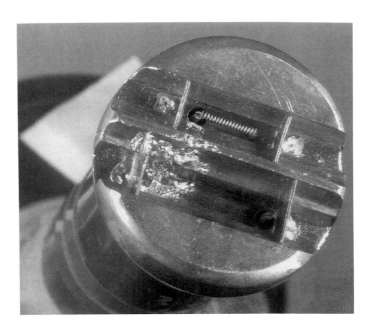

Fig. 2-9
CATHODE INJURY
A photograph of an x-ray tube in which filament evaporation has been caused by excessively high filament temperatures. The resulting accumulation of tungsten on the inside of the glass envelope due to this vaporization causes arcing of the electrom beam toward these sites and may cause a point of high temperature and resulting fracture of the glass envelope. Eventually filament evaporation causes a non-functioning tube.

Fig. 2-8
X-RAY TUBE HOUSING
Photographs of x-ray units with the tube housing covering the tube and the entire x-ray machine (A). A non-illuminating beam collimator (arrow) is attached at the exit port of the housing and creates an opening that permits the escape of the primary x-ray beam. A ceiling suspended x-ray tube has the tube housing covering only the x-ray tube (B). The controls for this unit are present on the tube head (arrows).

exposures are possible. If, however, the "boost-and-hold" technique is used, each exposure could easily reach a total of 5 seconds. This means that only 6,000 exposures are possible. The "boost-and-hold" method should be avoided if the patient is not correctly positioned or everything is not prepared for the examination.

One company that produces x-ray tubes has determined that 40% of all tube failures were because of thermal overloading that caused <u>anode cracking</u> in rotating anode tubes. This results from thermal shock caused by making a high temperature exposure on a cold anode. Anode cracking in the form of a large radial crack destroys the balance of the anode and resulting destruction of the tube. Warming up the tube in a way that the entire anode is slowly and evenly heated prevents this problem. Use warm-up procedures, for example, such as 3 exposures at 100 mA, 60 kVp and 1/10 seconds with a 10 second delay between each exposure. This will pre-heat the anode to a degree that pre-heating is required only once each day prior to the first radiographic study. When a maximum exposure is made, the anode is pre-heated and there is less chance of its cracking due to overheating. Although preheating the anode prior to exposure is of extreme importance when using a rotating anode, it is not necessary to preheat a stationary anode.

It is also possible that a single excessive exposure generates so much heat at one point on the anode surface that <u>anode melting</u> or <u>pitting</u> occurs at this spot regardless of preheating the anode (Fig. 2-10). These surface irregularities result in a tube that continues to function but with variable and reduced radiation output. This type of anode injury can be avoided by referring to the tube rating chart to avoid exceeding the maximum exposure settings for a single exposure. A basic rule in use of x-ray tubes is to use high kilovoltage and low milliamperage-seconds techniques since this reduces the heat units required per exposure. Anode pitting may also be due to concentration of heat in one spot on the anode due to a failure of the anode to rotate properly during an exposure because of bearing or circuitry failure that usually results from frequent thermal overloading of the tube and housing.

The metallic deposit on the glass envelope that results from filament melting is sufficient to create a secondary anode and arcing of the electron beam to the secondary anode causes a localized spot of high temperature resulting in a fracture of the envelope at this site. The cracking of the glass envelope that results from <u>secondary arcing</u> from the filament to the tungsten deposits on the glass envelope occurs usually at higher kilovolt range exposures. In addition, arcing of the electron beam toward the tungsten plated glass envelope removes a part of the selected electron beam and there is a varying decrease in the size of the primary x-ray beam between exposures. This results in intermittent radiographic underexposures that occur without any explainable cause. The arcing maybe be partially prevented by using an x-ray tube with a metallic insert in the tube so that the deposition of tungsten is on the metal insert and therefore it cannot create a focal region on the glass envelope for the arcing to occur.

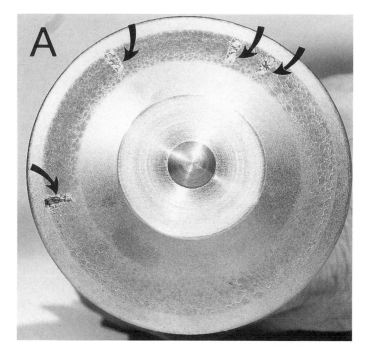

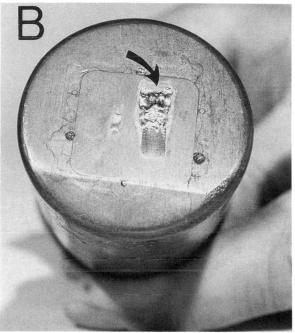

Fig. 2-10
ANODE INJURY
Photographs showing anode injury (arrows) to a rotating anode (A) and a stationary anode (B). This pitting was due to melting of the target surface caused by excessive heat during an exposure. This injury changes the surface characteristics of the target and creates x-ray photons that are misdirected or are absorbed by the roughened surfaces and are unable to escape from the target. In the stationary anode tube, the decrease in photon production is constant and can be partially accommodated for by increasing exposure settings. In the rotating anode tube, it is not possible to know the area on the disc where the electron interaction will occur, and, therefore, the level of production of x-rays varies with each exposure.

Anode <u>bearing wear</u> may result from several causes such as movement of the tube housing while the anode is still rotating or any form of tube overheating from several causes including holding the switch in a pre-exposure position for a long time. The "boost-and-hold" technique generates excessive bearing heat that is damaging to bearing surfaces. Bearing assembly wear can also be caused by changing milliamperage stations while the rotor is engaged.

F. TUBE RATING CHART

The tube rating chart is a composite graph with curves for mA, kVp, and exposure time settings, showing the maximum combinations that can be used safely for a single exposure (Fig. 2-11). Knowing two of the three variables makes it possible to use the chart to determine the maximum value of the third variable. Use of this chart is important in verterinary radiography. Anode cooling and housing cooling charts are also available but used only in the event of multiple exposures made during a short period of time. This is almost never important in veterinary radiography since it is difficult for patients to be positioned so quickly that a rapid series of exposures can be made.

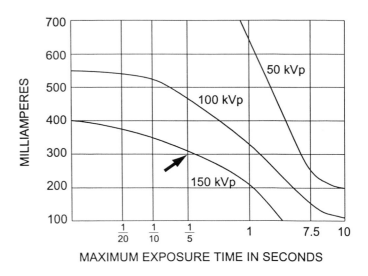

Fig. 2-11
TUBE RATING CHART
A drawing of a tube rating chart that permits the determination of the maximum kVp, mA, and exposure time that can be used safely in a single exposure to avoid injury to the x-ray tube from excessive heat production. Using this chart, a single 300 mA exposure can be made safely at 150 kVp for an exposure time of 1/5 second (arrow). Note that the chart is for a specific focal spot size.

REFERENCES

Rendano VT and Ryan G. Technical assistance in Radiology Part 1. Radiation equipment. Continuing Education 9:467-72, 1988.

Thompson TT. The abuse of radiographic tubes. Radio-Graphics 3:397-9, 1983

Trigg CN. X-ray tube failures and prevention: A preliminary report. Rad Tech 50;430-5, 1979.

Wallace R. Diagnostic x-ray tube failure and prevention. Radiol Techn 48:568, 1977.

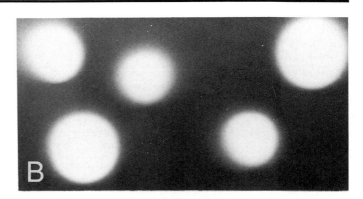

Radiographs of 5 coins made entirely with secondary radiation. A dog's abdomen was radiographed with a vertical x-ray beam. The technique used to expose (A) was 50 kVp and 10 mAs and the technique to expose (B) was 70 kVp and 10 mAs. The cassette with the coins taped on its face was held perpendicular to the floor and 1 meter outside the primary beam. Secondary radiation originated from the dog's body and the tabletop and traveled perpendicular to the primary beam and exposed the films.

3. X-RAY MACHINE

The quantity and quality of x-rays produced by an x-ray tube can be specifically controlled by altering certain variables in the x-ray machine in order to produce the desired radiograph. One of these controls alters the maximum speed of the electrons flowing across the x-ray tube and the speed is determined by the <u>kilovoltage potential</u>, or <u>kilovoltage peak</u> (kVp). This setting determines the maximum energy of the electron and thus the maximum energy of the x-ray photon produced. In addition the number of electrons that interact with the target in the tube is determined by the current flowing through the x-ray tube and is referred to as <u>milliamperage</u> (mA). The time of the exposure is another type of quantity control and when considered with an mA setting determines the <u>milliampere-seconds</u> (mA x sec = mAs). The combination of these variables used for a given imaging procedure is the basis of radiographic technique, and their specific selection influences the appearance of the final image. Their appropriate selection results in a radiographic image characterized by correct film density, contrast, and detail of anatomical features; their inappropriate selection compromises the information content of the image (Fig. 3-1). Later we will understand that selection of the focal spot size or selection of the distance between the x-ray tube and the patient also affect film quality.

There are a number of methods available for technique selection and they are commonly known as: (1) three factor, (2) two factor, and (3) one factor automatic exposure control system based on a sensor positioned beneath the patient or an anatomically related systems. The x-ray machine includes several major circuits and components that determine which of the technique selection methods is used. A review of the circuits provides for a better understanding of the operation of the exposure controls.

The <u>three factor system</u> of radiographic technique selection is the most common system found in clinics and in that system, the operator independently selects the kVp, mA, and exposure time for each radiographic image. The size of the mA setting automatically determines the size of the focal spot to be used. Such a system requires a high degree of operator interaction and a judgmental error on the part of the operator may result in a suboptimal radiograph. Adherence to carefully prepared technique

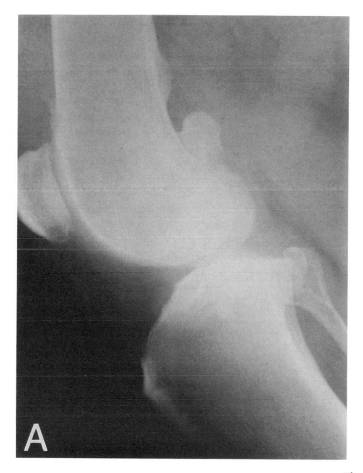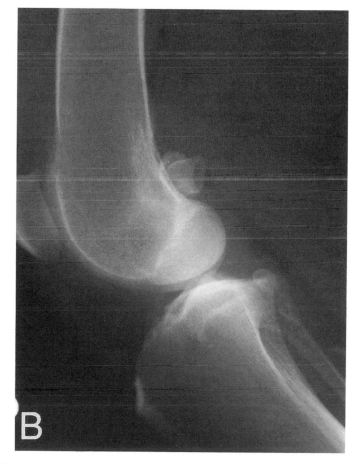

Fig. 3-1
FILM QUALITY
Two lateral radiographs of the stifle (femorotibial) joint of a dog show differences in film density with one radiograph (A) appearing less dense than the other radiograph (B). The increase density could be due to a higher kVp setting, higher mA setting, or a longer exposure time.

charts is essential.

In the two factor system of radiographic technique selection, the operator independently selects the kVp and mAs for each radiographic image. Size of the focal spot is selected automatically by the mA setting. Technique selection is simplified in that independent selection of mA and exposure time is no longer required. Rather, only their product must be selected. In this system, the mAs selector controls both the exposure time and tube current and is usually coupled to the kVp selector in such a manner that any combination of kVp and mAs results in a level of heating of the target compatable with the focal spot size is use. Usually the shortest exposure time is automatically selected. Adherence to carefully prepared technique charts is still required.

In the one factor system of radiographic technique selection, the operator independently selects only the kVp and tube current (mA) and time of exposure are automatically selected based on the selected kVp. Technique charts are still required but are simplified, necessitating specification of only the kVp and an automatic exposure control setting appropriate to the examination. Automatic exposure control systems result in a greatly simplified technique selection. In such systems, the radiation exiting the patient is sensed and used to control the duration of the exposure.The sensor maybe positioned either anterior or posterior (above or below) the image receptor (cassette). Selection must be made of the number of sensing areas or fields to accommodate certain anatomical areas. Another form of automatic exposure control systems is based on anatomical programming and is not usually appropriate for veterinary radiology because of the wide variety of body sizes and types that may be radiographed.

A line voltage compensator is a special feature that x-ray machines may have to assist in the control of x-ray exposures. Often an accurate measurement of the line voltage is not available and an undetected rise or drop in input voltage results in an overexposed or underexposed radiograph. To correct this problem, a meter on the control console permits determination of the level of the incoming line voltage and a control provides a method for adjustment of the line voltage so that it is constant at 110 or 220 volts at the time an exposure is made. This insures that a given kVp setting results in a film density that is reproducible. On some machines, the technologist must observe the needle on the meter and adjust the supply voltage with a control knob, however, in many newer machines, line compensation is automatic and a meter indicating the incoming line-voltage may not be required.

The autotransformer changes the voltage supplied to the x-ray machine to create the voltages of varying magnitude that are sent to the high voltage circuit of the x-ray machine. A transformer serves to alter electrical potential (voltage) inversely with the flow of electrons (amperage). It requires two separate windings of electrical wire around an iron core and functions because of electromagnetic induction because the flow of electrons changes direction (alternating current). The autotransformer is unique in that it has only one winding and one core and thus differs from the conventional transformer. It is possible for the autotransformer to increase or decrease the incoming voltage. The autotransformer can be designed to step up voltage to approximately twice the input voltage value thus increasing the range of kVp settings available on the machine.

The filament heat control circuit is responsible for providing the current to heat the filament which "boils off" the electron cloud (Fig. 3-2). A low current flows through the filament to warm it and prepare it for the thermal jolt necessary to produce x-rays. At this low filament current, there is insufficient heating for thermionic emission. By depressing the exposure button, the filament current is increased to permit thermionic emission and an exposure can occur. Remember, there is no current flow across the x-ray tube at the time of filament heating and therefore, no production of x-rays.

The degree of heat in the filament determines the number of electrons available to travel to the anode. The unit of measure of the number of electrons available is the milliampere (mA), or one-thousandth of an ampere. Most machines have a variable mA control; however, some small portable units have a fixed mA setting. In other small portable machines, the mA during an exposure can be set at 10, 15, or 20 while in the larger machines the mA settings vary between 100 to 1000. Since this is the measure of the number of electrons that flow across the x-ray tube, it is an indication of the number of x-ray photons that can be formed, and a general measure of the power of the x-ray generator.

Milliampere-seconds (mAs) is the relationship between mA and exposure time. A higher mA setting allows for a corresponding decrease in the exposure time and still achieves production of the same number of x-ray photons. An exposure obtained with a setting of 0.1 second and 100 mA would be 10 mAs (0.1 sec x 100 mA = 10 mAs). A second exposure could be obtained with a setting of 1.0 second and 10 mA and would also produce 10 mAs (1.0 sec x 10 mA = 10mAs). The product of milliamperage and time is called milliampere-seconds (mAs) and is a measure of the number of photons that are produced. Using the same machine, equal mAs settings produce radiographs of

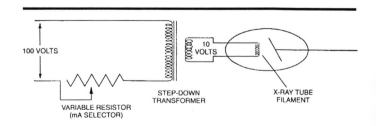

Fig. 3-2
LOW-VOLTAGE (FILAMENT) CIRCUIT
A constant voltage is delivered to a variable resistor that becomes the mA selector. The altered voltage then passes to the step-down transformer where it is altered to the correct amperage and voltage to heat the filament as desired.

equal density, assuming all other factors are constant. Use of this type of adjustment of exposure settings, in which the mA setting is increased and the exposure time is decreased, permits the use of short exposure times and partially alleviates the problem of patient motion during radiography. Another advantage of a machine with high mA settings is that the resulting greater amount of x-ray photons produced during the exposure permits radiographic examination of thicker patients.

kVp controls provide a method of precisely determining the required kVp setting for the radiographic exposure. The two selection knobs or dials, major and minor, represent two separate switches on the autotransformer. The voltage selected by the autotransformer becomes the input voltage to the high-voltage step-up transformer and it is subsequently increased in the high-voltage circuity and provides the kilovoltage required to move the electrons across the x-ray tube. The major control usually has 10 kVp differences between each setting and the minor control has 2 or 3 kVp differences between each setting. Other units have a single kVp control with 5 kVp differences between each setting. Newer machines have a digital readout and any kVp setting can be programmed. The kVp selectors are a form of quality control since they determine the energy of the photon beam which measures the penetrating ability of the x-ray beam. Higher kVp settings result in a higher percentage of x-ray photons penetrating the patient and reaching the film. On most consoles the kVp meter is a prereading voltmeter and allows determination of the kilovoltage to be monitored before the exposure.

The high-tension circuit is responsible for converting the voltage of the low-tension circuit into an appropriate kilovoltage of the proper electrical waveform. The high-voltage section contains three primary parts: (1) high-voltage step-up transformer, (2) filament transformer, and (3) current rectifiers. The high-voltage step-up transformer increases the voltage to kilovolts and produces the high potential across the x-ray tube so that the electron beam flows across the gap in the tube and interacts with the target to produce x-ray photons (Fig. 3-3). The number of windings of electrical wire around an iron core in the transformer on the primary side is less from the number on the secondary side in a step-up transformer and the ratio is referred to as the "turns ratio". This ratio determines how the voltage is changed. If the ratio between the windings is 1000, the voltage within the high-tension circuit is changed 90 volts to 90,000 volts (90 kVp). Now you can understand why the cables that lead to the x-ray tube are so heavily shielded, they carry voltages measured in thousands of volts. (The voltage in your apartment or house is between 110 and 120 volts.)

Transformers operate only on alternating current (AC), that means that the electrons alternate direction of flow in a predetermined manner. Thus, the only way to generate kVp is through the use of alternating electrical current. The voltage flowing through an AC line can best be pictured as a wave, steadily increasing from zero to a maximum peak, then falling to zero, then falling to a negative minimum, and then rising to zero again (Fig. 3-4). Electrical current in the U.S. has 60 such cycles per second. That means that

the flow of electrons changes direction 120 times per second. While alternating current is a requirement in the operation of a transformer, an x-ray tube produces x-rays only when the flow of electrons is from the cathode to the anode thus requiring direct current.

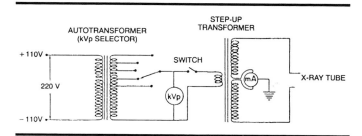

Fig. 3-3
HIGH-VOLTAGE CIRCUIT
The autotransformer selects an appropriate voltage that when passed to the step-up transformer is increased in potential to the kilovoltage level so that when expressed across the x-ray tube it provides the energy to cause the electron beam to strike the target producing the primary x-ray beam.

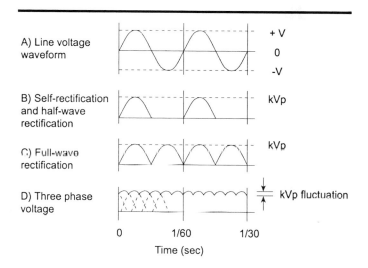

Fig. 3-4
ELECTRICAL WAVE FORMS
The line voltage alternating current has a waveform flow in one direction and then reverses the flow to the opposite direction. The time of electron flow in each direction is determined at the power source and is indicated in the number of electrical cycles/second. With an input waveform of 60 cycles/second, each cycle is 1/60 seconds in length (A). If this waveform is expressed across the x-ray tube, electrons pass across the tube only in one direction and the reverse flow is lost. The resulting waveform is called self-rectification or half-wave rectification and indicates that only one-half of the electrical energy is being used (B). If the current is fully rectified, the flow of electrons in both halves of the cycle across the x-ray tube is in the same direction and full use is made of the electrical energy. This is referred to as full-wave rectification (C). If three separate waveforms are superimposed, each 120 degrees out of phase, the voltage expressed across the x-ray tube has only minimal fluctation, and this is referred to as three phase voltage (D)

19

Rectification is a way of altering one of the characteristics of electrical energy. In alternating current, the electrons that want to flow from the anode to the cathode create a problem that can be solved by the appropriate design of the x-ray circuit that results in a type of current rectification, that is, some process by which the flow of electrons is changed so that the flow is always in the same direction across the x-ray tube. In the simplest x-ray circuit, the x-ray tube serves as the rectifier (self rectification), since current can only flow through the circuit when the target is positive with respect to the filament. In this form of rectification, only one-half of the current passes across the x-ray tube and it is termed a half-wave rectified current. In this form, the negative potential portion of the alternating current cycle is eliminated and the voltage remains at zero during the negative portion of the cycle and only one half of the electrical energy (electron flow) is used (Fig. 3-4). The resulting x-ray output from self-rectification or half-wave rectification is a pulsating x-ray beam with 60 x-ray pulses each second.

This loss of energy was the reason for development of full-wave rectified wave forms that are accomplished through appropriate placement of four diode tubes or more recently solid-state rectifiers. A full-wave rectified current is generated so that a positive voltage is always impressed across the x-ray tube in the correct direction (cathode to anode) during both halves of the alternating current (Fig. 3-4). This technique results in a current that is pulsating with 120 x-ray pulses each second and is employed in nearly all large stationary x-ray units.

The energy of the photons within the x-ray beam varies from a maximum to the lowest energy that can escape from the x-ray tube. If the energy of each electron passing across the tube could be increased, the average energy of the photon beam would be increased. In both half-wave and full-wave rectified circuits, the voltage applied to the tube fluctuates between zero and the peak kV, and is referred to as a pulsating potential so that the resulting x-ray energy spectrum varies over a period of time. In an effort to increase the average energy of the photon beam, a three-phase x-ray generator supplies a voltage to the tube that ranges from a peak voltage to a minimum voltage of only about 5 to 20% less than the maximum (Fig. 3-4). Through the added use of capacitors, it is possible to generate a near-constant potential that produces an almost constant energy electron beam that results in an x-ray energy spectrum that only varies < 5 % in its intensity. The higher average energy x-ray beam increases the efficiency of x-ray production and permits exposures to be made at shorter times requiring fewer photons.

The timer circuit is separate from the other main circuits and controls the exposure time through: (1) mechanical timers, (2) synchronous timers, (3) electronic timers, (4) mAs timers, and (5) phototimers. Mechanical timers operate by turning a knob that winds a spring that controls the exposure time by unwinding. Synchronous timers are based on a synchronous motor that relates to the frequency of the electric current (60 Hz in the United States). mAs timers monitor the product of mA and time and terminate the exposure when the desired mAs is attained. Phototimers measure the quantity of radiation reaching the film and automatically terminate the exposure when sufficient radiation to provide the required film density has reached the film.

A spinning top can be used to check the acurracy of timers on some x-ray machines. It is a heavy metal disc with a single hole that is rotated on a pedestal during the radiographic exposure (Fig. 3-5). Because x-rays are emitted in pulses from all but three-phase equipment, a half-wave-rectified machine produces 60 pulses per second and a full-wave-rectified machine produces 120 pulses per second. By knowing the type of current rectification and counting the resulting black dots on the radiograph, it is possible to determine if the timer is accurately controlling the length of the exposure time (Fig. 3-5). It is also possible to use the spinning top to determine the type of current rectification.

The relationship between kVp setting and mAs setting is an inverse relationship. The higher the kVp setting, the lower the mAs setting that is required to obtain a diagnostic radiograph of similar quality. This relationship, as it applies to the 70 to 100 kVp range normally used for diagnostic veterinary radiography, can be stated as follows. If you add 10 kVp and divide the mAs in half, a radiograph of comparable density is produced. Conversely, if you subtract 10 kVp and double the mAs, a radiograph of comparable density is produced. The following pairs of kVp and mAs settings, produced in the same x-ray machine and x-ray tube, result in radiographs of a similar quality.

• 70 kVp and 2.0 mAs
• 80 kVp and 1.0 mAs
• 90 kVp and 0.5 mAs

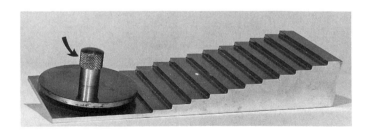

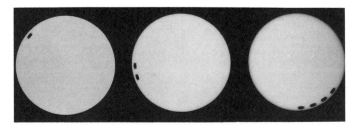

Fig. 3-5
SPINNING TOP
Photograph of the spinning top (arrow) and an aluminum step-wedge and radiographs made at 1/60 second, 1/30 second, and 1/15 second exposure. It is possible to evaluate the pattern of black dots produced and ascertain the type of current rectification and the accuracy of the timer. Is this machine half-wave rectified or full-wave rectified?

Knowledge of the kVp—mAs relationship can also be used in other situations. If the density of a radiograph is too high (overexposed) and thought not to be diagnostic, it is possible to correct the problem by decreasing the exposure factors by <u>either</u> decreasing the kVp by 10 <u>or</u> by halving the mAs. Conversely, if the density of a radiograph is too low (underexposed) and thought not to be diagnostic, it is possible to correct the problem by increasing the exposure factors by <u>either</u> increasing the kVp by 10 <u>or</u> by doubling the mAs.

Beyond the range of 70 to 100 kVp, the kVp-mAs relationship described above does not hold. In lower kVp ranges, the change in kVp setting required to compensate for a halving or doubling of the mAs is lower (4 to 6 kVp). In the higher kVp ranges, the change in kVp setting required to compensate for a halving or doubling of the mAs is higher (14 to 20 kVp).

REFERENCE

Rossi RP. Methods of Technique Selection in Radiographic Imaging. RadioGraphics 5:998-1001, 1985.

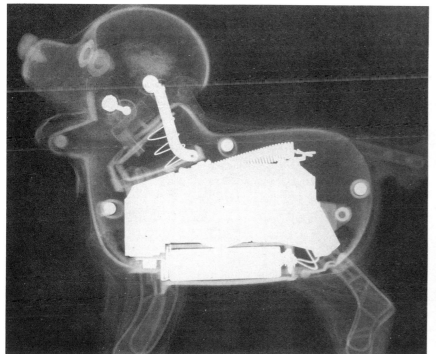

Batteries but no heart.

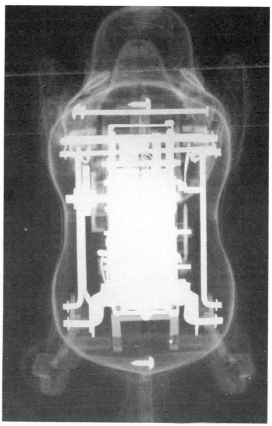

4. SECONDARY OR SCATTER RADIATION

Two types of radiation are responsible for the exposure of a radiograph and are thus important in diagnostic radiology. One of these is that part of the original x-ray beam that was generated at the tube anode and has passed through the patient unchanged and is recorded on the x-ray film (the remnant beam). The second type of radiation is referred to as secondary radiation or scattered radiation and results from three types of interaction between radiation and matter. The interactions result in variable degrees of absorption of the primary x-ray beam within the differing tissues of the patient. The probability of these types of interactions is dependent on: (1) the elements present, (2) the specific gravity of the tissues, and (3) the beam energy (kVp).

The first type of interaction between radiation and matter is classical or coherent scattering of the x-ray photon (Fig. 4-1A) and may occur with the photon interacting with an atom and being deflected in a new direction without a loss of energy. This type of interaction occurs with low kVp photons and is relatively unimportant in diagnostic radiology.

A more important interaction between x-ray and matter is photoelectric absorption (Fig. 4-1B). This type of interaction occurs when an incident photon enters an atom, ionizing the atom by imparting all of its energy to an inner shell electron which is ejected from its orbit. The ejected electron is called a photelectron, which has such low energy it cannot escape the patient. The interaction is called "capture" since all of the energy of the photon is given up. The remaining void in the electron shell is filled by an outer shell electron and produces a low energy characteristic photon with the energy dependent on the level of electron shell and the binding energy of that atom. Because the binding energies present in the body tissues are so low, the resulting photon is unlikely to escape the body. For practical purposes, all of the energy of a photon undergoing photoelectric absorption remains deposited in the patient. Photoelectric process occurs in a highly selective manner, the probability of absorption being much greater in higher atomic number (Z) tissues and when the energy of the incident photon exactly matches the binding energy of an inner shell electron. Since, the binding energies of elements in the body are low (< 20keV), this type of interaction is favored when low kVp settings are used. The probability of photoelectric absorption varies approximately as the third power of the atomic number (Z) of the absorbing tissue. This accounts for the high efficiency of lead (Z=82) in absorbing x-ray photons of diagnostic energies. If photoelectric absorption were the only mode of absorption in tissue, bone would be particularly prominent because of photon capture due to its large amount of calcium. The differential photoelectric absorption of bone as compared to an equivalent mass of soft tissue is almost 4 to 1. For equivalent thicknesses of bone and soft tissue, the differential is about 7 to 1 because of the greater density of bone.

Compton scattering (Fig. 4-1C) of a primary photon occurs within the patient when the photon imparts some of its energy to an outer shell electron, causing a loosely bound electron to leave its orbit, with the photon retaining sufficient energy to continue in a new direction with a lower energy level. At low x-ray energies, Compton scattered photons are likely to be scattered back toward the x-ray source or be of such low energy that they cannot escape the patient. In either situation, the scattered photons do not reach the film. At higher x-ray energies, the scattered photon is more likely to be directed at a forward angle, and may have enough energy to exit from the patient and reach the film. The probability of Compton interaction is

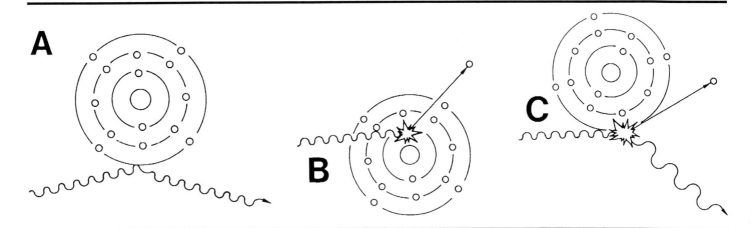

Fig. 4-1
INTERACTION OF RADIATION WITH MATTER
Classical or coherent scattering (A), photoelectric capture (B), and Compton scattering (C) are illustrated. In all examples, the photon enters from the left and interacts with the electrons of the atom. In classical scattering, the photon is simply redirected maintaining the same energy level. In photoelectric capture, the energy of the photon is transferred to a photoelectron. In Compton scattering, the photon gives up some of its energy but continues in a new direction. In both photoelectric capture and Compton scatter, characteristic photons are produced because of the removal of shell electrons, however, they are of such low energy that they fail to escape from the patient.

essentially equal for all materials on a gram-for-gram basis. This means that equal thicknesses of different materials absorb x-ray by this mode in proportion to their densities. Characteristic radiation may be released at the time of the interaction, with the energy dependent on the level of the electron shell and the binding energy of that atom. Usually, the characteristic radiation is of such low energy that it doesn't escape the patient.

It is possible for a released electron from either a photoelectric capture or Compton reaction to cause further interactions, however, the energy levels are all so low that any photons produced are unable to escape from the patient's body. The relative interaction as a function of atomic number of the absorbing medium and energy of the incident photons can be seen in different ways (Fig. 4-2).

Two terms pertaining to the interaction of radiation with matter are frequently misunderstood. Absorption of radiation refers to the local depositon of the radiation energy in the object being irradiated. However, when an x-ray beam interacts with an object, not all of the incident energy is absorbed locally, some photons are emitted as scattered photons. Therefore, attenuation is defined as the reduction in intensity of the primary x-ray beam as it traverses matter, by either absorption or scattering. Thus, absorption refers to the complete absorption of primary photons and attenuation refers to the reduction of energy of the primary beam by all interactions.

From the perspective of the radiographic film, an x-ray photon may have one of 4 possiblilities. First, it can pass completely through the patient without affecting the patient or being altered in any way and reach the film. Second, by undergoing classical scatter the direction of the photon can be altered without change in its energy level. Third, by undergoing photoelectric capture, the energy of the x-ray may be completely absorbed by atoms within the patient. Fourth, by undergoing Compton scatter, some residual energy of the x-ray photon may reach the film.

The combination of primary photons and scattered photons reaching the film results in film exposure or film density. To obtain radiographs of high quality, scatter radiation must be limited or film contrast, the comparison of different film densities, is markedly compromised producing a gray radiograph instead of one with a black and white appearance. There are three factors that influence the production of scatter radiation and all of these may be controlled at least partially. They are the; (1) kVp setting,

(2) field size, and (3) patient thickness.

As x-ray energy is increased through higher kVp settings, the relative number of x-rays that undergo Compton scatter increases also. This suggests that low kVp technique would result in production of minimal scatter radiation and thus produce a radiograph with high image quality. However, in using lower kVp technique, photoelectric absorption increases, resulting in markedly increased mAs technique that causes increased patient dosage and long exposure times. Because of the potential reduction in patient dose and the shorter exposure time that eliminates patient motion, high-kVp technique is preferred to low kVp technique.

The amount of scatter radiation from Compton scatter increases as the field size increases and restriction of beam size is important to control the amount of scatter produced and reduce the tendency for the radiograph to be gray without contrast.

Scatter radiation increases when radiographing body parts that are thicker. Unfortunately this is not easily altered by the technologist, however, it is possible to use compression devices to minimize tissue thickness and thus lessen the production of scatter radiation.

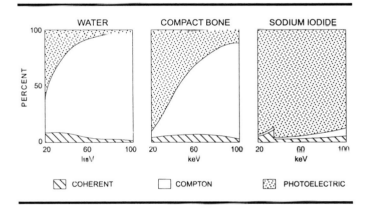

Fig. 4-2
FREQUENCY OF INTERACTIONS BETWEEN PHOTONS AND TISSUE
Major differences occur between the frequency of occurrence of coherent scatter, Compton scatter, and photoelectric capture dependent on energy of the incident photons and the nature of the interacting tissue. Increase in keV causes an increase in Compton scatter in water and bone, while photoelectric capture remains high in radiographic contrast agents. Coherent scatter plays a minimal role in interactions.

5. ACCESSORY EQUIPMENT

A. BEAM FILTRATION

The primary function of the filter is to reduce the radiation exposure to the patient. Filtration is the process of increasing the effective energy of the x-ray beam by passing it through an absorber. This increase in beam energy can occur only with a polychromatic beam or one that contains a spectrum of photons of different energies such as occurs in an x-ray beam. It may also be thought of as the technique of eliminating, through absorption, a disproportionately greater percentage of the lower energy portion of the x-ray beam that contributes little to production of the diagnostic radiograph (Fig. 5-1). Lower energy potons are absorbed in the first few centimeters of tissue within the patient and give no diagnostic information on the film, however, the patient's overall radiation dose is increased. Every object through which the x-rays pass on their way from the tube anode to the film acts as a filter (Table 5-1).

Filtration alters the characteristics of the primary beam by: (1) increasing the mean beam energy and (2) decreasing the overall beam intensity. The increase in the percentage of more penetrating photons in the beam is referred to as "hardening" of the beam and can be measured by evaluation of the half-value layer of the beam. Filtration is usually expressed in mm of aluminum equivalents, or mm of copper equivalent and is expressed in terms of the required thickness needed to absorb one-half of the x-rays.

Filtration of the primary x-ray beam is divided into inherent and added filtration (Table 5-1). Inherent filtration of the primary x-ray beam is due to the: (1) window in the glass envelope of the x-ray tube (1.4 mm thickness—0.78 mm Aluminum Equivalents), (2) insulating oil around the tube (2.36 mm thickness—0.07 mm Aluminum Equivalents), and (3) covering over the aperture in the tube housing (1.02 mm thickness—0.05 mm Aluminum Equivalents). It is easy to understand why the tube window might be especially constructed of berryllium (Z=4) or, more commonly, of plastic (Z=6) to avoid the absorption of the major portion of the x-ray beam. The materials responsible for inherent filtation equal approximately 0.9 mm aluminum equivalents (Trout, 1963).

Added filtration results from other materials placed externally in the primary x-ray beam and are in addition to the inherent filtration. External beam filters are usually selectively installed at the tube head and are not changed. Aluminum, (Z=13), is used as the added filtration in most low energy diagnostic x-ray machines. This element attenuates mostly by photoelectric absorption in the low energy region of the photon beam. Copper, (Z=29), is used for high-energy radiation producing units, such as therapy machines, because it results in removal of higher energy photons.

Recommendations of the National Council on Radiation Protection and Measurements for total filtration to be used in diagnostic radiography are found in NCRP II 36. When using an x-ray beam with a maximum energy of less than 50 kVp, the total inherent and added filtration should be 0.5 mm aluminum, with a maximum energy between 50 and 70 kVp, the total inherent and added filtration should be 1.5 mm aluminum, and with a maximum energy in excess of 70 kVp, the total inherent and added filtration should be 2.5 mm of aluminum. In most machines, the

Table 5-1
X-RAY BEAM ATTENUATOR*

Attenuator	% of Beam Remaining
Target	100
Inherent filtration:	
Tube glass envelope (0.78 mm Al equiv)	6.6
Tube housing insulating oil (0.07 mm Al equiv)	5.9
Bakelite tube window (0.05 mm Al equiv)	5.6
Added filtration:	
Added filter (0.5 mm Al equiv)	4.2
Collimator mirror and face plate (1.0 mm Al equiv)	2.4
Air between tube and patient (negligible loss)	2.4
30-cm patient	0.01
Grid (varies with type)	< 0.01
Beam interaction with film	< 0.01

*(Trout, 1963)

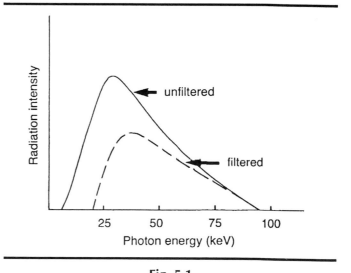

Fig. 5-1
EFFECT OF FILTRATION OF PHOTON ENERGY
Passage of the x-ray beam through tissue results in the selective absorption of the lower energy portion of the beam. Note that the effect of the filter is less prominent on the higher energy photons.

sum of the inherent and added filtration exceeds the recommended total filtration of 2.5 mm Al equivalents.

Many of the photons produced are low energy and, if they escape through the glass window of the tube, they are absorbed by the first few centimeters of patient tissue and contribute nothing to the exposure of the radiograph. All they do is contribute to the patient radiation dose. Therefore, a principle reason for utilizing beam filtration is to decrease the exposure level to the surface of the skin of the patient. Use of the recommended total filtration decreases the exposure dose to the patient by almost 80% (Table 5-2). Another study reported the dose reduction in milliroentgens (mR) per milliampere-seconds (mAs) when using appropriate filtration in the primary x-ray beam to be a dose reduction to the skin of 67%: 1) the exposure at 1 meter from the x-ray tube was 14.0 mR/mAs with 0.5 mm of aluminum total filtration: 2) the exposure at the same distance was 4.6 mR/mAs with 2.5 mm of aluminum total filtration. While patient dose is of extreme importance in radiography of man, it is of less interest in radiography of animals. Still, it is possible for an individual holding a cassette in veterinary radiography to accidently be in the primary beam during an exposure and the use of recommended filtration would decrease the skin exposure that person would receive.

Even though most of the reduction Is of lower energy photons, there is still the necessity of increasing the exposure time or mA setting to compensate for the loss of the higher energy photons (Table 5-3). The effect of 2.5 mm aluminum filtration on exposure times in the kVp range of 60 to 70 kVp, causes an increase of approximately 50% to compensate for this loss. The additional exposure required increases with an increase in the thickness of the filter and decreases as the kVp range increases. Therefore, it is possible that the use of added filtration in conjunction with a small portable unit using low kVp settings may cause the lengthen of the exposure time so that movement of the patient during the exposure results in the production of an unsatisfactory radiograph.

Your technique chart is developed with both the inherent and added filtration in place so it is not necessary to determine the effect of the filtration at the time of each radiographic study. However, it may be desirable to develop a separate low-energy technique chart made with the removal of the added filtration for use in radiography of birds.

Remember that the patient is also a form of filter with the rate of attenuation depending on the atomic composition of the anatomic structures encountered by the x-ray photons. These anatomic structures are classified according to their effective atomic numbers into three categories: (1) adipose tissues, (2) body fluids and soft tissues with the exclusion of fat, and (3) bone.

Table 5-2
EFFECT OF ALUMINUM FILTRATION ON PATIENT EXPOSURE*

Al Filter	Exposure Dose to Skin (mr)	% Decrease in Exposure Dose
None	2,380	—
0.5 mm	1,850	22
1.0 mm	1,270	47
3.0 mm	465	80

*(Trout et al, 1952)

Table 5-3
PERCENTAGE ADDITIONAL EXPOSURE REQUIRED AS COMPARED TO 1 MM AL FILTRATION*

		Filtration		
		2 mm Al	3 mm Al	4 mm Al
kVp range	50	38%	70%	120%
	80	21%	42%	58%
	100	17%	35%	52%
	140	9%	26%	38%

*(Mattson, 1955)

REFERENCES

National Council on Radiation Protection and Measurements: Medical X-ray and Gamma-Ray Protection for Energies up to 10 MeV. Washington, DC, U.S. Government Printing Office, Report No. 33, 1968.

Trout ED. The life history on an x-ray beam. Radiol Technol 35:161-70, 1963.

Trout ED Kelley JP and Cathey GA. The use of filters to control radiation exposure to the patient in diagnostic roentgenology. Am J Roentgenol 67: 942-52,1952.

Mattson O. Practical photographic problems in radiography. Acta Rad Suppl 120, 1955.

B. BEAM RESTRICTORS

X-ray beam restriction involves the use of devices that are attached to the opening in the x-ray tube housing that regulate the size and shape of the area of exposure by the primary x-ray beam. Their use is important in veterinary radiography since by limiting the size of primary beam exposure, they consequently: (1) decrease the potential exposure to the hands of an individual holding the cassette or patient, (2) improve radiographic quality through a decrease in the amount of scatter radiation produced, and (3) decrease the exposure to the patient. Every diagnostic x-ray machine should have a beam restrictor of some type. Preferably, it should have an adjustable field size and attach to the tube housing is such a manner that it can be rotated so that the field of exposure can match the shape of the cassette no matter how it is positioned on the tabletop. Every radiograph should have a border of unexposed film so that you can be certain that the field of exposure is smaller than the film.

Beam-restricting devices can be in the form of: (1) a lead aperature diaphragm, (2) a lead cone, (3) a lead cylinder, or (4) an adjustable lead aperature shutter. Aperature diaphragms are a type of x-ray beam restrictor and consist only of a sheet of lead with a hole in the center. The size and shape of the hole determines the size and shape of the x-ray beam at a given focal-film distance. This is obviously the simplest type of beam restrictor and may be the type of restrictor available with small portable x-ray units. The advantage is in its simplicity and low cost, while, the principal disadvantage is the necessity to physically change the aperature if the size of the field of exposure is to be altered. This may be difficult because there may not be a convenient method of attachment to the tube housing.

A second type of beam restrictor is a cone or cylinder. When using a cone, it should be understood that the flare of the cone is usually greater than the flare of the x-ray beam in which case the base plate that attaches the device to the tube housing is the only part of the device that restricts the size of the x-ray beam (Fig. 5-2). Thus, it is little more than an aperature diaphragm. Cylinders influence beam size and also may have the feature of being extended, thus helping in the determination of beam centering. The main disadvantages of these non-adjustable restrictors is the requirement of needing several sizes to provide the field sizes for each cassette size.

The field of exposure when using a cone or cylinder is a circle which places limitations on their use as a collimation device. When comparing the use of a rectangular field collimator, the area needed to cover an anatomical region is approximately 40% less than the area exposed by a circle. This is especially important when radiographing the bones of the horse's limbs or the spine of a dog, both fields which have great length but little width. The use of a cone as a collimating device does not accurately limit the area of irradiation in these examinations. Reduction in radiation dosage in dental radiography through the use of accurately restricted size radiation fields has been reported (Winkler, 1968).

The adjustable lead shutter beam limiting device with each shutter consisting of four or more lead plates, is the best beam restrictor. It provides an infinite variety of x-ray field sizes and shapes (Fig. 5-3). They are most commonly referred to as a collimator. Early types of collimators had the shutters operating together from one control so that the field could only be square partially limiting the value of the device. In more recent collimators, two pair of lead shutters operate independently providing the opportunity for unlimited field size and shape. By using shutters with more than 1 lead plate, they function together to clean up the pneumbra due to the scattering of primary radiation seen at the edge of the field.

To make use of the beam restrictor most practical, the area to be exposed should be illuminated (Fig. 5-4). The field is illuminated by a light beam from a light bulb in the collimator that is deflected by a mirror mounted in the path of the x-ray beam at an angle of 45°. If the target of the x-ray tube and light bulb are the same distance from the center of the mirror, the light beam as it passes through the second shutter opening is collimated to coincide with the x-ray beam. Collimators may have a back-up system to determine the exposure field size through use of a calibrated scale on the front of the collimator next to the knob that adjusts the shutter size. Collimator structures, including the exit plastic portal and the reflecting mirror provide added filtration and is one reason why high quality radiographs of birds cannot be produced through the use of a collimator and is a reason to remove the collimator and other added filtration prior to avian radiography.

Often the collimator has a metal tape box incorporated so that a measurement of focal-film distance can be easily made. Other collimators have two light beams, or laser beams, that use a parallax system to determine the selected

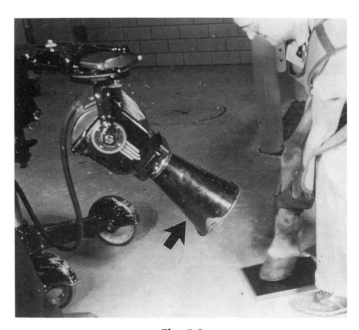

Fig. 5-2
BEAM LIMITING DEVICES
A large cone (arrow) is nonadjustable and creates a circular radiation field that provides little protection to the feet of the person holding the horse's foot. No method of illumination of the radiation field is available with this type of device.

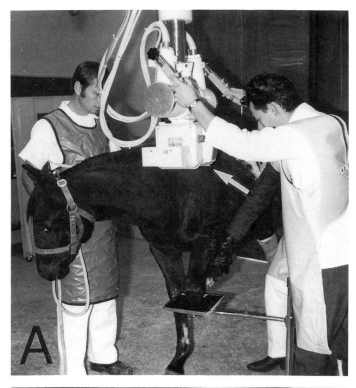

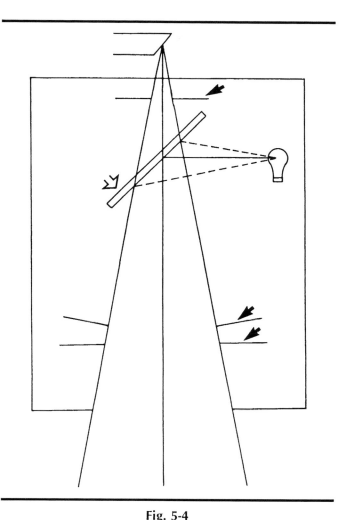

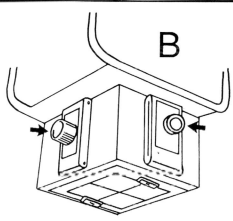

Fig. 5-3
ADJUSTABLE LEAD SHUTTER BEAM LIMITING DEVICE

A photograph of a beam limiting device (arrow) with two pairs of "L" shaped lead shutters that move independently to produce an unlimited number of square or rectangular shaped exposure fields (A). A drawing of a similiar type of beam limiting device with individual controls that are available for independent adjustment (arrows) (B).

Fig. 5-4
SCHEMATIC DRAWING OF A BEAM RESTRICTOR

The x-ray beam originates at the tube and is limited by a series of shutters (solid arrows). The beam passes through a mirror (hollow arrow) that reflects a light beam in such a way that the area irradiated by the x-ray beam is equal in size and location to the area illuminated by the light.

focal-film distance. The collimator may also provide a place to hold the beam filters. Many collimators have a thin light beam that is directed to the side of the table so that it can be seen when the bucky tray is pulled out. This light beam identifies the center of the field of exposure and permits more accurate alignment of the cassette with the central x-ray beam.

A technique is available to determine if the illuminated field and radiation field are similar in size and position (Curry 111, et al. 1984). A cassette is placed on the tabletop and a radiation field selected that is smaller than the size of the cassette. The lower right corner of the field is identified by a lead "R" and the corners of the illuminated field are identified by paper clips or other convenient metal strips. A low intensity exposure is made (40-50 kVp, 1-2 mAs). Without moving the cassette, metallic markers, or collimator position, the exposure field is increased and a second, similar, exposure is made that insures that the location of metallic markers is identified. By comparing the field of illumination determined by the metallic markers and the field of actual exposure as determined by the first exposure, it is possible to determine the correctness of the illuminated field. If a discrepency exists, it is possible on some collimators to correct the disparity by adjusting a set screw on the side of the collimator that changes the angle of the mirror (Fig. 5-5).

A problem in using beam limiting devices often exists when using a portable x-ray machine at short focal-film distances, such as 20 to 24 inches (50 to 60 cm). The collimator openings may be large enough to cover an 8 by 10 inch (18 x 24 cm) cassette, but are not sufficiently large to cover a larger 14 by 17 inch (35 by 43 cm) cassette. This limitation in cassette size due to the collimator should be clearly understood prior to use of the portable unit and should not be used as an excuse to remove the collimator from use. The collimator is the most practical radiation safety device available to the veterinarian and its use should not be compromised. The need to use an assistant in cassette positioning in radiography of large animals especially demands that a collimator be used so there is no possibility of a part of the assistant being within the primary x-ray beam.

During routine radiography, the film is exposed by both primary and scattered radiation. Thus, the density of the radiograph is increased as a result of the exposure by the scattered radiation. This increase in additional exposure continues to increase with field sizes up to 900 cm^2 (30 cm x 30 cm). At that size, the total quantity of scatter radiation is near its maximum (Curry 111 et al, 1984). If the collimator limits the field of exposure to a small area less than 100 cm^2 (10cm x 10cm), it may be necessary to increase the exposure technique by about 5 to 6 kVp to compensate for the loss of film density due to the decrease in scatter radiation reaching the film.

Sometimes the area of the film to be exposed can be limited by the use of lead sheets placed over the film rather than by the use of a collimator. This is often done when using tabletop techniques and in radiography of horses limbs where two views are to be made on a single radiograph. It should be understood that this method of beam restriction does not limit the amount of patient exposed or the amount of scatter radiation produced. Thus, there is scatter radiation generated outside of the field outlined by the lead sheets that is redirected toward the opening between the lead sheets. Therefore, the amount of scatter radiation reaching the film remains essentially the same.

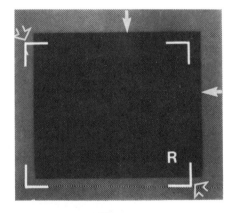

Fig. 5-5
SCHEME TO EVALUATE FIELD LOCATION
By making two superimposed radiographic exposures and identifing the corners of the illuminated field by metallic markers, it is possible to compare the location of the illuminated field with the actual field of exposure. In this example, the field of radiographic exposure (solid arrows) is shifted above and to the right of the illuminated field as indicated by the "paper clips" (hollow arrows).

REFERENCES

Curry T S III Dowdey J E and Murry R C. Christensen's Introduction to the physics of diagnostic radiology. 3rd ed Lea & Febiger, Philadelphia, 1984.

Reinsma K. The inherent filtration of x-ray tubes. Radiol 74:971-2, 1960.

Trout ED Kelley JP and Furmo EJ. A study of the inherent filtration of diagnostic x-ray tubes. Radiol 66:102-6,1956.

Winkler KG. Influence of rectangular collimation and intra-oral shielding on radiation dose in dental radiography. J Am Dent Assoc 77;95, 1968.

C. GRIDS

Scatter radiation, or secondary radiation, is probably the biggest single factor contributing to decreased film quality in radiographic studies and is the result of a redirection of part of the primary x-ray beam following Compton scattering in the patient. It has been shown that of the radiation reaching the film, the scatter fraction following passage of the x-ray beam through 5 cm of polystyrene is 50% and following passage through 10 cm of polystyrene is 70% (Motz, et.al., 1978). Others have reported the secondary radiation to be between 60% and 70% of the total radiation that reaches the film (Mattsson, 1956). The scatter or redirected radiation strikes the film from different directions, causing a generalized photographic fog that covers the film, and is present to some degree in each radiographic examination. If the thickness of the part radiographed exceeds 10 to 13 cm, the amount of scatter created becomes sufficient to cause a loss in quality of the radiograph by reducing the contrast between adjacent areas on the radiograph. The quantity, energy, and direction of the scatter radiation is directly dependent on: (1) patient density, (2) total volume of tissue irradiated, and (3) energy (kVp) of the primary beam of x-rays.

To correct this problem, the first grid was built in 1913 by Dr. Gustave Bucky of Germany who discovered the principle of "a system of lead foil strips placed on edge in the pattern of boxes" with the strips separated by x-ray transparent interspaces. By 1915, Bucky had a patent for a cross grid and thought that he could completely eliminate lines on the film. Dr. Hollis E. Potter of Chicago found that no method eliminated seeing the pattern of the squares on the radiograph when using the quadrangular network of Bucky's and therefore he outlined in 1920 a basic principle of a parallel pattern of lead strips that would travel a distance equal to a few inches during the exposure. The grid is frequently referred to as the Potter-Bucky diaphragm. Lysholm developed a grid in 1928 with only a few mm thickness to the lead strips and interspaces of about 0.4 mm and called this a fine-line grid and stated that motion of the grid wasn't necessary since the lines were so fine that their resulting pattern on the radiograph was not disrupting.

Today, a grid is a flat plate composed of a series of thin lead foil strips separated by x-ray transparent spacers that is positioned between the the source of the scatter radiation (patient) and the recording device (x-ray film). In studies of a large patient, use of a carefully fabricated grid is absolutely essential to limit potential loss of film contrast. By positioning the grid between the patient and the cassette, it is used to improve the diagnostic quality of radiographs by absorbing a portion of the scatter radiation (Compton scattering) that results from interaction of the primary x-ray beam with the patient (Fig. 5-6). The amount of secondary radiation decreases to approximately 30% of the total radiation that reaches the film when using a 5:1 ratio grid (Mattsson, 1956). Two factors are involved in describing the transmission of the scatter radiation. First, there is a certain percentage of scatter that has the same direction as the primary, or at least falls within the interior angle

defined by two lead strips. That amount of lower-energy scatter is attenuated by the interspace material only. The other factor deals with the percentage of higher-energy scatter radiation that has sufficient energy to penetrate the thickness of a lead strip in which they undergo only slight attentuation. The unaffected primary beam is slightly attenuated by the interspace material and is attenuated to a more significant degree by the lead strips, Therefore, use of the grid prevents a portion of the scattered radiation from reaching the film but it also attenuates, or absorbs, a portion of the primary x-ray beam causing a need for increase in exposure factors to make the radiographic study.

Construction of the grid is rather simple, appearing to be a flat plate with a series of lead foil strips approximately 0.05 mm in thickness and numbering between 500 and 1500 that are set on edge parallel to each other with interspaces filled either with aluminum or some organic

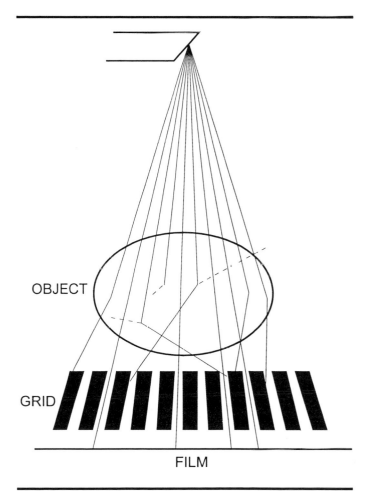

Fig. 5-6
GRID USE
A drawing shows interaction of the x-ray beam with a patient creating scatter radiation that results in generalized fogging of the film unless a device such as a grid is placed between the patient and the film where it absorbs a part of these newly directly photons. A part of the primary beam passes through the patient and radiolucent spaces in the grid and reaches the film. Other photons interact within the patient and alter their direction causing interaction with the lead strips in the grid.

compound (Fig. 5-7). The lead strips run parallel to the long dimension on most grids. The height, thickness, and number of strips per inch (cm) can vary. Radiolucent interspacers are placed between the lead foil strips to provide support. The interspacers are of fiber, plastic, aluminum, or some organic material of low density and are approximately 0.3 mm in thickness. The type of interspacer influences transmission of the primary beam. Use of aluminum with low kVp techniques may result in having to markedly increase the technique because of the increased absorption of primary photons by the aluminum interspacer. This problem is unimportant when using techniques greater than 100 kVp. Aluminum has the advantage of not absorbing moisture and has the greater ease in manufacturing. A binder is used to hold the strips of lead and interspacer together. A covering material, such as aluminum, provides strength and prevents damage to the interspacers and lead strips. Grids are made in various sizes to match the size of the film and cassette.

Grid pattern is determined by the orientation of the lead strips and permits construction of several types of grids (Fig. 5-8). A linear grid has all of the lead strips parallel to each other and is the simplest and most common type of grid. This type of grid has the advantage that the primary x-ray beam may be angled along the length of the grid without loss of primary radiation. Crossed (crosshatch) grids are made by sandwiching two linear grids together with the lead strips of one layer at right angles to the lead strips of the second layer. Crosshatched grids are much more expensive than the linear type, require use of much higher exposure factors, and require much more careful tube positioning to avoid grid cut-off. Cross grids are usually used in a stationary mode and are uncommonly used in radiology of animals.

Types of grids vary based on the relationship of the lead strips to the x-ray beam (Fig. 5-9). A parallel grid is constructed in such a way that all of the lead strips are perpendicular to the face of the grid and planes drawn through the strips continue to be parallel to each other and do not intersect in space. Use of this type of grid always results in some excessive absorption of the primary beam near the film edges (Fig. 5-10) and thus it is best used at long target-grid distances and with small x-ray fields. Centering with the primary beam is not as critical since all strips are perpendicular to the plane of the grid. However, the surface of the grid must be perpendicular to the central x-ray beam.

A focused grid eliminates peripheral grid cutoff which is the main disadvantage of linear grids. The design indicates that the lead strips are at angles that start at 90° to the surface at the center of the grid and progress to greater angles toward both edges of the grid (Fig. 5-9). The lead strips are angled in such a way that planes drawn through each lead strip, if continued beyond the surface of the grid, intersect at a specified distance from the surface of the grid. For this reason, the line is sometimes called a convergence line. The distance from the surface of the grid to the point of intersection of the planes is called the focal distance of the grid and describes the distance that the tube should be from the grid during use. An x-ray tube positioned at the intersection of the planes results in the most efficient use of the grid with the greatest amount of the primary beam passing through unimpaired to reach the film. Acceptable distances that can be used from tube to grid are referred to as the grid range, focal range, or focusing range and use of the grid within these distances permits the majority of the primary beam to pass through the radiolucent slots, or spaces, between the lead strips. The

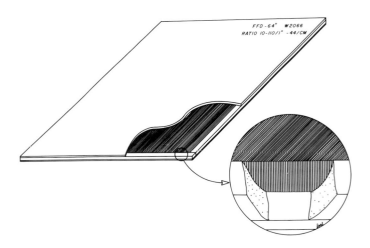

Fig. 5-7
GRID DETAIL
Detailed drawing of a grid shows the way in which the lead strips are positioned in the grid and protected on the sides and ends. Notice the identification on the face of the grid; FFD—64", ratio 10-1, 110 lines/inch (44 lines/cm)

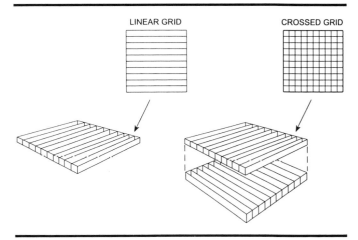

Fig. 5-8
GRID TYPES
Drawings of linear and crossed grids as seen "en-face" and at an angle that show the different alignment of the lead strips drawn as dark lines. Linear grids have lead strips only in one direction while crossed grids are usually constructed by placing one linear grid over another with the lead strips at right angles to each other.

focusing range is wider for a low-ratio grid and narrower for a high-ratio grid. A 5:1 grid focused at 40 inches (100cm) has a focusing range of approximately 28 to 72 inches, while a 16:1 grid focused at 40 inches (100cm) has a focusing range of only 38 to 42 inches. Focal ranges are indicated on the surface of the grid.

Both <u>linear</u> and <u>crosshatch</u> grids can be <u>focused</u> or <u>parallel</u>. Use of a focused grid that is linear requires that the central beam must intersect somewhere along the line marking the center of the grid and be perpendicular to the surface of the grid to avoid excessive absorption of the primary beam. Use of focused grids that are crossed requires that the central beam must intersect at a point marking the center of the grid. The point that represents the intersect

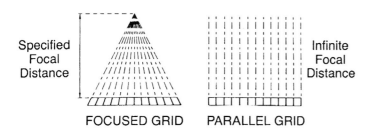

Fig. 5-9
GRID TYPES
Drawings of a focused and parallel grid as seen from on-end showing the different alignment of the lead strips drawn as dark lines within the grid. The dashed lines show a continuation of the lead strips into space where they met at a predetermined point in a focused grid or remain parallel and do not met in a parallel grid.

of the two convergence lines is called a convergence point. An understanding of this concept explains why in the use of a focused grid that is crossed, the tube must be in a single position in space so that the central beam can strike the exact center of the grid and the beam must be perpendicular to the surface of the grid to avoid excessive absorption of the primary beam.

There are several ways to characterize a grid in addition to linear or crossed and parallel or focused. One is by the <u>number</u> of lead strips per inch (cm) (Fig. 5-11). This number of lead strips, or lines, usually ranges between 60 to 133 lines per inch (24 to 53 per cm) and is described as <u>grid frequency</u>. An increase in the number of lines suggests that they are not as thick and do not cast as large a shadow on the radiograph if the grid is used in a stationary mode. Also as the number of lines increases, the width of the lead strips expectedly decreases and the grid is less efficient in the absorption of higher energy scatter radiation. A trend toward stationary, fine-line grids with 133 lines per inch (53 lines per cm) has not been successful because of the lower lead content. Number of lines may not be as important if the grid is used as a moving grid since the lines are not visualized on the radiograph.

<u>Grid-ratio</u> is another method to characterize a grid. The grid-ratio defines the relationship between the height of the lead strips to the width of the spacer between the strips (Fig. 5-11). If the lead strips are five times as high as the space between them, the ratio is 5:1. The grid-ratio partially expresses the efficiency of the grid in absorbing scatter radiation. Grid ratios range from 5:1 to as high as 16:1. The grid with the higher ratio absorbs scatter radiation to a greater degree than a grid with a lower ratio. The higher ratio grid has the disadvantage of: (1) requiring more perfect

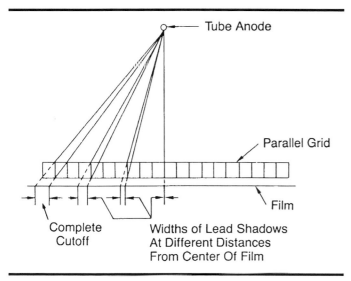

Fig. 5-10
GRID CUT-OFF USING A PARALLEL GRID
Lead strips directly under the tube cast a shadow the same width on the film. More laterally positioned lead strips cast shadows of increasing width as the photons move away from the center line of the grid. This causes a progressive increase in the absorption of the primary photons by the lead strips resulting in a decreasing film density toward the edge of the film

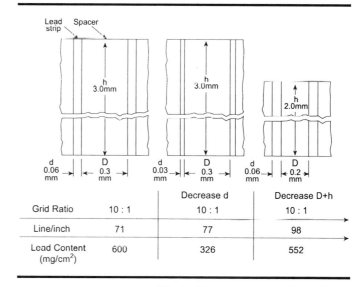

	Decrease d	Decrease D+h
Grid Ratio	10 : 1	10 : 1	10 : 1
Line/inch	71	77	98
Lead Content (mg/cm²)	600	326	552

Fig. 5-11
GRID RATIO, LINES PER INCH, AND LEAD CONTENT OF A GRID
Grid-ratio defines the relationship between the height of the lead strip and the width of the spacer. Lines per inch (cm) vary with the width of the lead strips on the spacers. Lead content is the weight of specified area of the grid (mg/cm2).

centering of the primary beam, (2) requiring a greater exposure because of increased absorption of the primary beam, and (3) having a much narrower focusing range. A 5:1 ratio grid is reported to clean up approximately 85% of the scatter radiation, whereas a 16:1 ratio grid may clean up as much as 97% (Bushong, 1984). It is assumed that the ratio of a crossed grid made up of two 5:1 linear grids functions about the same as a linear grid with a 10:1 ratio.

A third way to characterize grids is by the selectivity of the grid in permitting the transmision of all primary x-rays and the absorption of all of the scatter x-rays. Selectivity is related to grid-ratio, but the total mass of lead in the grid has a major influence on selectivity. The level of lead content is usually expressed in gm/cm^2 (Fig. 5-11). Consideration of lead content as a measure of selectivity is suggested as a better way to evaluate grid function; however, this numerical information is usually not available.

Despite the common use of grid-ratio as a method of evaluating the grid, grid-ratio does not accurately describe the ability of the grid to improve radiographic contrast. Contrast improvement factor is the best method of describing the value of a grid in improving film quality. It is the ratio of the contrast measured on a radiograph made with the grid as compared to the contrast measured on a radiograph made without using the grid (Fig. 5-12). Remember that it is the grid's ability to improve contrast that is its primary function. Unfortunately, this factor is not often available to the buyer of a grid. Generally, the contrast improvement factor is higher for high-ratio grids, however, other factors such as lead content greatly influence this measure of grid performance. A crossed grid has a higher contrast improvement factor than a linear grid of twice the grid ratio. That is, a crossed grid made up of two 5:1 ratio linear grids cleans up more scatter radiation than a 10:1 linear grid (Bushong, 1984).

A grid can be used in a moving or stationary mode. If the grid is used stationary, grid lines are identified on the resulting radiograph, while if the grid moves during the exposure, grid lines are blurred and are not distracting as the radiograph is evaluated (Fig. 5-13). Exposure factors need to be increased additionally when using a moving grid because of the unavoidable lateral decentering of the x-ray tube with subsequent reduction in transmitted primary radiation. Usually, because of the short excursion of the grid, this loss in film density is not greater than about 20% (Boldingh, 1964). A radiograph made using a stationary grid creates an x-ray image composed of shadows cast by the grid strips and in the interspace areas with a photon density slightly greater than in the radiograph made with a moving grid. Thus, the number of primary photons that are transmitted per unit area is the same, except that when using the stationary grid, these photons are "compressed" between the strips (Ter-Pogossian, 1967). Since, your technique chart is made using the grid in its expected manner, there is no reason to have to compensate for the differences between a moving or stationary grid. Grids that remain stationary during the exposure are used in the following situations: (1) positioned over the cassette on a tabletop, (2) fixed in position in a grid cabinet just beneath

the tabletop or between the tabletop and the cassette (Fig. 5-14), (3) attached to a holder (Fig. 5-15), used free in a vertical mode with horizontal beam radiographic technique, or (4) built into the face of the cassette. In these modes, the grid does not move during the exposure and grid lines are easily identified on the radiograph. Most cross grids are used in a stationary mode.

To make the exposure with the grid moving, a mechanical or electrical device is required. Moving grids are found most commonly in association with a permanent cassette holder that is beneath the tabletop or in a wall-mounted holder. The moving grid is often called a Bucky, Bucky tray, Bucky grid, Bucky diaphragm, or Potter-Bucky diaphragm. These names give reference to Dr. Gustave Bucky, who built the first grid in 1913, and Dr. Hollis E. Potter, who introduced a method of moving the grid in 1920 to avoid the presence of the lead strip shadows on the radiograph. Early movable grids were spring-loaded and traveled across the film once during the exposure and were called catapult grids. It was necessary to manually pull a

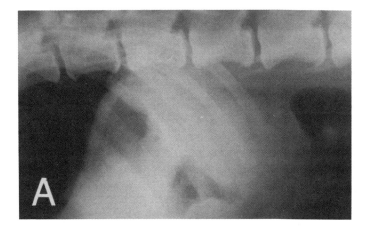

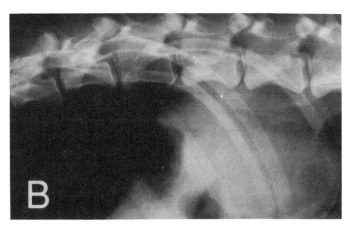

Fig. 5-12
COMPARISON OF RADIOGRAPHS MADE
WITH AND WITHOUT A GRID
Comparison of a radiograph made without use of a grid (A) easily shows the improvement in film quality that can be obtained through use of a grid (B). Radiographic contrast is compromised by fogging from scatter radiation if the grid is not used. It is important to recognize the increase in radiographic technique required when using a grid.

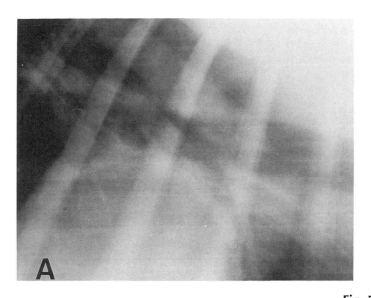
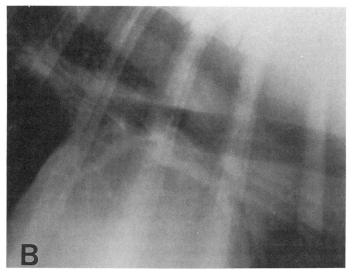

Fig. 5-13
COMPARISON OF RADIOGRAPHS MADE USING STATIONARY AND MOVING GRIDS
Grid lines are visible in the radiograph made with the grid in a stationary mode (A) and may slightly compromise the quality of the resulting radiograph. The radiograph made using the grid in a moving mode (B) does not permit the visualization of the grid lines and is a more pleasing radiograph to examine.

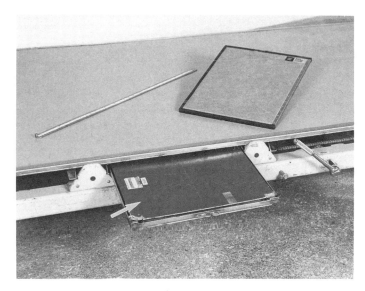

Fig. 5-14
GRID HOLDER
The grid (arrow) is positioned under a large animal table within a tray and is used in a stationary mode. The cassette fits under the grid.

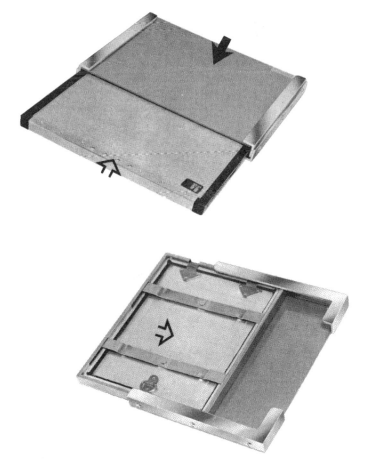

Fig. 5-15
GRID HOLDER
The grid (solid arrow) is within the face of the cassette holder and the cassette (hollow arrows) slides into the holder for use. The grid is used in a stationary mode.

level "cocking" the grid prior to use. Often a timer was set that determined the length of time required for the grid to travel across the film one time. This time was slightly longer than the exposure time to insure movement during the complete exposure time. Newer units have reciprocating grids that move continuously back and forth during the exposure. The most brief exposure times that can be used with this type of grid motion is usually 0.2 second. Since the reciprocating grid moves faster, it may be used with a more brief exposure time and it does not require manual resetting after each exposure. Motion of the grid must be fast enough relative to the exposure time or individual lines representing the blurred lead strips are seen on the radiograph. A third type of moving grid is an oscillating grid that moves in a circular fashion around the grid frame. It is obviously not possible to have a moving grid when manually holding the cassette.

Disadvantage to the use of a moving grid relate to the cost of the unit and the fact that it, like any other mechanical device, may be subject to malfunction. Also, a moving grid may produce noise during operation that is objectionable to the patient. The distance between the patient and the film is increased with use of a grid causing slight magnification and geometric unsharpness. Obviously, patient radiation dosage is markedly increased with the use of grids because of the increased exposure factors required to compensate for use of the grid. Still, the advantages of moving grids far outweigh the disadvantages and they are the technique of choice. A focused grid is most commonly used when moving grids are employed.

The bucky factor refers to the alteration in radiographic technique required due to: (1) the absorption of 20 to 30% of the primary beam and (2) absorption of 80 to 90% of the scatter radiation. The amount of absorption is dependent on: (1) grid ratio, (2) the number of strips/inch (cm), (3) grams of lead/sq.in.(cm.), (4) the thickness of the object, and (5) width of the beam (Boldingh, 1961). The affect of the grid is practically independent of kilovoltage (Matsson, 1956). Most bucky or grid factors are between 3 and 8 times the mAs required without use of the grid. That means that an exposure made with an mAs of 1.0 would need a new mAs of 3.0 to 8.0 if a grid were used in the same examination (Table 5-4). This change in technique is approximately the same whether a grid is used in a moving or stationary mode. If a portable machine is set on the highest kVp and mA possible, the only other method to increase the technique so that the grid can be used is through either an increase in exposure time or a decrease in focal-film distance. Increasing the exposure time results in the possibility of patient motion during the exposure, whereas decreasing the focal-film distance causes magnification and blurring of the image with loss of film quality.

A grid should be used in the radiography of any anatomical structure which is solid and is more than 11 cm thick. Radiography of the thorax in a normal healthy patient presents the possibility to not use the grid until radiographing a larger patient (>15cm) because the aerating lung causes much less attenuation of the primary x-ray beam and production of much less secondary radiation. However, in an obese patient with a thickened chest wall or one with pleural fluid or lung consolidation or collapse, there is an increase in tissue density and a need to use a grid technique to control the effect of the secondary radiation.

If the machine you use has capabilities in excess of 300 mA, it is possible to recommend use of a grid technique regardless of the tissue thickness. This is possible because the increase in radiographic technique can be made and still permit exposures with short time intervals. Thus, patient motion does not become a problem in causing decreased film quality. Still, it must be appreciated that the studies made using a grid require use of higher exposure factors and consequently, patient exposure and scatter radiation reaching a technician is increased.

Use of the grid in cross-table examinations introduces the problem of positioning the grid so that the surface is perpendicular to the central beam with the beam striking the center line of the grid. It must be understood that to use a grid correctly, it is necessary for the plane of the grid to be perpendicular to the central x-ray beam. This requires the use of some ingenious devices to insure that the grid is perpendicular to the beam and that the beam is centered on the grid. Problems with this type of positioning almost completely prevents use of a grid in any examinations where the grid is held freely.

The problem of grid positioning in radiography of larger animals is one of the reasons that overhead suspended tubes usually have a second lighter-weight suspended column that holds the cassette and grid. The columns that hold the tube and the cassette are connected overhead so that movement of the tube results in similar movement of the cassette and grid. This means that when the tube is locked in position, the x-ray beam is parallel to the ground and directed toward the center of the cassette holder. Any subsequent movement of the x-ray tube results in synchronous movement of the cassette holder and the x-ray beam remains centered on the cassette and grid. By the use of this arrangement, it is possible to rather easily radiograph the thorax or abdomen of a larger animal and improve the quality of the radiograph by the correct use of the grid.

Table 5-4
BUCKY-FACTOR TO COMPENSATE FOR EXPOSURE REDUCTION DUE TO GRID USE*

RATIO	at 70 kVp	at 95 kVp	at 120 kVp
no grid	1	1	1
5:1	3	3	3
8:1	3.5	3.75	4
12:1	4	4.25	5
16:1	4.5	5	6

*Characteristics and Applications of X-ray Grids. Leibel Flarsheim Co., 1968.

One major disadvantage that accompanies the use of x-ray girds is the increase in patient radiation dose of up to 8 times that exposure dose measured without the use of a grid (Bushong, 1984). In addition, the use of a moving grid instead of a stationary grid with similar physical characteristics causes approximately 15% additional radiation to the patient. However, grid selection should not be compromised so that failure to use the grid interferes with the diagnostic quality of the radiograph. The level of kVp used greatly influences patient dose. In general, the use of high kVp and high-ratio grids results in lower patient dose and radiographs of equal quality when compared with the use of low kVp and low-ratio grids.

INCORRECT GRID USE

One of the primary disadvantages associated with use of grids is the absorption of a part of the primary x-ray beam by the lead strips. Incorrect use of a focused grid can increase this absorption of the primary beam if the beam is not directed in such a manner that it passes between the lead strips with the least absorption possible. Grid cutoff is the term used to describe the situation in which an excessive amount of useful x-rays are prevented from reaching the film. This problem is primarily associated with focused grids but also exists with the use of parallel grids to a lesser degree. The grid cut-off may: 1) be equal on both edges of the radiograph, 2) may be uniform throughout the radiograph, or 3) may be more pronounced on one edge of the radiograph than the other.

A focused grid may be inadvertently used inverted and be positioned perpendicular to the central beam with the central beam centered (Fig. 5-16). Severe cutoff occurs on the two edges of the radiograph with a more normal exposure along the center of the grid (Fig. 5-17). The higher the grid ratio, the narrower is the strip of "nearly" normal exposed film. Focused grids are usually identified on one surface with the words "tube side" or "tube side up" indicating the side to be directed toward the tube. This type of error usually occurs only once and is immediately noted and corrected.

Lateral decentering occurs when the x-ray tube is positioned laterally to the center line on the grid but at a correct focus-grid distance and with the x-ray beam perpendicular to the surface of the grid (Fig. 5-18). The lead strips absorb the primary radiation equally across the entire radiograph. Three factors affect the degree of cutoff: (1) grid ratio, (2) focal-grid distance, and (3) the distance of decentralization. If you are using a grid with a ratio of 5:1 or 8:1 at a 40 inch (100 cm) focal-grid distance, it is possible to have the decentralization reach 1 inch (2.5cm) without compromising film quality. This type of error is common and is due to undetected lateral movement of the x-ray tube as it hangs over the tabletop. It is obvious that it is not possible to have this type of technical error when using a linear parallel grid.

If the central beam is directed on the central line but with the grid at an angle to the central beam, increased cutoff occurs (Fig. 5-19). This may occur due to the grid not level or the tube being tilted. Either of these may be referred to as an off-level grid and the cutoff is equal across the entire radiograph (Fig. 5-20). In radiography of small animals using an x-ray table, the most common cause for this type of grid misuse occurs with a tube housing that is loose that permits the x-ray tube to rotate within its holder. The centering light from the collimator directs the central beam onto the center of the grid making it appear that the beam is "centered" but does not indicate that it is at other than a right angle to the tabletop. Since the lines in a focused grid are commonly parallel with the long axis of the table, the angulation must be laterally directed to cause increased grid cutoff. If the angulation is longitudinal, there is no additional grid cutoff. In working with a horizontal beam, it is not uncommon to find that the surface of the grid is not

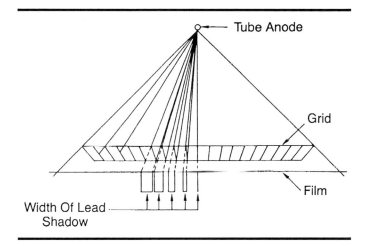

Fig. 5-16
GRID CUT-OFF AS A RESULT OF AN INVERTED GRID
Drawing illustrates beam cut-off caused by using a focused grid inverted. Film density decreases rapidly toward the edges of the radiograph.

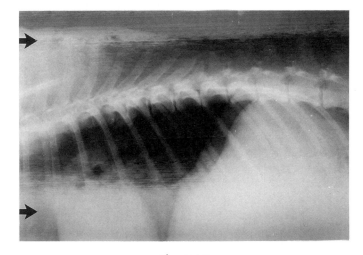

Fig. 5-17
GRID CUT-OFF AS A RESULT OF AN INVERTED GRID
Radiograph shows the grid cut-off (arrows) when using a focused grid in an inverted manner.

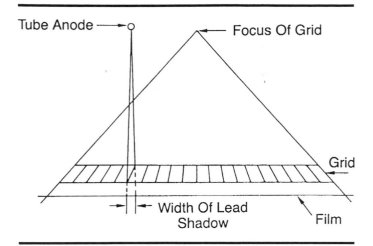

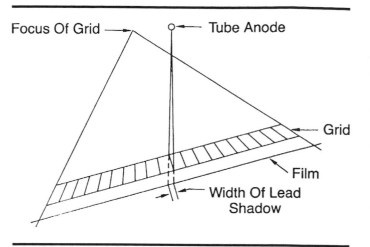

Fig. 5-18
GRID CUT-OFF AS A RESULT OF
LATERAL DECENTERING OF THE BEAM
Drawing illustrates beam cut-off caused by lateral decentering of
the beam. Film density is decreased equally across the entire radiograph.

Fig. 5-19
GRID CUT-OFF AS A RESULT OF A TILTED OR "OFF-LEVEL" GRID
Drawing illustrates beam cut-off caused by using an "off-level'
grid. Film density is decreased equally across the entire radiograph.

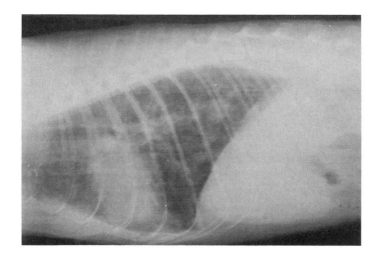

Fig. 5-20
GRID CUT-OFF
A lateral radiograph of the thorax of a cat with equal grid cut-off
across the entire film characterised by visible grid lines. This could be
the result of an off-level grid or lateral decentering of the tube.

perpendicular to the central beam as a result of their being no physical connection between the tube and grid holder.

Grid cutoff occurs if the grid is positioned closer to or further from the stated range of focal-film distance when the grid is perpendicular to the central beam and the central beam is centered (Fig. 5-21). This is referred to as an off-focus grid. The grid cutoff is more severe on the edges of the radiograph and is identified more prominently when using a high ratio grid in which the tube to grid range is very narrow.

Any combination of these errors is additive and the resulting grid cutoff becomes more severe. The situation of decentralization plus an increase or decrease in the distance from the tube to the film causes the cutoff to be more prominent on one side of the radiograph than on the other. A most severe combination of errors occurs with decentralization of a primary beam that is angled. A linear grid is forgiving if the centering is only slightly off mid-line and the resulting grid cut-off is minimal. A crosshatch grid requires perfect alignment of the x-ray beam with the center of the grid to avoid grid cutoff of any type. The central beam can be directed at any point on the surface of a parallel grid if the surface of the grid is perpendicular to the central x-ray beam.

Selection of the correct grid is difficult because of the usual requirement to purchase a single grid that is useful in as many different examinations as possible. Therefore, the first decision in purchase is to determine for which studies the grid is to be used. This is principally influenced by knowing whether it is to be used for radiography of small or large animal patients. In small animal radiography, the size should be maximum to include the thorax or abdomen of a large patient and should be focused at 40 inches (100 cm) or greater with a grid ratio of 8:1 or 10:1. A general rule is that grid ratios up to 8:1 are satisfactory at tube potentials below 90 kVp while grid ratios above 8:1 find application when potentials exceed 90 kVp (Dushong, 1984). The number of lines should be between 60 to 85 lines per inch (24 to 33 lines per cm). However, if the grid is to be used for studies of limbs of large animals, one that is 8 x 10 inch (18 x 24 cm), has a grid ratio of 5:1 or 8:1, and has 40 to 60 lines per inch (16 to 24 lines per cm) is recommended. If the grid is to be used for studies of the thorax of large animals, the characteristics may be similiar to those listed for the grid to be used in small animal studies. A grid used for large animal chests may be focused at a larger focal-film distance if it is to be used in conjunction with powerful x-ray equipment. It may be possible to use a linear grid when radiographing the feet of large animals since the width of the field of exposure is small. Modern grids are sufficiently well manufactured with a large enough number of grid lines that the presence of the lines caused by stationary usage is not objectionable. However, moving-grid mechansims rarely fail mechanically so they can be used without problems if the grid motion occurs in a short enough time period.

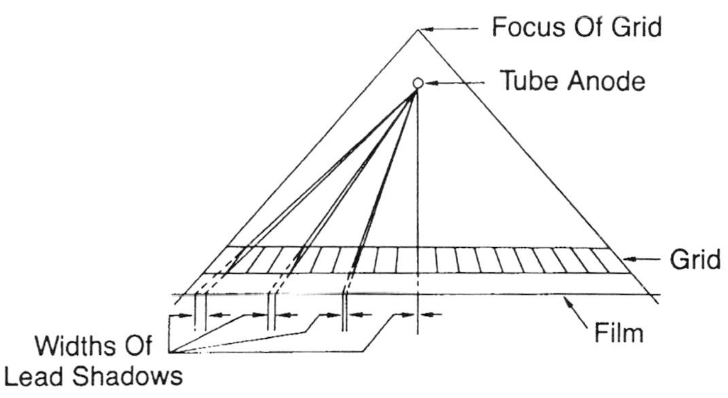

Grids installed in an undertable tray are well protected and require little care. Uncommonly, liquid contrast agents may flow onto the surface of the grid and present a repetitive pattern of artifacts on each subsequent radiographs. The grid can be detached from its position under the table and the surface wiped clean to correct this type of problem. Because of their location under the table, it is difficult to bend the grids and damage them in that manner. Stationary grids that are attached to a cassette are obviously more prone to damage as a result of being dropped or bent while in use. Construction of the grid is such that little force is needed to injure the grid by bending or separating the lead strips resulting in increased or decreased absorption of the primary x-ray beam and produces an overexposed or underexposed region on the radiograph (Fig. 5-22). This is one of the reasons for having a well constructed cassette/grid holder that protects the grid and is an inherent problem whenever you place the cassette and grid directly under a large patient. Care should be used in cleaning grids since excess water damages the filler material between the lead strips unless it is aluminum.

D. AIR-GAP

The air-gap technique is an alternative to the use of radiographic grids in the control of scatter radiation in certain situations. Moving the cassette away from an anatomical area to be radiographed creates an air-gap that provides an opportunity for some of the scatter radiation to escape and not strike the cassette causing fogging (Fig. 5-23). This technique can be used especially in radiography of the thorax, abdomen, or thoracic or lumbar spine of a horse or cow. It must be used with large focal-film distances such as those > 40 inches (> 100 cm) so that the added object-film distance doesn't cause objectionable magnification. The air gap can be between 4 and 6 inches (10 to 15 cm) but can extend up to 12 inches (30 cm). By selecting greater focal-film distances such as 60 to 70 inches (150 to 180 cm), discarding use of the grid, and adding the air gap, it is usually possible to obtain high quality radiographs of thick anatomical parts, such as the thorax in large animals, with use of a lessor amount of radiation (decreased machine

Fig. 5-21
GRID CUT-OFF AS A RESULT OF AN "OFF-FOCUS" GRID
Drawing illustrates beam cut-off caused by using an "off-focus" grid. Film density is equally decreased selectively on both edges of the radiograph.

settings) than would have been required if using a grid. Air-gap technique is not as effective with high kVp technique because of the greater percentage of x-rays that scatter in a forward direction. At settings below 90 kVp, more of the scattered x-rays are directed laterally and have a higher probability of being scattered away from the film. The air-gap should not be referred to as air filtration since this layer of air does not act as a selective filter of low-energy scattered x-rays (Gould and Hale, 1974). One disadvantage of the air-gap technique is image magnification with associated geometric unsharpness, however, an increased focal-film distance can compensate for the magnification.

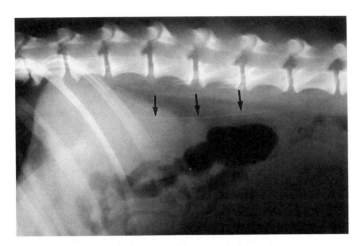

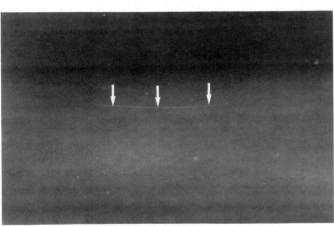

Fig. 5-22
GRID DAMAGE
If a grid is damaged, the relationship between the lead lines and the primary x-ray beam may be altered in some manner. In this grid, a focal injury seems to have bent only one or two lead strips that prevented the x-ray beam from reaching the film creating an unexposed line on the radiograph (arrows). A second radiograph made of only the grid shows the grid injury exactly as before (arrows) and rules out other artifacts as a cause. Note the possibility that the center of the grid is absorbing more of the primary beam than is the edges of the grid.

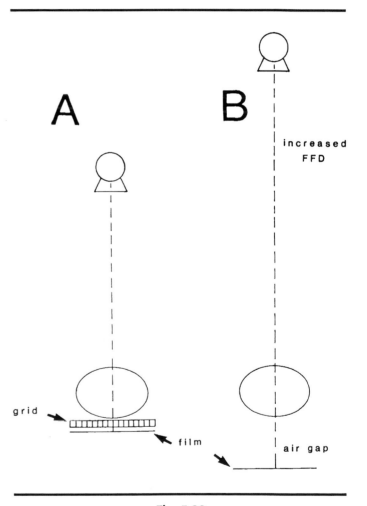

Fig. 5-23
AIR-GAP TECHNIQUE
Drawing showing the relationship of the tube, patient, grid (arrow), and cassette (arrows) in a conventional radiographic examination (A) and using an air-gap technique (B). Note that the FFD is increased, grid is not utilized, and patient-cassette distance is increased in the air-gap technique.

REFERENCES

Hondius-Boldingh W. Grids to Reduce Scattered X-ray in Medical Radiography. Phillips Research Reports Suppl. 1. Eindhoven, 1964.

Hondius-Boldingh W. Quality and Choice of Potter Bucky Grids. Part VI. Acta Radiol 56:202-8. 1961.

Bull K W Curry lll T S Dowdey J E and Christensen E E. The cutoff characteristics of rotating grids. Radiol 114-453-5, 1975.

Bushong S C. Radiologic Science for Technologists, 3rd ed C.V.Mosby Company, St. Louis 1984.

Characteristics and Applications of X-ray Grids, rev. ed. Liebel Flarsheim Company, 1968.

Curry T S 111 Dowdey J E and Murry R C. Christensen's Introduction to the physics of diagnostic radiology. 3rd ed Lea & Febiger, Philadelphia, 1984.

Dick C E Soares C G and Motz J W. X-ray scatter data for diagnostic radiology. Phy Med Biol 23:1076-85, 1978.

Gould R G and Hale J. Control of scatered radiation by air gap techniques: Applications to chest radiography. Am J Roentgenol 122:109, 1974.

Mattsson O. Some studies on primary and secondary radiation and on secondary screening in diagnosis. 1956.

Reiss KH. Scattered radiation and characteristic film curve. Radiology 80:663,1963.

Ter-Pogossian M M. Physical aspects of diagnostic radiology, Harper & Row , Publishers New, York, 1967.

Trout E D. The life history of an x-ray beam. Rad Tech 35:161-70,1963.

van der Plaats G J. Medical X-ray techniques in diagnostic radiology, 4th ed. Martinus Nijhoff, The Hague, 1980.

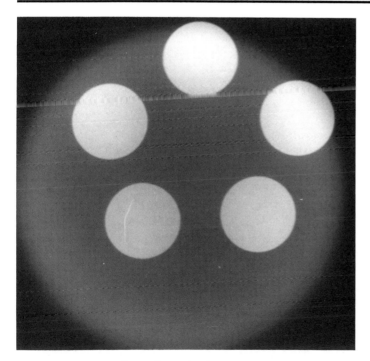 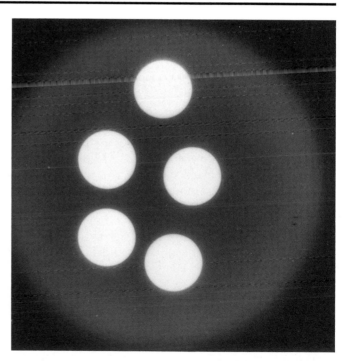

These are two radiographs made of 5 coins positioned relative to a 20cm paper cup filled with water. In one study, the coins are on top of the paper cup and in the other study, the coins are on the bottom between the paper cup and the film. Explain why one group of coins is larger than the other and why one group of coins is white and the other group is gray.

6. X-RAY FILM, FILM HOLDERS, INTENSIFYING SCREENS, AND FILM MARKERS

A. X-RAY FILM

The uniformily distributed photons in the useful beam at the time of production are altered in their distribution in space after passing through the patient and the beam of remnant x-rays varies according to the characteristics of the anatomic structure through which it has passed (Fig. 6-1). It is necessary to transfer the information obtained by the x-ray beam after it passes through the patient to some form that can be readily interpreted by the clinician. The most common type of image receptor used in veterinary radiography to record this information is the use of silver halide crystals mounted on a plastic support, this is a description of conventional radiographic film. Radiographic film is used: (1) to provide a permanent record containing the maximum amount of diagnostic information that can be recorded and (2) to permit its re-examination as is required or convenient. Other techniques used in information transfer include the: 1) fluoroscopic screen, 2) image intensifier, 3) television monitor, 4) video tape, and 5) multiformat camera.

X-ray film composition is similar to other types of conventional photographic film and basically has two parts, the base and the emulsion (Fig. 6-2). The film base, currently a polyester, provides support for the emulsion, and therefore it must be stable, inert, and uniformly transparent. The strength of the base has become more important with the use of automatic processors. Blue dye is added to the base to slightly tint the film resulting in less eyestrain for the viewer. A thin adhesive subcoat insures uniform adhesion of the emulsion layer to the film base. The emulsion consists of a homogeneous mixture of gelatin that provides mechanical support for the silver halide crystals. In a typical emulsion, most (90% to 99%) of the silver halide is silver bromide and the remainder (1% to 10%) is usually silver iodide. The emulsion is covered by a protective covering of gelatin that protects it from scratching, pressure, and contamination during use and processing. It permits rather rough handling of the film prior to exposure without production of film artifacts, however, the crystals are more sensitive following exposure and film artifacts occur more frequently. Most film commonly used in radiography has the silver halide crystals coated in an emulsion on both sides of a polyester base. However, some examples of single-emulsion film are available (OM-1, Kodak). The thickness of a sheet of radiographic film ranges from 0.20 to 0.30mm.

The emulsion in the film is sensitive to ionizing radiation or light and a latent image is formed on the film by the absorption of a photon of energy that reaches the film. The absorption is primarily by photoelectric interaction with the atoms of a silver halide crystal. The energy of the photon removes an electron from the silver halide atom creating a photoelectron that is temporarily caught by a sensitivity trap (positively charged silver ions) in the crystal caused by

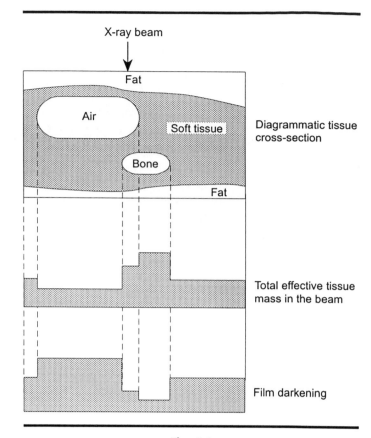

Fig. 6-1
RELATIONSHIP BETWEEN OBJECT MASS AND FILM DENSITY
Diagrammatically, the limiting effect of various tissues on the resulting number of photons that eventually reach the film can be shown. The x-ray beam interacts with a cross-section of tissue and the selective absorption of the primary photons is shown with the resulting film darkening at the bottom of the drawing. Note that the total effective tissue mass in the beam is dependent both of the thickness of the tissue and its composition.

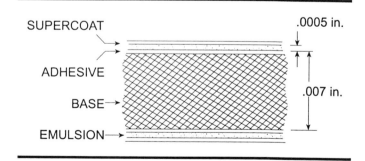

Fig. 6-2
CROSS-SECTION OF A DOUBLE EMULSION X-RAY FILM
The components of x-ray film are identified.

an imperfection created in the crystal at the time of film production. A number of photoelectrons congregate at the sensitivity speck producing a region of negative electrification that attracts positively charged silver ions that join to form a silver atom that grows to become large enough to form a developmental center or latent-image center that result in the change of an entire silver halide crystal to silver. Numerous tiny silver halide crystals in the emulsion are thus converted to metallic silver by exposure to the x-ray photons. The same pattern of latent image formation occurs in the event the film exposure is from visible light as when it is exposed by x-ray photons. The greater the number of silver halide crystals that have been transferred to metallic silver, the blacker is the film following developing and the greater is the film density. Processing is the term applied to the chemical reaction that transforms the latent image into a manifest radiographic image.

Radiographic film is characterized by film speed. The speed of the film determines the amount of x-ray or light photons required to produce a visible image on the film. Basically, a faster film has: (1) thicker emulsion, (2) larger silver halide crystals, (3) requires less exposure to light or x-ray photons to produce a given film density, (4) produces a grainier image that lacks in definition, and (5) has less latitude in exposure and processing. Slower film has: (1) thinner emulsion, (2) smaller silver halide crystals, (3) requires more exposure to light or x-ray photons to produce a given film density, (4) produces an image that is less grainy and has greater definition or detail, and (5) has greater latitude in exposure and processing. Film speeds are currently based on a system that assigns a numerical base value of 100 to an earlier film-screen system referred to as par-speed film when used in conjunction with par-speed intensifying screens. Slower film speed requires the use of increased machine settings in the form of increased mAs, which means an increase in exposure time or mA setting. The compensation in speed can also be made by increasing the kVp setting.

Another way of characterizing film is by describing film contrast. This is the difference between two densities noted on the radiograph. Contrast is determined in part by the character of the film, in part by the processing technique, and in part by kVp range used. Some films are manufactured to have higher contrast with images on the film appearing "black and white", whereas, other films have lower contrast and the images on the film have many detectable shades of grey. Descriptions of film characteristics are usually available from different manufacturers. Film speed, sensitivity, type of processing and level of contrast are usually included within their descriptions (Tables 6-1, 6-2).

Film may also be described by latitude, or the range of exposure techniques that produce an acceptable image. Latitude is usually inversely proportional to contrast. High latitude exaggerates subject contrast. By ploting the log of the photographic density that results from progressively increased radiographic exposures, a curve is developed that is described as a characteristic curve, or "H and D" curve, named after Hurter and Driefield who used it first in 1890. Film with more latitude has a more shallow slope on the H

Table 6-1
KODAK FILM CHARACTERISTICS

X-OMAT RP	High contrast Medium speed Blue- and ultraviolet-sensitive Automatic and manual processing
X-OMAT K	High contrast Medium speed Blue-sensitive Automatic and manual processing
X-OMAT L	Wide latitude Medium speed Blue- and ultraviolet-sensitive Automatic processing
X-OMAT G	Very high contrast Low speed Blue-sensitive Automatic and manual processing
X-OMAT TL	Fine grain Direct exposure film Excellent detail Good for specimen radiography Automatic processing
Ortho G	High contrast Automatic and manual processing Blue-, ultraviolet-, and green-sensitive Orthochromatic sensitivity
Ortho L	Wide latitude Approx. the same speed as Ortho G film Increased exposure latitude compared to higher contrast films Automatic and manual processing Blue-, ultraviolet-, and green-sensitive Orthochromatic sensitivity
Ortho H	Medium contrast Automatic processing Twice the speed of Ortho G film Blue-, ultraviolet-, and green-sensitive Orthochromatic sensitivity
Ortho M	Very high contrast Single-coated Blue, ultraviolet, and green-sensitive Orthochromatic sensitivity High definition Automatic or manual processing Approx. twice the speed of Min-R and NMB films For use with a single LANEX fine screen or double screen
Blue Brand	Blue-sensitive Medium speed High contrast Automatic (long cycle) or manual processing

Table 6-2
DUPONT FILM CHARACTERISTICS

Cronex 4	High contrast Full speed Blue-sensitive
Cronex 4L	Medium contrast Full speed Wide latitude Blue-sensitive
Cronex WDR	Wide latitude Full speed Blue-sensitive
Cronex 7	High contrast One-half speed Blue-sensitive
Cronex 7L	Medium contrast One-half speed Wide latitude Blue-sensitive
Cronex 10T	High contrast High resolution One-half speed Blue-sensitive
Cronex 10L	Medium contrast High resolution One-half speed Blue sensitive
Cronex 8	High contrast One-half speed Green-sensitive
Cronex 8L	Medium contrast One-half speed Green-sensitive
Cronex OTG	High contrast High resolution One-half speed Green-sensitive

Table 6-3
COMPARISON OF RELATIVE NUMBER OF X-RAY PHOTONS AND LIGHT PHOTONS AT VARIOUS STAGES FOR DIRECT AND SCREEN-FILM EXPOSURES*

Stage	Type of Exposure	
	Direct	Screen-film
Incident x-ray photons	1000	20
X-rays absorbed by film	10	(>1)
X-rays absorbed by screens	—	5
Light photons produced	—	5000
Light photons incident on film	—	3000
Light photons absorbed by film	—	1000
Latent images formed	10	10

Intensification factor = 1000/20 = 50

*Bushong, 1980

and D curve. Film with less latitude has a steep slope on the H and D curve and is often preferred by many because it has a more black and white appearance and "looks pretty" (Fig. 6-3).

There are two basic types of film that are used in radiography (Table 6-3). One is a screen type of film that is manufactured with crystals that are sensitive to visable fluorescent light that originates from the crystals in the intensifying screens within the cassette and results in exposure of the film. These crystals are less sensitive to x-ray photons. This type of film requires less exposure to produce an image than does direct exposure-type film because of the intensification factor due to the use of the fluorescent intensifying screens. Some loss in image definition or detail occurs because of this intensification process. Screen film is the type of film used with cassettes and is used most commonly in veterinary radiography.

Non-screen film or direct exposure film, is the second type of film and is exposed by direct action of the x-ray photon and may be used for examinations of the horse's foot where the requirement for detail is great and motion during the exposure can be controlled. Because tissue thickness is less, it can also be used for intra-oral studies in dogs and cats and in studies of the whole body of smaller birds and smaller exotic species. Non-screen film does not have the protection afforded by a strong cassette and some type of cardboard film holder or individually packaged paper wrappings is used to protect the film. (A lead-foil backing shields the film from back-scatter radiation.) Because there is no intensifying action by the intensifying screens, exposure times of non-screen film are much longer. Exposure times (mAs) are around 10 times longer than that required for screen film when used with intensifying screens. Dental film is a special form of non-screen film that is individually packaged. It comes in sizes ranging from 2 1/4 x 3 inches

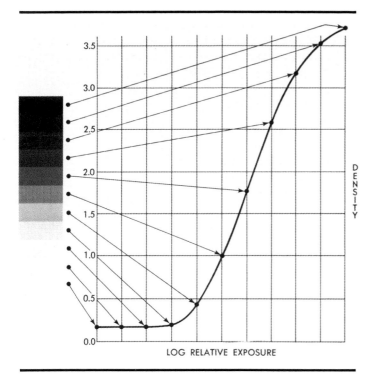

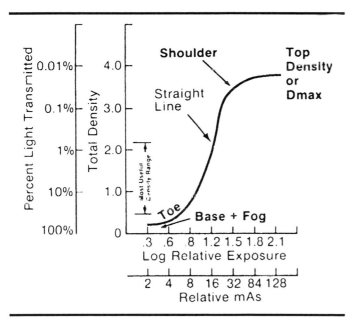

Fig. 6-3
CHARACTERISTIC CURVES

Relative exposure of the film is shown on the x-axis with the resulting film density shown on the y-axis. Note that the density of 0.18 ± 0.20 is usual for base density plus fog. The range of diagnostic densities is between 0.25 and 2.0. This curve is referred to as an "H and D" curve and it changes shape dependent on the latitude of the film.

(57 x 76mm) to 7/8 x 1 3/8 inches (22 x 35 mm). Some dental film packets have two films for the production of two identical radiographs with a single exposure permitting the production of a duplicate record. Many types of non-screen film have thicker emulsions and require processing in wet tanks.

Mammography film is a type of non-screen film that was originally an industrial-grade double-emulsion direct-exposure film. However, the radiation doses associated with use of the film in mammography were much too high requiring development of a new type of film. Newer types of non-screen film used for mammography examinations are faster and have a thinner but stronger base permitting processing in an automatic processor.

Duplicating film—Duplication of an existing radiograph requires the use of a different type of film that is a single-emulsion film that is exposed to ultraviolet light passing through the existing radiograph. Normally, film response is directly related to the amount of light received by the film so that the greater the exposure, the blacker the film becomes on processing. However, with increased exposure to light, the response of the duplicating film reverses and a positive copy is produced. This is obviously desired in the process of producing a duplication of an existing radiograph. The processing of the film is as with conventional radiographic film.

Spectral response—Screen-type film can also be classified by the nature of the visible light from the intensifying screens to which the films are sensitive. For many years, most x-ray film was "blue-sensitive," meaning that the primary photographic response of the film was to ultraviolet, violet, and blue light that originated from the intensifying screens. Calcium tungstate was commonly used as the phosphor in the intensifying screens because it efficiently converted energy of the x-ray photon into photographically usable ultraviolet, violet, and blue portions of the spectrum. Today, many films are produced that are sensitive to green light resulting from production of a new generation of intensifying screens that utilize rare-earth phosphors instead of the conventional blue light producing calcium tungstate. Approximately 60% of the emission from rare-earth phosphors is within the green portion of the spectrum and about 25% of the emission is within the ultraviolet, violet, and blue portions of the spectrum. Because of the wide range of energies of light produced by the intensifying screens, it is possible to use both blue and green light emitting screens with blue- or green-light sensitive films to create film-screen systems with markedly differing speeds. To obtain the greatest speed for a film-screen system, it is imperative that a film be used whose sensitivity to various colors of light is properly matched to the spectrum of light emitted by the screen.

The method of changing the sensitivity of the film is rather simple. By covering the silver halide grains in the film with a thin layer of dye that absorbs green light, the sensitivity of the film to green light can be increased. This type of "green sensitive" film is referred to as orthochromatic film or "ortho" film and is sensitive to all colors but those on the red end of the spectrum (panchromatic film). Film used with calcium tungstate crystal screens does not need to be dye-sensitized because the emission of light is in the wavelength (blue) that silver halide absorbs. Remember that the type of film that is utilized determines the type of filter that is required on the safelight in the darkroom (Fig. 6-4).

In commonly used x-ray film, a considerable fraction of film darkening is due to a factor referred to as <u>crossover exposure</u>. The primary cause of this crossover is the incomplete absorption by the adjacent film emulsion of all of the light emanating from the adjacent intensifying screen. In double-coated film used with a pair of intensifying screens, the crossover effect is attributed to additional exposure of the film emulsion to light emitted by the screen adjacent to the opposite side of the film. The light from the intensifying screen is emitted in all directions and spreads due to transmission, scattering, and reflecting in the film base and emulsion interfaces. The resulting image on the film does not have good detail, or is as "sharp" as it should be. The use of coating below both emulsion surfaces of the film absorbs some of this excess light and decreases the crossover. The coating is invisible during normal processing and is not seen on the processed radiograph. The presence of the coating reduces the relative speed of the film; however, the image quality is enhanced considerably.

<u>Film size</u>—Screen-film comes in different sizes that correspond to the size of the cassettes to be used (Table 6-4). Non-screen film or direct exposure film usually comes in a pre-packaged lightproof holder in the same sizes even though a conventional cassette is not used. Screen-type film comes in boxes usually without any interleaving paper and is available in 25, 50, 100, or 500 sheets per box. Screen-type <u>film costs</u> vary with the price of silver, but average prices are $1.00 for a sheet of small size film and $2.50 for a sheet of the largest film. The price of film is influenced by the number of films per box, the number of boxes purchased, and the brand of film purchased. Non-

Table 6-4
METRIC/U.S. CONVERSIONS

Film Size	
Metric	**U.S. Customary**
Sizes Equal	
35 X 43 cm	14 X 17 inches
35 X 35 cm	14 X 14 inches
Metric sizes slightly different from inch size	
18 X 43 cm	7 X 17 inches
Metric size without U.S. equivalent	
30 X 40 cm	
30 X 35 cm	
24 X 30 cm	
18 X 24 cm	
U.S. size without metric equivalents	
	8 X 10 inches
	10 X 12 inches
	11 X 14 inches

screen film is more expensive because of increased silver content and a small film is approximately $2.00 per sheet.

<u>Film storage</u>—Boxes of film should be stored on end to reduce the pressure on the film in a room that is cool and has a low humidity since moisture causes deterioration of the film. Therefore, storage should not be near a hot-water heater, radiator, or steam line. Obviously, the film should not be stored near the primary x-ray beam where it could receive repeated exposure to radiation. Film is dated and there is some risk of radiographic fogging if out-of-date film is used. If you determine that you are not likely to use film prior to its exposure date, it is suggested that the film be placed in a plastic bag within a refrigerator or freezer. Deterioration of the film is thus delayed, the film is kept dry, and it can be used satisfactorily after the expiration date. In an effort to prevent any problems in film storage, avoid purchase of large quantities of film that require long periods of storage time.

B. FILM HOLDERS (CASSETTES)

Two basic types of film holders are used in veterinary radiography. These correspond to the two basic types of x-ray film that are used. Since screen-type film requires the use of intensifying screens, it is placed in rigid <u>cassettes</u> that offer protection to both the film and the intensifying screens and insures close contact between the screens and the film (Fig. 6-5). It is important to understand the relationship between the cassette front and back, the intensifying screens, and the film (Fig. 6-6). Since non-screen film is a direct-exposure type film it is used in a nonrigid, lightproof paper, cardboard, or plastic holder. One of the advantages of non-screen film is that it may be purchased in a convenient lightproof envelope with a "ripstrip" that is

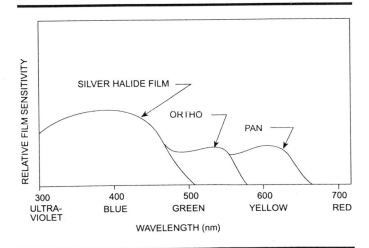

Fig. 6-4
**RELATIVE SPECTRAL SENSITIVITY OF SILVER HALIDE,
ORTHO, AND PANCHROMATIC FILMS**

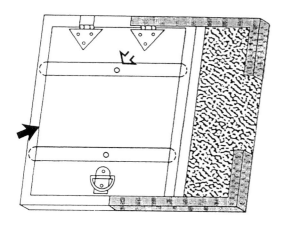

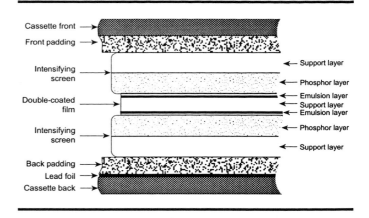

Fig. 6-6
CROSS-SECTION OF A CASSETTE
The parts of the cassette are labeled. Notice the relationship of the cassette, intensifying screens, and the film.

Cassette front
Front padding
Intensifying screen
Double-coated film
Intensifying screen
Back padding
Lead foil
Cassette back

Support layer
Phosphor layer
Emulsion layer
Support layer
Emulsion layer
Phosphor layer
Support layer

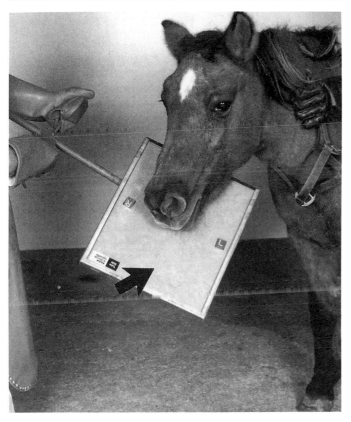

Fig. 6-5
CASSETTE
A cassette (solid arrows) is shown within a holder with a long handle that permits the assistant to be outside the primary x-ray beam. The fasteners pivot on the back of the cassette (hollow arrow).

discarded after use without any need to "reload" the film holder.

Cassettes that are used for screen-type film are made with a front composed of some type of relatively radiolucent material. Four available materials are commonly used in making up the front cover; 1) aluminum, 2) Bakelite, 3) polycarbonate, or 4) carbon-fiber. Comparison of the different types of cassettes has shown that carbon-fiber produces the least scatter, is capable of increased image contrast, requires the lowest machine settings, provides the lowest patient exposure, but is the most expensive (Shuping et al, 1980. Schmidt et al, 1983). The reduction of patient's exposure when compared with aluminum fronts ranged from 28% at 60 kVp to 17% at 120 kVp (Schmidt et al, 1983).

The back of the cassette is hinged in some manner so that the cassette can be opened and film removed for processing and reloaded for the next examination. One type of closure consists of stainless steel hinges with small slide catches. A more common type of hinge consists of steel crossbars that each pivot on a shouldered rivet with nylon washers attached in the middle of the cassette (Fig. 6-5).

A thin (0.5 mm) sheet of lead foil is placed on the back of the cassette (the non-exposure side) to absorb a part of the back-scatter radiation that is created when the x-ray beam interacts with the cassette. The Compton scattering, otherwise, causes a generalized fogging to the entire film. Assuming no protection from back-scatter, 5% to 10% of film density can result from the backscatter. The energy, direction, and amount of back-scatter is dependent on the material and thickness of the cassette backing and is increased by the positioning of the cassette on a heavy tabletop or on the ground during exposure. The Compton scatter increases with increased kVp, especially over 100 kVp level. A thicker lead sheet is needed under non-screen film to control the effect of the backscatter.

A pad of felt is placed around the periphery of the cassette between the cassette edges and the hinged back, forming a light-tight seal. The felt is often worn away in older cassettes causing a light-leak which causes a repeated blackened pattern on the edge of the radiograph.

Cassettes can be placed in holders for protection or to position and immobilize the cassette during exposure (Fig. 6-7). While most cassettes are flat, it is possible to purchase curved cassettes that utilize conventional film sizes. These might be helpful in many craniocaudal or caudocranial examinations in small animal radiography where it is impossible to obtain full extension of a limb.

It is helpful if cassettes used for an examination can be identified so that any artifacts noted on a radiograph can be easily traced to the cassette used for production of that radiograph. By writing a number on the top edge of one of the intensifying screens with a heavy black felt-tipped pen and covering the lettering with a piece of polyester tape or a thin coat of clear fingernail polish, it will appear on all subsequent radiographs made using this cassette. The same number can be written on the outside of the cassette.

The cost of cassettes is high, depending on their size and on whether they are of light-weight or heavy-duty construction. The average cost, without intensifying screens, for a light-weight small cassette is $60.00, a heavy-duty small cassette is $80.00, a light-weight large cassette is $100.00, and a heavy-duty large cassette is $140.00.

REFERENCES

Schmidt RA Chan H-P Kodera Y Doi K and Chen C-T. Evaluation of cassette performance: Physical factors affecting patient exposure and image contrast. Rad 146:801, 1983.

Shuping RE Fewell TR Phillips RA Gross RR and Showalter CK. Dose reduction potential of carbon fiber material in diagnostic radiology. Diag Rad p59, October 1980.

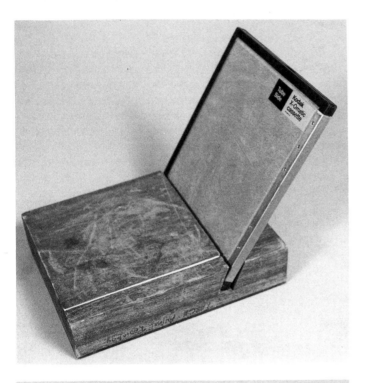

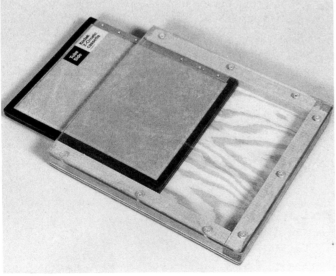

Fig. 6-7
CASSETTE HOLDERS
Many types of cassette holders are used to protect the cassette, position the cassette, and assist in positioning the patient.

C. INTENSIFYING SCREENS

Less than 1% of the remnant x-ray beam incident on radiographic film interacts with the film and contributes to the latent image. Because of this inefficiency, intensifying screens were used as early as 1897 and were built with calcium tungstate crystals. The purpose of the screens is to provide a mechanism through which a phosphor (Greek=light bearer) can be utilized that converts energy carried by an x-ray photon into visible light that results in exposure on the x-ray film and formation of the latent image is enhanced. Approximately 30% of the x-rays incident on an intensifying screen interact with the screen and with each such interaction a large number of visible-light photons are emitted (Fig. 6-8). Conseqently, the screens act as an amplifier of the remnant radiation reaching the screen-film cassette. This intensifying effect results in a savings of about 30 to 50 times the number of x-ray photons needed to produce the radiographic exposure comparing the use of screen-type film with screens sensitive to visible light to the use of screen type film alone (Table 6-5). Companies describe the characteristics of the screens they produce (Tables 6-6, 6-7).

Use of screens permits the use of lower mAs settings than would be necessary with non-screen technique permitting shorter exposure times and a decrease in unsharpness of the radiograph due to patient motion. In addition, patient exposure is reduced, scatter radiation to personnel assisting in the examination is reduced, use of a small focal spot is often possible, greater selection of kVp settings is possible, and tube life is prolonged.

A knowledge of the construction and function of the intensifying screens permits the most efficient usage of this important piece of accessory equipment. Screens have a thickness of about 0.4 mm and consist of four layers: (1) base or support, (2) a reflecting layer, (3) phosphor layer in a binder, and (4) a protective coat. The thin layer of tiny phosphor crystals is mixed with a suitable binder and coated in a smooth layer on the cardboard or plastic support. The base serves to attach the binder and phosphor crystals to the cassette. It is important that the binder is strong enough to protect the phosphor crystals from injury. The screen is covered by a protective coating that resists marking or abrasive wear, permits easy cleaning, and helps to eliminate the build-up of static electricity. The reflecting layer is made of a white substance such as titanium dioxide or magnesium oxide and is spread between base and binder in a thin layer so as to reflect any light photons not emitted in the direction of the film. This tends to prevent their loss as far as any photographic activity is concerned.

An efficient phosphor: (1) has a high absorption coefficient due to the high atomic number so that the probability of x-ray interaction is high (Fig. 6-9), (2) has a high conversion efficiency of absorbed x-ray to light, (3) causes a fluorescence in the region of the spectrum where the x-ray film emulsion is most sensitive (Fig. 6-10), (4) does not deteriorate under continued exposure to the radiation normally required, (5) remains stable with age, (6) withstands high temperature and high humidity, (7) has no afterglow, (8) has no delay in build-up, and (9) permits precise control

in manufacturing so that uniformity in the product can be guaranteed. Materials commonly used as phosphors are: (1) calcium tungstate, (2) zinc sulfide, (3) lead-activated barium sulfate, (4) strontium/europium-activated barium sulfate, (5) thalium-activated gadolinium oxysulfide, (6) terbium-activated gadolinium oxysulfide, (7) terbium-activated lanthanum oxysulfide, (8) terbium-activated yttrium oxysulfide, (9) thulium-activated lanthanum oxybromide, (10) niobium-activated yttrium tantalate, and (11) thulium-activated activated yttrium tantalate.

Differences in screen imaging characteristics are basically caused by differences in the composition of the phosphor and the resulting energy of the light produced. Calcium tungstate crystals emit a wavelength of 3600 to 4350 Ångstroms which is the blue-violet to ultraviolet range. They were first discovered in 1896 and served well until the 1960's, when a new group rare-earth phosphors were discovered that used elements of group III in the periodic table having atomic numbers of 57 to 71. The rare earth phosphors have peak wavelengths at 4200, 4400, and 5400 Ångstrom units, the majority occurring around 5400 Ångstrom units which is in the green spectrum. A second generation of rare earth screens contains rare earth components which also emit blue light.

All of these phosphors exhibit higher x-ray absorption efficiency and greater x-ray energy-to-light conversion efficiency than conventional calcium tungstate screens. Light emitted from these newly developed phosphors is within narrow bands of wavelengths as compared to the broad band emission of calcium tungstate screen (Fig. 6-10). This increase in speed results in a loss of detail on the radiograph, however, in situations where patient motion is of great concern, use of the higher speed systems must be considered (Pharr and Fretz, 1979).

Table 6-5
COMPARISON OF RELATIVE NUMBER OF X-RAY PHOTONS AND LIGHT PHOTONS AT VARIOUS STAGES FOR DIRECT AND SCREEN-FILM EXPOSURES*

Stage	Type of Exposure	
	Direct	Screen-film
Incident x-ray photons	1000	20
X-rays absorbed by film	10	(>1)
X-rays absorbed by screens	—	5
Light photons produced	—	5000
Light photons incident on film	—	3000
Light photons absorbed by film	—	1000
Latent images formed	10	10

Intensification factor = 1000/20 = 50

*(Bushong, 1980)

Table 6-6
DUPONT SCREEN CHARACTERISTICS

Quanta Detail (QD)	Slow speed, high resolution, blue-UV-emission (yttrium tantalate: thulium-activated)
Quanta Fast Detail (QFD)	Medium speed, high resolution, blue-UV-emission (yttrium tantalate: niobium-activated)
Quanta 111 (Q111)	Ultra speed, blue-emission (lanthanum oxybromide: thulium-activated)
Quanta V (QV)	Blue and green-emission (lanthanum oxybromide: thulium-activated plus gadolinium oxysulfide: terbium-activated)

Table 6-7
KODAK INTENSIFYING SCREEN CHARACTERISTICS

X-Omatic fine	Blue-and UV-emission (barium lead sulfate, yellow dye)
X-Omatic regular	Blue-and UV-emission (barium strontium sulfate; europium-activated, neutral dye)
Medium-speed-CaWO$_4$	Blue-emission (calcium tungstate)
High-speed-CaWO$_4$	Blue-emission (calcium tungstate)
Lanex fine	Green-emission (gadolinium oxysulfide: terbium-activated, neutral dye) 60 kV—extremity
Lanex fine	Green emission (gadolinium oxysulfide: terbium-activated, neutral dye) 80 to 120 kV—general purpose
Lanex medium	Green emission (gadolinium oxysulfide: terbium-activated, yellow dye)
Lanex regular	Green emission (gadolinium oxysulfide: terbium-activated)
Min-R	Rare earth screen, high detail for mammography

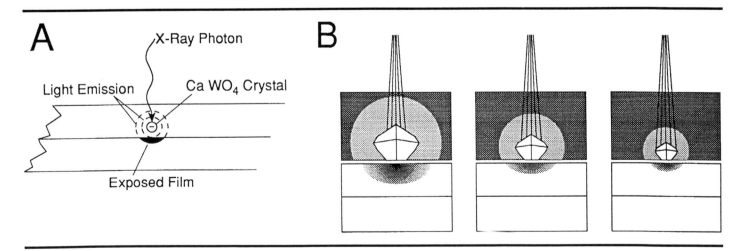

Fig. 6-8
EFFECT OF SCREEN CRYSTAL SIZE ON FILM DETAIL
An x-ray photon is shown to interact with a CaWO$_4$ crystal in the intensifying screen (A). The interaction with different sized crystals (B) in the intensifying screens results in fluorescence that exposes an area of film dependent on the size of the crystal. The smaller the crystal, the better is the radiographic detail, however, the exposure must be greater to produce the radiograph. Crystal size thus partially determines screen speed as well as film detail.

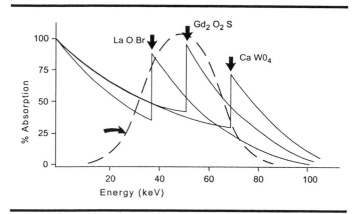

Fig. 6-9
PHOSPHOR ABSORPTION CURVES
Absorption curves of three phosphors used in intensifying screens of an 80 kVp x-ray beam attenuated by having passed through a patient's body. Note the increased absorption at the K-edge (straight arrows) of the predominant element (Lanthanum = 39 keV, Gadolinium = 50 keV, Tungsten = 69 keV). A higher level of absorption of the x-ray photons reflects a more efficient x-ray energy-to-light conversion by the intensifying screen. The background curve (curved arrow) represents the heterogenous character of the x-ray beam with energies of the photons ranging from less than 20 keV to the maximum of 80 keV.

At one time, the screens to be mounted in the front of the cassette had a thinner coat of phosphor than those to be mounted on the back, making their installation in a cassette non-interchangeable. The thicker phosphor coating of the back screen compensated for absorption of x-rays by the front screen and yielded a balanced exposure to both emulsion layers of the film. Today, most screen pairs have similar speed screens and are therefore interchangeable.

Care of the intensifying screens is important especially when working with animals, where there is a high possibility of dirt and dust being carried into the darkroom. If this debris is deposited on the surface of the screens inside the cassette, it creates artifacts on every film exposed in that cassette. Exposure of the film is dependent on visible light reaching the film from the screens and any piece of hair or dirt absorbs that light creating a white artifact on the radiograph (Fig. 6-11). Small pieces of dust and dirt eventually are forced into the surface of the screen and cannot be removed and produce a permanent artifact. Regular cleaning of the screens is not difficult and can be performed through use of a commercial screen cleaner or mild soap and warm

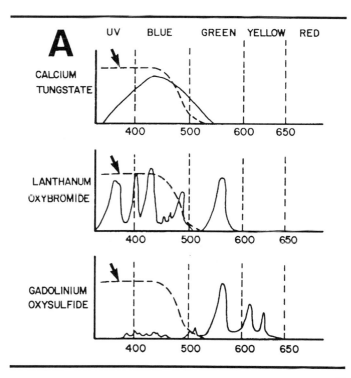

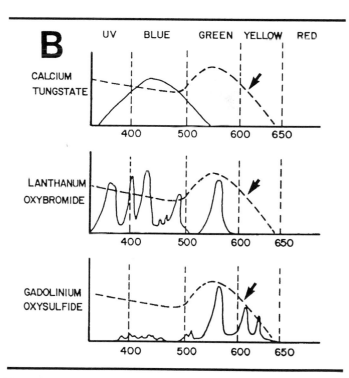

Fig. 6-10
PHOSPHOR SPECTRAL EMISSIONS
Spectral emission from three intensifying screens utilizing different phosphors. Note the narrow bands of wavelengths in the rare-earth phosphors as compared with the wave length emission from calcium tungstate. The background curves (arrows) represent the spectral sensitivity of standard silver halide radiographic film (A) and orthochromatic film (B). Comparison of the curves for the spectral emission of the phosphors and the sensitivity of the crystal used on the film permits you to make a determination of the efficiency, and thus the general level of speed, of the film-screen system.

water. Most screen cleaners have antistatic agents incorporated so that regular cleaning also helps to control the production of static electricity. Avoid using denatured alcohol or any abrasive product to clean the screens since they permanently injure the protective coating of the screens. Depending on frequency of usage, screens should be clean-ed every two weeks. If screens are cared for, they have a long lifetime measured in years. Most companies suggest replacement of the screens after 8 to 10 years, but many screens remain in active use for 20 to 30 years and perform satisfactorily. Screens having a yellow tinge should be discarded since this coloration affect the speed of the screens.

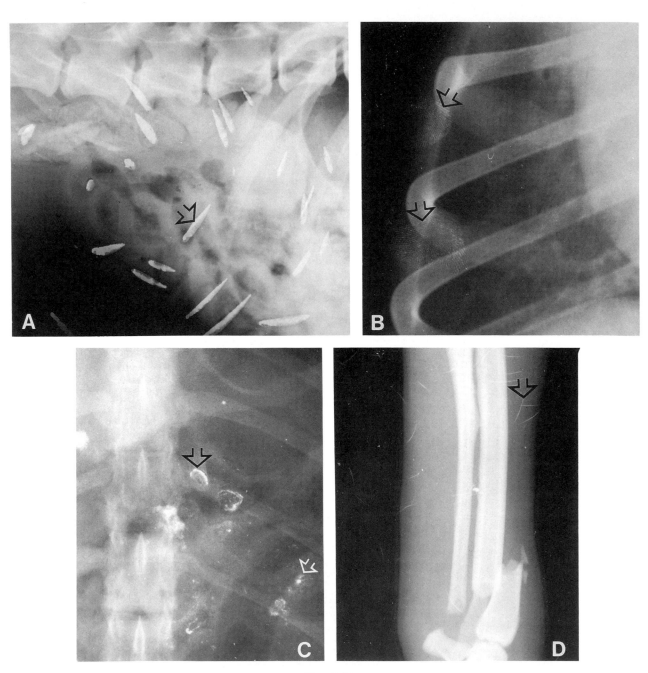

Fig. 6-11
FILM ARTIFACT
Any defect on the surface of the intensifying screen causes an artifact on the film (arrows) characterised by underexposure due to the prevention of visible light from passing from the screen to the film. The artifact may be the result of dirt on the screen (A), dirt on fingers resulting in "finger prints" (B), a chemical spill on the screen (C) or foreign material such as hair (D).

REFERENCES

Pharr JW and Fretz PB. X-ray-intensifying screen technology for improving veterinary field radiography. J Am Vet Med Assoc 175:1103, 1979.

Strömberg B Olsson S-E and Lundgren M. Rare earth intensifying screens in veterinary radiology. J small Animal Pract 19:689, 1978.

Sackett MH. Caution: speed ahead—rare earth imaging systems. Rad Tech 48:537, 1977.

Burgess AE and Hicken P. Comparative performance of x-ray-intensifying screens. Radiology 143:551, 1982.

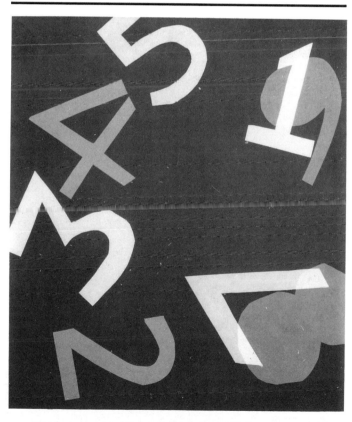

Numbers were cut from typing paper and the uneven numbers (1,3,5,7) were placed between the film and the lower intensifying screen. The even numbers (2,4,6,8) were placed between the film and the upper intensifying screen. The screen intensity was not balanced and the upper screens produced greater light intensity than the lower ones. Notice that when the numbers were overlapping, no light reached the film and the radiograph was unexposed. This demonstrates how a thin piece of paper can prevent light from the screens from reaching the film resulting in an unexposed region.

D. FILM-SCREEN SYSTEMS

Older film-screen systems were blue systems and used film sensitive to ultra-violet, violet, and blue light and used phosphors such as calcium tungstate and barium lead tungstate. Orthochromatic systems are more common today and refer generally to green systems and use film sensitised by covering it with dye that changes the absorbed color principally to green light but also to ultraviolet and blue light. The phosphors are generally rare-earth type.

With the development of new phosphors in the intensifying screens and faster films, there is an increasing number of possible combinations of film and screens. In particular, rare earth screens are available in many combinations with different films, resulting in varying relative speeds. When calcium tungstate is used with blue sensitive film of par speed, the speed of the system is usually rated at 100. Newer film-screen combinations have speeds as slow as 20 and as high as 1200. (Tables 6-8, 6-9, 6-10).

A major factor in the selection of a film-screen system is the determination of the most desirable system speed that best satisfies the needs of your clinic. If you are using a small portable x-ray unit with minimal power, the use of a faster film-screen system assists you in production of radiographs with a relatively short exposure time (low mAs). To obtain the fastest speed for the system, rare-earth screens must be used in conjunction with film emulsions that have absorption characteristics matched to the emission of the screen. This high speed also enables you to use a longer focal-film distance that results in improvement of film definition or detail. If you have a higher powered x-ray machine, the need for a faster film-screen system is not as great and you may wish to utilize two film-screen combinations. One could be a slower system for use on extremities to obtain a higher level of definition or detail and the second system could be a faster system for use on the thorax and abdomen to obtain radiographs with

Table 6-8
RELATIVE SPEEDS OF KODAK FILM-SCREEN COMBINATIONS

FILM	X-OMATIC Fine Extremity	LANEX Fine Screen Pair Extremity	LANEX Fine Screen Pair General	$CaWO_4$ Medium Speed	LANEX Medium Screen Pair General	$CaWO_4$ High Speed	X-Omatic Regular	Lanex Regular
Blue-sensitive:								
X-OMAT RP	30	—	—	100	—	250	200	250
X-OMAT K	30	—	—	100	—	250	200	—
X-OMAT L	30	—	—	100	—	250	200	250
X-OMAT S	50	—	—	150	—	400	300	400
Blue Brand	40	—	—	120	—	250	200	250
Green-sensitive:								
X-Omat G	20	—	—	60	—	120	100	120
Ortho G	—	60	100	—	250	—	—	400
Ortho L	—	60	100	—	250	—	—	400
Ortho C	—	—	80	—	250	—	—	400
Ortho H	—	150	200	—	500	—	—	800
T-Mat G	—	80	100	—	300	—	—	400
Ortho-M		50						250

Table 6-9
RELATIVE SPEEDS OF DUPONT FILM-SCREEN COMBINATIONS

		Film									
Screens		4	4L	WDR	7	7L	10T	10L	8	8L	OTG
QD	250	250	250	80	80	80	80				
QFD	500	500	500	250	250	250	250				
Q111	800	800	800	400	400	400	400				
QV								400	400	400	

Table 6-10
RELATIVE SPEEDS OF
KONICA FILM-SCREEN COMBINATIONS

Screens	Film			
	MG	MGH	MGL	MGC
KF	125	125	125	125
KM	250	250	250	250
KR	400	400	400	400

adequate definition but less chance for film quality compromise due to patient motion. You should not use a system faster than you need for your particular requirements because of the loss of film quality that is inherent in the faster systems. Because of the availability of high speed systems at a relatively low cost, many practices have acquired systems whose speed is totally inappropriate for the type of x-ray machine in use.

The speed of the system is inversely related to the magnitude of the mAs setting that is required to produce an exposure. If you change to a different film-screen system, you should expect to alter the mAs settings used with the first system inversely by a factor similar to the factor representing the difference between speeds of the two film-screen systems. If you change from a 400 speed system to an 800 speed system, this is an increase in speed by a factor of 2. Therefore, you need to decrease the mAs setting to one-half to compensate for changing to the new system. When comparing film-screen systems that are produced by different manufacturers, there are probably slight differences that require minimal changes in your technique chart in addition to those expected.

A major drawback to fast radiographic systems is the quantum noise, or statistical noise in the system. Today's fast, efficient screens produce in the range of 500 to 2000 light photons for each absorbed x-ray photon. These light photons scatter in all directions, but do not migrate far before ultimately exposing the contiguous film creating a deposit of developed silver centered at the location of the absorbed x-ray photon. The more efficient the conversion of absorbed x-ray energy into useful light energy and the greater the absorption of the light photons by the film, the larger is the density deposit for any photon. As a result, the larger each deposit, the fewer deposits that are needed to produce a given film density. The photon count may be low enough that point-to-point statistical fluctuations in the distribution is visually evident as graininess and is referred to as quantum mottle.

Another disadvantage of rare-earth systems is that the relative speed of the system is dependent on the energy of the x-ray photon. This means that as the kVp level increases, the response is not linear. In addition, careful determination of radiographic technique conversion factors must be made when switching from calcium tungstate to rare earth screens. Additional disadvantages are the increased emulsion sensitivity to the average darkroom safelight illumination found with green-light-sensitive film that necessitates safelight modification. Also, there is a possible increase in cost of rare earth screens compared to calcium tungstate (Rossi et al, 1976). However, even when considering these disadvantages, rare-earth systems are recommended for any clinic with a low-rated x-ray generator.

Advantages in use of rare-earth systems also include the reduction in patient radiation exposure that is affected by the speed of the film-screen system. Skin entrance dose reductions of 52% and 68% have been achieved using the faster systems relative to the par-speed standard film-screen combinations (Buchanan et al, 1972, Wagner and Weaver, 1976, Smathers et al, 1984). If this reduction in patient exposure can be accomplished with acceptable loss in image detail or image mottle, this is another reason that the use of the faster systems must be strongly considered. In addition, the use of faster systems allows for the use of smaller focal spot for increased resolution of the radiographic image (Arnold et al, 1976).

REFERENCES

Arnold BA Eisenberg H and Bjarngard BE. The LST and MTF of rare-earth oxysulfide intensifying screens. Radiology 121:473, 1976.

Buchanan RA. An Improved X-ray Intensifying Screen. IEEE Trans Nucl Sci, NS-19:81, February, 1972.

Buchanan RA Finkelstein SI and Wichersheim KA. X-Ray Exposure Reduction Using Rare-Earth Oxysulfide Intensifying Screens. Radiol 105:185, 1972.

Fearon T Vucich J Hoe J McSweeney WJ and Potter BM. A comparative evaluation of rare-earth screen-film systems. Invest Radiol 21:654, 1986.

Rossi RP Hendee WR and Ahrens CR. An Evaluation of Rare Earth Screen Film Combinations: Radiol 121:465-71, 1976.

Smathers RL Alford BA Messenger J Agarwal SK and Taylor TS. Radiation dose reductions in the neonatal intensive care unit. Invest Radiol 19:578, 1984.

Wagner RF and Weaver KE. Prospects for X-Ray Exposure Reduction Using Rare Earth Intensifying Screens. Radiol 118:183, 1976.

E. FILM IDENTIFICATION

Every radiograph should be marked in a manner that permits later positive identification of: (1) the patient radiographed, (2) the date of the examination, and (3) who performed the examination. Additional information can include the owner's name as well as the patient's age, sex, and breed and the radiographic study performed. Some clinics or hospitals use patient identification numbers that further clarify the identity of the patient. It is not difficult to imagine the loss of value of a radiographic study when there is no identification on the radiograph or when multiple radiographic studies of the same patient cannot be evaluated correctly because of the absence of dates of examination. There is a mistaken idea that a radiograph not identified cannot be used in litigation against the veterinarian. This assumes that the litigation centers around the poor quality of the radiographic study. More often the problem centers around the veterinarian facing malpractice charges because of the quality of the patient's record. Frequently, there is no written evidence to prove that the radiographic examination was performed irrespective of the quality of the radiographic study.

Several methods can be used to permanently identify radiographs. These include: (1) lead markers, (2) identification cards used with lead blockers, and (3) lead-impregnated tape. Lead markers are easy to use since film identification results at the time of the exposure. Lead numbers or letters are placed in a holder or taped directly to the face of the film holder (Fig. 6-12). The lead letters completely attenuate the primary x-ray beam so that the film directly under the lead is unexposed and appears transparent on the radiograph. It is possible to purchase prepared identification markers with lead letters that have the name and address of the clinic or hospital spelled out permanently. It is then necessary to only change the date of the examination and identification of the patient. The greatest difficulty in use of these markers is associated with the tendency for the markers to slide or fall off the cassette prior to the exposure. Another problem results from a failure to include the part of the cassette with the markers in the primary beam because of close collimation of the primary x-ray beam.

A second technique for film identification uses blockers of some type to prevent exposure to a small corner of the film. This can be done by: (1) lead blockers placed on the outside of the cassette, (2) thinner lead foil blockers placed on the inside of the cassette, or (3) removal of a corner of the intensifying screens (Fig. 6-13), all of which insure that there is no exposure, or only minimal exposure, of the film in this area at the time of the radiographic examination. Following removal of the film in the darkroom, but prior to processing, a typed or written card is placed between this portion of the film and a light source. The light is "flashed" and the written information on the card is recorded on the previously unexposed or underexposed film (Fig. 6-14). This occurs because the ink or typewritten information prevents the visible light from reaching the film, leaving the film under the identification information unexposed. Some of the flashing devices are automatic and terminate the time of the exposure of the card. Other flashers are manual and the light remains on as long as the switch is depressed making it possible to overexpose the film during the marking. The size of the lead blocker is 1 x 3 inches (2.5 x 7.5 cm), and the size of the card is usually a standard 3 x 5 inches (7.5 x 12.5 cm).

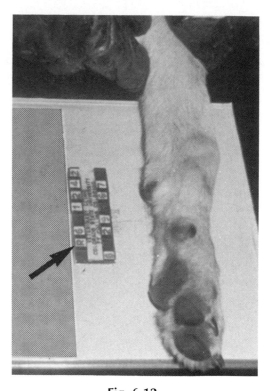

Fig. 6-12
FILM IDENTIFICATION SYSTEM
Lead numbers and letters placed in a holder (arrow) and taped to the cassette prior to exposure provide positive film identification.

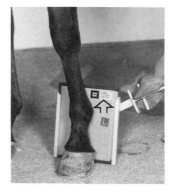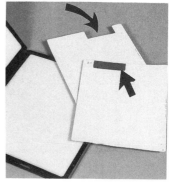

Fig. 6-13
FILM IDENTIFICATION SYSTEM
Exposure of a corner of the film is prevented in any of three ways: (1) a lead shield may be placed on the outside of the cassette (open arrow), (2) a thin lead shield may be placed on the intensifying screen (solid arrow), or (3) a corner of the intensifying screen may be cut away (curved arrow). This "protected" area on the film can then be exposed in the darkroom "printing" the data that identifies the patient and the day of examination.

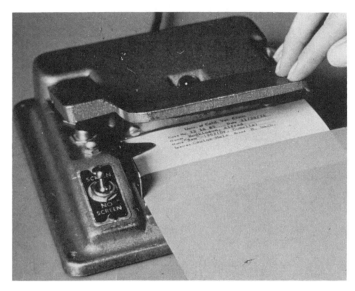

Fig. 6-14
FILM IDENTIFICATION SYSTEM
After protecting a corner of the radiograph during exposure, a typed card is placed between a light source and the film, a lever (fingers) is depressed turning on a light, and the film is "flashed". The duration of the exposure is pre-determined and is different for screen and non-screen film.

New cassettes should be ordered with all blockers in the same predetermined location on the face of the cassette. With the blockers all placed in the same location in all cassettes, it is easy to know the corner of the film that is to be "flashed" prior to developing. There are 8 different corner positions available for positioning the lead blocker (Fig. 6-15). The upper left corner as seen when the cassette is lying on its front surface with the back opened is the most common location since that makes it the easiest for a right-handed person to remove the film and flash the upper left corner without having to change the position of the film within the right hand. It should be realized that this small section of the film is not exposed by the primary x-ray beam, and thus no part of the patient's body should be placed over this area, especially an area of clinical interest. The identification cards can be filed after use in identifying the radiograph and provide the clinic with an alphabetical card record of all radiographic examinations. It is also easy to reuse a card by writing a new date or other information on it, thus reminding you that you have earlier radiographs of this patient.

A less commonly used, but satisfactory, technique utilizes disposable, lead-impregnated tape that is placed on the outside of the cassette at the time of exposure (Fig. 6-16). Tape is placed on a "holder blocker" to which is permanently attached the name and address of the hospital in lead letters. By "writing" on the tape with a ball-point pen or other suitable smooth tip, the powdered lead within the tape is displaced and a difference in density results that permits the primary x-ray beam to be selectively absorbed. Any information can be written on the tape and it is easy to cross out dates or other information and write

in new information. The tape is available in 50-foot or 100-foot rolls or in precut 3-inch (7.5 cm) strips packaged 300 strips in a dispenser carton. Tapes can be thrown way after use or can be attached to a filing envelope for use at a later date. These can be obtained from most x-ray dealers.

F. FILM MARKERS

Patient Orientation markers are needed to identify the limb being examined or the side of the body. These right and left markers are made of lead and are taped to the cassette face or are in the form of a clip and fastened to the edge of the cassette (Fig. 6-17).

Medial and lateral markers are important in identifying the medial or lateral aspect of the limb, especially in those studies where no identifiable anatomical features are present. These markers are necessary distal to the midshaft of the metacarpal or metatarsal bones in large animals. It is a good plan to consistently position all identification markers and orientation markers laterally. This insures that you can identify the lateral side of the patient on the radiograph in a situation in which only a part of the identification marker can be seen. This often results when a marker: (1) is covered by a lead glove, (2) was accidently left off, or (3) fell off unnoticed prior to the exposure. However, it is still important to use all markers in all examinations, since it provides a more positive method to determine this important information.

Fore- and hindlimb markers are required in radiography of horses and cattle to identify the radiographs of the distal parts of the fore and hind limbs. These are usually done with a "F" or "H" lead marker placed on the cassette face prior to exposure. It is also possible to make the identification on the ID card; however, it is necessary to keep the cassettes separated until "flashing" the film, since they may include studies of different limbs. Also, the ID card must be changed during film processing to indicate which limb was examined. It is better to have the film identified at the time of exposure and to not be required to perform any special identification in the dark room.

Positioning markers indicate the nature of the direction of the x-ray beam that was used for the exposure. Lead markers with an arrow (Fig. 6-17), lead markers with a mercury bubble (Fig. 6-17), or a suspended arrow that points vertically toward the ground all indicate that the cassette was erect during the study. Other markers can be purchased that indicate if the patient is "recumbent" or "erect" and are important for examinations of the head, thorax, and abdomen. Special markers have been produced that indicate the direction of the x-ray beam as it passed through a horse's limb, i.e., CrCa (craniocaudal), CaCr (caudocranial), etc.

A lead marker or forceps attached to the hair coat can be used to identify an area on the patient that is of special clinical interest, such as the site of a puncture wound or point of greatest pain, or crepitus as noted on palpation. To limit the size of the marker and prevent it from covering an area of interest, lead or steel "B-B"s can be taped over an area of interest.

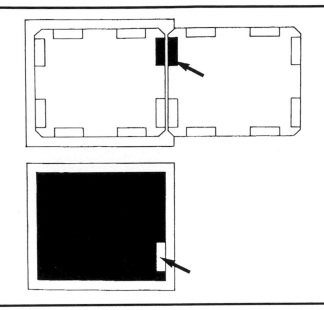

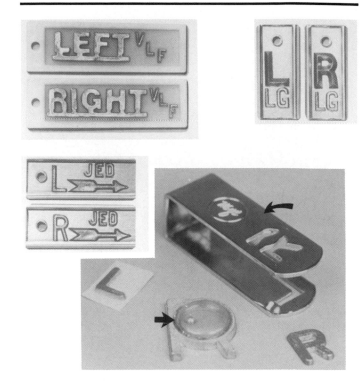

Fig. 6-15
FILM IDENTIFICATION SYSTEM
Drawing of an opened and closed cassette shows the recommended position of the blocker (arrows) to be utilized in film identification. The other available positions are seen in the drawing of the open cassette.

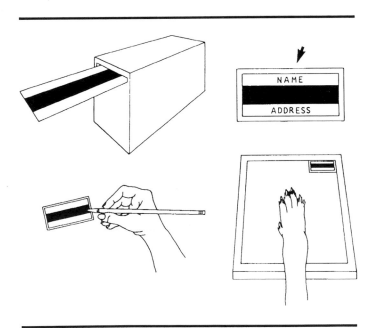

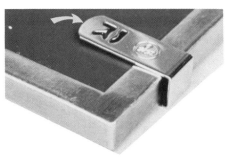

Fig. 6-17
FILM MARKERS
Most forms of right and left markers are taped on the surface of the cassette except for the "clip" variety (curved arrows). The Mitchell markers have a mercury "ball" (straight arrow) that moves relative to how the marker is positioned during the study and is helpful in determining if a radiograph was made using a horizontal x-ray beam. Note the use of initials on some markers to identify the person conducting the examination.

Fig. 6-16
FILM IDENTIFICATION SYSTEM
This film marking system utilizes metallic impregnated tape that is available in a continuous strip or in precut lengths. Identification data is written on the tape with a pencil or pen. The tape is then placed on a holder (arrow) with pre-set lead letters that identify the practice. The holder and tape are then placed on the cassette front.

Technician identification markers are of value if you have more than one person making radiographic examinations. By having the initials of the individual on the film, it is easy to know to whom you should direct questions about the examination later (Fig. 6-16).

Time or sequence of exposure markers are important in special procedures such as excretory urography or barium sulfate studies of the gastrointestinal tract (Fig. 6-18). In addition, if you re-examine a limb after further patient preparation or after a surgical procedure, it is of value to know the sequence of the examinations. Radiographs made after injection of a contrast agent should be identified as a second study and the sequence of exposures during the study indicated. Intra-operative radiographic studies are most accurately evaluated if sequentially numbered. A sequence of films is usually indicated by lead numbers taped onto the face of the cassette. The time of exposure is also important if more than one study was made during the same day as might be the case in examination of the thorax in a patient with severe pneumonia or pleural effusion accumulation. Some "flashers" used to make the identification of the film also expose the film showing both the date and time of processing the film (Fig. 6-14).

It should be remembered that it is possible to write on the film in the event that other identification devices have not worked satisfactorily. This can be done when the film is still in the wash since the emulsion scraps off easily as the information is "written" on the film. However, you must be careful to avoid scratching the emulsion in the same region as a significant lesion. When the film is dry, it is possible to use several types of pens to write directly on the film. Another technique is to write on a paper label that is then attached to the film. None of these are as satisfactory as the other techniques described, but any form of identification is better than nothing. Avoid the system of relying on the identification of the patient through information written on the film envelope instead of identifying each individual film, since once a film is separated from the envelope, that identification is lost.

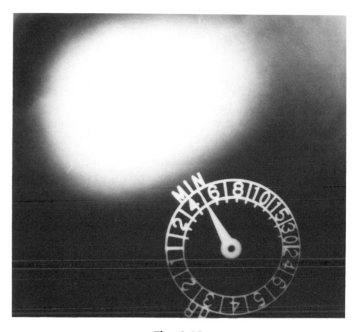

Fig. 6-18
FILM MARKER
This type of marker permits identification of a time sequence in which the radiographs were exposed. It is used most commonly following the injection or feeding of a contrast agent.

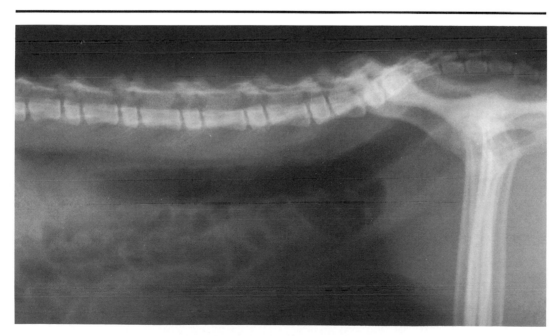

How can this cat have so many lumbar vertebrae?

7. FILM PROCESSING

The most common technical errors made in veterinary radiography occur during film processing. It seems strange that there is great consideration given to purchase of a powerful x-ray machine and new screened cassettes and the continued use a darkroom for film processing that is a partially remodeled toilet, still being used occasionally for its original purpose. The clinician interested in using radiology as a diagnostic technique should strongly consider construction of a separate darkroom since the use of a dry and clean separate processing area eliminates many of the artifacts commonly found on both automatically and manually processed film. A major cause of errors in film processing is associated with the continued use of wet tanks and there is no question that the purchase of an automatic film processor upgrades radiographic quality remarkably.

Study of the history of film processing during the last 40 years reveals great change in the photographic processing of medical radiograph. Prior to the mid 1950's, all medical x-ray film processing was done by hand using rack and tank processing (wet-film tanks). This cycle took over 1 hour to provide a dried radiograph which could be interpreted accurately. Films were particularly manufactured for 68° F processing. During the early 1950's, automatic tank processor systems that moved the film, still attached to a holder, became available from several manufacturers including Pako. In 1957, Eastman Kodak introduced the first roller transport automatic film processor called the Model M. This unit was 10 feet long, weighed nearly 1500 pounds and sold for over $33,000.00. The processing cycle was approximately 6 minutes and developer temperatures were increased to about 81° F. Film emulsions were changed from an acetate base to a polyester base to improve their transport through the automatic processor. In 1965, Eastman Kodak marketed a processor that produced a dry film in approximately 90 seconds using a developer temperature of 95° F. The size of the unit decreased to 38 inches long, 650 pounds, and sold for $9,000.00 to 12,000.00. Today many table-top automatic processors with cycle times between 2 and 3 minutes are available for between $4,000.00 and $6,000.00.

The character of the darkroom is similar regardless of whether automatic or manual processing is used. One-half of the darkroom is maintained as the dry side and the other half as the wet side (Fig. 7-1). This arrangement provides a clean, dry place to unload and load cassettes separate from the area where the wet-tanks or film processor are located. Cleanliness of the room is important since this is the one place where both intensifying screens and films are repeatedly exposed to the air. If the counter tops are dirty, it is easy for the dust to be blown into the cassette with resulting film artifacts and eventual permanent damage to the intensifying screens. If wet-tank processing is used, there is a special need for a wet-film examining area (Fig. 7-1). The darkroom may also provide storage space for unused film, loaded cassettes, and a thermometer and hangers if using wet-tank processing. The level of humidity in the darkroom should be controlled since this is usually where you store the unexposed film, and it stores best at 30% to 50% humidity.

Use of a lead-lined film storage bin insures that the unexposed films are protected from scattered radiation and light. However, this does not guarantee that someone is never going to open the door to the darkroom with the film bin opened and gives a good reason for putting a lock or latch on the door or using a film bin with a weighted front that closes automatically when you take your hand from the handle (Fig. 7-1).

Light leaks around the door cause fogging of the film as does a safe-light that does not functioning correctly. These are important points because of the increase in sensitivity of the x-ray film to visible light following exposure. The darkroom light must be chosen to match the light sensitivity of the film in use (Fig. 7-2). A Wratten #6B filter (amber) is used in processing of blue-sensitive film only, while a Kodak GBX filter (red) is used in processing of green-sensitive film. Blue-sensitive film can be handled safely in filtered light that is also safe for green-light sensitive film.

Safelights must be used with the correct wattage bulb, usually 6 1/2 to 15 watts and be located at least 4 feet (120 cm) from the film on the counter top. The following technique is recommended to evaluate the effect on film of safe-light illumination or leakage of light around the door

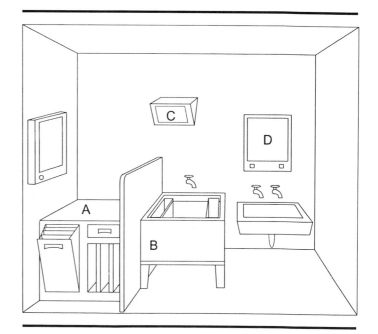

Fig. 7-1
DARKROOM LAYOUT FOR WET-TANK PROCESSING
Schematic drawing of the three areas in a darkroom using wet-tank processing. Processing occurs from left to right. The cassette is opened on the counter top (A) where the film is placed on a hanger. The film is placed consecutively in a series of tanks containing developer, rinse, fixer, and wash water (B). Safelights are mounted on the wall (C). A viewbox (D) with a drip sink is available for wet-film viewing. A film bin located below the counter (A) stores unused film prior to its being used to reload a cassette.

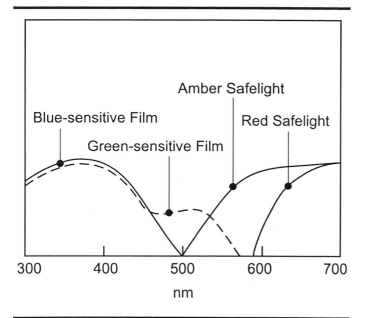

Fig. 7-2
RELATIONSHIP OF FILM SENSITIVITY
TO SAFELIGHT TRANSMISSION

The light from an amber safelight does not expose blue-sensitive film but does expose ortho, or green sensitive, film. A red safelight has a light emission toward the red end of the spectrum and does not expose either type of film. Wavelengths are listed in nanometers (nm).

into the darkroom. Place a film on the counter top in a location where you normally unload the cassette and use a piece of cardboard or the film box to cover the film. Position the covering so that 1/4 of the film is exposed to the normal illumination of the room under darkroom conditions for 1 minute. Shift the cardboard so that 1/2 of the film is exposed for 1 additional minute, and then shift the cardboard so that 3/4 of the film is exposed for 1 additional minute. Remove the cardboard so that the entire film is exposed for 1 additional minute or a total 4 minutes. Process the film in a routine manner. Any fogging causes the film to be blackened and allows you to detect the amount of any light leak.

It is usually not necessary to have radiation shielding in the walls of the darkroom, even when it is adjacent to the x-ray room, because in most situations the personnel responsible for processing the films are also the ones helping to restrain the patients during radiography. The average weekly dose rate to personnel from scatter radiation at a distance of 5 feet and with a workload of 62.5 milliamperage-minutes per week at 100 kVp does not require any shielding as described in NCRP Report No. 36 (Watters, 1982). However, some consideration can be given to shielding film stored in the darkroom.

A. WET-TANK FILM PROCESSING

Wet-tank film processing presents unique features the first of which is having to attach the film to the film hanger (Fig. 7-3). The primary function of the developer solution is to reduce the exposed silver halide crystals to elemental silver ($Ag^+ + e^- = Ag$) and in wet-tank processing, the time of developing may be from 2 to 7 minutes depending on the type of film being used (Table 7-1). Use of longer developing times permits use of the lowest mAs settings in the production of the radiograph. Shorter developing times require the original exposure of the film be greater in an effort to achieve the same film density as you would have with a longer developing time because of failure to use the developer to reduce exposed silver halide crystals to its full extent. Use of higher developing temperatures permits the use of shorter developing times or the use of less radiation exposure. Developer temperatures may range from 68° to 80°F (20° to 26.5°C). A water temperature regulator is not essential but is highly recommended. The longer developing times are usually used with the lower temperatures. Agitate the hanger slightly to remove any air bubbles from the surface of the film at the time of placing the film in the developer. Film processing chemistry follows the same principles whether it is by wet-tank or automatic processor.

It is recommended that you use developer solution manufactured by the same company that made the film currently in use or that you follow the recommendations of the film company. The level of the developer solution is maintained by adding fresh replenisher solution. It is easy to spot those films processed in tanks in which the developer solution is low (Fig. 7-4). Eventually, the developing solution becomes exhausted from age and the developer solution appears yellowish or brown or the processed radiograph fails to have the expected density or contrast. Thoroughly clean the developing tank when changing solutions to avoid mixing the old chemical with the fresh solutions resulting in immediate oxidation of the chemicals and shortening of the life of the new solution. The size of the developing tank is governed by the volume of work. For a small clinic, a stainless steel tank with 5 gallon removable inserts and a 10 to 15 gallon wash space is probably satisfactory (Fig. 7-1).

When you remove the hanger from the developer, lift it quickly from the developer tank and drain the exhausted developer into the rinse bath and **not** back into the developer tank. The film should be in the rinse bath at 60° to 85°F (15.5° to 29.5°C) for 30 seconds with continuous agitation. The rinse bath removes the excess developer solution prior to placement of the film in the fixer tank. However, developer solution in the film emulsion continues the developing process until the film is placed into the fixer. This rinse bath is not used in the automatic processors because of the constant replacement of fresh chemicals and the film passes directly from the developer solution to the fixer solution. The tank for the rinse bath in wet-tank processing is often the same tank as used for the final wash. A tank containing a separate stop bath solution retards the development process faster and more uniformly than rinsing the film and can be used prior to a water rinse.

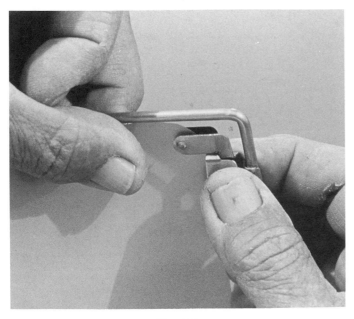

Fig. 7-3
FILM HANGERS
One of the time consuming parts of wet-tank processing is fastening the film onto the film hanger.

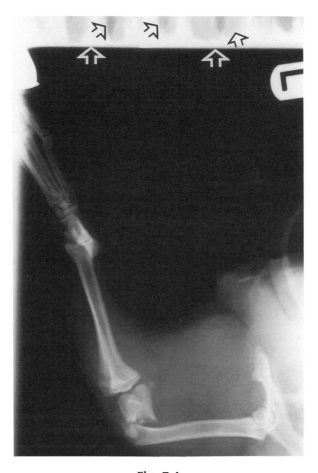

Fig. 7-4
FILM ARTIFACT
The lines across the top of the film indicate the level of the developer solution (white arrows) and splashing of the fixer solution (black arrows).

Table 7-1
DEVELOPER CHEMISTRY FOR MANUAL PROCESSING

General Function	Chemical	Special Function
Developing agents	Metol	Quickly builds up gray tones in the image.
	Hydroquinone	Reducing agents convert silver bromide crystals into metallic silver. Slowly builds up black tones and contrast in the image.
Activator	Sodium carbonate	Swells and softens emulsion so that reducing agents may work more effectively. Provides required alkalinity for reducing agents.
Restrainer	Potassium bromide	Restrains reducing agents keeping unexposed silver halide from being developed.
Preservative	Sodium sulfite	Prevents rapid oxidation of developing agents
Solvent	Water	Provides liquid in which to dissolve chemicals.

Often algae forms in the rinse water tanks and its growth can be controlled by adding bleach to the rinse water. This must be done carefully since the chlorine in the bleach can remove the silver from the radiograph forming what is referred to as "horn silver". If the bleach contaminates the fixer solution, it forms a percipitate resulting in a marked decrease in radiographic density. If algae is a particularly bad problem in your clinic, it can be partially eliminated by filtration of the incoming water using a filter with a pore opening of not more than 35 microns.

As you move the hanger from the rinse water to the fixer solution, let the excess water drain into the rinse instead of draining the water into the fixer solution and causing its dilution. However, a small amount of carry-over water and developer is not detrimental to the action of the fixer solution. The sodium thiosulfate (hypo) in the fixer converts the undeveloped silver bromide crystals into soluble compounds and dissolves them away in addition to preserving the emulsion to prevent its eventual deterioration (Table 7-2). The fixer solution should be from 60° to 85°F (15.5° to 29.5° C) and the film should be fixed for 2 to 4 minutes. Agitate the hanger in the fixer solution intermittently. Fixing leaves the silver image on the film as a permanent record. If the fixer is at full strength and the temperature is near the development temperature, the film is ready to be first viewed after 10 to 15 seconds in the fixer solution. The total time in the fixer in wet-tank processing is not critical as long as the films are left for 2 to 4 minutes with intermittent agitation. However, do not leave the film in the fixer longer than 30 minutes since this requires a longer final wash time because the emulsion swells and holds an increased amount of fixer solution. The level of the fixer solution does not drop as quickly as the developer solution because of the water continually added to the fixer tank by each film as it moves from the rinse tank. Still, you remove some fixer solution as you move each film into the wash and the fixer solution regularly needs addition of fixer replenisher solution. Change the fixer solution when the time required for the film to change from a cloudy appearance to a clear appearance exceeds 5 minutes. This is referred to as the clearing time and normally should be less than 2 minutes. It is easy to spot those films processed in tanks in which the fixer solution is low (Fig. 7-4).

As you move the hanger from the fixer solution into the wash water do so in such a manner that the fixer solution is carried over and drains into the wash water. The final washing should be in clean running water with approximately 8 volume changes per hour at 60° to 85°F (15.5° to 29.5°C) for 5 to 30 minutes. The time of washing in wet-tank processing is not critical and is dependent on the time in the fixer solution and the rate of replacement of the wash water. Generally the wash time should be 10 minutes, assuming clean running water. The wash removes the remaining silver complexes and the excess fixer.

The films in wet-tank processing should be dried in a clean place (Fig. 7-5) prior to cutting the corners and filing the films into a permanent storage envelope. It is possible to use a wetting agent for a final wash that reduces surface tension and reduces drying time and minimizes drying water marks. The basic steps required for processing films in wet tanks are outlined (Table 7-3).

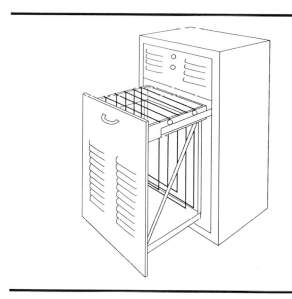

Fig. 7-5
AUTOMATIC FILM DRYER
The wet film still attached to the hanger is hung in the dryer. The time and temperature may be controlled automatically.

Table 7-2
FIXER CHEMISTRY FOR MANUAL PROCESSING

General Function	Chemical	Special Function
Fixing agent	Sodium or ammonium thiosulfate	Clears away unexposed silver bromide crystals.
Acidifier	Acetic or sulfuric acid	Stops development by neutralizing developer. Provides required acidity.
Hardener	Ammonium chloride or sulfide	Restrains swelling of gelatin and hardens emulsion.
Preservative	Sodium sulfite	Prevents oxidation and discoloration of fixing agents.
Solvent	Water	Provides liquid in which to dissolve chemicals.

Table 7-3
BASIC STEPS IN PROCESSING X-RAY FILM IN WET TANKS

1. Stir solutions to equalize their temperatures using separate paddles for developer and fixer tanks.

2. Check temperature of solutions since this influences the time of developing

3. Load film on hanger avoiding bending or scratching the film.

4. Set timer for developer time based on temperature of developer.

5. Place loaded film hanger into developer with slight agitation of the hanger to remove air bubbles and completely immerse the film.

6. Remove film from developer tank quickly at the appropriate time draining the excessive developer solution into the rinse tank (do not drain expended developer solution back into developer tank).

7. Rinse film thoroughly for 30 seconds agitating the hanger vigorously (do not scratch film emulsion on other films hanging in the rinse tank). Rinse developer solution from film hanger by submersing hanger.

8. Lift hanger from rinse tank and let the excess water drain into the rinse tank. When no more water is running from the film, place the film hanger into the fixer tank agitating the hanger to remove air bubbles. Completely immerse the film.

9. Film can be lifted from fixer solution and viewed briefly after 10 to 15 seconds. Replace hanger in fixer solution for a total of 2 to 4 minutes.

10. Place hanger into final wash tank (this may be the same tank as used for the rinse) for at least 30 minutes depending on the rate of replenishing of the wash water.

11. Place hanger in drier or hang on outside rack for film to dry. Avoid dusty area.

12. Remove dried film from hanger and trim corners.

13. Place films into storage envelope checking identification of film.

B. AUTOMATIC FILM PROCESSING

As the name implies, automatic processors control the processing of the films in an automatic manner and make the often tedious job of film processing a real joy (Fig. 7-6). The name is probably misleading since it implies that all of the actions are "automatic" and do not require your attention. Actually, mechanized film processor is a more accurate term, since this suggests that you need to observe the process. The transfer of the film, time the film is in the individual tanks, control of the temperature of the solutions, and concentration and replacement of the solutions at a predetermined rate are all handled automatically. This insures that there is a constant treatment of each film and once there is confidence in the use of the technique chart, all radiographic exposures should be satisfactory in terms of exposure and processing. All of this assumes that the automatic processor functions correctly. Processing times range from 90 seconds to 8 minutes. Developer temperatures range from 77° to 96°F, with the temperature inversely related to the length of processing times. The price range of automatic processors begins at $4,000.00 and goes to over $24,000.00. The processor can be installed entirely within the darkroom or may extend through the wall and releases the dry film into an adjacent area. The unit may be freestanding within the darkroom or may be a mobile installation. The type of installation is usually made dependent on the cost and availability of an area in an adjacent room that can be made into a film examination area. Many questions need to be considered prior to installation of an automatic processor (Table 7-4).

The processing chemicals for automatic equipment differ from conventional wet-tank chemicals since they are especially concentrated and adapted to high-speed roller operation at higher temperatures, however, the basic chemical reactions are similar (Tables 7-5, 7-6). Care of the rollers in the automatic processor is important to avoid film artifacts and the roller racks should be removed from the processor and washed clean at the end of the day (or week) and allowed to dry with the top removed. The cross-over rollers should be wiped wet at the beginning of the next day.

Processing and replenisher chemicals are available for use in both manual and automatic processors. Almost all come in concentrated liquid form and require mixing and/or dilution with tap water to prepare the developer or fixer solution. Developer for an automatic processor probably is described as "Rapid X-ray Developer" and is more chemically active and requires less developer time. The developer for wet-tank processing is described as "Developer and Replenisher" and is less-active chemically and requires a longer developer time. It is probably better to use processing chemicals prepared by the same company that produces the x-ray film you are using. Use caution in the disposition of used chemicals since they are toxic and most local regulations do not permit the deposition of these chemicals into ordinary sewer lines.

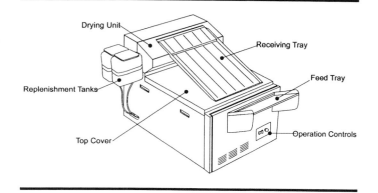
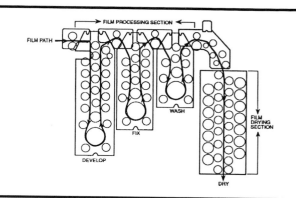

Fig. 7-6
AUTOMATIC FILM PROCESSOR
A drawing shows the major parts of a tabletop processor. A schematic drawing of the roller transport system illustrates the film pathway through an automatic processor where the three tanks and film drying section are identified.

Table 7-4
QUESTIONS TO CONSIDER PRIOR TO
PURCHASE AND INSTALLATION OF AN AUTOMATIC FILM PROCESSOR

1. What is the length of the processing cycle?

2. Can you change the length of the processing cycle?

3. What is the processing capacity per hour?

4. What is the size of film accommodated?

5. What types of film can be processed?

6. When can you turn on the room light during processing?

7. Does the unit automatically turn off the safelight during film feed?

8. Is the operation standby or continuous?

9. If a standby unit, does the solution temperature remain ready for processing without warm-up time?

10. Is there a signal advising operation at the correct processing temperature?

11. Are replenisher tanks supplied? Is the size adequate for your clinic?

12. Is the unit a floor or tabletop model?

13. Is the unit installation permanent or mobile?

14. Is the filter and cartridge on the incoming water line supplied?

15. What is the water requirement in gallons/minute?

16. Are there ducting requirements for the dryer section?

17. Is the unit installed through a hole in the wall or is it contained entirely within the darkroom?

18. What are the drain requirements? Is draining into an open sink? Is there a problem of odors?

19. Can a septic tank system accept drainage from the unit? (Depends on volume and local regulations.)

20. Does the unit require an electrical capability not provided by a standard 110- or 230-volt wall outlet?

21. Is the amperage requirement in excess of standard 15 Amp current?

22. Is grounding of the unit required? Are grounding wires provided?

23. Can you easily remove the transport system for cleaning? Where will you clean the racks?

Table 7-5
DEVELOPER CHEMISTRY FOR AUTOMATIC PROCESSING

General Function	Chemical	Special Function
Developing agents	Phenidone	Quickly builds up grey tones in the image.
	Hydroquinone	Reducing agents convert silver bromide crystals into metallic silver. Slowly builds up black tones and contrast in the image.
Activator	Sodium carbonate	Swells and softens the emulsion so that reducing agents may work more effectively. Provides required alkalinity for reducing agents.
Hardener	Gluteraldehyde	Controls emulsion swelling to allow better transportation of films through the processor.
Restrainer	Potassium bromide	Restrains reducing agents keeping unexposed silver halide from being developed.
Preservative	Sodium sulfite	Prevents rapid oxidation of developing agents.
Solvent	Water	Provides liquid in which to dissolve chemicals.

Table 7-6
FIXER CHEMISTRY FOR AN AUTOMATIC PROCESSOR

General Function	Chemical	Special Function
Fixing agent	Ammonium thiosulfate	Clears away unexposed silver bromide crystals.
Neutralizer	Acetic acid	Neutralizes alkaline developer carried over from developing solution.
Hardener	Aluminum chloride	Restrains swelling of gelatin and hardens emulsion.
Preservative	Sodium sulfite	Prevents oxidation and discoloration of fixing agents.
Solvent	Water	Provides liquid in which to dissolve chemicals.

REFERENCES

Gray JE. Light log on radiographic films—how to measure it properly. Radiology 115:225,1975.

Watters JW. The x-ray room and equipment. Comp on Cont Ed 2: 873-82, 1980.

Watters JW. The radiographic darkroom and film processing. Comp on Cont Ed 4: 311, 1982.

8. COPYING RADIOGRAPHS

Radiographic duplicating film has a single emulsion and is available in a size similar to that of diagnostic film and offers a fast, simple, and relatively inexpensive way to copy radiographs. It does this through the technique of solarization where it is possible to produce a copy which is identical to the original radiograph (Curry III et al, 1984). Normally, as x-ray exposure increases, so does the resulting density of the film, up to a maximum limit of approximately 2 seconds. This is seen regularly in diagnostic radiography as techniques are increased by change in the mA, kVp, or time settings. However, if the exposure is increased considerably beyond the 2 seconds that produces the maximum density, a subsequent decrease in film density occurs. The downswing curve that represents this decrease in film density is called the solarization curve and is the result of very high film exposures (Fig. 8-1). It means that the increased exposure has actually destroyed the developable state of the film that had been induced by the earlier part of the exposure. The film's characteristic curve can be evaluated and it is noted that as the curve extends beyond the toe, straight line and shoulder it reaches a region of solarization where increased exposure results in decreased film density. The increased exposure required for copying film must be great when compared to that commonly used in diagnostic radiography.

Solarization can be partially explained by rebromination which is a currently favored hypothesis. Bromine gas is formed when silver bromide decomposes in the photolytic process at the time of original exposure. The bromine passes from the silver halide crystal into the surrounding gelatin. The gelatin neutralizes the small qualities of bromine formed in the normal latent-image formation. However, gelatin is easily saturated with bromine. The amount of bromine liberated during the large exposures of light used in the solarization process cannot be destroyed by the gelatin and large quantities of bromine build up in the spaces between emulsion grains. When the exposure is completed, this excess bromine reacts with metallic silver at the latent-image centers on the surface of the grain and coats the latent-image center with a layer of silver bromide which effectively isolates it from the action of the developing solution. Thus the grain, even though it contains one or more latent-image centers, does not develop.

The emulsion on copy film has been solarized prior to use. The technique of solarization is usually done with light or done chemically in the preparation of duplicating film. It is possible for you to solarize conventional diagnostic film by exposing the film to daylight for 30 to 90 seconds prior to placing it next to the film to be copied. However, it is difficult to control the degree of solarization produced in the film and copy film should be used where possible.

Following solarization commercially or in your darkroom, the emulsion is exposed with an ultraviolet light source in the process of making the copy radiograph. These lamps mounted in a standard radiographic illuminator serve as a good light source and it is possible to produce your own copy machine easily. A cassette with the front removed and replaced with glass may be used to hold the original radiograph and copy film in close contact. The emulsion side of the copy film must face the original radiograph. The pair of films is then exposed to the ultraviolet light. Recommended time of exposure is about 6 seconds with the view box about 2 feet from the cassette and must take place within the dark room. Following exposure, the exposed copy film is processed as a routine x-ray film. To change film density, permit more light to reach the solarized film to decrease the resulting film density. Commercially available duplicating film is available on a blue-tinted base for copying routine radiographs and a clear base designed for copying images produced by ultrasound. Commercially available copiers are now routinely used to prepare full-sized copies of radiographs (Fig. 8-2).

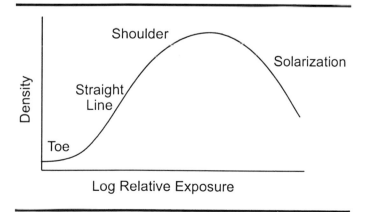

Fig. 8-1
SOLARIZATION
The characteristic H and D curve shows film density extending into the region of solarization following prolonged film exposure where the increased exposure results in decreased film density. The increased exposure required for copying film is great when compared to that commonly used in diagnostic radiography.

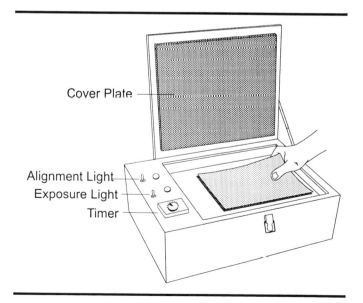

Fig. 8-2
X-RAY FILM COPIER
Some copiers accept all film sizes up to and including 14" x 17" and use 110 volts. Some units can do subtraction work. Photo furnished by Techno-Aide/Stumb Metal Products Co, Nashville, TN 37209.

9. RADIOGRAPHIC QUALITY

Radiographic quality is that feature of a diagnostic radiograph that describes to what degree the shadows identified on the film clearly depict the anatomical features under investigation. Factors affecting radiographic quality are separated by the stage in production of the radiograph where the loss in film quality occurred and which of the features of radiographic quality is affected.

Radiographic (film) density refers to the darkness of the radiograph and is determined by the number of x-ray photons that reach the film and by the developing process that causes conversion of the silver halide crystals into metallic silver. It is possible to measure radiographic density on any part of the radiograph by measuring the amount of light that can pass through at that site. Density has a precise numerical value that can be calculated if the level of light incident (Io) on a processed film and the level of light transmitted (It) through the film are measured. Density is defined as the log 10 of Io/It. Radiographic film contains densities ranging from near 0 to 4, however the useful range of densities is approximately 0.25 to 2.5.

The density of the margins on the radiograph outside of the shadow of the patient is determined by the quantity of x-ray photons produced for the study and is independent of the photon energy. No tissue is present to stop the x-ray photons and, therefore, all photons that are produced reach the film (screens) and contribute to the radiographic density. However, the presence of a bone within the x-ray beam increases subject density resulting is a decrease in film density since more of the photons are absorbed and prevented from reaching the film. Radiographic density at the site of a bone is also determined by the quality of the x-ray photons in the beam since only the higher-energy photons pass through the bone and reach the film (screens). Factors that influence radiographic density are listed (Table 9-1).

Radiographic contrast refers to the observed differences in radiographic density (photodensity) between any two anatomical structures in the radiograph. These differences permit identification of the various body organs and structures on the film. A radiograph that has sharp differences in density, in which a structure "stands out" more, is called a high-contrast radiograph (has greater contrast). On the other hand, if the density differences are small and not distinct, the radiograph is of low-contrast. Contrast is influenced mostly by the level of the kVp setting used, the amount of film fog, and the character of the patient. Higher kVp settings produce a radiograph with a longer scale of contrast with less difference between each

Table 9-1
FACTORS INFLUENCING RADIOGRAPHIC DENSITY

Machine factors
    mA setting
    kVp setting
    exposure time
    incoming line voltage

Physical factors
    subject density
    subject thickness
    use of contrast agents
    focal-film distance
    film speed
    intensifying screen speed
    grid factor
    beam filtration

Processing factors
    developer time
    developer temperature

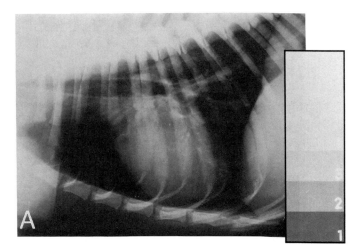

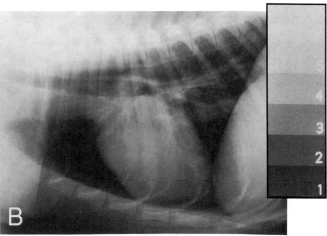

Fig. 9-1
RADIOGRAPHIC CONTRAST
Film A was made with an exposure of 40 kVp and 40 mAs while film B was made with an exposure of 100 kVp and 1.5 mAs. The resulting radiographs of a dog's thorax and of an aluminum step-wedge show how the scale of contrast is dependent on kVp settings.

step on the scale, while lower kVp settings produce a radiograph with a shorter scale of contrast and more obvious differences between each step on the scale (Fig. 9-1). Film fog erases the areas of minimal film density and shortens the contrast scale. Subject contrast influences radiographic contrast in that a patient with an abdomen filled with fluid has much less radiographic contrast than an abdomen filled with fatty tissue. It is possible for you to influence subject contrast by the use of either positive or negative radiographic contrast agents and through the use of "paddle" or compression techniques that decrease patient thickness. In determining the film to be used in your clinic, it is advisable to inquire into the contrast level of various films.

The usual method of representing the response of a film to radiation is by the use of the characteristic curve (H and D curve, after Hurter and Driefield). This curve expresses the relationship between radiation exposure to the film and the resulting film density. It is obtained by exposing film to a graded series of exposures and plotting the resultant density measurements as read from a densitometer on the vertical axis versus the logarithm of the exposure on the horizontal axis. The underexposure region is represented by the straight line portion where the density is in proportion to logrithmetic exposure, and the region of heavy densities where the curve flatterns. The curve is approximately linear between densities of 0.4 and 2.0 and the gradient of the slope defines the difference in

density that results from a known difference in exposure. This brings together the concept of film density and film contrast. Film contrast refers to the gradient of the characteristic curve of the film and determines the ultimate radiographic contrast that can be achieved with a given subject contrast. The tangent of the angle which the straight line portion of the curve forms with the log exposure axis is the "gamma" and is a measure of contrast for that film. The labeling of a film as "high" or "low" contrast is based partially on the value of the average gradient (Fig. 9-2).

The lower-most film density is partially due to the base density and therefore the curve does not extend to zero. Base density is the density inherent in the base of the film and is due to the composition of the base and the tint added to make the radiograph more pleasing to the eye. This normal background density of an unexposed film decreases the transmitted light by 37%, yet appears to be almost transparent.

If the exposure of the radiograph results in densities that are in the toe or shoulder of the H & D curve film contrast will be lost.

Contrast is also affected by mAs settings that shifts all of the radiodensities up or down the H&D curve but does not alter their relative position on the x-axis. In other words, at a given mAs, if the film beneath a muscle receives twice the exposure of the film beneath the adjacent bone (a 2:1 ratio), doubling the mAs does not alter this relationship but

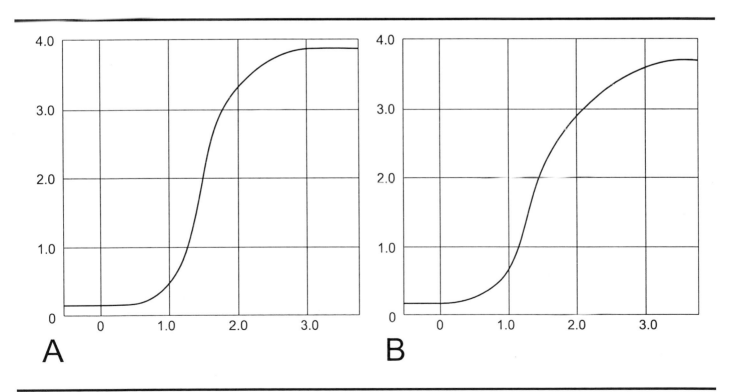

Fig. 9-2
CHARACTERISTIC CURVES
Relative exposure is shown on the x-axis with resulting density shown on the y-axis. Film A has higher contrast while Film B shows wider latitude.

simply changes the photodensity of both the muscle and bone on the radiograph.

Contrast is influenced by two additional factors: (1) the nature of the film contrast that is inherent in the film and (2) the influence due to the processing of the film. These can be controlled by the selection of the film purchased and the nature of film processing in your clinic.

Latitude is the range of exposure levels that can be imaged on the film and still have a diagnostic radiograph. Latitude and contrast are inversely related. A high contrast, low latitude film requires a more accurate exposure setting but provides the greatest contrast between similar tissues. A low contrast, high latitude film permits a greater range of exposure settings in the production of a diagnostic radiograph. Appreciate that if a radiograph is badly over- or underexposed that both contrast and latitude are reduced and information is lost.

Film fogging is defined as unwanted exposure to a part or all of the film. This degradation in film quality may be the result of: (1) radiation exposure, (2) light leak while in the cassette, (3) exposure to light during loading and unloading of the cassette, (4) exposure to light while in the film bin, (5) chemical fogging, (6) scatter radiation, or (7) aging of the film. This increased amount of silver deposited on the film eliminates the lower density steps and thus takes away the contrast in the minimally exposed regions on the radiograph. Thus, the radiograph has no "white" or transparent areas that freely transmit light from the view box. Contrast can be measured by use of an aluminum stepwedge that shows the differences in film density produced between successively thicker aluminum steps. It has been suggested that 50% of all darkrooms cause film fogging (Gray and Haus, 1978). A way to control fogging should begin with an examination of the dark room. Another way to control film fogging is to limit the amount of scatter radiation that reaches the film by using a grid and by controlling the amount of tissue irradiated through use of a collimator. Factors influencing radiographic contrast are listed (Table 9-2).

Radiographic detail refers to the sharpness of the shadows seen on the radiograph. It is sometimes called definition. Geometric unsharpness is due to the: (1) focal-spot size, (2) focal-film distance, (3) object-film distance, and (4) screen-film contact. These are all physical features that can be controlled to some extent. Motion unsharpness is theoretically due to movement of the object, cassette, or tube during the exposure. Most loss of detail is due to movement of the patient and/or cassette. Structure mottle refers to the construction of the phosphor of the intensifying screens and is a cause of loss of radiographic detail and is due to the speed of intensifying screens used in production of the radiograph. The faster the speed of the screen, the greater the loss of detail and the lower the resolution on the film. Film graininess refers to the distribution in size and space of the silver halide grains in the emulsion. The faster the speed of the film, the greater the loss of detail and the lower the resolution on the film. Quantum mottle refers to the random nature in which x-rays interact with the image receptor. If an image is produced with just a few x-ray photons, there will be an undesirable fluctuation in the optical density of the image. Factors influencing radiographic detail are listed (Table 9-3). Terms such as: (1) resolution, meaning the ability to image two separate objects and visually detect one from the other, and (2) radiographic noise, including film graininess, structure mottle, and quantum mottle, are also used to describe radiographic quality.

Table 9-2
FACTORS INFLUENCING RADIOGRAPHIC CONTRAST

Machine factors
  kVp setting

Physical factors
  beam filtration
  beam collimation
  subject contrast
  use of contrast agents
  scatter radiation
  radiation fog
  light fog

Processing factors
  age of film
  developing time
  developing temperature
  developer age
  fixer time
  fixer age

Table 9-3
FACTORS INFLUENCING RADIOGRAPHIC DETAIL OR DEFINITION

Machine factors
  focal spot size

Physical factors
  focal-film distance
  object-film distance
  film-screen contact
  patient thickness
  patient motion
  film speed
  intensifying screen speed

REFERENCES

Gray JE and Haus AG. Protocol for Basic Photographic Processor Quality Control. Applied Radiology, pp. 115-8, January/February, 1977.

Gray JE and Haus AG. Lecture RSNA-1978.

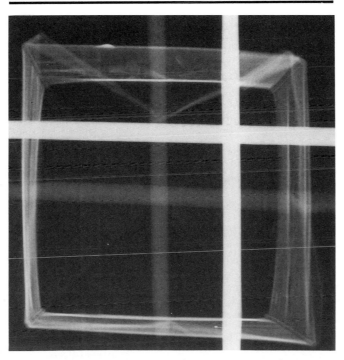

A radiograph was made of a large paper milk carton that was empty. Small holes were made in the sides of the carton near the top that would just accept paper straws. Three paper straws were placed to go from the top to the bottom of the radiograph and three additional paper straws were placed to go from side to side. Two straws are filled with iodinated contrast agent, two are filled with water, and two are empty. Why are you unable to identify the straws that were empty?

10. TECHNICAL ERRORS

X-ray film is not only sensitive to light and radiation, but also is very sensitive to extraneous pressure, fumes, temperature, humidity, and rough handling. Because of this, unexpected artifacts, technical errors, appear on processed films every day with both manual (wet-tank) processing and automatic film processing. These artifacts cause retake rates of 10% or more in many clinics using diagnostic radiology and probably cost the average clinic several thousands of dollars each year, since it is estimated that the average cost of retake films is estimated to be over $4.00 per sheet if the cost includes all personnel and fringe benefits, generating equipment, film chemistry, supplies, and other expense (Lindstrom, 1979). Yet, little attention is given to correcting this obvious waste of money and technician time.

Technical errors may destroy the diagnostic qualities of the radiograph. Sometimes the film is made completely unusable, but more often a decision is made that the radiograph is compromised, but "usable", and it is accepted as though it were a radiograph of high technical quality. This ultimately compromises the diagnostic quality of the entire study. Some of the technical errors are sporadic in their appearance while others are noted repeatedly on every film. Consideration of the patterns of occurrence assists in arriving at a decision of the cause and what the corrective action should be.

It is possible to classify artifacts based on their general appearance on the radiograph (Table 10-1). That is, determination of whether the error is focal in location or is general throughout the entire radiograph and whether the resulting artifact is clear (radiolucent), dark (radiopaque), or only cloudy. Some artifacts effect the character of the surface of the film emulsion, while others affect the manner in which the silver halide crystals were exposed or processed. By a classification of this type, most artifacts can be recognized and their cause correctly determined.

Some artifacts affect film density and are characterized by having caused too great or too little exposure of the film by visible light from the intensifying screens on screen-type film or direct x-radiation on non-screen film and result in an alteration in the number of silver crystals throughout the film (Fig. 10-1). Other conditions can artifically affect the number of the silver crystals on only a portion of the film. This change in film density, whether focal or generalized, is detected by noting the amount of transmitted light from the viewbox and can be easily seen when viewing the radiograph. Problems in film density that affect the entire film are usually solved by correcting exposure settings. Focal errors in film density are due to other problems.

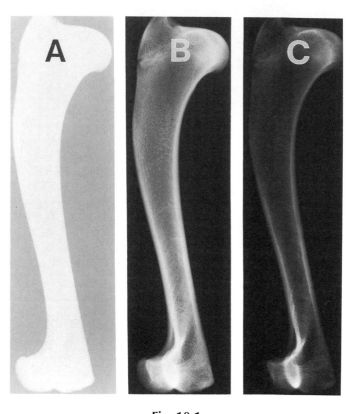

Fig. 10-1
FILM DENSITY
A radiographic study made using changing mAs factors that result in: (A) under exposure, (B) correct exposure, and (C) over exposure of the film.

Table 10-1
QUESTIONS TO ASK WHEN DEALING WITH PROBLEMS OF FILM ARTIFACTS:

1. has the artifact occured in the past? what corrective action was taken that time?
2. is the artifact periodic?
3. is this the first time for this particular artifact?
4. was the film handled in an unusual manner?
5. did the problem occur just after replacing chemicals?
6. if there a difference in temperature and humidity in the darkroom?
7. did the artifact occur after changing film type?
8. does the artifact occur in the same location on the film?
9. does the artifact have a directional tendency (parallel pattern)?
10. does the artifact affect both sides of the film?
11. can the artifact be viewed with relected light?

Loss of radiographic contrast is another artifact that results from a general fogging of the film and usually affects the entire film and may be due to causes such as radiation fog, chemical fog, and light fog. The solution to the problem is based on the specific cause. Fogging by scatter radiation can be at least partially controlled by the use of a grid or tighter collimation (Fig. 10-2). Chemical fogging can be corrected by insuring that processing solutions are fresh and by using recommended processing times and temperatures. Light leaks can be from errors in exposing the film during loading or un-loading or from light leaks while the film is in the cassette (Fig. 10-3). A film may be fogged by placing it under the safelight for a prolonged period, handling it at a close distance from the safelight, by exceeding the recommended level of the wattage of the bulb in the safelight, or by having a light leak around the filter holder. In addition, the type of safelight filter may not be suitable for the spectral sensitivity of the film.

Fogging can also be caused by film storage over an extensive period of time in an area with high-temperature and high-humidity. The higher the speed of the film, the more sensitive is the film to fogging. Film should not be stored at a temperature greater than 68°F (20°C) which means that film should not be left inside a motor vehicle in the summer.

Static electricity causes a type of fogging that often appears as a "tree", "branch", "star-burst", "crown", "swamp", "smudge", "spot", or "dots". These static marks are particularly seen during a dry season on films that are mistreated (Fig. 10-4). This is the same electrostatic charge phenomenon seen when our feet move quickly across carpeting. When the film is negatively charged, the static appears in a branch form. When the film is positively charged, the static marks appear in the dot or smudge form. Specific causes of static marks include: (1) drawing the film quickly out of the storage box, (2) sliding the film across the intensifying screen in the cassette when loading or unloading, (3) using an intensifying screen recently wiped by a dry cloth, (4) static discharge from a chemical-fiber glove or cloth, or (5) working on a charged work bench. Eliminate static electricity in the darkroom by: (1) raising the humidity inside the room, (2) handling the film carefully and not sliding it across another suface, (3) cleaning intensifying screens with a cleaner that contains an antistatic agent, and (4) using cotton instead of chemical-fiber cloths or gloves.

Certain technical errors cause focal defects on the film. One of these errors results from the influence of pressure applied to the film through partially bending the film or at a site of finger-nail pressure. Both the "bend" and the "nail" mark have a characteristic appearance. The appearance of the pressure mark varies relative to whether the pressure is minimal or strong and whether the film has been exposed or not. Minimal pressure causes a desensitized (white) mark prior to exposure and a sensitized (black) mark following exposure (Fig. 10-5). A strong pressure causes a sensitized (black) mark both prior to and following exposure.

Splashed drops of developer, fixer, or water falling on the film before its processing cause white (desensitized) marks or blackened (sensitized) marks. If developer is splashed, the marks are blackened, more so after film exposure. If fixer is splashed, the marks appear as wash-off marks in which the

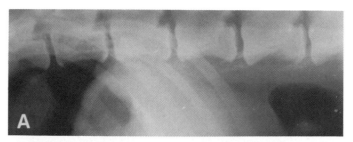
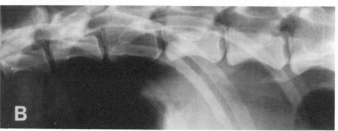

Fig. 10-2
RADIOGRAPHIC CONTRAST
A radiographic study made without use of a grid (A) and with use of a grid (B) shows the effect of the grid as it lessens the amount of scatter radiation that reaches the film improving the radiographic contrast. The exposure factors were altered to compensate for the use of the gird.

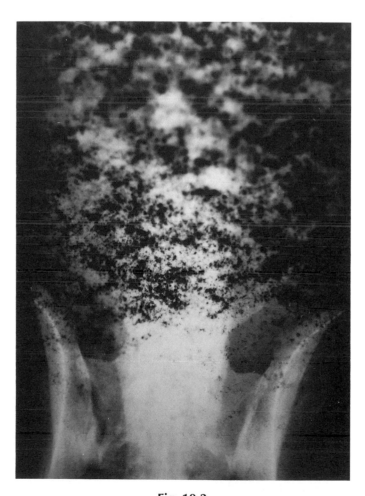

Fig. 10-3
FILM ARTIFACTS DUE TO LIGHT EXPOSURE
A radiograph exposed to light passing through the course interleaving paper prior to loading the film into the cassette causing numerous black artifacts.

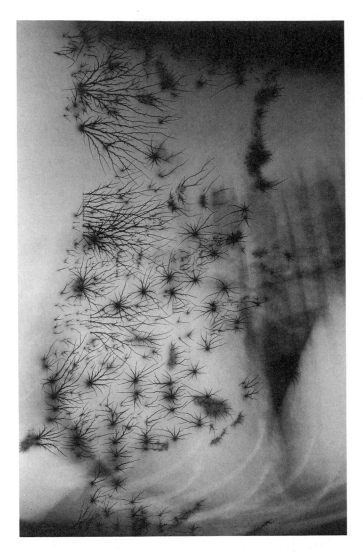

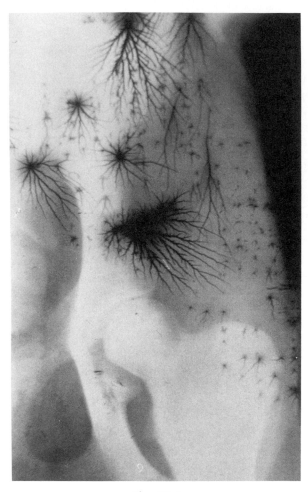

Fig. 10-4
FILM ARTIFACTS DUE TO STATIC ELECTRICITY
Radiographs with different patterns of heavy focal black
areas due to exposure due to static electricity.

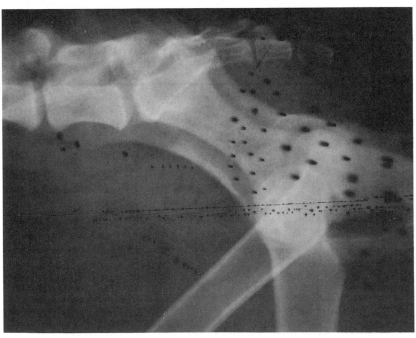

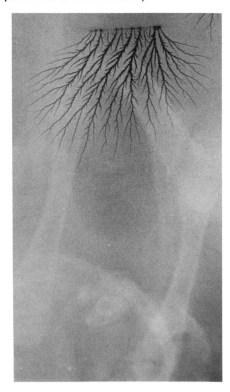

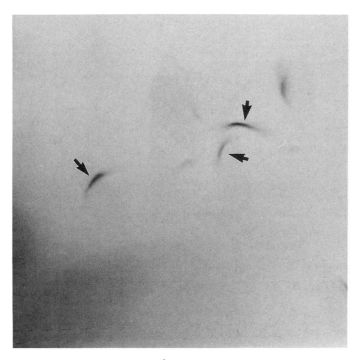

Fig. 10-5
FILM ARTIFACTS DUE TO PRESSURE DEFECT
A radiograph illustrates the effect of pressure on the film causing black cresent marks (arrows).

The type of film processing influences the nature of the radiographic technical errors. Manual processing permits errors associated with processing times and temperature of solutions that are usually not-repeated, while automatic processing may cause certain repeated problems that are reproducible and regular in their appearance and are due to improper film loading or film handling by the processor. Transport problems result in pressure marks and are parallel and in a horizontal or vertical pattern and occur with the same pattern on different sheets of film. Developer rollers or developing-fixing crossover rollers may have a rough surface and cause a pressure artifact (Fig. 10-10). Artifacts of this type may also be found if the pressure by the opposite rollers is too strong, or if eccentrically rotating pressure is applied unevenly to the film as it passes through the rollers. Misalignment of a guideshoe in the cross-over assembly cause "shoe marks" that can be eliminated by their adjustment. Accumulation of any type of sediment on the rollers produces artifacts as the

crystals are removed from the emulsion. Wash water causes slightly white marks before exposure and slightly blackened marks after exposure.

Dirty or damaged intensifying screens cause desensitized (white) artifacts that appear on all films made using that cassette-screen combination (Fig. 10-6). Clean the screens periodically and examine the surface looking for damage. Avoid touching the screen surface with bare hands when loading or unloading the cassettes because of the oil and dirt on fingers that is transfered to the screens. Avoid splashing water on the film that causes it to stick to the screens causing damage to the screen when the film is removed. Avoid wearing any jewelry while working in the darkroom that can scratch the surfaces of the screens. Never leave cassettes open permanently in the dark room, but reload and close them immediately, to avoid injury or soiling of the screens. Any repeated artifact that is white (desensitized) should make you think of a screen artifact.

Film artifacts resulting from failure to remove all of the collars, halters, and metallic or plastic identification discs from patients are common. These, in addition, to dirt, debris, or radiopaque contrast agents on the hair coat cause many retakes (Figs. 10-7, 10-8, 10-9).

Distorted, magnified, or blurred radiographic images are often due to physical problems of motion during an exposure or the way in which the cassette is held adjacent too the patient. Increased object-film distance, especially if not equal, causes an unequal loss in film detail. The distance of an object from the film can often be estimated by the appearance of the object on the radiograph.

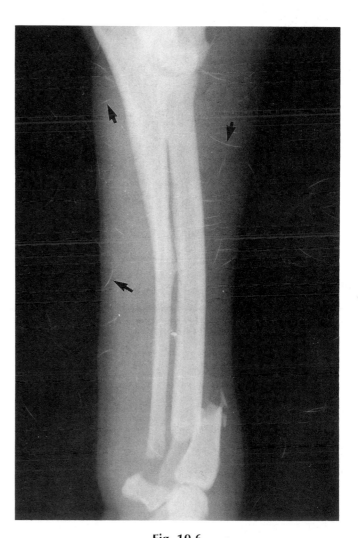

Fig. 10-6
FILM ARTIFACTS DUE TO CONDITION OF INTENSIFYING SCREENS
Any type of dirt or debris on the screens prevents the visible light originating from the screens from reaching the film and causes a pattern of underexposure (arrows).

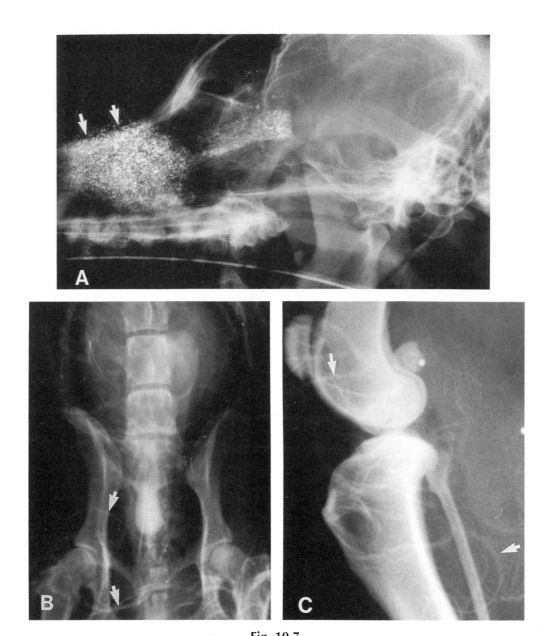

Fig. 10-7
FILM ARTIFACTS DUE TO ERRORS IN PATIENT PREPARATION
Radiographs with a pattern of underexposed areas (arrows) due to radiopaque contrast agent on a positioning sponge (A), radiopaque contrast agent on the hair coat (B), and wet hair coat (C).

74

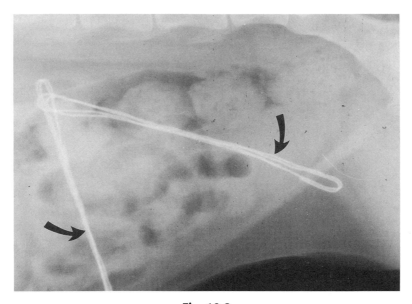

Fig. 10-8
FILM ARTIFACTS DUE TO ERROR IN PATIENT PREPARATION
Radiopaque markers in surgical sponge (arrows) placed under the cat during post-surgical radiographic study of the abdomen cause a prominent white film artifact.

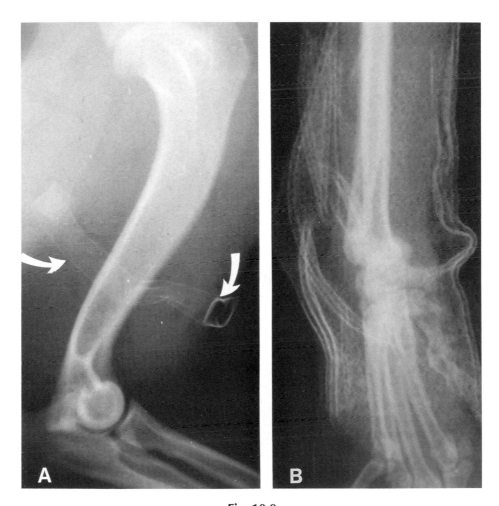

Fig. 10-9
FILM ARTIFACTS DUE TO ERROR IN PATIENT PREPARATION
A rubber surgical drain (arrows) in the foreleg of a dog (A) and a foreleg plaster bandage of a cat (B) both cause prominent white film artifacts.

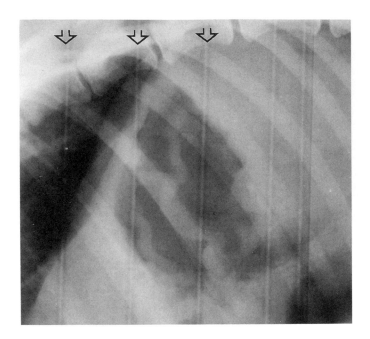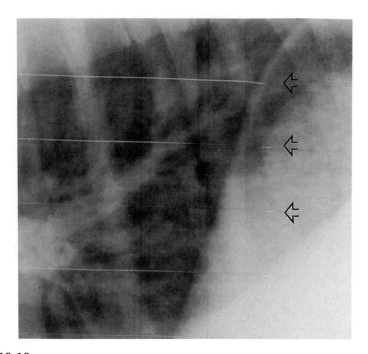

Fig. 10-10
FILM ARTIFACTS DUE TO AUTOMATIC PROCESSOR ROLLER MARKS
Evenly distanced parallel linear marks on the film (arrows) may be due to rollers with rough surface, rollers that are not cleaned regularily, or rollers set at a pressure that was too high.

particles come into contact with the film and can be corrected by cleaning the rollers. Films may not be able to move smoothly through the processor causing rollers to spin over the film surface.

As the film passes through the detector rollers of the processor, it normally activates a microswitch assembly that in turn starts the developer and fixer replenishment pumps. Failure of this switch leads to the film being processed by weakened solutions. If the developer solution temperature is too high, pressure artifacts become increased because the film is more sensitive. If the pressure by the rollers is insufficient to remove the developer solution, streaky marks are found on the processed film. This also occurs if fixer solution attaches to the developing-fixing crossover rollers.

Examples of film artifacts are described below.

Increased film density may be due to: (1) incorrect machine settings with too high a setting of the kVp or mA or the exposure time being too long (Fig. 10-1), (2) decreased focal-film distance, (3) use of a faster film-screen system, (4) overestimation of thickness or density of the part to be examined, (5) surge in incoming line voltage, (6) missing beam filter, (7) increased developer time, (8) too high developer temperature, (9) safelight leak, (10) safelight too close to working surface, (11) safelight stronger than 25 watt bulb, (12) safelight filter not compatible with film sensitivity, (13) exposure timer inaccuracy, or (14) change in film-screen combination.

Decreased film density may be due to: (1) incorrect machine settings with too low a setting of the kVp or mA or the exposure time being too short (Fig. 10-1), (2) lengthened focal-film distance, (3) use of slower film-screen system, (4) underestimation of thickness or density of the part of be examined, (5) drop in incoming line voltage, (6) an increase in the beam filter thickness, (7) x-ray tube anode failure, (8) decreased developer time, (9) too low developer temperature, (10) exhausted developer, (11) failure to hold the exposure switch closed for the length of the exposure time, (12) exposure timer inaccuracy, (13) change in film-screen combination, or (14) loading two films in a cassette.

Loss of film contrast, or gray films, may be due to: (1) film exposed to light either preceeding or following exposure, (2) film exposed to scatter radiation due to failure to use a grid (Fig. 10-2), (3) film exposed to back-scatter during exposure, (4) film out-of-date, (5) film not stored properly, (6) combination of developer time too short and temperature too high, (7) developer chemistry exhausted, contaminated, or diluted, (8) temperature developer solution too high, (9) combination of overexposure and underdeveloping, or (10) inherent character of the film-screen combination.

Localized areas of increased density on the film may be due to: (1) developer dust or liquid splashed on film, (2) linear scratch on film, (3) bending film (Fig. 10-5), (4) static electricity due to rough handling or friction (Fig.10-4), (5) exposure of film edge to light while film is stored in film bin, (6) exposure of film border to light while in the cassette, (7) exposure of film to light escaping from a damaged safelight filter that deteriorated due to use of a high-wattage bulb, and (8) film exposure by light passing through the sheet of interleaving paper (Fig. 10-3).

Localized areas of decreased density on the film may be due to: (1) fixer or water splashed on film before developing, (2) foreign material on screen (Fig. 10-6), (3) bending film, (4) radiopaque material on hair or skin (Figs. 10-7, 10-8, 10-9), (5) film not developed because stuck to other film or wall of tank while being developed, (6) crystals not reduced because of air bubbles next to film while in fixer solution, (7) emulsion scratches, (8) poor film-screen contact, (9) positive contrast agents that have spilled on the tabletop or cassette fronts or absorbed onto the hair coat or into positioning sponges (Fig. 10-7), (10) rolls of fatty tissue in the patient especially in the cervical region, (11) perivascular injection of iodinated contrast agent, and (12) bullet fragments or shotgun pellets.

Poor detail (unsharpness, distorted, magnified, or blurred radiographic images) may be due to: (1) patient motion, (2) cassette motion, (3) tube motion, (4) increased object-film distance, (5) decreased focal-film distance, (5) beam not perpendicular to cassette, (6) poor film-screen contract, (7) fast screens with large cystal size, or (8) double exposure of the film.

Grid faults cause heavy parallel lines across the radiograph due to improper use of a grid and result from: (1) use of grid outside of the focal range of the grid, (2) grid positioned not perpendicular to central beam, (3) central beam not centered on midline of grid, (4) grid used inverted, (5) bent grid, or (6) cassette with a grid in the face used with another grid.

Stains on the film may result from: (1) developer not mixed completely, (2) film underdeveloped, (3) solutions dripping on film from dirty hanger clips, (4) warm developer or wash water causing film emulsion to soften and "run", (5) inadequate fixation, and (6) inadequate washing.

Crescent marks that are either black or white are usually due to bending the film while handling.

Reticulation is a cobweb-like pattern of white lines on the film due to a breakdown or cracking of the surface of very old intensifying screens. It may also present with a "filigree" pattern. Reticulation pattern can also result from swelling of the film emulsion and subsequent shrinking of the emulsion that occurs when the film is subjected to wide variations in temperature during processing.

Miscellaneous artifacts include: (1) brownish-yellowing on the film where fixing was not complete or (2) cloudy and sticky film due to inadequate wash. When the discoloration appears only in the area of the blackened silver, it is an example of exhausted fixer and inadequate washing.

Special artifacts are due to use of automatic processors include: (1) black lines or scratch marks on films due to pressure marks from rollers or bent cross-over shoes (Fig. 10-10), (2) streaks or staining on film due to dirty rollers, and (3) underdeveloped films due to developer not replenishing.

REFERENCES

Cullinan JE and Cullinan AM. Illustrated guide to x-ray technics. 2nd ed JBLippincott, Philadelphia, 1980.

Gray JE. Light fog on radiographic films—how to measure it properly. Radiology 115;225,1975.

Keats TE. An atlas of normal roentgen variants that may simulate disease. Year Book Medical Publishers, Chicago, 1975.

Lindstrom RR. Design of a shared radiology quality assurance program. Rad/NucMed June 1979, p51.

Olnick HM Weens HS and Rogers JV. Radiological diagnosis of retained surgial sponges. JAMA 159:1525, 1955.

Spiegel SM and Palayew MJ. Retained surgical sponges: Diagnostic dilemma and an aid to their recognition. RadioGraphics 2:53,1982.

Sweeney RJ. Radiographic artifacts: Their cause and control. J B Lippincot Company, Philadelphia, 1983.

Williams RG Bragg DG and Nelson JA. Gossipyboma the problem of the retained sponge. Radiology 129:323,1978.

11. TECHNIQUE CHARTS

A technique chart is a table with predetermined x-ray machine settings that enables the radiographer to select the correct machine settings based on the thickness of the tissue and the anatomical portion of the body that is to be radiographed. A correctly designed technique chart used in a correct manner regularly produces a diagnostic radiograph. It is obvious that you must enter the chart with the correct measurement of the part to be radiographed and you must accurately place the correct settings on the machine (Fig. 11-1).

Items that need to be standardized at the time of developing a technique chart include: (1) speed of x-ray film, (2) speed of intensifying screens, (3) focal-film distance, (4) amount of inherent and added filtration, (5) type and quality of developer solution, (6) temperature and time of film developing, (7) use of a grid, (8) type of grid, and (9) character of the incoming line voltage. Once these are established, the chart can be constructed. Since these factors are not changed frequently, the chart remains functional for a rather long period of time. If you should change any of the factors, such as deciding to utilize a different speed film, the technique chart requires modification. Certain factors such as: (1) focal spot size, (2) object-film distance, and (3) cassette size do not affect film quality and can be changed without having to make a change in exposure settings.

Because of basic differences between x-ray machines, it is not possible to use a technique chart developed for one x-ray machine on other machines without some modification. Separate technique charts must be used for determining exposures for screen or non-screen film technique and for determining exposures for tabletop (non-grid) technique and grid technique.

Unfortunately, the size and density of many of the anatomical regions examined in veterinary radiography vary widely in size, shape, and density. Thus, even if all of the other variables are standardized, it remains difficult to develop a technique chart that functions adequately for all studies. Therefore, it may be necessary to recognize that the technique chart provides the operator with a standard technique that may need to be altered because of unique features inherent in this patient. An understanding of some of these situations enables you to recognize them and make required changes to the recommended techniques prior to their use.

A series of general rules influence exposure factors and knowledge of these rules is required in the development of a technique chart (Table 11-1).

One category of problems causes the resulting radiographic density to be less than expected. This occurs if there is marked soft tissue swelling after trauma or due to obesity or in the presence of any type of casting or splinting material. It also occurs commonly in the presence of pleural fluid or abdominal fluid. Any of these situations increases the amount of tissue to be penetrated by the primary beam and it is necessary to compensate by increasing the kVp setting by 10 or double the mAs setting.

Another category of problem occurs in patients in which there is an unusual loss of tissue and radiographic density is greater than expected. This occurs when disuse osteopenia has occurred because of long-standing non-weightbearing disease or patients in which the bone density is not as great as expected or because of the young age of the patient. It is also found in the thoracic study of a cachetic patient. This loss of expected tissue can be compensated for by decreasing the kVp setting by 10 or by halving the mAs setting.

A flow chart for the development of a technique chart is provided (Table 11-2). There are recommendations for specific anatomical regions. Low contrast is required for the thorax and the chart should require high kVp (>90 kVp) and fast exposure time settings. A medium contrast is recommended for the abdomen and the chart should require medium kVp settings (80 to 100 kVp) and higher mAs settings. Higher contrast can be used for skeletal structures using lower kVp settings (<70 kVp) and higher mAs settings.

Reasons why techniques charts fail to provide the correct machine settings are summarized (Table 11-3).

REFERENCES

Ticer JW. Radiographic Technique in Practice, 2nd ed., WB Saunders, Philadelphia. 1984.

Watson JC. Considerations in Formulating X-Ray Exposure Factors. Vet Med 49:435, 1954.

Watters JW. Development of a Technique Chart for the Veterinarian. Compend on Cont Ed 2:568, 1980.

Technique Chart For Use With Grid

Grid ratio: _____

Lines per inch: _____

FFD: _____

cm Thickness	kVp Settings														
	1	2	3	4	5	6	7	8	9	10	11	12	13	14	15
11						60	62	64	66	68	70	72	74	76	78
12					60	62	64	66	68	70	72	74	76	78	80
13				60	62	64	66	68	70	72	74	76	78	80	83
14			60	62	64	66	68	70	72	74	76	78	80	83	86
15		60	62	64	66	68	70	72	74	76	78	80	83	86	89
16	60	62	64	66	68	70	72	74	76	78	80	83	86	89	92
17	62	64	66	68	70	72	74	76	78	80	83	86	89	92	95
18	64	66	68	70	72	74	76	78	80	83	86	89	92	95	98
19	66	68	70	72	74	76	78	80	83	86	89	92	95	98	
20	68	70	72	74	76	78	80	83	86	89	92	95	98		
21	70	72	74	76	78	80	83	86	89	92	95	98			
22	72	74	76	78	80	83	86	89	92	95	98				
23	74	76	78	80	83	86	89	92	95	98					
24	76	78	80	83	86	89	92	95	98						
25	78	80	83	86	89	92	95	98							
26	80	83	86	89	92	95	98								
27	83	86	89	92	95	98									
28	86	89	92	95	98										
29	89	92	95	98											
30	92	95	98												
	mAs	mAs	mAs	mAs	mAs	mAs	mAs	mAs	mAs	mAs	mAs	mAs	mAs	mAs	

Figure 11-1

TECHNIQUE CHART

Columns #1 to #12 provide different kVp settings for variations in cm thickness of the patient

Table 11-1
GENERAL RULES THAT INFLUENCE EXPOSURE FACTORS

1. Influence of mA
   a. film density is directly proportional to mA setting
   b. mA does not appreciable alter film contrast if the film density is correct

2. Influence of length of exposure time
   a. film density is directly proportional to exposure time
   b. length of exposure time does not appreciably alter film contrast if the film density is correct

3. mAs concept
   a. the product of mA and exposure time in seconds is commonly considered as a single factor
   b. milliamperage x exposure time in seconds equals milliampereseconds (mA x seconds = mAs)

4. Influence of focal-film distance (FFD)
   a. film density is inversely proportional to the focal-film distance squared
   b. change in focal-film distance results in a change in film density
   c. minimal change in focal-film distance does not appreciably alter film contrast if the film density is correct

5. Influence of kVp setting
   a. low kVp settings produces a film with high scale of contrast
   b. high kVp settings produce a film with low scale of contrast
   c. change in film density results with change in kVp setting

6. Relationship of patient thickness (cm) and kVp setting
   a. change in thickness of patient required a change in kVp setting
   b. for each additional cm thickness of patient, add 2 kVp (under 80 kVp)
   c. for each additional cm thickness of patient, add 3 kVp (in the 80-100 kVp range)
   d. for each additional cm thickness of patient, add 4 kVp (over 100 kVp)

7. A general relationship exists between mAs and kVp settings
   a. if you double the mAs setting and subtract 10 kVp, the film density remains essentially the same in the 70 to 90 kVp range
   b. if you halve the mAs setting and add 10 kVp, the film density remains essentially the same in the 70 to 90 kVp range
   c. if film density is dark, halve the mAs setting or subtract 10 kVp to correct the error
   d. if film density is light, double the mAs setting or add 10 kVp to correct the error

Table 11-2
FLOW CHART FOR DEVELOPMENT OF A TECHNIQUE CHART

A. Technique chart for studies of a dog over 11 cm in thickness requiring use of a grid

1. Selection of model dog
   a. Mature
   b. Moderate muscling
   c. Not obese
   d. Not thin
   e. Hair coat clean and not unduly heavy or long
2. X-ray machine
   a. Evaluate incoming line voltage (if not possible, be certain that there is no heavy voltage drain on the circuit)
   b. Set tube-film distance at 90 cm to 100 cm (36" to 40")—if unit 100 mA or higher
      OR Set tube-film distance at 60 cm to 75 cm (24" to 30")—if unit 30 mA or less
   c. Position beam filter (2 mm al. equivalent)
   d. Position collimation device commonly used
3. Cassette and film
   a. Select cassette with intensifying screens that represent the speed and age of other screen pairs (speed recommended is dependent on mA capability of x-ray machine)
   b. Select film that is not out of date or damaged (speed recommended is dependent on mA capability of x-ray machine)
4. Grid
   a. Position grid over cassette if exposure is to be on the tabletop
      OR Check position of grid if under table and used with a bucky tray or grid cabinet or holder
   b. Ensure grid is clean and without artifacts
5. Darkroom
   a. Manual wet tank processing
      1) Standardize developer solution temperature (preferably 20°C (68°F)
      2) Ensure solutions are of average strength (not contaminated or exhausted but not necessarily freshly mixed)
      3) Check timer clock for accuracy and establish developer time (preferably 5 minutes)
   b. Automatic processor
      1) Check developer replenisher rate with recommendations on unit
      2) Check solution temperature with recommendations on unit
6. First test exposures of abdomen of a dog measuring over 11 cm thickness
   a. Divide cassette by lead sheets or use collimator shutter position
   b. Position dog on side for lateral abdomen study
   c. Measure carefully the width of the portion of the abdomen to be radiographed—record this measurement
   d. Make three test exposures on one film of 70 kVp and 2.5, 5.0 and 10.0 mAs (use mAs as near as possible to these recommendations)
   e. Process film   —if underexposed, go to #7 below
                        —if overexposed, go to #8 below
                        —if one of the exposures is correct, go to #9 below
7. Subsequent test exposures if film is underexposed
   a. Make three test exposures of 70 kVp and 10, 20 and 40 mAs
      OR Make three test exposures of 80 kVp and 5, 10 and 20 mAs
   b. Process film—if underexposed, reevaluate speed of intensifying screens and film and consider a faster combination
      OR Re-evaluate the character of the grid and select one that permits use without as great an increase in exposure factors
      OR Decrease the focal-film distance
                        —if one of the exposures is correct, go to #9 below
8. Subsequent test exposures if film is overexposed
   a. Make three test exposures of 70 kVp and 0.6, 1.2 and 2.5 mAs
      OR Make three test exposures of 60 kVp and 1.2, 2.5 and 5.0 mAs
   b. Process film—if overexposed, re-evaluate speed of intensifying screens and film and consider a slower combination
      OR Re-evaluate the character of the grid and select one that permits use with a greater increase in exposure factors
      OR Increase the focal-film distance to 100 cm (40°)
                        —if one of the exposures is correct, go to #9 below

(Table 11-2 continues on next page)

81

9. Correct exposure (correct film density)
  a. Note the kVp and mAs of the best exposure
  b. Consider altering the exposure to achieve the best kVp and mAs combination for your machine using rules given in the previous discussion
    1) If a 100 mA maximum unit, try to use the shortest exposure time and highest mA settings possible for your machine
    2) If unit has capability of over 100 mA, try to use the additional latitude available in selection of kVp and mA ranges in which you can work
  c. Go to the technique chart on the following page
    1) Complete the chart in the upper right corner concerning the grid and focal-film distance used
    2) Find the cm thickness of the trial dog on the left side of the chart
    3) Move across the chart on that line until you reach the kVp value closest to the one used for the trial exposure
    4) Mark that column at the bottom of the chart "abdomen" and record the mAs value used. This is a constant mAs-variable kVp technique for the abdomen!
  d. Test exposures of other parts of the dog over 10 cm in thickness
    1) Repeat the procedure for the thorax, extremities, pelvis, vertebral column, and skull
    OR
    2) Use the following estimated values and complete the technique chart. Assume for the purposes of this example that column #9 is the column you have selected for the abdominal studies.
      a) Select the next higher column (#10) and this is the technique chart for "extremities"
      b) Select the column that is two columns higher (#11) and this is the technique chart for the "vertebral column" and the "skull"
      c) Select the column that is three columns higher (#12) and this is the technique chart for the "pelvis" and "hip joints"
      d) Select the column that is five columns lower (#4) and this is the technique chart for the "thorax"
      e) Remember that the mAs is the same for all columns

B. **Test exposures to establish a technique chart for parts of the dog that measure less than 11 cm thickness**
  1. Follow the same procedure as described above *except*
    a. Remove the grid from use
    b. Select a different dog that has an abdomen that measures 10 cm or less
  2. Evaluate the film used to establish the technique chart to be used with a grid to estimate the exposure range to be used to produce the test films for the chart to be used without a grid.
  3. Make a new technique chart for use without a grid by determining the correct columns for all anatomical parts. This chart is also appropriate for the anatomical parts of a larger dog that measure 10 cm or less

C. **Test exposures to establish a technique for cat**
  1. Follow the same procedure as described above *except*
    a. Remove the grid from use
    b. Select a cat that has an abdomen that measures less than 10 cm
  2. Evaluate the film used to establish the technique chart to be used without a grid to estimate the exposure range to be used to produce the test films for the chart for the cat.
  3. Make a new technique chart for the cat for use without a grid. Determine the correct columns for all anatomical parts. This chart is appropriate for all parts of the cat that measure 10 cm or less. In cats in which the area to be radiographed measures over 11 cm in thickness, use the dog chart.

D. **Test exposures for non-screen technique chart**
  1. Follow the same procedure as described above *except*
    a. Limit tissue thickness to 1cm to 5 cm
    b. Use an extremity such as the paw as a model exposure
  2. Make a new technique chart for extremities of 1 cm to 5 cm thickness, intra-oral studies, and avian studies. This chart is less exact than the others and requires more correction as you use the chart.

E. **Correct the technique charts to suit your individual desires and to permit you to obtain the most from your x-ray machine**
  1. Shift columns as you discover that a particular examination is consistently over- or underexposed
  2. Shift columns to lower kVp settings to permit you to utilize your machine to the best advantage. (Remember that adding 10 kVp to a technique and dividing the mAs in half produces a comparable radiograph.) If you shift columns to utilize a different kVp range be sure that you alter the mAs setting.

Table 11-3
TECHNIQUE CHART FAILURE

Under certain circumstances, technique charts fail to provide the machine settings that produce a radiograph of satisfactory film quality. Some conditions cause a decrease in tissue density or a decrease in the amount of fluid or fat present within a body cavity and a resulting overexposed radiograph. By recognizing some of this conditions prior to performing the study, it is possible to compensate by <u>decreasing the kVp setting by 5 to 10</u>.

1. focal destructive bone disease
2. generalized bone disease
3. emphysematous soft tissues
4. pneumothorax
5. air filled megaesophagus
6. massive pulmonary air trapping
7. aerophagia with dilated air filled stomach
8. gastric dilation/torsion syndrome
9. obstructive ileus with dilated air-filled small bowel
10. pneumocolon following enema
11. pneumocystogram
12. soft tissue atrophy or weight loss on a follow-up radiographic study
13. pneumoperitoneum

Some conditions cause an increase in tissue density or an increase in the amount of fluid present within a body cavity and a resulting underexposed radiograph. By recognizing some of this conditions prior to performing the study, it is possible to compensate by <u>increasing the kVp setting by 5 to 10</u>.

1. pleural effusion
2. pulmonary fluid
3. pneumoconiosis
4. pulmonary fibrosis in an older patient
5. bronchiectasis
6. post-surgical thoracic study
7. cardiomegaly
8. pericardial fluid
9. ascites
10. large abdominal mass
11. ingesta filled gastro-intestinal tract
12. soft tissue edema
13. soft tissue calcification
14. barium sulfate contrast study
15. positive contrast cystogram

12. RADIATION SAFETY

In the almost 100 years since the discovery of x-rays, considerable information has become available concerning the characterization and quantification of radiation and its interaction with matter. One thing learned is that ionizing radiation is an environmental or occupational hazard. More is probably known about the consequences of exposure to x-rays than from any of the other hazards faced by a population of people. Paradoxically, the increase in knowledge about the consequences of radiation exposure has increased its ranking as an issue of serious concern to society.

The owner of a veterinary practice, clinic, or hospital is responsible for radiation safety in that practice and is responsible for assuring that any radiation source under his or her control is used only by persons competent to use them. In addition, the owner is responsible for providing the instruction of personnel on safe operating procedures, for promulgating rules for radiation safety, and for designating the location and limits of areas to be used for x-ray examination. Levels of radiation to workers should be kept to as low a level as is practical and still obtain the diagnostic radiographs required. The recommendations for exposure level must consider the ALARA ("as low as reasonably achievable") concept which is based on the knowledge that there is no threshold dose for radiation injury, that is, all radiation exposure entails some degree of risk.

It is important that everyone understand that we live in a "field of radiation" throughout our lives. This is referred to as background radiation and varies throughout the country and the world. New calculations of this background radiation have been recently increased because of the inclusion of the effects of radon gas that is found within certain houses (Table 12-1). Currently this background exposure is estimated to be 360 millirem for an average person living in America. This is small compared with the federal safety standard for allowable occupational exposure, which is 5000 millirem per year. This information is contained in Ionization Radiation Exposure of the Population of the United States, NCRP Report No. 93 and can be purchased for $15 from the National Council on Radiation Protection and Measurements, 7910 Woodmont Ave., Suite 1016, Bethesda, Md 20814.

One of the most common methods of measuring x-radiation is to measure the charge the photons produce by ionizing air. The quantity that expresses the ionization produced by x-rays in a specific volume (e.g., 1cc) in air in known as the exposure. The unit for expressing this exposure is the roentgen. It is used for both x and gamma radiation in the energy range from a few KeV to a few MeV. The roentgen was originally defined as the amount of x-radiation that produces 1 electrostatic unit (esu) of either positive or negative charge that resulted from interactions in 1 cc of dry air at 0° C and 760 mm pressure. It is defined currently in equivalent units as 2.58×10^{-4} coulombs/kg of air. This amount of radiation imparts an amount of energy equal to 5.4×10^{7} meV per gram of air, or 0.87 rad (radiation absorbed dose). A roentgen of x-radiation in the energy levels used in diagnostic radiology also produces 0.96 rad in tissue. Thus, for most purposes, it can be seen that values of exposures in roentgens can be considered essentially numerically equal to absorbed doses in rads and to tissue irradiated to dose equivalents in rem (radiation equivalent mammal).

A Rad or Radiation Absorbed Dose is a unit of absorbed dose for any ionizing radiation having energy transferred to the irradiated material. The energy transfer is equal to 100 ergs/gram of material. One Roentgen is equal to 0.93-0.98 Rad. The new unit of absorbed dose is the Gray (Gy) in which 100 rads equal I Gy or 1 rad equals 1 cGy. Rem (Roentgen equivalent in man or mammals) is a measurement of radiation of any type which produces the same biological effects in man as would result from absorption of 1 rad of x or gamma radiation. The new unit of dose equivalence in the Sievert (Sv) in which 100 rem = 1 Sv.

Radiation injures tissues by the ionization of vital molecules within the cell and may be referred to as somatic injury that is related to both physical and chemical injury caused by the radiation. The biological effects are determined by the rate of delivery of the radiation, the area of the body exposed, the sensitivity of the individual and the variation of sensitivity of body cells.

The time interval in which the radiation is received is very important in determining its affect. A total of 650 rads administered at one time to the whole body of a person would be expected to cause a death rate of 50% of the individuals receiving that radiation dosage even though receiving best medial care. This is called the LD50 (lethal dose to 50%). Yet, the same 650 rads administered in smaller dosages of 1 rad per month over a period of 50 years would not result in a detectable injury to the people. This difference in response to the same total dose recognizes the ability of the body to repair tissues injured by the radiation. It is this feature that permits those who work in the radiation field to receive low levels of radiation each month and not show any untoward results from this low-level radiation.

Table 12-1
SOURCES OF BACKGROUND RADIATION EXPOSURE PER YEAR FOR PERSONS LIVING IN AMERICA

Source	Millirem
Radon gas	200
Cosmic radiation	27
Rocks and soil	18
From inside human body (K_{40})	40
Medical x-rays	39
Nuclear medicine	14
Consumer products	10
Other	< 3
Total:	360

Source: National Council on Radiation Protection and Measurements.

The amount of the body exposed to the radiation beam is another factor strongly influencing radiation effects. In the use of ionizing radiation for the treatment of tumors, a local tumor site might receive a total of 6000 rads. This total dosage might be administered in fractions three times each week for a four week period using a depth dose of 500 rads for each fraction. This high level of exposure can be administered to a small portion of the body, whereas the same exposure to the entire body would most certainly result in the death of the animal.

Certain cells within the body are more radiosensitive with the sensitivity increased in tissue characterized by rapid cell division and lack of differention. Thus, the lymphocyte, immature white and red blood cells, and all immature germ cells are highly sensitive to radiation injury. The cells lining the gastrointestinal tract have a turnover time of 36-48 hours making them particularly sensitive to radiation. The hematopoietic tissue shows signs of radiation injury, such as leukopenia or anemia, that occurs between 10-15 days after whole-body exposure, with the appearance of the radiation effect determined by the half-life of the cells. The thyroid gland is particularly sensitive to radiation effects. The lens of the eye has also been shown to be susceptible to injury to irradiation, but it takes many years for the resulting cataracts to be identified. Extremities can withstand much higher doses of radiation than the blood-forming organs because of the decreased sensitivity of epithelial, muscle and nerve tissue. The use of lead gloves or mittens is still important because of the greater opportunity for exposure to the hands.

Radiation injuries may be acute and be noted within days following whole-body irradiation, or may be chronic and take years for the effects to be demonstrated. Also, the effects may be short term such as erythema to the skin, or long term such as injury to the lens of the eye. The acute radiation syndrome is relatively easy to describe and consists of a prodromal period, a latent period, and manifest illness. The illness is characterized by epilation, hemorrhage, fever, infection, diarrhea, cardiovascular collapse, and a central nervous syndrome. These manifestations are determined by the level of whole body exposure. With exposure of 100 to 600 rads a hematopoietic form occurs, with exposure over 600 rads a gastrointestinal form occurs, and with exposure over 10,000 rads an always fatal central nervous system form occurs. Various acute radiation effects have been recorded (Table 12-2). The lethal dose from whole body radiation to 50% of the population in 30 days ($LD_{50}/30$) for various species is recorded (Table 12-3).

Since we all live within a radiation field, referred to as background radiation, and certain members of society work in areas in which the level of exposure are increased, it is appropriate that a concept of permissible exposure be developed. The limits of greatest concern to those working with diagnostic radiology relate to whole-body dose which means exposure to any major portion of the whole body, head and trunk, gonads, lens of the eye, active blood-forming organs, or the whole body. Inclusion of the lens of the eye means that any personnel monitoring device need be worn on the outside of a lead apron and near the neck to more accurately measure exposure to the eye. An occupationally exposed individual over 18 years of age may receive at this time, on the average, a maximum whole-body dose equivalent of 5 rems per year (MPD—maximum permissible dose). In addition, there is a provision which permits an occupationally exposed individual over 18 years of age to receive 3 rems per calender quarter but remain within the 5 rems per year limit. The maximum possible long-term accumulated dose equivalent can be calculated on the basis of 5 rems per year starting with age 18; that is, the maximum accumulated whole-body dose equivalent is equal to 5(N-18), where N is the age in years. An individual 58 years of age could have accumulated 200

Table 12-2
ACUTE EFFECTS OF WHOLE BODY IRRADIATION
MEASURED IN REM (RAD EQUIVALENT IN MAN OR MAMMAL)

REM	Effecty
5-20	possible late effect; possible chromosomal aberration
20-100	temporary reduction in leukocyte count
100-200	"mild radiation sickness" with vomiting and diarrhea,
200-300	"serious radiation sickness" with bone marrow syndrome and hemorrhage $LD_{10-35}/30$ *
300-400	"serious radiation sickness" with the addition of intestinal mucosa injury $LD_{50-70}/30$
400-1,000	acute illness $LD_{60-95}/30$
1,000-5,000	acute illness $LD_{100}/10$
>5,000	acute illness with central nervous syndrome $LD_{100}/2$
ALSO	
>50	temporary sterility in men
>300	permanent sterility in women

*($LD_{10-35}/30$ = lethal dose within 10 to 35 percent of the population within 30 days) (Goldman, 1982)

Table 12-3
LETHAL DOSE IN REM FOR WHOLE BODY RADIATION FOR VARIOUS SPECIES (LD$_{50/30}$)

Species	REM
Sheep	155
Swine	195
Goat	230
Guinea pig	255
Dog	265
Human	400
Monkey	400
Rat	900
Gerbil	1059
Desert mouse	1520

rems (58-18 x 5 = 200) and remain within what is assumed to be a safe level of radiation exposure.

It is interesting to note that this maximum permissible dose of 5 rem per year has only been a standard since 1958. In 1931 the standard was 50 rem per year, lowered in 1936 to 30 rem per year, lowered in 1948 to 15 rem per year, and finally lowered in 1958 to 5 rem per year.

There are specific dosages for certain parts of the body for radiation workers. The maximum permissible dosage per year for the hands is 75 rem (25 rem per quarter) and 30 rem annually for the forearm (10 rem per quarter).

The levels of radiation commonly encountered in performing radiographic examination on animals are not of a level to consider potential genetic injury. The use of lead aprons effectively shield the gonads of both men and women. It is important to recognize that the whole body exposure required to cause abortion of a human fetus is an exposure that would cause the death of the fetus and would also cause serious injury or death to the mother. The frequency of spontaneous fetal abnormality can be due, in part, to a variety of toxic environmental causes, thus, it is not possible to recognize when a particular fetal abnormality is the result of radiation or if that radiation was produced by an x-ray tube.

Basic rules can be used to decrease your exposure to radiation in the course of a radiographic examination. First, remember that the radiation exposure to an operator of an x-ray machine may result from the following components: (1) the useful beam consisting of photons coming directly from the target through the collimating devices and interacting with the patient's body, (2) scattered radiation originating primarily in the body of the patient, and (3) leakage radiation which penetrates the x-ray tube housing and collimator and is not part of the useful beam. It is important to remember all three types of radiation when thinking of radiation protection.

The first rule is radiation safety is to limit the time of exposure. This can be done by insuring that only the necessary number of exposures are made and that repeat views are not required because of technical errors. The

elimination of repeat views is one of the best ways to decrease your exposure to radiation and is often affected by how you approach the patient to be examined (Figure 12-1). This limitation of exposure also might be achieved through acquisition of faster film-screen systems that require less radiation but still produce diagnostic radiographic studies. Adoption of higher degrees of filtration of the useful beam and use of higher tube voltages make it possible to reduce the surface dose to the patient, and incidentally, the scattered dose to the radiological workers (Binks, 1955).

The second method of decreasing radiation exposure is by increasing the distance between you and the source of radiation (Fig. 12-2). The examination of sedated patients permits you to step further away from the primary beam.

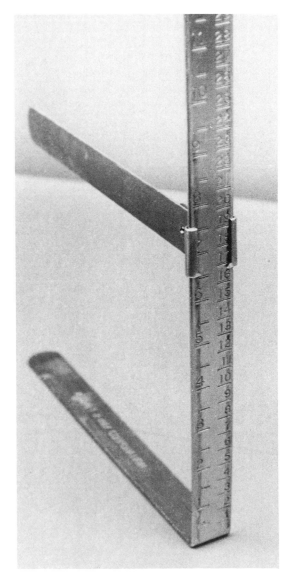

Fig. 12-1
CALIPERS
By correctly measuring the patient prior to the radiographic examination you can select the correct technique from the technique chart and avoid many repeat studies. This is one of the most important methods available to reduce radiation exposure to both patient and technician.

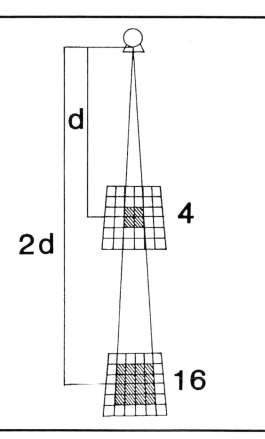

Fig. 12-2
INVERSE SQUARE LAW
By doubling the distance from the x-ray tube (d to 2d) the photon field must cover an area 4 times as large (4 to 16). This means that if you can double the distance from a radiation source, the exposure level you receive is only 1/4 as much.

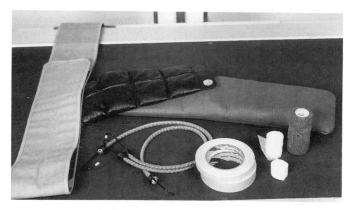

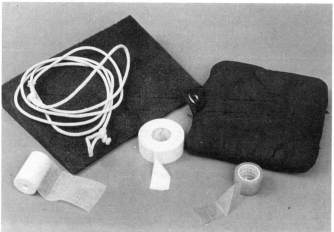

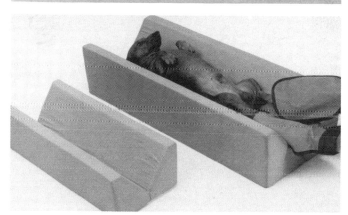

Fig. 12-3
POSITIONING AND RESTRAINING DEVICES
Gauze, tape, and rope are commonly used restraining devices while foam wedges and sandbags are used in positioning. (Foam positioning devices courtesy of Radiation Concepts Inc. Ft. Lauderdale FL 33314)

Other patients can be positioned through use of tape, ropes, gauze, sandbags, or foam wedges or devices (Fig. 12-3). The use of a film or cassette holders moves you a greater distance from the primary beam and secondary radiation (Figs. 12-4). Collimation of the x-ray beam controls the size of the radiation field and also lets you be positioned a greater distance from the field of the primary beam (Fig. 12-5). Much of the source of radiation is from scatter radiation that originates from the patient and table. A gap of 3-4 feet (1 meter) between the unit and a wall decreases the exposure by scatter radiation to an assistant in the room. The dose to the wall is unchanged, but the radiation that scatters back and reaches the person is greatly decreased.

Direct body shielding is the third and most important method of decreasing your exposure to the ionizing radiation. This shielding is accomplished through the use of lead gloves, lead aprons, and lead shields behind which you can stand (Figs. 12-6, 12-7). Lead aprons, when worn correctly, protect the major blood-forming organs within the body. These aprons must be treated carefully to avoid damage to the lead shielding (Fig. 12-8). The addition of a 0.5 mm lead equivalent collar to the apron shields the

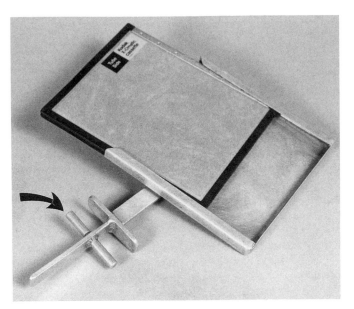

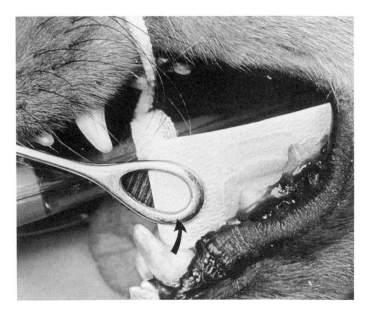

Fig. 12-4
CASSETTE HOLDERS
A hand-held cassette holder with a "grip" (arrow) that insures that it can be positioned without motion during the exposure. Use of film holders such as the forceps (arrow) increases the distance of the assistant from the primary x-ray beam.

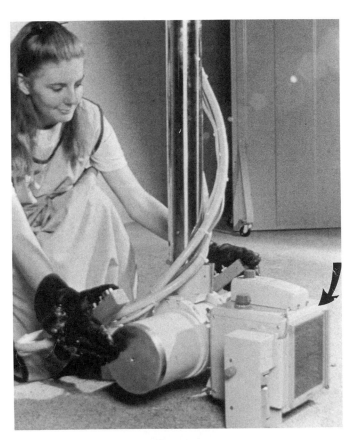

Fig. 12-5
COLLIMATOR
Use of a beam limiting device (arrow) is one of the most important radiation protection devices that can be used in diagnostic radiology.

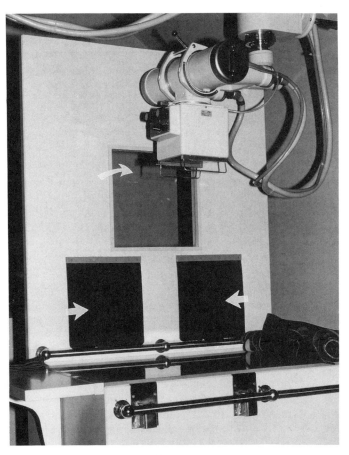

Fig. 12-6
RADIATION SHIELD
Two lead covered openings for hands (straight arrows) and the single leaded glass opening through which to watch the positioning of the patient (curved arrow) are seen. Combined with the use of lead gloves, this makes small animal radiography much safer from radiation exposure.

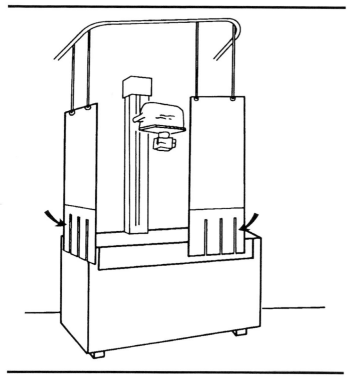

Fig. 12-7
RADIATION SHIELD
Drawing showing lead impregnated acrylic shielding that has been ceiling mounted on a track that permits movement as needed. Fenestrated lead shielding has been attached to the bottom of the shields (arrows).

thyroid gland. Lead glasses with a 0.35 mm lead-equivalent protection can be worn to protect the lens of the eye. Usually, regular prescription glasses have a lead content (Fig. 12-9). Lead aprons and gloves are usually sold as containing 0.5 mm lead equivalent. Both should be tried on prior to purchase to insure that they are comfortable and that you can still assist in immobilization of the patient when wearing the gloves.

It is recommended that aprons and gloves be physically examined or radiographed periodically to determine the character of the lead lining (Fig. 12-10). These protective devices can be evaluated for defects by placing them on a large cassette and making a routine radiographic exposure. If you detect any breaks in the aprons or gloves, they should be replaced. Use a 90 kVp exposure at 50 mAs to 250 mAs at a 40 inch (100cm) focal-film distance. Gloves and aprons are made to shield a person from scatter radiation and should not be placed within the more energetic primary beam (Figs. 12-11, 12-12). The exposure within the scattered beam for which the aprons and gloves provides protection, ranges between 0.1 mr to 0.4 mr/exposure.

Up to the present time, protection of personnel from radiation has been difficult because of the inability of seeing through most shielding materials. Now, transparent, lead-plastic viewing panels offer a simple, cost-effective way to achieve protection to workers. The shielding material is a lead-impregnated plastic that is transparent, lightweight,

shatter-resistant, and easy to handle. It can be suspended by chains from a ceiling-mounted track (Fig. 12-7), can be built into a movable shield on wheels, or can be built into a permanent radiation shield. The panels are available in a choice of sizes and usually have a 0.5 mm lead equivalency but may have increased protection with a 0.82 mm lead equivalency.

Another important radiation safety practice is to remove as many people as possible from the examination area. This number can often be decreased through the use of sedating or anesthetizing the patient. Those not directly involved in restraint of the patient, should be removed from the radiation area. Everyone who cannot be removed from the examination room should be positioned at as great a distance from the source of the radiation as is practical. Use of restraining devices and cassette holders permits you to reposition people away from the area of the primary beam. This rule includes the complete removal from the examination area of all pregnant women, women unsure of the status of possible pregnancy, and individuals under the age of 18 years. They should not receive any level of radiation. Basic radiation safety rules should be understood by all who work with the diagnostic radiographic equipment under your control (Table 12-4).

New fiber and foam extrusion technology has presented an alternative material in the form of carbon conjugate that provides significant reduction in radiation dose to the patient while maintaining high resolution images. Only recently is carbon available in a form sufficiently stable to support body weight required for a tabletop or to form the front for a cassette. By using carbon conjugate in tabletops and cassette fronts, mA requirements are reduced and the radiation exposure to the patient can be reduced almost 30%. Obviously, there are savings in anode erosion, bearing failure, and filament evaporation resulting from the reduction in heat. (Budin, 1980)

Another method of reducing radiation exposure to the patient is to consider the relationship between kVp settings and the mR received by the patient. Comparable exposure settings producing similar film density using screen techniques show that the radiation exposure to the patient can be halved by using high kVp techniques. The dose required to produce unit density on the film using intensifying screens at 50 kVp is 300 mR on the surface of the patient while 100 kVp produces a surface dose on the phantom of 80 mR. This affect is not noted as prominently in the use of non-screen techniques (Table 12-5). Radiation intensity is also dependent on beam filtration and character of the anode.

There are certain publications that are important to the Veterinarian in the determination of what is required in a practice relative to radiation safety. These include NCRP Report No. 33. Medical X-ray and Gamma-Ray Protection for Energies up to 10 MeV -Equipment Design and Use (1968) and NCRP Report No. 36. Radiation Protection in Veterinary Medicine (1970).

Recent studies have shown a low radiation exposure to veterinary clinicians. The results determined from radiation detection devices distributed to a randomly selected sample

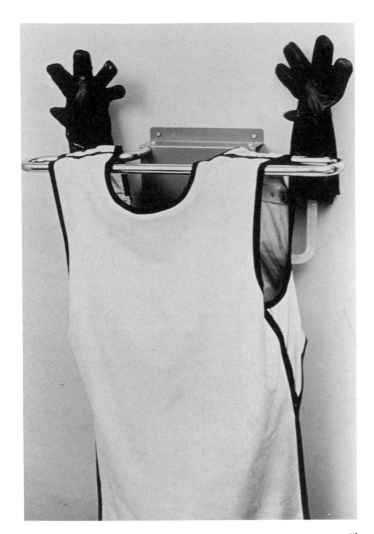
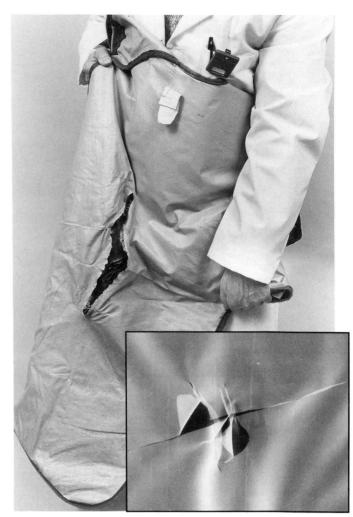

Fig. 12-8
LEAD APRON
Lead aprons should be carefully hung on racks to avoid leaving them folded for long periods of time resulting in cracking of the covering and the lead shielding.

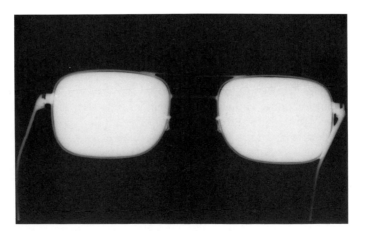

Fig. 12-9
SAFETY GLASSES
A radiograph of glasses show the absorption of the primary beam
by the lens in prescription glasses at 90 kVp and 10 mAs.

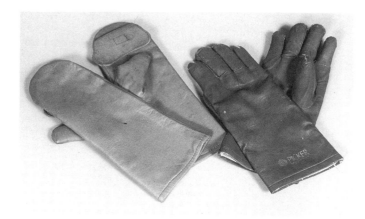

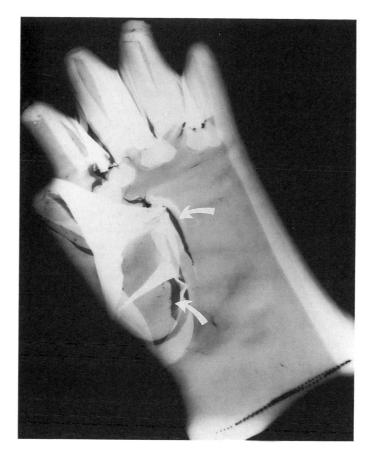

Fig. 12-10
LEAD GLOVES
The external appearance of the lead gloves or mittens may not indicate the character of the lead shielding. A radiograph of a lead glove demonstrates severe damage to the lead lining (arrows).

Table 12-4
BASIC RADIATION SAFETY RULES FOR DIAGNOSTIC RADIOGRAPHY

1. Remove personnel from the examination area who are not involved in the procedure.

2. Never permit anyone under the age of 18 in the examination area during the procedure.

3. Never permit pregnant women in the examination area during the procedure.

4. Rotate personnel who assist with the radiographic examination.

5. Use patient tranquilization whenever possible.

6. Never permit any part of the body to be within the primary beam.

7. Always wear lead aprons when assisting in the examination.

8. Always wear lead gloves when holding a cassette.

9. Use beam collimation to limit the size of the primary beam.

10. Never position your feet within the primary beam when holding a cassette.

11. Use the fastest film-screen system compatible with obtaining diagnostic radiographs.

12. Use full strength developer and proper solution temperatures to insure that the processing procedures allow for the use of minimum exposures.

13. Always wear film badges.

14. Always plan your radiographic procedure carefully to avoid unnecessary retakes.

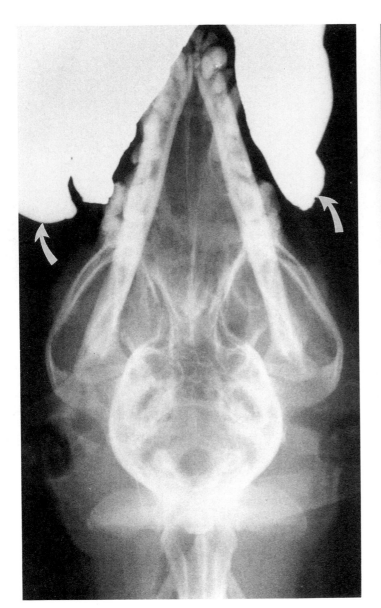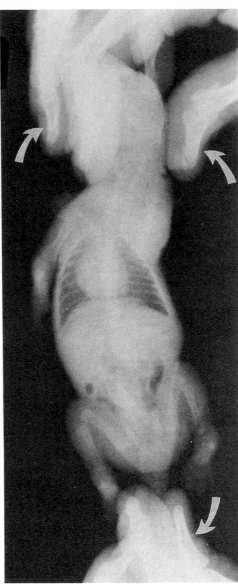

Fig. 12-11
RADIATION SAFETY
The practice of hand holding patients even with a gloved hand can not be considered an acceptable procedure. The appearance of these radiographs offers rather incriminating evidence.

Table 12-5
COMPARATIVE EXPOSURES

Exposure required to produce film density = 1.0 using par speed film-screen system and calcium tungstate screens using a 16 cm phantom varying kVp settings and the resultant change in mR received by the patient

kVp	mAs	mR
40	40	5.9
60	8	
80	3	4.0
100	1	3.3
120	0.8	
140	0.5	2.8

(Mattsson, 1955)

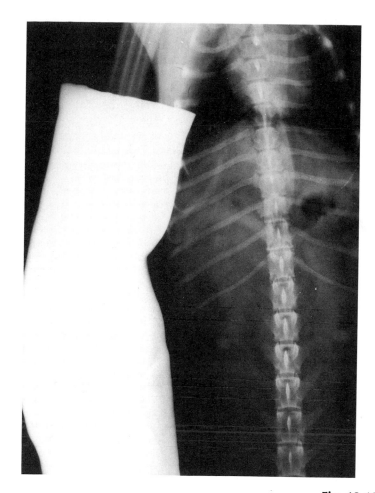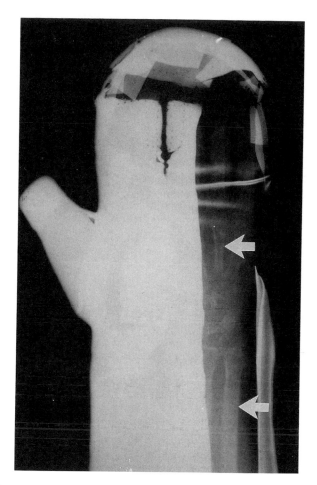

Fig. 12-12
RADIATION SAFETY
It is unsafe to have a lead glove within the primary x-ray beam as seen on this abdominal radiograph of a dog. The second radiograph is made with one-half of the glove cut-away showing that while the glove may be thought to shield the arm from the primary beam, this is not the situation. Notice the bones in the forearm (arrows).

of 118 women veterinarians showed that only 14.4% had documented exposures >15 mrem/month during the monitoring period measured under a lead apron. The maximally recorded whole-body dose for one veterinarian was 44.2 mrem/quarter-year which was well below the maximal permissible doses of 1250 mrem/quarter-year (Moritz et al, 1989).

Personnel monitoring detectors are used in long-term monitoring of low levels of radiation such as would be expected in a veterinary clinic. It is more important to know the total dose accumulated over an extended period, say a month. It is understood that if you are to make a radiographic examination, there is the probability that you may receive a small amount of radiation exposure. If you practice good safety procedures, this level of exposure does not cause injury that is detectable. Because of the "invisible" nature of x-rays, it is required that some form of detector be used to evaluate the radiation safety procedures that you are using. There are several different types of detectors which are suitable for personnel and environmental monitoring.

The most widely used personnel monitor for both x-

and gamma radiation and charged particles is the <u>nuclear emulsion monitor</u>. It consists of a piece of film that is inserted in a special plastic holder which can be clipped to your clothes, and is more commonly known as a <u>film badge</u>. (Fig. 12-13). The effect of radiation exposure appears as a darkening of the developed film. The amount of darkening is read with a densitometer and is proportional to the absorbed dose to the film. It provides a reasonably accurate means of determining x-ray exposure during radiographic examinations and also can detect beta and gamma irradiation. The badge also contains a variety of filters that selectively absorb radiation of varying energies so that both the amount and energy of the radiation can be estimated. The films are developed on a periodic basis and evaluated by measuring the density of the blackening on the film. The same film may be worn for a week, or more commonly a month. The length of time between evaluations depends on the amount of radiation to which the worker is probably exposed. The density on the film is compared to standard films that have been exposed to known radiation doses. Generally, film badges are capable of measuring doses from

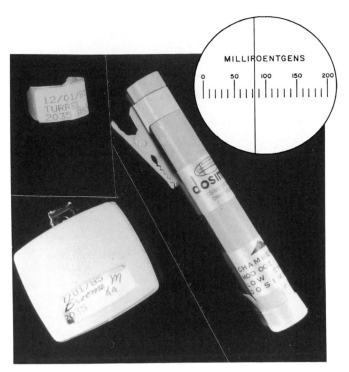

Fig. 12-13
RADIATION DETECTION DEVICES
A photograph shows a film badge, a ring badge, and a pocket ionization chamber. The chamber provides immediate information of the level of radiation received. The level of radiation must be written in a log book for permanent recording. The film badge and ring badge are sent to a service that processes the films and returns a permanent record. A drawing shows the quartz fiber hairline on the scale of the self-reading dosimeter.

10 mR to 500 mR. All exposures noted on monitoring devices are carefully recorded.

The film badge is usually worn on the pocket, lapel, or collar on the outside of the lead apron. This seems inappropriate on first thought, however, the lens of the eye and the thyroid gland may not be protected from x-radiation by the lead apron, and it is the exposure to those organs that becomes the critical exposure. It should be understood that the exposure to your body that is beneath the lead apron is much less than the reading on the film badge.

Because of the potential exposure to the hands, it may be advisable to wear a monitoring badge in the form of a ring (Fig. 12-13) as a detection devise. This ring is worn within the lead gloves and determines the exposure to the skin of the hands. These are not used as often as indicated in radiography of horses with the wide-spread practice of hand-held cassettes. The use of film badges is available for a small cost and serves as an indicator of the type of radiation safety program practiced within your practice. The cost of the film badges depends on the number of film packets per shipment and ranges from $10.00 to less than $5.00 per film. One current price is $108.00 per dozen film packets.

A second form of personnel monitor is a thermoluminescent (TLD) dosimeter. These TLD detectors are well suited to general personnel and environmental monitoring of x and gamma radiation. The principle of operation is that energy absorbed from the radiation raises the molecules of the detector material to metastable states. They remain in these excited states until they are heated to a temperature high enough to cause the material to return to its normal state with the emission of light. The amount of light emitted is proportional to the energy absorbed, hence it is proportional also to the dose to the detector. The emitted light is measured with a photomultiplier tube. A TLD material used in personnel dosimetry is lithium fluoride.

An immediate, direct reading, method of determining radiation exposure is through the use of a pocket ion chamber (Fig. 12-13). The chamber consists of a small capacitor, charged prior to use, and connected to a glass fiber electroscope. The unit is mounted in a pen-type housing which can be clipped into the pocket of a shirt or laboratory coat. Exposure of the chamber to ionizing radiation results in loss of charge proportional to the amount of exposure and a corresponding deflection of the fiber. The deflection can be viewed directly by means of a lens and a scale built into the instrument. The disadvantage of these chambers is that while they are convenient to use and are fairly accurate, they must be handled carefully. If they are exposed to excessive moisture, leakage across the insulator results and causes deflection of the fiber and resulting erroneous readings. Rough handling also produces spurious results. Another serious disadvantage is the absence of a permanent record of exposure as is available if using the film badges.

A summary of the personnel monitoring detectors is provided (Table 12-6).
See REFERENCES on page 96.

Table 12-6
PERSONNEL-MONITORING DETECTORS*

Detector	Radiation Detected	Range	Minimum Energy Detected	Advantages	Possible Disadvantages
Film	gamma beta thermal neutron fast neutron	0.001 to 10,000 rem	20 kev for gamma rays, 200 kev for beta rays	1. Inexpensive 2. Gives estimate of integrated dose. 3. Provides permanent record.	1. A moderate directional dependence. 2. Strong energy dependence for low-energy x-rays. 3. False readings produced by heat, pressure, and certain vapors. 4. Information not immediately available.
Pocket Ionization Chambers	gamma beta minus gamma thermal neutron fast neutron minus gamma x-rays	0.001 to 2000 R	30 kev for gamma rays, 20 kev for fast neutron	1. Yield fairly accurate information. 2. Small size. 3. Information available immediately. 4. Reasonably uniform in response to radiation in the energy range of 50 kev to 2 mev. 5. Require little maintenance 6. Reusable.	1. There is no permanent record. 2. Frequent reading, tabulation, and recharging may be required. 3. Subject to accidental discharge through shock and sometimes, electrical leakage). 4. Range of measurement is limited: full scale ranges from 0.2 to 2000 R available. 5. Economical only for long-term use.
TLD	gamma beta thermal neutron fast neutron x-rays	5 to 10^5 Rad	20 kev	1. Indefinite shelf life within the useful range. 2. Small size. 3. Small energy dependence 4. Reusable 5. Inexpensive 6. Give estimate of integrated dose over long periods.	1. Limited TLD systems supplied as commercial service. 2. Cancellation of dose upon reading. 3. Dose range depends on the sensitivity of the reader. 4. Radiations detected depend on type of TL material.

*Modified from CRC "Handbook of Radioactive Nuclides" Part III, Nuclear Instrumentation

REFERENCES

Binks W. Some aspects of radiation hygiene. Brit J Rad 28:654, 1955.

Budin E. Radiation dose reduction with carbon material for tabletops and cassettes. Diag Rad p 46. Feb 1980.

Goldman M. Ionization radiation and its risks. West J Med 137:540-547, 1982.

Moritz SA Hueston WD and Wilkins, JR. Patterns of ionizing radiation exposure among women veterinarians. J Am Vet Med Assoc 195:737-39. 1989.

Osborn SB. Radiation doses received by diagnostic x-ray workers. Brit J Rad 28:650,1955.

Rendano VT Ryan G and Bassano. Radiation Safety—Transparent leaded-plastic panels: A product evaluation, J Am An Hosp Assoc 23:141-4 1987.

Rendano VT and Ryan G. Technical assistance in Radiology Part 11. Basic consideration and radiation safety. Comp Contin Ed 9:547-51,1988.

Van Hise JR. Lead-impregnated acrylic shielding for a diagnostic x-ray unit. J Am Vet Med Assoc 184:95-6,1984.

Watters JW. Radiation protection in veterinary hospitals. Comp Contin Ed 1:455-8,1979.

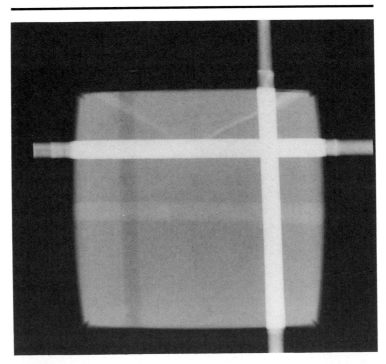

A radiograph was made of a large paper milk carton one-half filled with water. Small holes were made in the sides of the carton near the top that would just accept paper straws. Three paper straws were placed from the top to the bottom of the radiograph and three additional paper straws were placed from side to side. Two straws are filled with iodinated contrast agent, two are filled with water, and two are empty. Why are you unable to identify one straw filled with water and one straw that was empty?

13. ECONOMICS OF VETERINARY RADIOGRAPHY

An understanding of the separate costs of radiographing patients is necessary to determine the appropriate cost to recover from the owner for performing an examination. It is obvious that any discussion of costs may include figures that are quickly outdated. Many of the replacement costs listed represent national averages and vary, depending on the supplier and region of the country. Personnel and building costs differ greatly with the locality and your particular situation. If you are making all of your examinations in-the-field with a portable unit, you obviously have lower building and equipment costs. However, the number of re-take examinations is probably much higher than the in-house operation using an automatic film processor.

The cost analysis is based on the cost of a radiographic examination instead of the cost per single film. The major costs for radiographing a patient are involved in the cost of the equipment and in paying the personnel used to immobilize the patient and position it on the examination table. These costs should not be broken down into costs per single film but should be costs per examination. Most clinicians do not charge per suture to close an incision, why should radiology charges be made on the basis of each film. The cost of the film is the smallest portion of the cost of radiography.

The prices listed represent the cost based on purchase of new items (Table 13-1). These costs can be appreciably lowered by searching for used equipment, however, it may be difficult to obtain a guarantee relative to the operation of this used equipment. Remember that the cost of used equipment might be lower, but you must also consider the cost of delivery and installation. Bear in mind that radiographic equipment is physically large and may have specific electrical requirements if it is a stationary or ceiling-suspended unit. An individual who is mechanically and electrically inclined and likes bargain hunting may cut the investment cost of new equipment by 50%.

The purpose of this section is not so much to tell you the exact cost of each item, but has greater value in reminding you of the comparative role that each of the separate items plays in determining the total cost of operating a radiographic diagnostic service. The cost of the equipment depreciates over a period of time representing the estimated life span. Costs for each examination are based on a 10 to 15-minute examination with the assumption that the practice provides two people for examinations. A "professional fee" for the examination of the radiographs is not included.

Study of the figures shows how the cost of the radiographic film and personnel incurred in repeated views influences the total cost of the study. The cost of repeat studies because of errors in technique adds an appreciable cost to your practice. You should try to correct this loss. Random sampling of unsatisfactory radiographs suggests that 10% of the films are underexposed, 40% are overexposed, 22% are improperly positioned, 14% have motion artifacts, and 14% have film fogging of some type.

While a film-counting system that evaluates unsatisfactory films is not difficult to maintain, it probably is unnecessary. Assume a "retake" level at 10% to 25%, which is probably an accurate figure for most clinics, and an examination rate of 10 examinations per day. This means that you are repeating approximately 2 to 5 films/day which totals between $1200.00 to $3000.00 worth of film per year. If you include the cost of the equipment and personnel to perform the retakes, the total cost to your practice is probably $2400.00 to $6000.00 per year.

It is possible to decrease the cost of radiography by taking advantage of some commercial offers. Converting to rare-earth imaging systems can be done with the screens made available on a leasing program that includes installation of the screens or the loan of cassettes with screens. There is usually an associated obligation to purchase film from the company.

REFERENCES

Griffiths A O. Methods for Setting Fees for Services. Vet Econ 30:1982.

Wilson J F. Establishing a Realistic Fee Schedule. Compend on Cont Ed 5:262-70, 1983.

Table 13-1
RADIOGRAPHIC LABORATORY COST ESTIMATES

1. Equipment costs	
X-ray machine	
Portable	$4000-6500
Stationary	>$12000
Ceiling-Mounted	>$18000
Film processor	$4500 to $24000
Cassettes and screens (10)	$1200 to $1500
Aprons and gloves	$200 to $500
Grid	$300 to $1200
Positioning devices	$250
Film markers	$50
2. Darkroom equipment costs	
Film storage cabinet	$175
Imprinter	$200
View boxes	$500
3. Cost of space in building (per mo.)	variable
4. Fixed operation costs (per mo.)	
Utilities	$100
Building maintenance	variable
Processor maintenance	$40
Chemicals	$20
Equipment maintenance	variable
Film badge service ($12/person/mo.)	$12 to $48
5. Cost of labor per examination	
Radiology technician	$5
Assistant(s)	$0 to $10
6. Cost of film per examination	$10
7. Cost of Veterinary services	not included

14. RADIOGRAPHS AS A PART OF THE MEDICAL RECORD

The veterinary profession has always been vulnerable to malpractice actions because of the incomplete nature of its medical records. The absence of adequate records in such actions almost ensures an unfavorable outcome for a veterinarian because he has no convincing way to substantiate service provided. This occurs even though the service rendered may have been satisfactory. By definition, the medical record includes all information which a veterinarian might compile about a client's animal. It is a compilation of the pertinent facts of a patient's illness including history, clinical and laboratory findings, and treatment. These records serve as evidence of the ability of the veterinarian to promptly and accurately record basic information concerning the patient. It is important to recognize that radiographs and radiographic reports are also a part of the medical record and that the legal rulings concerning medical records apply to them as well. A part of record-keeping is the use of a systematic method of filing so that retrieval is convenient (Rumore et al, 1981). In the case of McCarry v. Merceir County, the courts determined: "Radiographs are part of the history of the case, like notes made by the physician, and are therefore a part of the medical file on the patient. They represent a professional service involving skill and judgment like anything else the physician does. They have extraordinary value to the physician. They are meaningless to most lay persons and are useful only when associated with other factors in the case and when expertly interpreted" (Hannah, 1991). Although this case dealt with a human patient the reasons behind the ruling apply equally to radiographs of animals. Some states have legal requirement as to the exact period of time that radiographs should be maintained, regardless of this requirement, it is a good practice to keep radiographs as long as other medical records are kept. Much has been written about the admissibility of veterinary medical records in court and there seems to be no difference between veterinary medical records and other medical records. Computerized veterinary medical records are admissible in courts of law provided that certain standards are met. It is the position of the AVMA Professional Liability Insurance Trust that "all original radiographs should remain in the custody of the animal hospital that took them because they provide a basis for a diagnosis and for the treatment rendered. In the event of a malpractice claim, the radiographs could be extremely valuable in building a strong defense. If they are given to the owner and subsequently lost, the defense of a case may also have been lost" (Professional Liability, 1992).

The owner has a right to know what is contained in these records and has the right to an abstract or explanation of the medical record. Ownership of radiographs in a veterinary practice in California was the subject of an opinion No. CV 74/168IL dated September 27, 1974 by the Attorney General of the State of California. That opinion stated that "it is our conclusion that, absent an agreement to the contrary, a veterinarian who takes x-ray films of an animal owns them,...". However, the opinion further stated that "the veterinarian may be under a moral or ethical duty to give these films or copies thereof to another veterinarian if the animal's owner so desires."

Requests to review radiographs may arise from people other than the owner of the animal who ordered the radiographic examination. This is a particular problem in confidentiality in a veterinary practice in which you have a request from a new owner or another veterinarian to review the results of a radiographic study performed earlier. Though there may be no state law regarding the confidentiality of veterinary medical records, a so-called "right of privacy" law might have application. This type of problem might arise when information is sought about a newly-purchased horse that was radiographed when it belonged to a previous owner, your client. Another area of question involves the desire by a veterinarian who is presently serving a potential owner to review a series of radiographs you made for the current owner prior to a sale. The problem in these cases deals with your response to a request from someone other than the owner, or agent, who ordered you to perform the radiographic examination. It is possible that your willingness to assist in one of these situations might provide information concerning the animal that would give reason to cancel a proposed sale or suggest that information concerning the clinical status of the patient was available and was not made known to a potential owner at the time of a sale. To be safe, you should divulge the findings from a radiographic examination only to the owner or his agent who ordered the study. Other veterinarians, even those now providing for the health needs of a patient, do not have the right to receive a medical record except with the express permission of the owner. This should always be handled with a properly prepared release form. A recent discussion of legal considerations of veterinary medical records states that although the ethical position seems clear, the legal position is not as clear and varies by jurisdictions. Generally the "physician-patient" privilege that exists between physician and patient does not exist between veterinarians and their clients.

Because the radiographic study is a part of the medical record, it is important that you have a clear policy of recording the loaning of the radiographs if they are released to a third party. You should have a signed release from the person requesting the transfer of the radiographs stating that they are the owner or agent of the patient describing in detail the name, breed, age, and sex of the patient. They should state the purpose for which they wish to have the radiographic study and to whom the radiographs are to be sent. This release statement must then be filed with the rest of the medical record. If your practice is large enough, it is worth obtaining a film copying unit that permits the easy copying of radiographs. Many copiers are priced between $495 and $1345, with smaller units that copy films up to 10 x 12 inches priced at less than $400. It is acceptable to charge a minimal cost for making these radiographs available to owners and that can rather quickly repay you for the cost of the copier and its operation.

Radiographic examinations are often used for evaluation of disease present at the time of sale of an animal or potential disease that might develop later in the life of the animal. These examinations often involve the musculoskeletal system but can involve the respiratory system also. These prepurchase examinations are often of horses and are a part of soundness examinations. In dogs they often involve the examination for dysplasias in the bones or joints. These examinations represent potential legal problems unless the nature of the examination requested is fully appreciated. Therefore, it is suggested that it is the responsibility of the veterinarian to determine that an adequate number of technically acceptable radiographs are obtained of the areas to be examined. The radiographs should be properly identified. The decision of who is qualified to evaluate the diagnostic nature of the radiographs is not a matter to be discussed here.

Radiographs as a component part of a case record are of only questionable value unless they are identified in such a way that there is no question concerning the identity of the animal examined, the anatomical part examined, and the date on which the examination took place. There is a mistaken idea that medical records only have a value in support of an allegation brought against a veterinarian. This negative attitude is erroneous. It should be realized that a good radiographic study along with a complete medical record, may provide the evidence necessary to clearly disprove an allegation and refute any possible charges of malpractice.

REFERENCES

Hannah HW. Veterinary medical records—some legal considerations. J Am Vet Med Assoc 198:67-9,1991.

Pritchard W R. Legal aspects of the medical record. Presented at the 10th annual meeting of the Amer. Assoc of Vet Medical Record Librarians. Anaheim CA July 16, 1975.

Rumore JJ Al-Bagdadi FK and Titkemeyer C. Medical records and the law. J Am Vet Med Assoc 178:202,1981.

Professional Liability—A report of the AVMA Professional Liability Insurance Trust. Vol 11, number 3, July 1992.

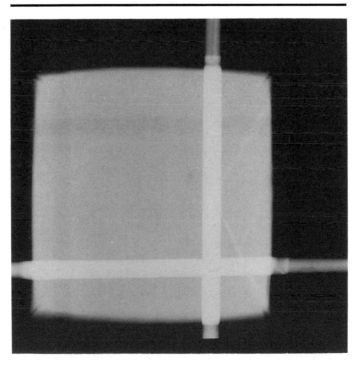

A radiograph was made of a large paper milk carton filled with water. Small holes were made in the sides of the carton near the top that would just accept paper straws. Three paper straws were placed from the top to the bottom of the radiograph and three additional paper straws were placed from side to side. Two straws are filled with iodinated contrast agent, two are filled with water, and two are empty. Why are you unable to identify the straws filled with water?

15. RADIOGRAPHIC EQUIPMENT

A. SMALL ANIMAL

Units for use in radiography of small animals fall generally into one category, that is a fixed table with an x-ray tube positioned over the table (Fig. 15-1). While some small animal clinics may continue to use small portable x-ray units with minimal mA capabilities, this cannot be recognized as an acceptable diagnostic unit today. Variations are found in the types of movement of the tube and table. The tube stand may be floor (Fig. 15-2), wall, or ceiling mounted (Fig. 15-1) with varying degrees of tube and stand motion. Those mounted on the floor may be fixed or have the capability of horizontal motion behind the table. The x-ray tube usually can move on the stand across the tabletop. With the tube stand mounted on the wall, the same type of horizontal and vertical movement is possible. The ceiling mounted tube is more expensive but has greater capabilities for vertical movement as well as horizontal movement in both directions. All forms of tube stands have a stable enough tube housing so that a heavy collimator with illumination of the radiation field can be utilized.

Instead of providing for tube head movement, it is possible to have a tabletop that is a floating-top variety. This assists in the positioning of the patient within the x-ray beam without having to move the patient on the tabletop. This is a great advantage when working with a large dog. It is possible for the tabletop to elevate and depress making it easier and more convenient to transfer a heavy patient onto the table (Fig. 15-3). Following positioning of the patient on the tabletop, it is elevated for the examination. Following the examination, the tabletop is then depressed and the patient more easily returned to the floor or guerney.

It is possible for the x-ray tube to rotate within its holder so that a horizontal beam can be produced. This may be directed toward a handheld cassette or toward a wall mounted cassette holder that may include a grid holder (Fig. 15-1).

The maximum mA and kVp settings and the shortest exposure time need to be known prior to the purchase of an x-ray unit. For a small animal stationary unit to be satisfactory, it needs to have a minimum capability of 100 mA and 100 kVp and a minimum exposure time of 1/20 second. Higher mA and kVp settings and shorter exposure times increase the possible use of the unit. Because of differences in construction and installation, there is some lack of consistency in the quality of exposure, but this is not a great problem. Studies have shown that even in high-quality machines the exposure consistency is only ± 5% to 8%. This is one reason why it is necessary to have an exposure chart developed for each x-ray machine and to use any other technique chart only as a guide for the development of your technique chart.

B. LARGE ANIMAL

Units for use in radiography of large animals fall generally into three categories: (1) small portable x-ray units with minimal mA capabilities (Fig. 15-4), (2) mobile x-ray units with high mA capabilities (Fig. 15-5), and (3) ceiling- or wall-mounted x-ray units with high mA capabilities (Fig. 15-6). With an understanding of these categories, it is rather easy to imagine the limitations that might be placed on the user of portable units and the advantages available in the use of larger units.

In the comparison of x-ray units, the maximum mA, kVp, and shortest exposure time are always considered. This is a satisfactory way of evaluating the potential use of an x-ray machine since these settings determine the thickness of tissue that might be examined as well as the shortness of exposure times that can be used. It must be understood, however, that because of differences in construction and installation, there is a great lack of consistency in the quality of exposure obtained with identical machine settings when focal-film distances and film-screen systems are constant. Studies have shown in some portable units that the exposure consistency is ± 18% to 75%, in medium-priced portable units the exposure consistency is ± 25%, and even on high-quality machines the exposure consistency is only ± 5% to 8%. This is one reason why it is so important to have an exposure chart developed for each x-ray machine and to use any other technique chart only as a guide for the development of your technique chart.

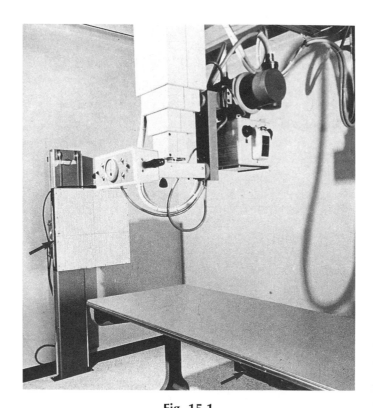

Fig. 15-1
SMALL ANIMAL RADIOGRAPHIC EQUIPMENT
A ceiling mounted tube positioned over a table with an undertable bucky tray (arrow) and a wall mounted cassette holder with movable grid (arrow) for "cross-table" radiography using a horizontal x-ray beam.

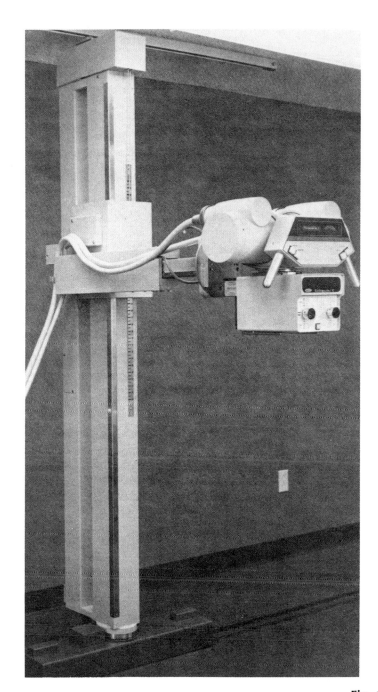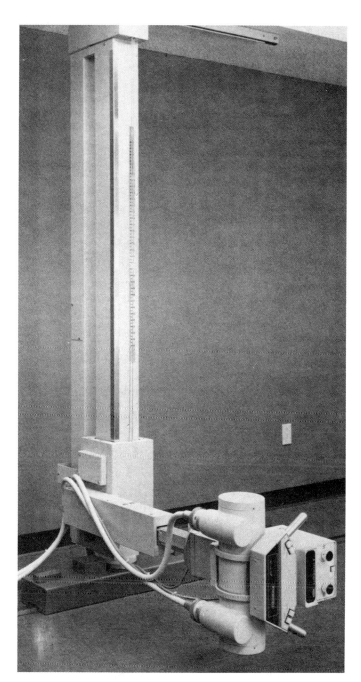

Fig. 15-2
SMALL ANIMAL RADIOGRAPHIC EQUIPMENT
A floor-to-ceiling mounted x-ray tube has the ability to move in all directions providing great flexibility for the operator. The unit can function over a table or could be used for horizontal beam studies of a standing patient.

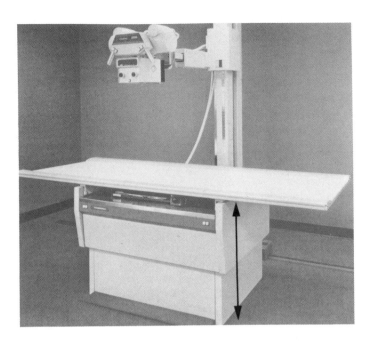
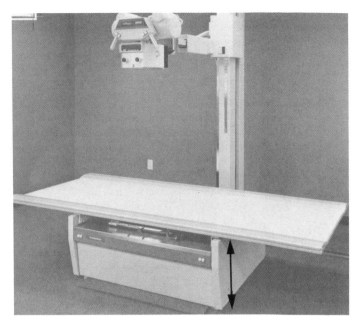

Fig. 15-3
SMALL ANIMAL RADIOGRAPHIC EQUIPMENT
A floor-to-ceiling mounted x-ray tube over a stationary table with a tabletop that elevates and depresses (arrows). This makes it much easier to position heavy patients onto the table from a guerney or from the floor.

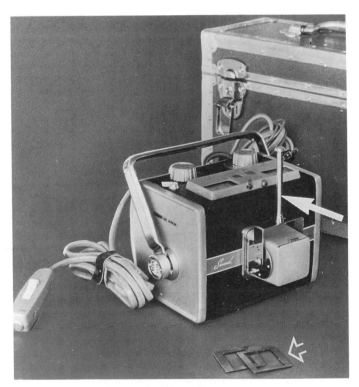
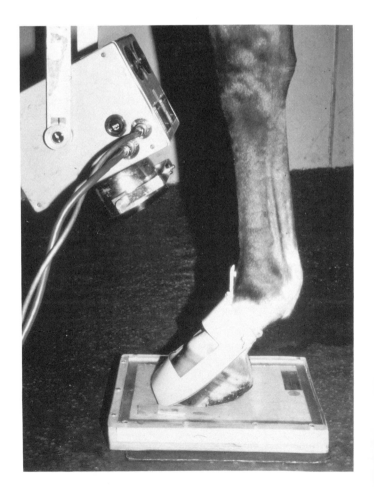

Fig. 15-4
PORTABLE X-RAY MACHINE
A "box portable" type of x-ray machine shown prior to use and being used for a navicular study of a horse. This unit has a beam restricting device consisting of lead aperature diaphragms (hollow arrow) and a pointer that moves into position for determining the direction of the central x-ray beam (solid arrow). This unit is commonly used for radiography of the extremities of large animals.

SMALL PORTABLE X-RAY UNITS

These are often referred to as <u>box portables</u> since their physical appearance is that of a small box (Fig. 15-4). They are light-weight, usually weighing around 15 to 20 kg, have a stationary anode type x-ray tube, are easily transported to a ranch or farm, and are easily carried to the stall or paddock in which the patient is housed. The majority of these units have a capability of 10 mA with a corresponding maximum kVp setting of 80 to 100 kVp. At lower kVp settings, the mA setting can be increased to 20 mA. There is one unit that has a capacity of 20 mA and 80 kVp. Exposure time is usually a minimum of 1/20 second and this is adequate to stop motion of the patient in most examinations of the extremities. It is possible to arrange a tube support system for these small units, but most are usually hand-held during exposures. Portable support systems that can be used in the field were the topic of a recent report (Koblik and Toal, 1991). A tripod-like system of support usually has adjustable-height legs and a gear-driven center post. In some units, the x-ray tube hangs in the center of the tripod or can be mounted above the legs. This unit is cumbersome to move quickly and difficult to position close to the patient. Four-legged stands use a pair of adjustable-height A-frame legs connected by a top bar. The tube is mounted to the connecting bar. This style of support is also cumbersome for most field application because it is difficult to move short distances, making adjustment of focal-film distance awkward. It is not easily adjusted for height, is difficult to position close to the patient and is nearly impossible to use underneath a standing animal. Two-legged stands use two curved or straight legs that attach to a baseplate. Casters may be provided for the baseplate, support legs or both. The tube may be supported by a round or square back-post or have a hinged extension arm. These units are mobile and easy to use on most distal limb studies, however, they remain difficult to move and position on uncertain surfaces.

Newer units are being produced that meet the description of a portable x-ray unit, but have capabilities of 50 mA at 100 kVp and 100 mA at 75 kVp. The lowest exposure time is 0.04 seconds. One such unit is available as a free standing unit mounted on a tripod with wheels and is complete with a light beam diaphragm.

These portable units are popular because of their ease in transportation; however, the limitations of such units must be understood. Often they are used at a great distance from an electrical power source at the end of a long extension cord. This compromises the electrical power available to the unit and often results in production of an underexposed radiograph. Studies have shown that an extension of 25 feet from the power source is acceptable, but a cord longer than 50 feet can cause a loss of up to 30% of the electrical energy. It is not difficult to use an inexpensive ($10.00) voltmeter that provides you with an immediate reading of the line voltage.

Because of the portable nature of the unit, all of the accessory equipment must be carried to the site of the examination. This includes heavy lead aprons, lead gloves, and positioning devices for the horse's foot or the cassette.

If the distance is great, it is possible for these positioning devices as well as radiation safety devices to not be utilized, thus compromising the quality of the examination as well as creating a radiation hazard.

While most portable units have collimators, only a few have a light that illuminates the field of exposure. Since these exposures may be made in the open, the illuminated field is often not bright enough to make use of it in identifying the field of exposure. Thus, the field of exposure is opened wide or the collimator is removed to insure that the entire film is exposed on each examination. This discards one of the best methods of reducing radiation exposure to those assisting in the examination. Because of the use of shorter focal-film distances, field-limitation devices often do not create a radiation field that covers the entire film. This leads to discarding the collimation device.

These portable x-ray units are often limited in their use to examinations of the extremities from the carpus and hock distally. They can be used for limited studies of the head and neck. In immature animals or in small ruminents, use of the portable units can be expanded to include studies more proximal on the limb.

LARGE MOBILE X-RAY UNITS

Another type of x-ray unit less commonly used for radiography of large animals is one that is mounted on wheels and is thus relatively easy to move within a clinic or hospital (Fig. 15-5). Because of this type of mounting, a relatively level, smooth surface is required for the unit to be moved safely. It is possible to arrange for a unit of this type to be moved in a trailer. The machine provides the

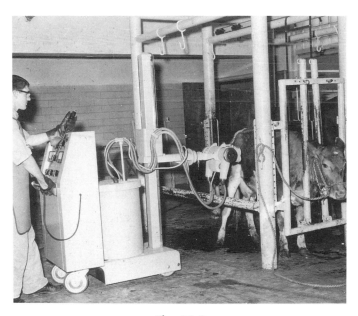

Fig. 15-5
MOBILE X-RAY MACHINE
A large mobile x-ray machine has capabilities that exceed the small portable units, and can be moved rather easily on a smooth surface. The unit is used here to radiograph the abdomen of a cow. The grid and cassette are suspended from the stocks on the opposite side of the cow.

advantage of moving the control panel, transformer, and tube unit to the site of the examination. The capabilities can include 100 to 300 mA, 100 to 120 kVp, and a timer with limitations at 1/60 to 1/120 seconds. Often the kVp readout is via a digital display. The increased capabilities are due to the use of a rotating anode type of x-ray tube and a large transformer. The tube head is such that it has a high-quality collimator with illumination of the radiation field. The large size causes difficulty in positioning the machine near the patient and being able to accurately and quickly position the x-ray tube. The weight of the unit makes it impossible to move into a stall or paddock because of the soft uneven surface. The tube-support system often does not permit positioning the tube very high and during radiography of the head the height of the tube position may create problems in stability of the unit. Usability of the unit is greatly enhanced by the presence of a pantographic type of arm support that holds the x-ray tube. This enables an easier positioning of the x-ray tube in any plane of motion.

The best use for this type of machine is in a clinic or hospital that has need of both large and small animal radiographic capabilities. A mobile unit can be: (1) easily moved to the area used for examination of lameness in horses, (2) moved to the surgery room for intra-surgical studies, (3) used to study a patient that cannot be moved from the back of a truck, (4) moved to a recovery stall for a post-surgical study, and (5) positioned over a stationary x-ray table for examination of small animals. It is this mobility that makes it a good solution for a large clinic that has need for a radiographic capability in examination of both large and small animals.

CEILING-MOUNTED X-RAY UNITS

These large, permanently mounted x-ray units have become popular in larger equine clinics and hospitals because of the ease and safety of operation and the increased capabilities (Fig. 15-6). The tube head support is ceiling-mounted and can be freely moved horizontally throughout the room and vertically from floor level to a height of 5 feet (1.6 m). This means that the tube head can be dropped to the floor level for a study of the horse's foot or can be raised quickly in the event of potential danger to the tube. However, since the standard tube crane only has a maximum of 5 feet (1.6 m) of vertical movement, the counterbalance system needs to be lowered for the tube head to reach the floor. With this arrangement it may not be possible to elevate the tube so that examinations of the head and neck can be performed. If the x-ray tube is connected to a second suspension column, it is possible to have the x-ray beam always directed to the grid-holder regardless of how the tube is moved (Fig. 15-7). Tube arms are also available which provide for movement of the tube beneath the patient (Fig. 15-8).

These units have a range of 100 to 1000 mA, 30 to 150 kVp, and exposure times as short as 1/60 to 1/120 second and have a rotating anode type of x-ray tube. Because the unit is used inside the clinic, it is possible to limit room light so that the collimator light that indicates the field of exposure can be easily seen. It is best to have the exposure controls at the tube head so that the exposure can be made at the time of tube positioning. Laser beam sources can be attached to the tube head in a parallax manner so that the correct focal-film distance can be immediately determined when the two beams coincide. A ceiling-mounted unit can be utilized with an x-ray table and would be of value in working with small ruminants.

A summary of the characteristics of the various types of large animal x-ray machines is provided (Table 15-1)

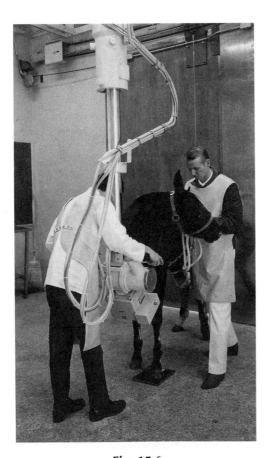

Fig. 15-6
CEILING-MOUNTED X-RAY TUBE
High capacity ceiling-mounted x-ray tube has great ease in positioning and safety when working with high-spirited animals. In this figure they are making a dorso-palmar view of the distal phalanx.

REFERENCES

Koblik PD and Toal R. Portable veterinary x-ray support systems for field use. J Am Vet Med Assoc 199;186-8, 1991.

Olsson S-E and Giers E. A multipurpose x-ray unit for veterinary use. J Am Vet Rad Soc 6:82-94, 1965.

Phillips DF. Radiology in your practice: choosing the right equipment. Vet Med 1987, pp587.

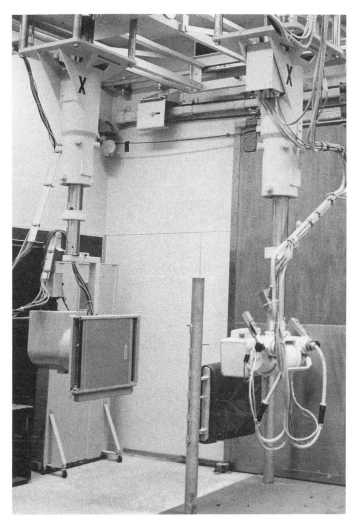

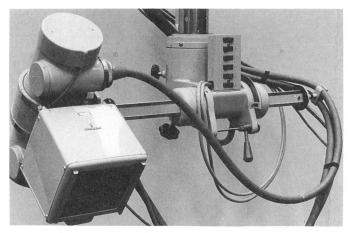

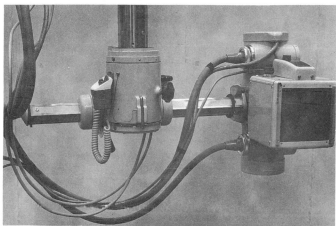

Fig. 15-7
CEILING-MOUNTED X-RAY TUBE
High capacity ceiling-mounted x-ray tube offers great ease in positioning and safety when working with high-spirited animals. The x-ray tube is interconnected to a cassette holder hung on a second ceiling suspended column.

Fig. 15-8
CEILING-MOUNTED X-RAY TUBE
Ceiling suspended x-ray tube with a special tube positioning device that makes it possible to rotate the tube or to shift the tube laterally to position it beneath the patient. (Courtesy of Veterinaire Rontgenologie, Utrecht)

Table 15-1
TYPES OF LARGE ANIMAL X-RAY MACHINES

Factors	Small Portable	Large Mobile/Stationary	Ceiling-Mounted
Cost	low ($4-6500)	high (>$12000)	high (>$18000)
mA capability	10-20	100-300	100-500
kVp capability	75-90	100	120
Exposure time (min.)	0.04	1/120	1/120
X-ray tube type	stationary anode	rotating anode	rotating anode
Number of focal spots	single	dual	dual
Focal spot size:			
small		0.5 mm	0.3 mm
large	1.5 to 3.0 mm	1.5 to 2.0 mm	1.5 to 2.0 mm
Machine mobility	high	high	none
Directing x-ray beam	difficult	very difficult	excellent
Exam limitation	distal limbs	due to tube head	minimal
Radiation hazard	high	minimal	minimal
Collimator	difficult to use	yes	yes
Exposure consistency	poor to good	good	good

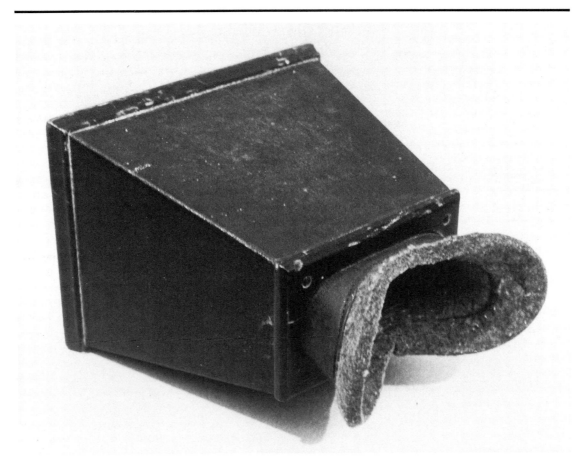

Hand-held fluoroscopic device used in the early years of radiology. This unattached unit was used as a fluoroscopic device by holding it in the primary x-ray beam and looking directly at the x-ray tube. The picture shows the felt-lined eye-piece that fit tightly against the face. The back side of the box contained the fluorescent screen and, hopefully, a leaded glass shield. These units are not in use today.

16. SPECIAL RADIOGRAPHIC EQUIPMENT

A. XERORADIOGRAPHY

The imaging technic of <u>xerography</u> was developed by Chester F. Carlson in 1939 as a method of duplicating manuscripts (Roach and Hillabae, 1955). He discovered that an electrostatic image of an object could be formed on a sensitive photoconductor surface when exposed to light. A uniform cloud of discrete particles (powder) could then be applied to the electrostatic image and the resulting "powder" image transferred to paper for a permanent image print. Experimentation revealed that the photoconductor material was also sensitive to conventional x-rays. Hence, in xeroradiography, an electrostatic latent image of an object can be formed during x-ray exposure comprised of varying charge densities determined by the differential absorption of the x-ray photons. An electrostatic charge is applied initially to a photoconductor plate of selenium. These photoconductor plates are placed in plastic cassettes which prevent light exposure. For exposure, the object is place between the plate and the tube. Once the plates are exposed, the print of the object can be produced in the development process. In developing the electrostatic image, the plate receives multiple bursts of colored powder and the resulting powdered images are then transferred to paper. The final print, therefore, consists of a powered image fixed to paper by heating and subsequent hardening of a plastic based emulsion. The process for medical imaging was not commercially available until 1956.

The <u>photoconductor material used is selenium</u> which behaves in the dark as an insulator, but, when exposed to light or x-rays, becomes a conductor of electrons. It is coated, with a controlled thickness of 130 μm, on an aluminum base plate, 9 x 14 inches (23 x 36 cm) that is used for stability, with a positive charge accumulated along the surface of the selenium layer and negative charges accumulated in equal numbers in the metal base plate. With exposure, the selenium becomes a conductor and the potential is discharged by the free flow of electrons in the selenium with loss of the positive surface charge. The latent image which is formed on the selenium surface is comprised of varying residual charge densities depending on the differential absorption of x-rays by the various structures in the radiographed specimen. Hence, the selenium surface below areas of high density, such as bone, retain proportionately greater charge potential than the surface before surrounding soft tissues (Boag, 1973).

The <u>electrostatic latent image</u> on the selenium plate is developed by dusting the page with charged plastic toner particles which are blue in color. During the dusting process, a build-up of toner particles occurs at each interface of charge density difference on the latent image. Both positive and negative charged toner particles are available for development.

The equipment consists of two separate units, a <u>conditioner and a processor</u>. The conditioner stores the selenium plates and removes the residual latent charge from the previous exposure by momentary heating in the relaxation oven. Just prior to loading, the surface charge is applied to the selenium plate by an air-ion generating device. From the plate-charging station the image reception is automatically loaded in the cassette. The conditioner is independent of the processor. Decay of the surface charge on the selenium plate occurs with noticeable loss of resolution in the final image in 15-20 minutes if the x-ray exposure has not been completed. Rough handling of the cassette can result in artifacts from unintentional surface discharge. Up to one-half hour after exposure, the cassette is placed in the processor and the selenium plate is removed automatically and advanced to the development chamber where a fine cloud of charged, blue particles is blown onto the plate. Because the particles are charged, they adhere to the plate in approximately the same distribution as the electrostatic charge pattern. The powder image is then transferred to plastic coated paper by direct contact and is fused by heating. The final print is cooled for permanent fixation and is suitable for examination. The plate is returned to the storage box. Note that the xerographic process is completely dry from start to finish requiring no photographic chemicals or water.

Individual plates are usable for about 6 months. Artifacts may occur due to excessive pressure being applied to their plastic cassette during positioning. Generally, the exposure latitude is wide and large variation in exposure (± 10kVp) do not alter image quality significantly. A long scale of contrast exists permitting both dense and lucent structures to be seen on the same print.

Xerography is best known for its use in mammagraphy in women where it provides good resolution, a wide range of perceptible densities, and prints in which the different densities are so well delineated that they are readily identified. Images of the extremities reveal exquisite soft tissue detail with enhancement of muscle planes, subcutaneous vasculature, individual lymph nodes, and connective tissue structures (Wolfe, 1969). The technique of xeroradiography has also been employed extensively in soft-tissue imaging of the pharynx and larynx (Osterman et al, 1977) and has been utilized for examination of thin cadaveric slices (Meschan et al, 1979). Each boundary of density difference in the radiographed subject is graphically demonstrated due to "edge enhancement". This inherent physical property accounts for the high resolution of density differences. This is due to toner being shifted from one side of the edge and laid down more heavily on the other side. This amplifies the contrast at the edge and causes an apparent density difference on each side of the edge.

The <u>radiation exposure</u> received by the patient is <u>higher</u> using xeroradiography than using non-screen technique and approximately 10 times higher when using conventional screen technique.

B. CONDENSER TYPE X-RAY APPARATUS

In most x-ray generators for diagnostic purposes, a system is used in which input from a commercial power source is supplied to a high voltage transformer, and x-rays are generated by loading the x-ray tube directly with the output of the high voltage transformer via high voltage rectifiers. This is referred to as the transformer type of x-ray production. It requires a large power source in order to generate the x-rays, and, is difficult to use is regions where a sufficiently large power source is not available.

The condenser type x-ray generator uses a condenser in which the electric energy for loading the x-ray tube comes from the discharging of the high energy electric charge from the condenser through the x-ray tube. To charge the condenser, only a small output current from the high voltage transformer is required. Consequently, the power source supplying the generator need have only a very low current rating. The tube has a grid-control device that controls the x-ray production within a period of several micro-seconds. The condenser is rated in microfarrads and the exposures are measured so that 1 mAs = microfarrad x kV setting. This determines the time to complete the charging.

The advantages of condenser type x-ray generators are: (1) good radiographs even when the power source has a low current rating, (2) tube voltage pre-indicated with great accuracy, (3) exposure times are short, (4) no danger of overloading the tube, and (5) equipment can be mounted in a truck and used in areas without a commercial power source.

REFERENCES

Boag JW. Xeroradiography. Phys Med Biol 18:3, 1973.

Meschan I Walter JB and Krueger WA. The utilization of xeroradiography for radiography of cross-section of thin cadaveric slices. Invest Rad 14:97, 1979.

Osterman FA James AE Heshike A Ryan JM Novak G Rao GUV and Bush M. Xeroradiography in Veterinary Radiography: A preliminary study. J Am Vet Rad Soc 16:143, 1975.

Roach JF and Hillabae HE. Xeroradiography. Am J Roentgenol 73:5, 1955.

Wolfe JN. Xeroradiograph of bones, joints, and soft tissues. Rad 93:583,1969.

17. TERMINOLOGY TO DESCRIBE RADIOGRAPHIC POSITIONING

The accepted method for naming radiographic projections describes the pathway of the x-ray beam from through the body. This is called the point-of-entrance to point-of-exit method. A radiograph of the thorax or abdomen made with the patient laying on the film in ventral recumbency (prone) with the x-ray tube above the patient is referred to as a dorsoventral (DV) view. The radiograph made with the patient laying on the film in dorsal recumbency (supine) is referred to as a ventrodorsal (VD) view. The directional terms dorsal and ventral are also used on the radiographs of the neck. Oblique views of the body are named by the entry and exit of the beam, however, now at least two descriptors are required; for example, right dorsal-left ventral oblique of the thorax (RD-LV). These terms can be used on a standing patient in the same manner.

For views of the limbs proximal to the carpus and proximal to the tarsus in a standing large animal patient, the view made with the x-ray tube in front of the limb and the film behind the limb is referred to as a craniocaudal view. If the beam is reversed and the x-ray tube is placed behind the limb, the view is referred to as a caudocranial view. In the recumbent small animal patient, the craniocaudal view is made with the limb extended forward on the tabletop with the x-ray tube above the limb and the film beneath the limb on the tabletop. The caudocranial view can be made with the limb extended behind so that the x-ray beam enters the caudal aspect of the limb and strikes the film under the limb. The lateral views of the limbs in either a standing or recumbent patient are usually referred to as only a lateral view and not as a lateromedial or mediolateral view, although, this terminology of indicating the location of the tube and film is appropriate.

Views of the carpus and distally on the forelimb in the standing large animal patient are called dorsopalmar views if the tube is in front of the limb and the film behind. Views with the tube placed behind the limb and the film in front are called palmarodorsal. Views of the tarsus and distal on the pelvic limb are called dorsoplantar views if the tube is in front of the limb and the film behind while they are referred to as plantarodorsal if the tube is behind the limb and the film in front. In the recumbent small animal patient with the forelimb extended in front with the tube above the limb and the film under the limb, the view of the carpus and distally is referred to as dorsopalmar while in the pelvic limb the view is called a dorsoplantar. If the forelimb is extended behind the recumbent small animal patient with the tube above the limb and the film under the limb, the view of the carpus and distally is referred to as palmarodorsal while on the pelvic limb the view is called a plantarodorsal.

Oblique views of the limbs are described in greater detail. The first part of the description locates the tube and the second part of the description locates the film. Thus, if the tube is cranial and lateral and the film is caudal and medial, the oblique is referred to as a craniolateral-caudomedial oblique. If the oblique is distal to the carpus, and the tube is dorsal and lateral and the film is palmar and medial, the oblique is referred to as a dorsolateral-palmaromedial oblique.

Another method of designating oblique views is to call them medial or lateral oblique views. The term indicates that portion of the dorsal or cranial aspect of the limb that is best visualized. Thus, the medial oblique of the carpus most clearly shows the dorsal aspect of the radial carpal bone and the second carpal bone. It might otherwise be called the dorsolateral-caudomedial oblique view. Some difficulty exists in understanding the naming for the oblique view for the medial or 2nd metacarpal bone on a horse. The view that would best show this bone would be the dorsomedial-palmarolateral view, or the lateral oblique view. Thus, the lateral oblique view best shows the medial splint bone. It is possible to add specific angles to these oblique views, but such lengthy description are impractical in daily use. The oblique views in the smaller patient examined on the tabletop are best described as medial and lateral obliques.

Many other special views achieve a descriptive term rather than a careful explanation of the location of the tube and film. Many of these views are used in examination of the head. A "frontal view" of the dog's or cat's head is made with the patient in dorsal recumbency and the noise pointing toward the tube. Because of the differences in the morphology of the head in various breeds, the exact positioning of the head and the exact angle of the x-ray beam vary and make specific descriptions of angles impractical and useless. It may be possible to use the term rostral in the description of some views, in an attempt to locate the tube.

Some views are made with the x-ray beam directed proximodistally and are generally classified as flexor views. They might be more specifically described as proximo-distal views. The flexor view of the navicular bone of the horse is made with the x-ray beam directed distally toward the film with the beam parallel to the flexor surface of the navicular bone. Obviously, the positioning of the foot and the positioning of the tube determine the angle of the beam and diagnostic studies can be made in a range of beam angles. In the horse, flexor views can be made of the proximal sesamoid bones, distal cranial aspect of the third metacarpal (tarsal) bone, olecranon process, patella, and os calcis.

Erect studies are made with a horizontal beam, however, the patient may be standing, in dorsal recumbency, in ventral recumbency, in lateral recumbency, or held erect with forelimbs extended in a rostral direction. The beam may be directed dorso-ventrally (ventrodorsally) or may be a laterally directed beam.

Some of the terminology used in describing radiographic positioning are illustrated (Figs. 17-1, 17-2).

REFERENCE

Nomina Anatomica Veterinaria 3rd ed., Ithaca, New York 1983.

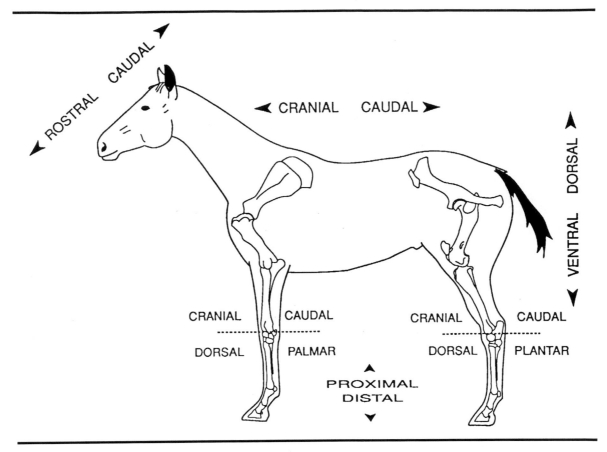

Fig. 17-1
LATERAL VIEW OF A HORSE WITH LABELS DESCRIBING RADIOGRAPHIC PROJECTIONS.

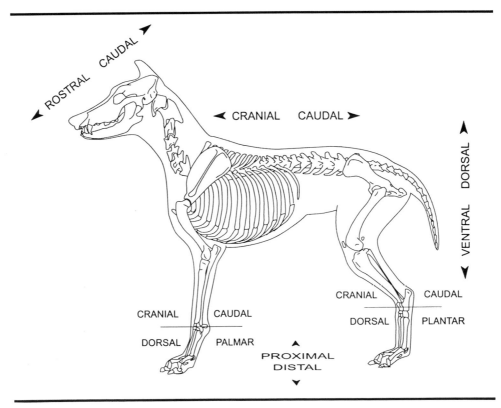

Fig. 17-2
LATERAL VIEW OF A DOG WITH LABELS DESCRIBING RADIOGRAPHIC PROJECTION.

SECTION B

RADIOGRAPHY OF THE DOG

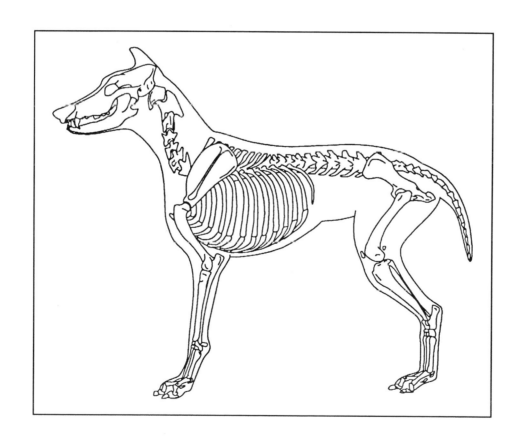

1. INTRODUCTION

Radiography of the dog is a common diagnostic procedure in most small animal clinics throughout the world. The indications for radiography range from determination of the cause of lameness for a puppy to an examination of the older patient with suspect pulmonary metastasis. Thus, the studies are used to benefit patients that present with a variety of clinical signs. There are no contraindications for radiography of the dog, only unique circumstances present with certain patients that result in a required change in a routine protocol. These circumstances may affect how sedation or anesthesia may be used or may affect the positioning that is possible to use in obtaining the study. Patient preparation is essentially the same for all studies and consists in cleaning and drying the hair coat as wet hair and debris cause confusing artifacts on the radiographs. Leashes and collars are removed prior to radiography to avoid compromising shadows on the radiograph. Remove bandages, splints, casts, or tape when possible prior to radiography since they all affect exposure of the film and create some type of film artifact.

Restraint can be provided using a variety of techniques. Anesthesia is the most desirable form of patient restraint since it means that optimal positioning can be obtained without technician exposure during the radiographic examination. Anesthesia is an unrealistic goal for all patients considering the nature of the disease, the age of the patient, or the nature of a traumatic injury. It is always possible to use sandbags, compression bands, positioning troughs, sponges, as well as tie-down ropes, tape, and gauze to assist in positioning of the dog either alone or in conjunction with chemical restraint. As in most things, a compromise can usually be reached in which there can be use of some positioning devices so that few technicians must remain within the room during the examination and they can be positioned at a greater distance from the x-ray beam. It is expected that radiation safety practices, such as beam collimation, use of as fast a film-screen system as practical, and lead aprons and gloves are to be used in all examinations.

Two views are required for almost all radiographic examinations and are preferably made at right angles to each other. Beam direction is described by terms that indicate the entrance and exit of the x-ray beam. Thus a dorsoventral beam enters dorsally and exits ventrally. Some terms are required if the beam is not vertical to the tabletop. Certain terms used to describe a view reflect the anatomical structure that is to be evaluated on the radiograph.

Identification markers are required for each radiograph and the name or clinic number of the patient, name of the owner, date of examination, and name of the clinic are the minimal information required. Right and left markers are needed.

Measurement of the patient prior to radiography is important to obtain the correct machine settings from a technique chart. Avoid making the measurements when the dog is standing but instead wait until it is positioned on the table. Remember that correct measurement and use of a correct technique is one of the best radiation safety rules since it eliminates repeat examinations.

Focal-film distances need to be standardized prior to development of the technique chart. Most radiographic units permit the use of 40 inches (100 cm) distance from the tube to the film. This distance can be used for all views of the dog, even those using a horizontal beam. Grids are usually positioned in undertable trays where they are used rather easily. Since the overhead tube is usually fixed to the table, the central beam remains centered on the gird thus avoiding the technical error of grid cut-off.

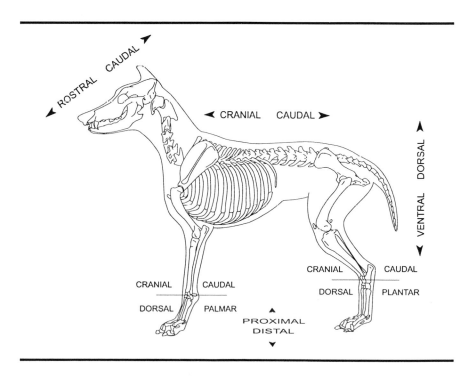

2. THORACIC RADIOGRAPHY

INTRODUCTION

Radiology is the most important diagnostic test in the investigation of thoracic diseases. Radiology usually reveals more specific information than physical examination and can be performed relatively cheaply, quickly, and safely, providing immediate results on which to base the next set of decisions. Radiographs reproduce the character of the patient's body on film and can be examined both at the time of the original examination as well as being available for review at another time. The x-ray image is a transillumination of the body at the moment the film is taken. It is this ability to see a representation of the interior of the patient, impossible by palpation or auscultation, that accounts for the great value of thoracic radiography. This is primarily due to the good contrast provided by the air in the lungs that opens up a window to the thoracic organs on non-contrast radiographs to an extent not possible with the abdominal radiographic study. In addition, radiographic examination provides a temporal dimension that permits evaluation of changes as you observe the progression of a disease. The study permits evaluation of parts of the trachea and lungs, pleural space, heart and great vessels, esophagus, lymph notes, diaphragm and ribs, sternum, and thoracic spine.

INDICATIONS

The clinical situations suggesting the use of thoracic radiography vary from a search for specific information such as a check for metastases, an evaluation of congenital heart disease, or an evaluation of a patient whose most specific clinical sign is dyspnea. Thoracic radiography often aids in making the decision of what other clinical examination or test should be performed next. Rarely does the radiographic study provide a definitive diagnosis at the time of the first film evaluation. Some general indications for thoracic radiography are listed (Table 2-1).

CONTRAINDICATIONS

The only contraindications for radiographs of the thorax is in a patient in which the rate of respiration creates movement of the thorax that cannot be stopped by a short exposure time. Sometimes it is possible to stop respiration by placing a hand or glove over the patient nose and mouth. This provides a short window of opportunity in which to make the exposure. If your x-ray machine permits an exposure of 1/30 second or shorter, you can radiograph the thorax in most dogs.

Presence of a large amount of pleural fluid or an intrathoracic mass increases the level of dyspnea when the dog is placed in certain positions. Usually, ventrodorsal positioning is the most stressful if the patient has pleural disease because of the difficulty in lung expansion. Thoracocentesis followed by drainage of pleural fluid may permit more comfortable positioning of the patient and production of a more diagnostic radiograph. The exposure factors need to be increased by 10 kVp or by doubling the mAs if pleural fluid or an intrathoracic mass is present.

Table 2-1
GENERAL INDICATIONS FOR THORACIC RADIOGRAPHY

1. suspect upper respiratory disease (acute or chronic)
2. suspect lower respiratory disease (acute or chronic)
3. recurrent non-responsive respiratory disease
4. presence of cough
5. presence of dyspnea
6. known or suspected thoracic trauma
7. known or suspected non-cardiogenic edema
   —electrical shock
   —near-drowning
   —head trauma
   —near-asphyxiation
   —allergy
8. preanesthesia study because of
   —patient's older age
   —post-trauma status
   —presence of associated respiratory disease
   —presence of associated cardiac disease
   —presence of malignant disease
9. evaluation for pulmonary metastases
10. postoperative study in the event of respiratory complications
11. suspect cardiac disease, either congenital or acquired
12. suspect swallowing dysfunction
13. survey examination in an older patient without specific clinical signs

---

PROTOCOL

Thoracic studies usually consist of a single lateral view and a dorsoventral view, although, the opposite lateral view may routinely be included in the study. A ventrodorsal view may be substituted for the dorsoventral view. Studies made especially for the heart should consist of a right lateral and dorsoventral view to obtain the most correct evaluation of the heart shadow (Table 2-2). Exposures are made near the completion of inspiration and should include the thoracic inlet and the diaphragm. With certain clinical signs, it is desirable to include additional views of the larynx and cervical trachea within the study. High kVp technique (90-110 kVp) provides a longer scale of contrast on the radiograph and is highly recommended for the best evaluation of the lung fields. Grid technique may not be required until the thoracic cavity measures greater than 15cm. Thoracic radiography in the anesthetized patient is usually not successful unless the lungs are fully inflated by positive pressure ventilation just prior to exposure.

Positioning for thoracic studies requires elevation of the sternum from the tabletop to insure lateral positioning. Extension of the forelimb removes the muscle mass of the forelimbs from over the precardiac lung field. Attempt to superimpose the sternum and spine in the dorsoventral or ventrodorsal views. Flexion of the shoulder and elbow when the dog is in a lateral view positions the olecranon process over the heart and provides a method of determining a point for centering the x-ray beam. Otherwise, there is a tendency to center the x-ray beam caudally on the lateral view, while the beam is often centered too far cranially on the dorsoventral view. The positioning for radiography of the thorax using a horizontal beam is found in the section on special procedures. The use of an esophageal swallow of barium sulfate suspension prior to exposure provides information useful in the diagnosis of mediastinal disease characterized by displacement of the esophagus.

Table 2-2
PROTOCOL FOR THORACIC RADIOGRAPHY

Routine views
    lateral
    dorsoventral (ventrodorsal)
Additional views
    opposite lateral
    dorsoventral or ventrodorsal oblique made at 20° to 30°
    transaxial tracheal inlet
    pulmonary metastasis—both lateral views
    mediasinal mass—increase exposure by 10 kVp
    pleural fluid—increase exposure by 10 kVp
        —consider using horizontal beam radiography

VIEWS
THORAX—LATERAL VIEW

Patient preparation: None required except to clean the hair coat and remove any collars or leashes.

Patient positioning: Place the dog in either right or left lateral recumbency. Selection of the side is dictated by ease of handling the patient, comfort of the patient, and location of lesion. Pull the forelimbs together and extend them cranially placing sandbags over the feet. Elevate the sternum using a wedge-shaped sponge. Avoid placing the head and neck in either a hyperextended or hyperflexed position because of the effect on tracheal position and diameter. Place sandbags over the pelvic limbs or use ropes to tie the feet to the table, if necessary.

X-ray beam direction: The vertically directed beam is centered on the heart at the 5th intercostal space.

Comments: Make the exposure at or near full inspiration.

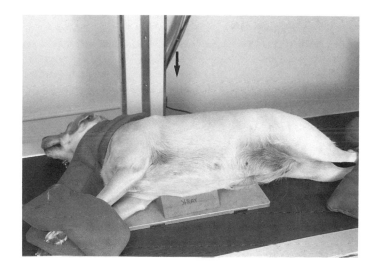

THORAX—DORSOVENTRAL VIEW

Patient preparation: None required except to clean the hair coat and remove any collars or leashes.

Patient positioning: Place the dog in sternal recumbency with the spine superimposed over the sternum. Pull the forefeet cranially and try to hold the elbows together under the neck. This positions the scapulae lateral to the lung field. If this is not convenient, place the forelimbs lateral with the elbows lateral to the thoracic inlet. This provides for easier positioning but positions the scapulae over the cranial lung fields. Use sandbags over the forelimbs and use ropes to tie the feet to the table. Use a trough or sandbags to help in positioning the abdomen. Leave the pelvic limbs in a near normal flexed position.

X-ray beam direction: The vertically directed beam is centered on the midthoracic spine.

Comments: Make the exposure near full inspiration.

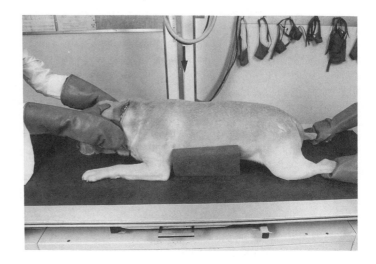

THORAX—VENTRODORSAL VIEW

Patient preparation: None required except to clean the hair coat and remove any collars or leashes.

Patient positioning: Place the dog in dorsal recumbency with the spine superimposed over the sternum. Pull the forefeet cranially positioning them lateral to the head keeping the nose on the midline. Use sandbags or ropes to tie the forefeet to the table. Use a trough, sandbags, or a compression band to stabilize the positioning of the abdomen. Leave the pelvic limbs in a frogleg (flexed) position.

X-ray beam direction: The vertically directed x-ray beam is centered on the midthoracic spine.

Comments: Make the exposure near full inspiration.

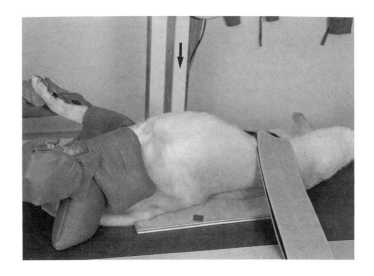

THORAX—DORSOVENTRAL—
THORACIC INLET VIEW

Patient preparation: None required except to clean the hair coat and remove any collars or leashes.

Patient positioning: Place the dog in sternal recumbency and pull the head into a marked hyperextended position. Pull the forefeet cranially and use sandbags to position the forelimbs or use ropes to tie the feet to the table. Use a trough or sandbags to help in positioning the abdomen. Leave the pelvic limbs in a near normal flexed position.

X-ray beam direction: The vertically directed beam is angled in approximately a 45° craniocaudal angle and centered on the thoracic inlet.

Comments: Make the exposure on expiration. Decrease the radiographic technique because of the decrease in tissue thickness.

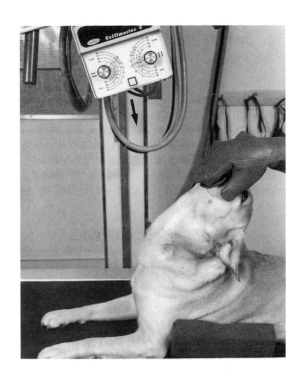

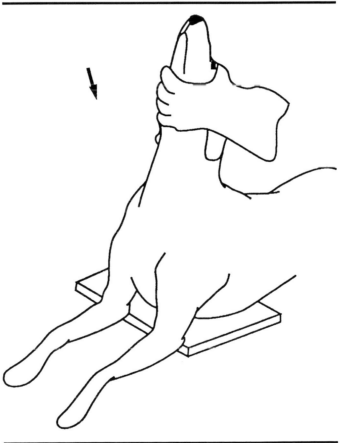

3. ABDOMINAL RADIOGRAPHY

INTRODUCTION

Abdominal radiography in the dog is frequently used as a survey study since it permits evaluation of a part of the gastrointestinal tract, urinary tract, a portion of the musculoskeletal system, as well as the peritoneal cavity. It has its greatest value in the detection of mass lesions that often cause shifting of adjacent abdominal organs. The routine abdominal study is often followed by a special radiographic study of the gastrointestinal or urinary system using contrast agents.

INDICATIONS

Since the study is a form of a survey study, the indications for examination are widespread and relate to the body systems that can be evaluated (Table 3-1). Any sign of anorexia, vomiting, or diarrhea suggests gastrointestinal disease. Problems of hematuria, dysuria, or crystalluria suggest urinary disease. A painful abdomen may relate to peritoneal disease, trauma to the abdominal wall, or a spinal injury. The clinician should not hesitate to use abdominal radiography as a routine in the establishment of a data base in many patients.

CONTRAINDICATIONS

Poor patient preparation affects the quality of abdominal radiographs. The presence of large amounts of food in the stomach, ingesta in the small bowel, feces in the colon, or a full urinary bladder often obscures areas of interest and reduces the value of the examination.

PROTOCOL

The amount of patient preparation varies with the nature of the examination. Suspect urinary bladder disease only requires cleansing of the terminal colon while a study of a suspect mid-abdominal mass requires that the entire gastrointestinal tract be emptied. If it is possible, consider fasting the patient for 12 hours prior to the examination, however this amount of time may not be available. In many patients with vomiting and diarrhea, the hollow viscera are empty at the time of presentation. Sedation or anesthesia is not commonly used for this study.

The entire diaphragm and pelvic region on the radiograph needs to be evaluated in most patients. This is relatively easy if the patient is a small or medium sized dog. If it is a large dog, a decision must be made of which portion of the abdomen is most important to include on a single radiograph, or whether two overlapping radiographs should be made to include both cranial and caudal aspects of the abdomen. Remember that greater exposure factors may be needed on the thicker cranial portion of the abdomen as compared with the thinner caudal portion.

The patient can be positioned in either right or left lateral recumbency for the lateral projection. While the right lateral is more commonly used, the left lateral may be of greater value since it allows stomach gas to move into the pylorus and proximal duodenum and permits radiographic evaluation of this more clinically important region.

The ventrodorsal view is preferred over the dorsoventral view for routine studies of the abdomen since positioning of the dog can usually be more easily controlled in dorsal recumbency. Ventrodorsal positioning is difficult in trauma patients with pelvic or hindlimb injuries because it is not possible to apply traction to the pelvic limbs because of pain. The dorsoventral view may be used if patients cannot tolerate dorsal recumbency because of respiratory distress or have pelvic injury (Table 3-2).

Table 3-1
INDICATIONS FOR ABDOMINAL RADIOGRAPH

those suggesting gastrointestinal disease
    anorexia
    vomiting
    diarrhea
    known ingestion of foreign body
    melana
    dyschezia
those suggesting urinary disease
    hematuria
    pyuria
    dysuria
    stranguria
    frequent urination
post trauma
findings on physical examination
    palpation of abdominal mass
    abdominal tenderness or pain
    abdominal wall tense
suspect malignancy

Table 3-2
PROTOCOL FOR ABDOMINAL RADIOGRAPHY

Routine
    right lateral view
    ventrodorsal view
Optional
    left lateral view
    dorsoventral view
    compression paddle views
    horizontal beam views
        lateral view in sternal recumbency
        lateral view in dorsal recumbency
        ventrodorsal view in left lateral position
        ventrodorsal view in right lateral position
        lateral view in erect position
        ventrodorsal view in erect position

The kVp scale selected should be in the medium range (75-90 kVp) since this provides a scale of contrast that is most diagnostic. Exposures are made at the end of expiration. Exposure times need not be shorter than 1/20 second since that speed stops motion of the diaphragm and the resulting motion of the abdominal organs. Measure the patient to determine the appropriate technique after the dog is positioned on the tabletop. In a patient that is large, obese, or has abdominal fluid, the measurement is often incorrect if measured standing on the floor or table prior to being positioning on the radiographic table.

The beam is centered in the mid-portion of the abdomen at a point just caudal to the last rib, or over the specific area of interest. A grid is required for dogs over 11 cm thick.

Certain special techniques can be used to increase the value of the abdominal study. These include the use of: (1) oblique views or a view made using a compression paddle that shifts overlying abdominal organs and permits better visualization of those organs beneath, (2) ingestion of a small amount of air or barium sulfate suspension into the stomach to permit evaluation of the cranial abdominal organs, (3) injection of a small amount of rectal air to permit evaluation of the caudal abdominal organs, and (4) special flexed positioning of the pelvic limbs in the male dog to permit evaluation of the urethra for possible calculi. Use of a horizontal beam technique with the dog in left lateral recumbency to detect free peritoneal air is discussed in the section on Special Procedures.

VIEWS
ABDOMEN—LATERAL VIEW

Patient preparation: No particular preparation is required except to clean the hair coat. Often the possibility that the contents of the gastrointestinal tract or urinary tract might compromise the quality of the study is not known until the first radiographs are evaluated. The patient should be encouraged to defecate or urinate prior to the study if this is possible.

Patient positioning: Most commonly the lateral view is made with the dog in right lateral recumbency. The forelimbs can be positioned cranially being held with sandbags or tied to the table, while the pelvic limbs need to be extended slightly where they are held using sandbags or are tied to the table. Sandbags can be placed across the neck to hold the head in an extended position. It may assist is positioning an obese patient to place a sponge beneath the sternum or beneath the pelvic limbs to ensure a more lateral positioning of the abdomen.

X-ray beam direction: The vertically directed x-ray beam is centered on the middle of the abdomen just caudal to the last ribs. It is possible to center the beam on the urinary bladder if this is of clinical importance.

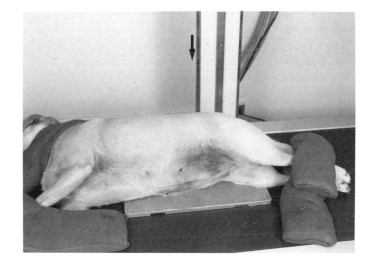

ABDOMEN—VENTRODORSAL VIEW

Patient preparation: No particular preparation is required except to clean the hair coat. Often the contents of the gastrointestinal tract or urinary tract are not known until the first radiographs are evaluated. The patient should be encouraged to defecate or urinate prior to the study if this is possible.

Patient positioning: The ventrodorsal view is used frequently because it is easier to position the dog by extending the forelimbs and tying them to the tabletop or holding them with sandbags. Sandbags may be placed lateral to the chest in a small or medium-sized dog to assist in positioning. The pelvic limbs are extended and held or tied to the tabletop. Palpation of the sternum insures that a correct positioning is obtained. If the patient is laying on a cassette, it may be helpful to place a small sponge over the edge of the cassette to make the positioning more comfortable.

X-ray beam direction: The vertically directed central beam is centered on the middle of the abdomen just caudal to the last ribs. It is possible to center the beam on the urinary bladder if this is of clinical importance.

ABDOMEN—DORSOVENTRAL VIEW

Patient preparation: No particular preparation is required except to clean the hair coat. Often the contents of the gastrointestinal tract or urinary tract are not known until the first radiographs are evaluated. The patient should be encouraged to defecate or urinate prior to the study if this is possible.

Patient positioning: The dorsoventral view is less frequently used because of the difficulty in achieving good positioning of the dog. It is a more desirable positioning than the ventrodorsal technique because it permits a more normal positioning of the abdominal viscera. It is relatively easy to extend the forelimbs and tie them to the tabletop, however, the pelvic limbs are flexed and may be more difficult to position. Usually the feet or hocks are held to insure the dog does not move during the exposure. Sandbags may be placed lateral to the chest in a small or medium-sized dog to assist in positioning. If the patient is dyspneic or sustained certain injuries, dorsoventral positioning may be required.

X-ray beam direction: The vertically directed x-ray beam is centered on the middle of the abdomen at L2 or L3.

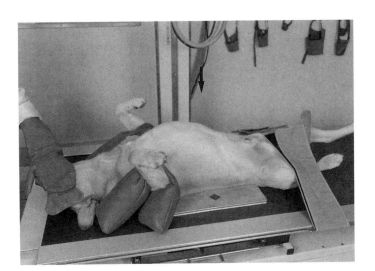

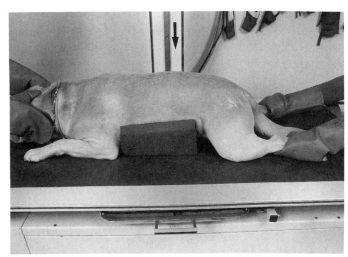

4. RADIOGRAPHY OF THE HEAD

INTRODUCTION

The anatomy of the skull and mandible is complicated causing radiography of the head to be difficult. When you consider the range in size of patients from a Chihuahua to a giant Irish Wolfhound as well as consider the variations in the shape of the head, this can be partially understood. Add to this the anatomical differences that are present when comparing the head of a bulldog with that of a collie and some of the problems in radiography of the dog's head can be appreciated. While a frontal study in a boxer would be relatively easy, the same study in a borzoi would be impossible because of the differences in the morphology of the frontal bone. There are certain regions that can be evaluated radiographically, while other areas cannot be studied. Some of these separate areas have special radiographic views.

A decision needs to be made at the time of radiography of the purpose of the study. It is possible to divide the studies of the head into the following: (1) routine skull and mandible, (2) nasal cavity and sinuses, (3) maxilla and maxillary teeth, (4) mandible and mandibular teeth, (5) temporomandibular joints, and (6) tympanic bullae.

INDICATIONS

The indications for radiography of the head include: (1) congenital abnormalities involving the bones or teeth, (2) trauma usually resulting from being hit by a car, (3) inflammatory lesions causing rhinitis or sinusitis, (4) tumors originating within the nasal region or in the overlying bone, and (5) degenerative changes associated with the periodontal region. Specific clinical signs include: (1) inability to pick-up food and swallow, (2) pain on examination of the head, (3) soft tissue or bony swelling, and (4) nasal discharge or epistaxsis.

CONTRAINDICATIONS

There are no contraindications to performing the survey study. It is necessary to anesthetize the patient for completion of the study.

PROTOCOL

Positioning becomes very difficult to standardize with the lateral views being the easiest to accomplish and the views of the temporomandibular joints and the basilar region of the skull the most difficult.

Radiographic techniques need to be varied due to the differences in thickness of bone. The German Shepherd Dog has a much thicker temporal and parietal region than the beagle dog. These differences can be partially detected by accurate measurements, but the techniques also need to be adjusted for suspected differences in bone thickness.

A survey study consisting of lateral and dorsoventral views can be made in a survey manner on an awake patient. However, anesthesia is needed if a detailed study of the head with special views is to be accomplished. The use of anesthesia also permits the use of slower speed film-screen systems or even the use of non-screen film. The presence of an endotracheal tube must be recognized and it should be removed from the field of exposure if possible.

Studies of the teeth are a special problem because the difficulty in positioning of the head and placement of the film to obtain the most diagnostic lateral views. Non-screen dental film is used in some practices to assist in solving these problems (Table 4-1).

The tongue creates a dense soft tissue shadow that often confuses interpretation of shadows in the nasal cavity and it should be placed laterally so that it is removed from the field of interest. The location of the external ears (pinnae) is important since they cast a prominent mixed density shadow on the radiograph.

Table 4-1
PROTOCOL FOR
RADIOGRAPHY OF THE HEAD

PROTOCOL FOR SURVEY STUDY
Routine views
    lateral
    dorsoventral
Optional views
    opposite lateral
    lateral obliques
    ventrodorsal
    frontal
    fronto-occipital for foramen magnum
    basilar for tympanic bullae
    basilar for odontoid process
    open-mouth ventrodorsal (extraoral film placement)
    closed-mouth dorsoventral (intraoral film placement)
    lateral oblique for temporomandibular joints

PROTOCOL FOR MAXILLA
Routine views
    lateral with mouth open
    lateral oblique with mouth open
    open-mouth ventrodorsal (extraoral film placement)
Optional views
    closed-mouth dorsoventral (intraoral film placement)

PROTOCOL FOR MANDIBLE
Routine views
    lateral with mouth open
    lateral oblique with mouth open
    dorsoventral
Optional views
    ventrodorsal
    ventrodorsal with intraoral film placement

PROTOCOL FOR DENTAL STUDIES
Routine views
    lateral
    dorsoventral
    lateral oblique of upper arcade
    lateral oblique of lower arcade

Optional views
    dorsoventral of maxillary incisors with intraoral film
      placement
    ventrodorsal of mandibular incisors with intraoral film
      placement

VIEWS

HEAD—LATERAL VIEW

Patient preparation: No special preparation other than cleaning the haircoat and removing any halter or collar.

Patient positioning: Place the patient in either right or left lateral recumbency dependent on the location of the lesion. The affected side is positioned next to the cassette unless the injury is of a nature that prevents this positioning. Place a foam wedge under the mandible to elevate the nose so that it is parallel to the tabletop and the rami of the mandible are superimposed. A line drawn through the medial canthus of the eyes should be perpendicular to the tabletop. It may be helpful to slightly open the mouth to separate the teeth. The pinnae (ears) must not be superimposed over areas of interest and are better positioned dorsal and caudally. Especially examine for the position of the dependent ear. A sandbag placed against the top of the head helps in positioning. The endotracheal tube may remain in position if the dog is anesthetized. The forelimbs are drawn back and held with sandbags or tied to the table. It is possible to a wooden spoon or paddle to help in the positioning.

X-ray beam direction: The vertically directed beam is perpendicular to the tabletop and centered at a point on the zygomatic arch midway between the eye and the ear. If interest is in the more rostal portion of the head, center the beam rostral and ventral to the eye. If the interest is in the mandible or teeth, center the beam on the point of interest.

Comments: Generally the radiographic technique is chosen to provide proper penetration of the thicker parts of the skull. Therefore, the nasal passages are over-exposed and require a bright light for evaluation of the radiograph. If the study is a dental study, increase the kVp setting because of the increase density of the teeth. Grid technique may be necessary in radiography of only the largest dogs.

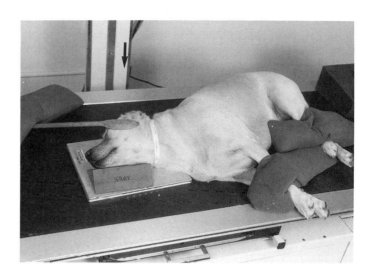

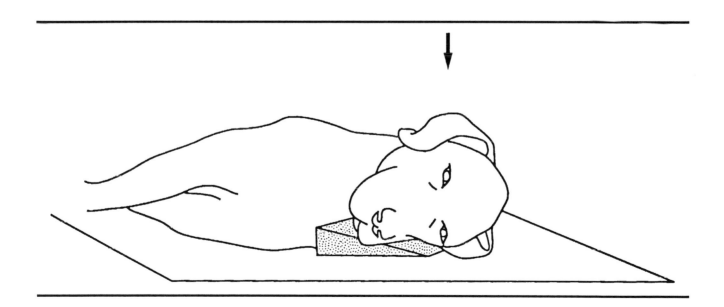

HEAD—DORSOVENTRAL VIEW

Patient preparation: No special preparation other than cleaning the haircoat and removing any halter or collar.

Patient positioning: Place the patient in sternal recumbency. The nature of the body of the mandible make positioning for this study relatively easy since it rests evenly on the tabletop. Ventral soft tissue swelling or the presence of a tumor mass might make this positioning more difficult. The head is held in position by putting pressure on the dorsum of the neck through use of a sandbag or through use of a gloved hand. The pinnae (ears) must not be superimposed over areas of interest and are better positioned laterally. The endotracheal tube casts an objectionable shadow but may remain in position if the dog is anesthetized. The forelimbs are held with sandbags. The body may be placed in a trough to assist in positioning.

X-ray beam direction: The vertically directed beam is perpendicular to the tabletop and centered between the eyes. If interest is in the more rostal portion of the head or in the teeth, center the beam just rostral to the eyes.

Comments: Generally the radiographic technique is chosen to provide proper penetration of the thicker parts of the skull. Therefore, the nasal passages are over-exposed and require a bright light for evaluation of the radiograph. If the study is a dental study, increase the kVp setting because of the increase density of the teeth. Grid technique may be required in only the largest dogs.

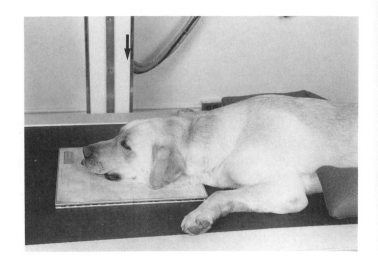

HEAD—VENTRODORSAL VIEW

Patient preparation: No special preparation other than cleaning the haircoat and removing any halter or collar.

Patient positioning: Place the patient in dorsal recumbency. Place a sponge so that it elevates the nose slightly. The size of this sponge varies with the conformation of the head. Try to position the head so the occipital bone is perpendicular to the tabletop and the nose points slightly upward. Resting the head on the occipital ridge makes positioning for this study difficult since the head tends to roll to one side or the other. Dorsal soft tissue swelling or the presence of a tumor mass might make this positioning more difficult. The head is held in position by using tape or a compression band across the mandible. The forelimbs are positioned lateral to the chest cavity and can be held by sandbags or tied. The pinnae (ears) are hidden under the head and must not be folded so they are superimposed over areas of interest. They are better positioned laterally where they can be used as handles in achieving correct positioning. The endotracheal tube casts an objectionable shadow but may remain in position if the dog is anesthetized. Notice the location of the dogs tongue so that it does not cause a shadow on the radiograph that is objectionable. The body may be positioned by using sandbags lateral to the thorax or by using a trough.

X-ray beam direction: The vertically directed beam is perpendicular to the tabletop and centered between the two parts of the mandible. If interest is in the more rostal portion of the head or in the teeth, center the beam just rostral to the eyes.

Comments: Generally the radiographic technique is chosen to provide proper penetration of the thicker parts of the skull. Therefore, the nasal passages are over-exposed and require a bright light for evaluation of the radiograph. If the study is a dental study, increase the kVp setting because of the increase density of the teeth. Grid technique may be required in only the largest dogs.

Brachycephalic breeds have a comparatively wide distance between the temporomandibular joints relative to the rostocaudal length of the nasal cavity. Also, the hard palate is located relatively nearer to the temporomandibular joints and the halves of the mandible converge far rostral to the tip of the nose. All of these factors serve to place the mandible over the nasal cavity at a location where its halves are widely separated suggesting that a closed mouth ventrodorsal view should be used to study the nasal cavity since it is free of mandibular superimposition. This view in brachycephalic breeds permits visualization of the frontal sinuses and the nasal area and is made with the skull rotated so that the nose is depressed 30° toward the tabletop. The shadow of the mandible is lateral so that it does not cast an overlying shadow except to cover the maxillary sinus recesses.

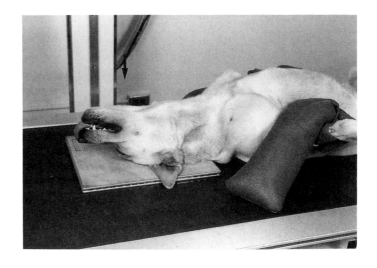

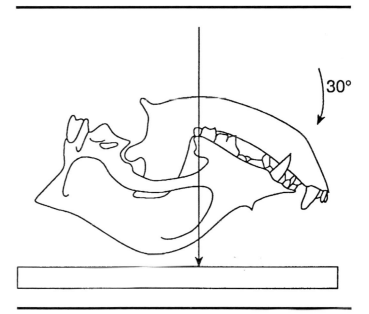

HEAD—FRONTAL VIEW

Patient preparation: No special preparation other than cleaning the haircoat and removing any halter or collar.

Patient positioning: Place the anesthetized patient in dorsal recumbency with the head positioned with the nose pointing upward. Place sandbags lateral to the head and next to the top of the head. The forelimbs are positioned lateral to the chest cavity and can be held by sandbags. The pinnae (ears) are positioned laterally. The endotracheal tube does not cause an objectionable shadow and may remain in position if the dog is anesthetized. Position the dogs tongue laterally so that it does not cause a shadow on the radiograph that is objectionable. Place sandbags to hold the forelimb lateral to the thorax. Tie the limbs if necessary. Place the body in a trough if thought to be helpful.

X-ray beam direction: The vertically directed beam is perpendicular to the tabletop and centered between the eyes. If the skull is positioned correctly, the beam is parallel to the bridge of the nose.

Comments: The kVp is decreased for this study because the thickness of the tissue to be penetrated is minimal. Therefore, the remainder of the radiograph is greatly underexposed.

This study is difficult or impossible in those breeds without prominent frontal bones such as the collie. The flatter the head the greater the limitation to visualize the frontal sinuses clear of the cranial vault.

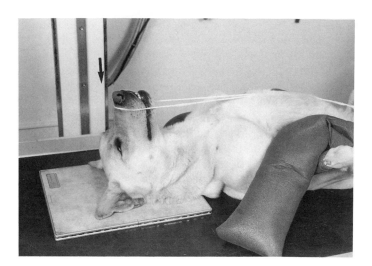

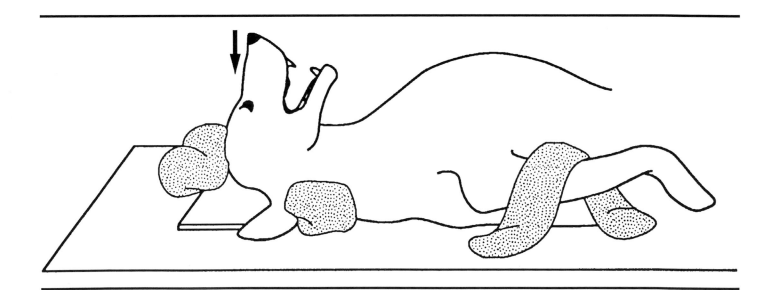

HEAD—FRONTO-OCCIPITAL VIEW

Patient preparation: No special preparation other than cleaning the haircoat and removing any halter or collar.

Patient positioning: Place the anesthetized patient in dorsal recumbency with the head positioned with the nose pointing upward but angled in a caudal direction between 30° and 45°. Place sandbags lateral to the head and next to the top of the head to achieve a degree of stabilization. The pinnae (ears) are positioned laterally. The forelimbs are positioned lateral to the chest cavity and can be held by sandbags. The endotracheal tube may cause an objectionable shadow but may remain in position if the dog is anesthetized. Position the dogs tongue laterally so that it does not cause a shadow on the radiograph that is objectionable. The dog's body can be positioned within a trough.

X-ray beam direction: The vertically directed beam is perpendicular to the tabletop and centered between the eyes. If the skull is positioned correctly, the beam intersects at an angle with the bridge of the nose.

Comments: Use the same technique as used for the routine views of the skull. The thickness of the tissue to be penetrated is slightly decreased, but the calvarium has a greater thickness of bone.

This study can be performed in all dogs and permits evaluation of the foramen magnum and the surrounding occipital bone.

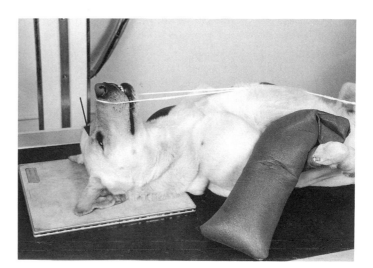

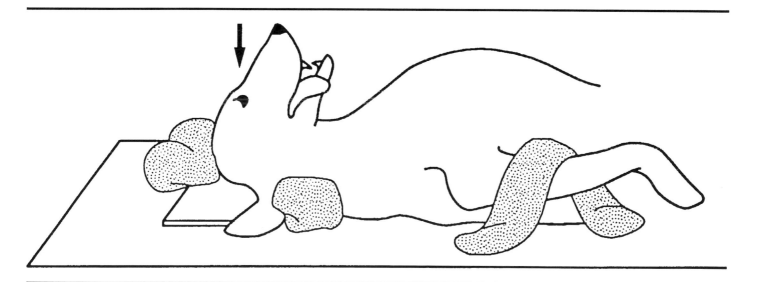

HEAD—BASILAR VIEW

Patient preparation: No special preparation other than cleaning the haircoat and removing any halter or collar.

Patient positioning: Place the patient in dorsal recumbency with the head positioned with the nose pointing upward. By placing gauze around the upper canine teeth and pulling rostrally and placing gauze around the lower canine teeth and pulling caudally the mouth can be held open. It is also possible to open the mouth by using a roll of gauze bandage or other suitable mouth speculum. Position the head so that the central beam bisects the angle created by the open-mouth (the hard palate and the horizontal rami of the mandible) realizing that this positioning is breed dependent. Place sandbags lateral to the head and next to the top of the head to achieve a degree of stabilization. The forelimbs are positioned lateral to the chest cavity and can be held by sandbags. The pinnae (ears) are positioned laterally. The endotracheal tube may cause an objectionable shadow and may be removed for this view if the dog is anesthetized. Position the dogs tongue laterally so that it does not cause a shadow on the radiograph that is objectionable. Use a trough to position the body if necessary.

X-ray beam direction: The vertically directed beam is perpendicular to the tabletop and bisects the angle created by the open-mouth.

Comment: Decrease the kVp technique used for the routine views of the skull since the thickness of the tissue to be penetrated is slightly decreased.

This study can be performed in all dogs and permits evaluation of the tympanic bullae and the odontoid process.

Brachycephalic breeds require use of a larger palatial angle (approximately 21°) than the mesaticephalic breeds (approximately 9°) and the dolichocephalic breeds (approximately 4°).

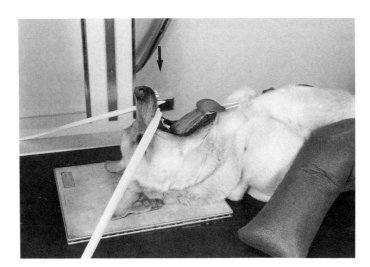

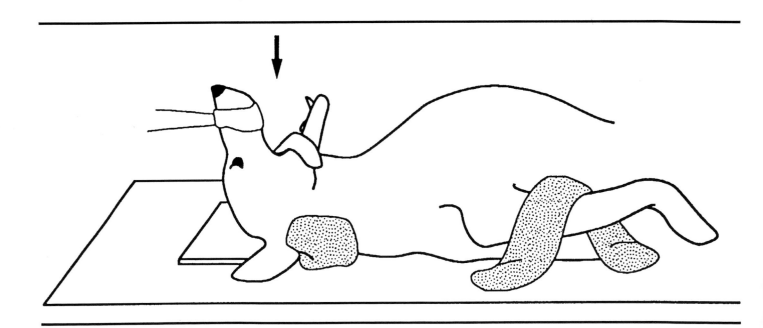

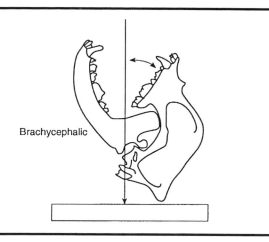

Brachycephalic

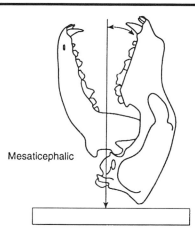

Mesaticephalic

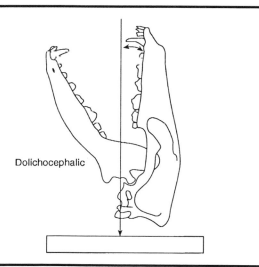

Dolichocephalic

HEAD—OPEN MOUTH VENTRODORSAL VIEW
(with extraoral film placement)

Patient preparation: No special preparation other than cleaning the haircoat and removing any halter or collar.

Patient positioning: Place the anesthetized or sedated patient in dorsal recumbency with the nose elevated slightly by placement of a foam wedge beneath the nose and the tabletop so the hard palate is parallel with the tabletop. The nose and mandible are held in position by tape to the tabletop. The mouth is opened as widely as possible with gauze placed around the lower canine teeth and pulled caudally. Include the dogs tongue within the gauze so that it does not cause an artifact on the radiograph. Place sandbags lateral to the head to achieve a degree of stabilization. The forelimbs are positioned lateral to the chest cavity and can be held by sandbags. The pinnae (ears) are positioned laterally. The endotracheal tube is held tightly next to the lower jaw.

X-ray beam direction: The vertically directed beam is angled between 20° and 30° to the tabletop in a rostrocaudal direction. The angle of the beam is somewhat dependent on the conformation of the head and how wide open is the mouth.

Comment: Decrease the kVp technique used for the routine views of the skull since only the nasal tissue is to be penetrated.

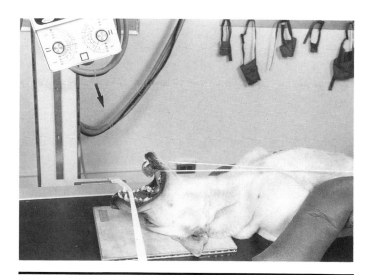

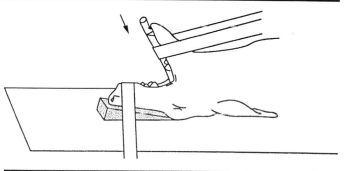

HEAD—CLOSED MOUTH DORSOVENTRAL VIEW
(with intraoral film placement)

Patient preparation: No special preparation other than cleaning the haircoat and removing any halter or collar.

Patient positioning: Place the anesthetized patient in sternal recumbency with the mandible resting on the tabletop. The mouth is opened as widely as possible to enable positioning of one corner of the cassette into the mouth. Non-screen film may be used. Place a sandbag over the neck for positioning. The pinnae (ears) are positioned laterally. The endotracheal tube is removed for this view. The dog's tongue is positioned beneath the cassette so that it does not cause a shadow on the radiograph. The forelimbs are positioned lateral to the thorax and can be held by sandbags.

X-ray beam direction: The vertically directed beam is perpendicular to the tabletop for the routine view. Angle the beam at a rostrocaudal angle to the film between 10° and 15° to better evaluate the incisor region and also obtain a view of the more caudal portion of the nasal region.

Comment: Decrease the kVp technique used for the routine views of the skull since only the nasal tissue is to be penetrated.

Non-screen film can be used effectively for this study since it can be positioned further into the mouth than can a bulky screened cassette.

HEAD—CLOSED MOUTH VENTRODORSAL VIEW
(with intraoral film placement)

Patient preparation: No special preparation other than cleaning the haircoat and removing any halter or collar.

Patient positioning: Place the anesthetized patient in dorsal recumbency. The mouth is opened to enable positioning of one corner of the cassette into the mouth. Non-screen film may be used. Hold the head in position by tape fastened to the tabletop. Place a sandbag over the neck and beside the head for positioning. The pinnae (ears) are positioned laterally. The dogs tongue is positioned laterally so that it does not cause a shadow on the radiograph. The forelimbs are positioned lateral to the thorax and can be held by sandbags.

X-ray beam direction: The vertically directed beam is perpendicular to the tabletop for the routine view and centered in the intermandibular space.

Comment: Decrease the kVp technique used for the routine views of the skull since only the mandible is to be penetrated.

Non-screen film can be used effectively for this study since it can be positioned further into the mouth than can a bulky screened cassette.

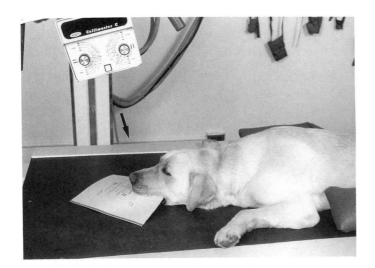

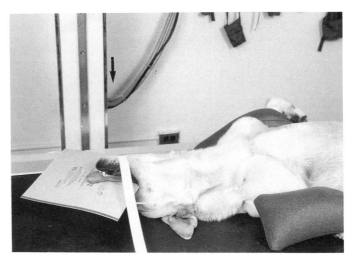

HEAD—LATERAL OBLIQUE VIEW FOR TEMPOROMANDIBULAR JOINTS

Patient preparation: No special preparation other than cleaning the haircoat and removing any halter or collar.

Patient positioning: Place the anesthetized patient in lateral recumbency with the joint to be studied dependent. Elevate the nose using a wedge shaped sponge. The angle created by the sponge is dependent on the conformation of the head. The angle required to radiograph the dolichocephalic breeds is approximately 10°, the angle for the mesaticephalic breeds is approximately 15°, and the angle for the brachycephalic breeds is between 25° and 30°. In addition, rotate the head dorsally, regardless of conformation, 10° so that the joint to be studied is positioned ventrally. The mouth is held partially open by a speculum. Place a sandbag over the neck to assist in positioning. The pinnae (ears) are positioned laterally. The endotracheal tube can be left is position for this view. The dogs tongue is positioned so that it does not cause a shadow on the radiograph. The forelimbs are positioned lateral to the thorax and can be held by sandbags.

X-ray beam direction: The vertically directed beam is perpendicular to the tabletop. This directs the beam along the articular surfaces of the medial portion of the dependent joint.

Comments: Use the kVp technique used for the routine views of the skull since it is necessary to penetrate the heavy portion of the calvarium

Usually both joints are radiographed.

The tympanic bullae are also identified on this oblique lateral view to good advantage.

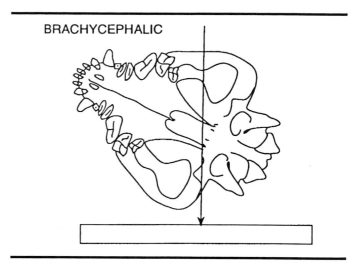

BRACHYCEPHALIC

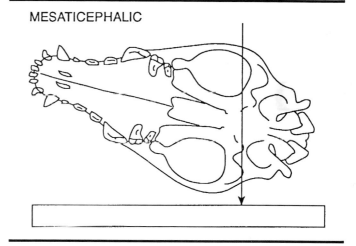

MESATICEPHALIC

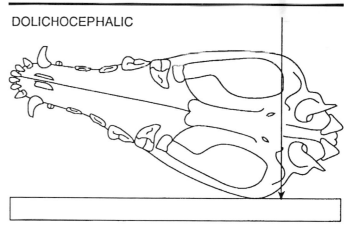

DOLICHOCEPHALIC

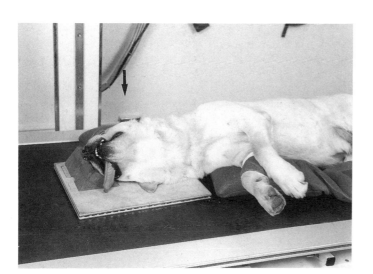

HEAD—OBLIQUE VIEW
FOR THE UPPER DENTAL ARCADE

Patient preparation: No special preparation other than cleaning the haircoat and removing any halter or collar.

Patient positioning: Place the anesthetized patient in right or left lateral recumbency with the affected side positioned next to the cassette. Place a foam wedge under the mandible to elevate the nose slightly and rotate the head. The degree of obliquity should be between 30° and 45°. Open the mouth using a speculum to separate the dental arcades. The pinnae (ears) must not be superimposed over areas of interest and are better positioned dorsal and caudally. Especially examine for the position of the dependent ear. The endotracheal tube may remain in position if the dog is anesthetized. The dogs tongue is positioned so that it does not cause a shadow on the radiograph. Use sandbags against the top of the head to assist with positioning. The forelimbs are held with sandbags or are tied to the table.

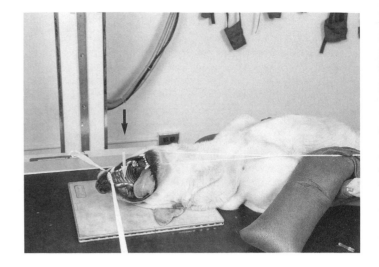

X-ray beam direction: The vertically directed beam is perpendicular to the tabletop and centered on the 4th premolar.

Comments: Generally the radiographic technique is chosen to provide proper penetration of the thicker parts of the skull. Therefore, the nasal passages are over-exposed and require a bright light for evaluation of the radiograph. Because the study is a dental study, it may be helpful to increase the kVp setting because of the increase density of the teeth. Grid technique may be necessary in radiography of only the largest dogs.

For those views in which only the roots of the premolars and molars need to be evaluated, the degree of rotation of the head can be between 25° and 35°. The orientation of the head required to visualize the entire upper canine tooth is 50° from lateral for dolichocephalic breeds, 45° for mesaticephalic breeds, and 35° for brachycephalic breeds. If only the roots of the upper premolars and molars needs to be evaluated, the rotation for dolichocephalic breeds and mesaticephalic breeds in 35° and is 25° for brachycephalic breeds.

Usually a roll of gauze or tape is used as a speculum since a metal mouth speculum is undesirable because of its opacity.

Usually oblique views of both upper dental arcades are made.

This study also provides evaluation of the bony lesions of the upper maxilla.

HEAD—OBLIQUE VIEW
FOR THE LOWER DENTAL ARCADE

Patient preparation: No special preparation other than cleaning the haircoat and removing any halter or collar.

Patient positioning: Place the anesthetized or sedated patient in lateral recumbency with the dental arcade to be studied on the dependent side. Open the mouth widely using a speculum of some type. The angle created by the sponge is dependent on the conformation of the head. Try to obtain an angle of approximately 30° to 45°. The pinnae (ears) are positioned caudally. The endotracheal tube can be left in position for this view. The dogs tongue is positioned so that it does not cause a shadow on the radiograph. The forelimbs are positioned lateral to the thorax and can be held by sandbags.

X-ray beam direction: The vertically directed beam is perpendicular to the tabletop and centered on the fourth lower premolar tooth.

Comments: Use the kVp technique used for the routine views of the skull since the dental structures are dense.

Usually oblique views of both lower dental arcades are made.

Usually a roll of gauze or tape is used as a speculum since a metal mouth speculum is undesirable because of its opacity.

This study also provides evaluation of the bony lesions of the mandible.

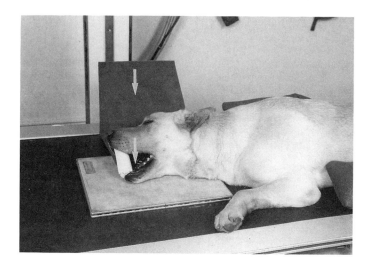

5. RADIOGRAPHY OF THE SPINE

INTRODUCTION

The average hospital or clinic has radiographic equipment of sufficiently high quality to perform spinal radiography. Since almost all patients are sedated or anesthetized, unusually brief exposure times or high kVp settings are not required. Even film-screen systems of average speed are satisfactory.

INDICATIONS

Most patients requiring spinal radiography have suffered acute spinal injury and present with paresis or paralysis that is partial or complete. Another group of patient include those in which less severe neurological signs are chronic but progressive and they are finally brought into the clinic. Because of the requirement that each of the vertebral segments and adjacent intervertebral discs be examined, requirements for radiographic positioning are somewhat more demanding than needed for radiography of the long bones.

Specific indications include: (1) acute disc disease, (2) chronic disc disease, (3) discitis/spondylitis/discospondylitis, (4) fracture/luxations, (5) congenital lesions, (6) degenerative changes, (7) tumors, and (8) vertebral instability.

CONTRAINDICATIONS

There are no contraindications for spinal radiography. Even if the patient cannot be carefully positioned because it cannot be sedated or anesthetized, it is possible to make a survey type study of the spine by making multiple lateral views. The problem associated with this type of survey examination is that the radiographs are accepted as a study of high quality instead of evaluating them for only prominent injury or disease and completing the study at another time.

PROTOCOL

Positioning is important and the following rules may help as you deal with the patient with a possible injury to the spinal cord. When possible, the patient should be sedated or anesthetized. A specific protocol should be followed when radiographing the parts of the spine (Table 5-1).

Use sponges in positioning the body so that the spine is parallel to the tabletop and so that the body is not rotated. Center the beam over the spine. Use smaller cassettes and include several views of the spine so that the inter vertebral disc spaces are parallel to the central beam and can be more accurately evaluated. The lateral views can be made with either side of the dog dependent, but are most easily made with the patient in right lateral recumbency because most right-handed workers find it more comfortable to work with the dog in that position. Ventrodorsal views are usually easier to make than dorsoventral views. It may not be possible to position the patient in dorsal recumbency because of the nature of the injury or because of pain. Under these circumstances, it may be helpful to use a horizontal cross-table beam and permit the dog to remain in lateral recumbency. This is not a high-quality radiograph, but may suffice for a survey study. Coned-down views may be helpful once a suspect lesion has been located. By using strict collimation and centering over the area of interest, the resulting radiograph may be of surprisingly high quality.

Dynamic radiography of the spine is possible especially in the cervical and lumbosacral regions. Lateral views are made with the patient in hyperflexion and hyperextension. If the patient is anesthetized, it is relatively easy to achieve these dynamic positions and it is possible that the spinal cord may undergo further compression caused by these dynamic movements. This is of greater concern in the smaller dogs.

Table 5-1
PROTOCOL FOR SPINAL RADIOGRAPHY

Anatomical location	Radiographic views
Survey study	
large dog	lateral center on C3-4, T6-7, T-L, L3-4, L-S
small dog	lateral center on C3-4, T6-7, L3-4
Occipitoatlantoaxial Spine	lateral neutral position hyperflexed position hyperextended position head rotated for odontoid process ventrodorsal open-mouth fronto-occipital open-mouth basilar
Cervical spine	lateral center C3-4 and C6-T1 ventrodorsal center C3-4
Thoracic spine	lateral center T6-7 ventrodorsal center T6-7
Lumbar spine	lateral center L3-4 ventrodorsal center L3-4
Lumbosacral spine	lateral neutral position hyperflexed position hyperextended position ventrodorsal beam angled caudo-cranially

A. CERVICAL SPINE

CERVICAL SPINE—LATERAL VIEW

Patient preparation: None required except for cleaning the haircoat and removing a collar.

Patient positioning: Place the sedated or anesthetized dog in lateral recumbency using sponges beneath the cervical spine to make the spine parallel to the tabletop. Use sponges beneath the sternum if necessary to achieve lateral positioning. Achieve lateral positioning of the entire body even though you intend to only radiograph the cervical spine. It is especially important that the head be in a perfect lateral position as well since obliquity of the head influences the position of the cranial cervical vertebrae. Sandbags can be used to position the head and can be placed on the limbs. Extend the head slightly. The forelimbs can be positioned caudally and pelvic limbs can be in neutral position placed one over the other tied to the tabletop or held with sandbags.

X-ray beam direction: The vertically directed beam is perpendicular to the tabletop and centered on C3-4.

Comments: Measurements should be made across the shoulder region at the level of C6 to insure adequate penetration of the beam of this region. The remainder of the film may be slightly overexposed but can be evaluated using a bright light.

Coned-down views can be made as desired.

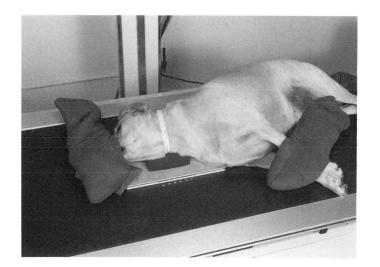

CERVICAL SPINE— LATERAL HYPEREXTENDED VIEW

Patient preparation: None required except for cleaning the haircoat and removing a collar.

Patient positioning: Place the sedated or anesthetized dog in lateral recumbency using sponges to make the spine parallel to the tabletop. Sandbags can be used to position the head and a sponge can be placed ventral to the mandible to maintain the hyperextended position. Use sponges beneath the sternum to help achieve lateral positioning of the body, if necessary. Position the head in a perfect lateral position since obliquity of the head influences positioning of the cranial cervical vertebrae. The forelimbs may be separated by sandbags and held so the body is in a lateral position and not obliqued. The pelvic limbs can be in neutral position placed one over the other tied to the tabletop or held with sandbags.

X-ray beam direction: The vertically directed beam is perpendicular to the tabletop and centered on C3-4

Comments: Measurements should be made across the neck at the level of C3-4. Views are usually well collimated and serve as coned-down views.

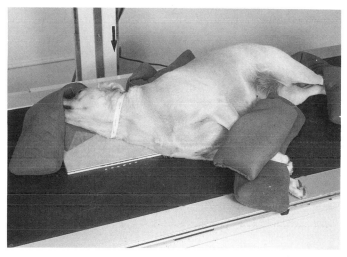

CERVICAL SPINE— LATERAL HYPERFLEXED VIEW

Patient preparation: None required except for cleaning the haircoat and removing a collar.

Patient positioning: Place the sedated or anesthetized dog in lateral recumbency using sponges to make the spine parallel to the tabletop. Elevate the nose using a sponge. Sandbags can be used to position the head and can be especially placed dorsal to the nose to maintain the hyperflexed position. Use sponges beneath the sternum to achieve lateral positioning of the body. It is especially important that the head be in a perfect lateral position as well since obliquity of the head influences the cranial cervical vertebrae. The forelimbs may be separated through the use of sandbags and are positioned caudally. The pelvic limbs can be in neutral position placed one over the other tied to the tabletop or held with sandbags.

X-ray beam direction: The vertically directed beam is perpendicular to the tabletop and centered on C3-4.

Comments: Measurements should be made across the neck at the level of C3-4. Views are usually well collimated and serve as coned-down views.

CERVICAL SPINE—LATERAL OBLIQUE VIEW FOR THE ODONTOID PROCESS

Patient preparation: No special preparation other than cleaning the haircoat and removing a collar.

Patient positioning: Place the anesthetized patient in lateral recumbency. Permit the head to assume a naturally obliqued position. The pinnae (ears) are positioned laterally. The endotracheal tube can be left is position for this view. The dogs tongue is positioned so that it does not cause a shadow on the radiograph. The forelimbs are positioned lateral to the thorax and can be held by sandbags.

X-ray beam direction: The vertically directed beam is perpendicular to the tabletop and centered on C1.

Comments: The cervical spine is positioned in lateral position and the head and the first cervical segment are oblique making the odontoid process visible.

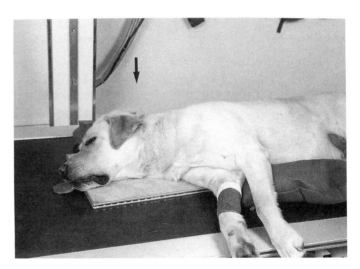

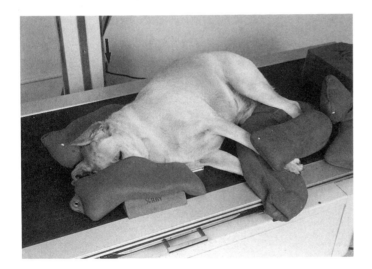

CERVICAL SPINE—VENTRODORSAL VIEW

Patient preparation: None required except for cleaning the haircoat and removing a collar.

Patient positioning: Place the sedated or anesthetized dog in dorsal recumbency using sponges placed under the more rostral portion of the neck to make the cervical spine parallel to the tabletop. Position the head so that the nose is pointing upward. If the head if fully extended, the occipital bone lies superimposed under C1-2. Sandbags may be positioned lateral to the head and neck. The body may be placed in a trough or stabilized by a compression band. The forelimbs are pulled caudally and held by sandbags or ropes. The pelvic limbs can be in neutral position.

X-ray beam direction: The vertically directed beam is angled slightly in a caudocranial direction to the tabletop and centered on C3-4.

Comments: This is often the last view made of the study of the cervical spine and it is convenient to remove an endotracheal tube prior to this view. Measurements should be made at the level of C6. This results in adequate exposure of the caudal cervical segments but minimal overexposure of the first cervical segments had may beed to be evaluated using a bright light. Collimate as necessary in obtaining coned-down views.

With the dog in this position, it is possible to open the mouth and make an open-mouth view of the odontoid process as described in the section on radiography of the head.

It is possible to rotate the patient's body and make oblique views of the cervical spine. Try to achieve 30° of obliquity with the ventrodorsal views. The endotracheal tube need not be removed for the oblique views.

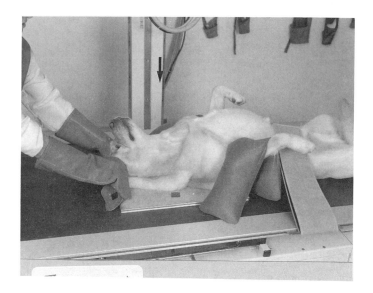

B. THORACIC SPINE

THORACIC SPINE—LATERAL VIEW

Patient preparation: None required except for cleaning the haircoat.

Patient positioning: Place the sedated dog in either lateral recumbency using sponges to make the spine parallel to the tabletop. Use a sponge beneath the sternum to achieve lateral positioning. Attempt to achieve this lateral positioning of the entire body even though you intend to only radiograph the thoracic spine. Sandbags can be placed on the neck to help position the dog. The forelimbs are extended and can be held with sandbags or tied to the table. The pelvic limbs are in neutral position or extended being placed one over the other and tied to the tabletop or held with sandbags.

X-ray beam direction: The vertically directed beam is perpendicular to the tabletop and centered on T6-7.

Comments: Measurements should be made across the mid-thorax. Coned-down views can be made as desired.

THORACIC SPINE—VENTRODORSAL VIEW

Patient preparation: None required except for cleaning the haircoat.

Patient positioning: Place the sedated dog in dorsal recumbency. Sandbags may be positioned lateral to the thorax and abdomen. The body may be positioned so the abdomen is in a trough or held by a compression band. The forelimbs are pulled cranially and held by sandbags or ropes. The pelvic limbs can be in neutral position either held or tied to the table.

X-ray beam direction: The vertically directed beam is centered on T6-7.

Comments: Collimate as necessary in obtaining coned-down views.

It is possible to rotate the patient's body and make oblique studies of the thoracic spine. Try to achieve 30° of obliquity with the ventrodorsal views.

This study can be made with a dorsoventral beam and the dog in sternal recumbency. Positioning may be more difficult.

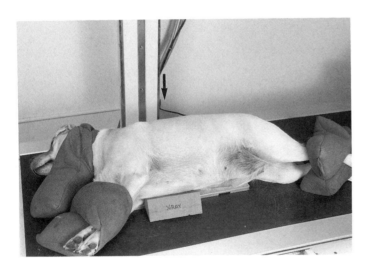
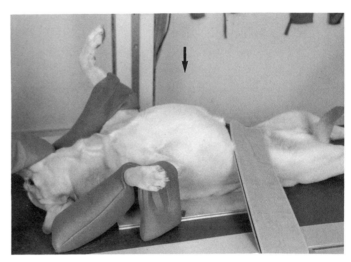

C. LUMBAR SPINE

LUMBAR SPINE—LATERAL VIEW

Patient preparation: None required except for cleaning the haircoat.

Patient positioning: Place the dog in lateral recumbency using sponges beneath the sternum or abdomen to achieve lateral positioning of the body. The forelimbs are extended slightly and are held with sandbags or tied to the tabletop. The pelvic limbs can be in neutral position or slightly extended and placed one over the other tied to the tabletop or held with sandbags. It may be helpful to place a sponge between the hindlegs

X-ray beam direction: The vertically directed beam is perpendicular to the tabletop and centered on L3-4.

Comments: Measurements should be made across the abdomen at the level of L6-7 to insure adequate penetration of the beam for the entire lumbar spine. Coned-down views can be made as desired.

LUMBAR SPINE—VENTRODORSAL VIEW

Patient preparation: None required except for cleaning the haircoat.

Patient positioning: Place the sedated dog in dorsal recumbency. Sandbags may be positioned lateral to the thorax. The body may be positioned so the thorax is in a trough or held by a compression band. The forelimbs are pulled cranially and held by sandbags or ropes. The pelvic limbs are fully extended and either held or tied to the table.

X-ray beam direction: The vertically directed beam is centered on L3-4.

Comments: Collimate as necessary in obtaining coned-down views.

It is possible to rotate the patient's body and make oblique studies of the lumbar spine. Try to achieve 30° of obliquity with the ventrodorsal views.

This study can be made with a dorsoventral beam and the dog in sternal recumbency. Positioning may be more difficult.

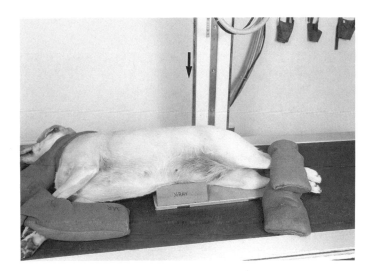

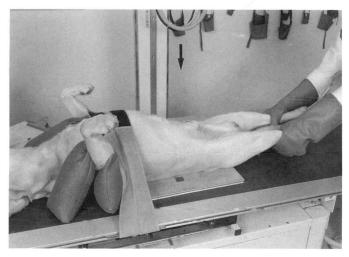

D. LUMBOSACRAL SPINE

LUMBOSACRAL SPINE—LATERAL VIEW
(neutral positioning)

Patient preparation: None required except for cleaning the haircoat.

Patient positioning: Place the dog in lateral recumbency using sponges beneath the abdomen to achieve lateral positioning of the body. The forelimbs are extended slightly and are held with sandbags or tied to the tabletop. The pelvic limbs are in neutral position or extended and placed one over the other tied to the tabletop or held with sandbags. Place a sponge between the hindlegs

X-ray beam direction: The vertically directed beam is perpendicular to the tabletop and centered on L-S junction

Comments: Use the technique for pelvic studies to insure adequate penetration.

LUMBOSACRAL SPINE—LATERAL VIEW
(hyperflexed view)

Patient preparation: None required except for cleaning the haircoat.

Patient positioning: Place the dog in lateral recumbency using sponges beneath the abdomen to achieve lateral positioning of the body. The pelvic limbs are pulled into a hyperflexed position and placed one over the other and tied to the tabletop or held with sandbags. Place a sponge between the hindlegs. The forelimbs are extended slightly and are held with sandbags or tied to the tabletop.

X-ray beam direction: The vertically directed beam is perpendicular to the tabletop and centered on L-S junction

Comments: Use the technique for pelvic studies to insure adequate penetration.

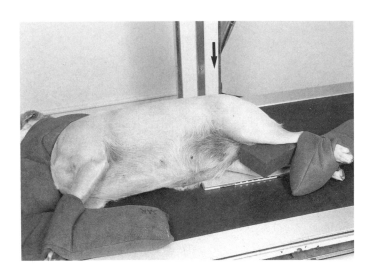

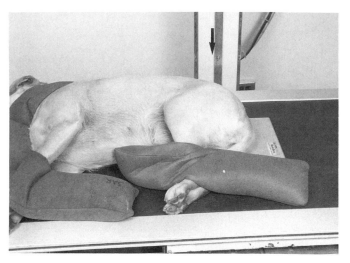

LUMBOSACRAL SPINE—LATERAL VIEW
(hyperextended view)

Patient preparation: None required except for cleaning the haircoat.

Patient positioning: Place the dog in lateral recumbency using sponges beneath the abdomen to achieve lateral positioning of the body. The pelvic limbs are pulled into a fully extended position and placed one over the other tied to the tabletop or held with sandbags. Place a sponge between the hindlegs. The forelimbs are extended slightly and are held with sandbags or tied to the tabletop.

X-ray beam direction: The vertically directed beam is perpendicular to the tabletop and centered on L-S junction

Comments: Use the technique for pelvic studies to insure adequate penetration.

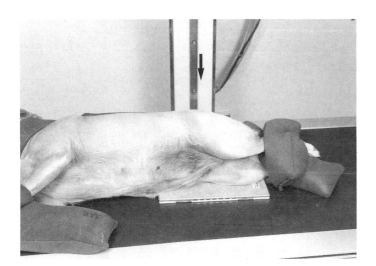

LUMBOSACRAL SPINE—
VENTRODORSAL VIEW

Patient preparation: None required except for cleaning the haircoat.

Patient positioning: Place the dog in dorsal recumbency. Position the body with the forelimbs pulled cranially and held by sandbags or ropes. The body may be positioned so the thorax is in a trough or held by a compression band. Sandbags may be positioned lateral to the thorax and abdomen. The pelvic limbs are partially extended and may be in external rotation.

X-ray beam direction: The vertically directed beam is angled 30° in a caudocranial direction and centered on the L-S junction

Comments: Collimate as necessary in obtaining coned-down views.

It is possible to rotate the patient's body and make oblique studies of the lumbosacral junction.

This study can be made with a dorsoventral beam and the dog in sternal recumbency, however, use a vertical beam that is obliqued 20° to 30° craniocaudally.

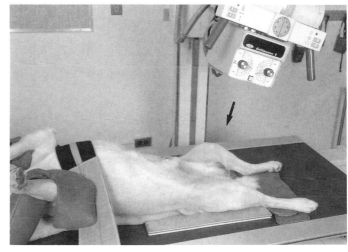

6. RADIOGRAPHY OF THE PELVIS AND HIP JOINTS

INTRODUCTION

Radiography of the pelvis is common because of frequent trauma involving both the pelvic bones and the hip joints and because of abnormal development of the hip joints that leads to a deforming arthrosis. Usually the trauma patient can be radiographed without sedation or anesthesia but the study for hip dysplasia usually requires some form of chemical restraint. It may be advisable to protect the testicles from radiation by covering them with a lead gonadal shield. Multiple views can be used especially when examining the hip joints (Table 6-1).

Table 6-1
PROTOCOL FOR RADIOGRAPHY OF THE PELVIS AND HIP JOINTS

Views for routine pelvis
    lateral
    ventrodorsal with limbs extended
    ventrodorsal with limbs in flexed position
Views for routine hip joint
    lateral hip joint
    lateral pelvis
    ventrodorsal with limbs flexed
Ventrodorsal views for hip dysplasia study
    with pelvic limbs extended
    with pelvic limbs flexed
    with pelvic limbs extended using a fulcrum
    with pelvic limbs flexed using a distraction technique

VIEWS
PELVIS—LATERAL VIEW

Patient preparation: The only preparation required is to clean the hair coat since this is often a film made following trauma.

Patient positioning: The dog is placed in lateral recumbency with the affected side next to the tabletop. The pelvic limbs are placed in a neutral position with the down limb slightly forward and are held in position by sandbags or tied. Notice the position of the tail, especially if it is long. If the dog is obese it may be necessary to place a sponge under the sternum and one between the pelvic limbs to position the pelvis in a true lateral position. The forelimbs are either held by sandbags or tied. A sandbag may be placed across the neck.

X-ray beam direction: The vertically directed beam is centered on the hip joint.

Comments: The radiographic technique is increased over than used for the spine because of the increase amount of bony tissue.

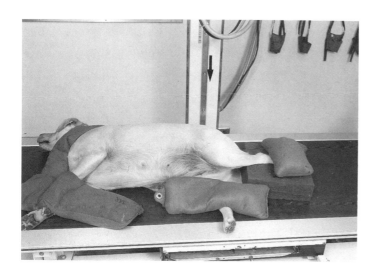

PELVIS—VENTRODORSAL VIEW
(with limbs extended)

Patient preparation: Nothing is required other than cleaning the hair coat. It may be desirable to sedate or anesthetize a large dog.

Patient positioning: The dog is placed in dorsal recumbency using a trough to assist in positioning, especially with a large dog. It is possible to use a compression band across the body in positioning or place sandbags lateral to the body, The pelvic limbs are in an extended position and can be tied to the table or held.

Attempt to place the pelvic limbs in internal rotation so the patellas are on the midline to provide the best positioning for a dysplasia examination. The forelimbs are extended forward and held by sandbags or tied to the table.

X-ray beam direction: The vertically directed beam is centered on the hip joints.

Comments: This is the position commonly used for a conventional hip dysplasia view and the dog is usually sedated or anesthetized so that the best positioning can be obtained. If the view is made following trauma or for another reason, the perfect positioning may not be required.

It should be understood that in attempting to extend the pelvic limbs fully, the femurs are not parallel to the tabletop but are approximately at a 30° angle with the tabletop.

Use a cassette large enough to include the femurs.

Often two films are placed within the cassette and the technique increased by 10 kVp so that two radiographs are produced at the time of a single exposure so one is available for referral for evaluation of the hip joints and the other can be retained by the practice. Instead of doing this, it is recommended that two separate exposures be made with the possibility of producing one film that is more diagnostic than the other.

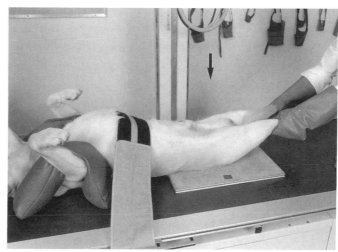

PELVIS—VENTRODORSAL VIEW
(with limbs flexed—frogleg view)

Patient preparation: Clean the hair coat.

Patient positioning: The dog is placed in dorsal recumbency using a trough to assist in positioning, especially with a large dog. It is possible to use a compression band across the body to assist in positioning or place sandbags lateral to the body. The pelvic limbs are held lateral to the pelvis forcing the limbs into a tight flexed position. It is possible to use sandbags over each foot to hold the pelvic limbs in position in a smaller dog. The forelimbs are extended forward and held by sandbags or tied to the table.

X-ray beam direction: The vertically directed beam is centered on the hip joints.

Comments: This view can be used in a hip dysplasia study. It also is the position used to obtain a study of the pelvis, especially of the hip joints, following trauma in which there is great pain associated with extending one of the limbs. The goal is to position both hip joints equally so that comparison can be more easily made on the radiograph.

Because of positioning, the cassette may be positioned crosswise.

PELVIS—VENTRODORSAL VIEW
(with limbs extended—fulcrum positioning)

Patient preparation: Clean the hair coat. It may be desirable to sedate or anesthetize the dog. Position a device between the dogs limbs that serves as a fulcrum. The size of the fulcrum varies with the size of the dog.

Patient positioning: The dog is placed in dorsal recumbency using a trough to assist, especially with a large dog. It is possible to use a compression band across the body to assist in positioning or place sandbags lateral to the body. The pelvic limbs must be hand held or the distal limbs wrapped together to obtain the inward pressure necessary to create the fulcrum effect. Attempt to place the pelvic limbs in internal rotation so the patellas are on the midline to provide the best positioning for a dysplasia examination. The forelimbs are extended forward and held by sandbags or tied to the table.

X-ray beam direction: The vertically directed beam is centered on the hip joints.

Comments: This position is used in a hip dysplasia study to obtain additional information that can be compared with the conventional hip dysplasia view. The dog is usually sedated or anesthetized so that good positioning can be obtained. The view has its greatest value in attempting to determine the degree of laxity within the hip joints.

Use a cassette large enough to include the femurs.

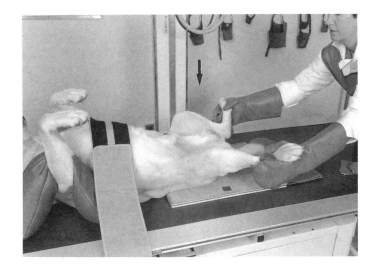

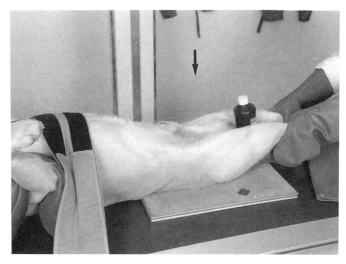

PELVIS—VENTRODORSAL VIEW
(with limbs flexed—distraction positioning)

Patient preparation: Clean the hair coat. It may be desirable to sedate or anesthetize the dog. Position a device around the dog's pelvic limbs that serves as a distraction device. It is also possible to achieve the same affect by placing a device between the pelvic limbs to force the limbs apart. ·

Patient positioning: The sedated or anesthetized dog is placed in dorsal recumbency using a trough or a compression band across the body to assist in positioning especially with a large dog. Sandbags may be placed lateral to the body. The pelvic limbs must be hand held or tied in a position so they are perpendicular to the tabletop. The distraction device is positioned so that there is a force attempting to subluxate the femoral heads. The forelimbs are extended forward and held by sandbags or tied to the table.

X-ray beam direction: The vertically directed beam is centered between the pelvic limbs.

Comments: This position is used in a special hip dysplasia study that demonstrates the exact amount of femoral head distraction that is possible. The dog is heavily sedated or anesthetized so that good positioning can be obtained. Increase the kVp by 10 because of the necessity of penetrating additional tissue because of the position of the pelvic limbs.

Use a cassette large enough to include the femurs.

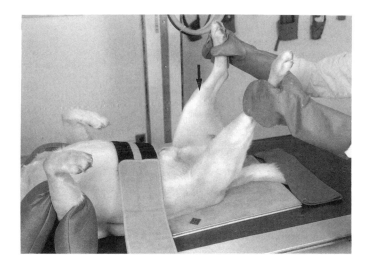

PELVIS—LATERAL VIEW OF THE HIP JOINT

Patient preparation: No special preparation required.

Patient positioning: Place the dog in lateral recumbency with the limb to be studied next to the table using sandbags to hold the limb in position. Abduct the unaffected leg and remove it from the field of view by tying or by use of sandbags. Use sandbags to stabilize the head and forelimbs.

X-ray beam direction: The vertically directed beam is centered on the dependent hip joint.

Comments: If pain prevents the complete abduction of the upper limb, it is possible to angle the x-ray beam in a distoproximal direction to project more of the hip joint. This can be easily done using tabletop technique without a grid.

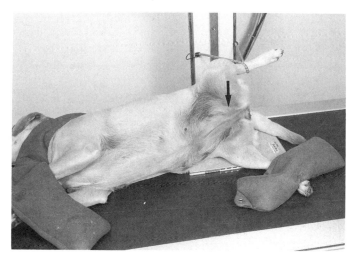

7. RADIOGRAPHY OF THE FORELIMB

A. INTRODUCTION

The lateral views of the forelimb are relatively easy to make, while the craniocaudal views in the proximal portion of the limb are more difficult because of the problem of being unable to position the bones parallel to the tabletop so they can be radiographed without geometric distortion. Oblique views are often made of the elbow and carpus, metacarpus, and digits and are helpful in diagnosis. Most of the views are made in patients with lameness or pain in the forelimb. Usually sedation or anesthesia is not required. Most studies except for the scapula in a large dog are made with tabletop technique without a grid. Often a comparable view of the opposite limb is helpful in diagnosis, especially if the growth plates have not closed. If the study is proximal on the limb, the lateral view of the opposite limb is the most easy comparison study to make. If the lesion is thought to be more distal, the craniocaudal view is the most easy comparison study to make. No special preparation of the limb is necessary for the studies except to clean the haircoat.

A survey study can be made rather easily that includes the entire limb and is of value in study of a skeletally immature patient. Usually the study is made using a craniocaudal beam and includes the elbow joint distally. If a lateral study is made, it can include the shoulder joint distally. These studies are usually made in a young dog suspected of having developmental bone or joint disease (Table 7-1).

Table 7-1
PROTOCOL FOR RADIOGRAPHY OF THE FORELIMB

SCAPULA
Routine views
    lateral
    caudocranial
Optional views
    lateral (dorsally displaced)

SHOULDER JOINT
Routine views
    lateral
    caudocranial
Optional views
    lateral
    extended
    flexed
      in internal rotation (supination)
      in external rotation (pronation)

HUMERUS
Routine views
    lateral
    craniocaudal
Optional views
    caudocranial
      with horizontal beam
      with vertical beam

ELBOW JOINT
Routine views
    lateral
    craniocaudal

Optional views
    craniocaudal
      internal oblique (supination)
      external oblique (pronation)
      with horizontal beam
    lateral flexed
    caudocranial with horizontal beam

RADIUS AND ULNA
Routine views
    lateral
    craniocaudal

CARPUS VIEWS
Routine views
    lateral
    dorsopalmar
Optional views
    dorsopalmar
      internal rotation (supination)
      external rotation (pronation)
    stress views
      lateral view with hyperextension
      lateral view with hyperflexion
      dorsopalmar view with lateral stress
      dorsopalmar view with medial stress

METACARPUS AND DIGITS
Routine views
    lateral
    dorsopalmar
Optional views
    dorsopalmar
      internal oblique (supination)
      external oblique (pronation)

B. SCAPULA

SCAPULA—LATERAL VIEW

Patient preparation: Remove dirt and debris from the hair coat.

Patient positioning: Place the patient in lateral recumbency with the affected limb down. Extend the limb cranially and place traction on it. The limb can be tied to the table. The opposite unaffected limb is removed from the x-ray beam by flexing the limb and pulling it caudally

X-ray beam direction: The vertically directed beam is centered on the neck of the scapula.

Comments: This view permits good evaluation of the neck of the scapula.

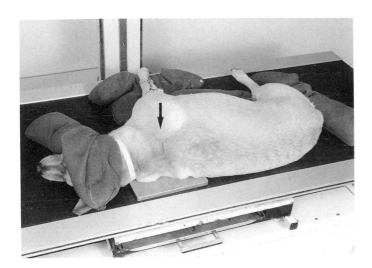

SCAPULA—LATERAL VIEW
(with dorsal displacement)

Patient preparation: Remove dirt and debris from the hair coat. The patient may require sedation.

Patient positioning: Place the patient in lateral recumbency with the affected leg down. Forcefully push the limb in a dorsal direction displacing the scapula dorsal to the vertebral column. Do this by grasping the limb firmly below the elbow joint, fixing it is extension, and pushing the shoulder upward until the scapula can be seen bulging the surface of the skin dorsal to the spinous processes of the thoracic vertebrae. At the same time pull the upper limb distally and in a caudal direction. This may create a slight rotation of the thorax but it isolates the scapula dorsal to the spine.

X-ray beam direction: The vertically directed beam is centered dorsally over the body of the scapula.

Comments: This technique cannot be used if the patient is painful and may be of value only with the use of chemical restraint.

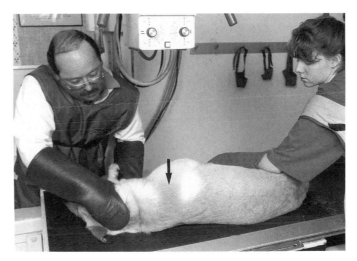

SCAPULA—CAUDOCRANIAL VIEW

Patient preparation: No special preparation.

Patient positioning: Place the patient in dorsal recumbency. Use a trough to support the abdomen or use a compression band. Extend the affected limb cranially as far as possible and hold it in position using sandbags or tie the limb to the table. Permit the dog's body to fall slightly away from the scapula, shifting the position of the ribs so that they are not superimposed over the scapula leaving the blade of the scapula perpendicular to the table. Tie the pelvic limbs to the tabletop or use sandbags to hold them in position.

X-ray beam direction: The vertically directed x-ray beam is centered on the scapula which can be rather easily palpated.

Comments: The technique used is the same as that uses for the dorsoventral view of the thorax.

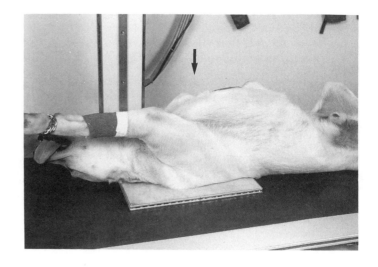

C. SHOULDER JOINT

SHOULDER JOINT—LATERAL VIEW

Patient preparation: No special preparation is required.

Patient positioning: Place the patient in lateral recumbency with the affected leg next to the tabletop. Forcefully pull the leg downward and cranially in order to position the shoulder joint ventral to the sternum and air-filled trachea and to separate the joint sufaces making evaluation of the joint easier. Arch the head and neck dorsally using sandbags to hold it in position. Pull the unaffected leg caudally and hold it with sandbags or tie it to the tabletop.

X-ray beam direction: The vertically directed x-ray beam is centered on the prominent acromion process

Comments: It is important to position the limb so the shoulder joint is not superimposed over the air filled trachea or the radiodense manubrium of the sternum. In attempting to extend the limb, it is often easy to rotate the dogs body by elevating the sternum from the tabletop. Avoid rotating the dog's body in this manner since it places the limb in an abducted position and positions the shoulder joint in an oblique position making evaluation of the articular surfaces of the shoulder joint difficult.

Correct positioning requires extension of the limb and may be difficult should the patient have a painful lesion. Sedation or anesthesia may be required.

This basic positioning can be altered slightly to make oblique views of the humeral head by turning the limb into a position of pronation or supination.

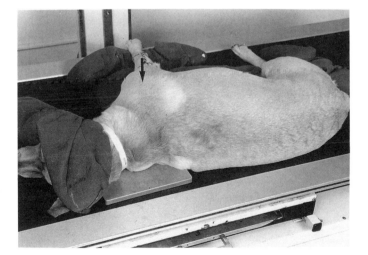

SHOULDER JOINT—CAUDOCRANIAL VIEW

Patient preparation: No special preparation is required.

Patient positioning: Place the patient in dorsal recumbency. Use a trough to support the abdomen or use a compression band over the thorax. Extend the affected limb as far as possible and hold it in position using sandbags or tie the limb to the tabletop. The dog's body falls slightly away from the scapula, shifting the ribs so that they are not superimposed over the shoulder joint leaving the blade of the scapula perpendicular to the tabletop. Tie the pelvic limbs to the tabletop or use sandbags to hold them in position.

X-ray beam direction: The vertically directed x-ray beam is centered on the shoulder joint which can be palpated.

Comments: The technique used is the same as that used for the dorsoventral view of the thorax.

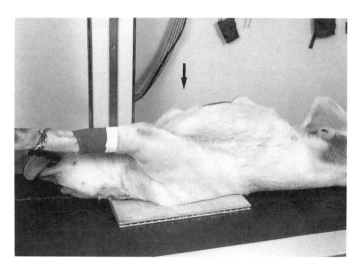

D. HUMERUS

HUMERUS—LATERAL VIEW

Patient preparation: Remove dirt and debris from the hair coat.

Patient positioning: Place the patient in lateral recumbency with the affected leg down. Extend the affected limb cranially and place traction on the limb. The opposite unaffected limb is removed from the x-ray beam by flexing the limb and pulling it caudally. Pull the dog's head dorsally so that it is not within the x-ray beam and use sandbags to hold the head in position. Place sandbags on the pelvic limbs or tie them to the table.

X-ray beam direction: The vertically directed beam is centered on the midshaft of the humerus

Comments: This view permits good evaluation of the humerus and the elbow joint. Usually the technique used does not penetrate the shoulder joint adequately.

HUMERUS—CRANIOCAUDAL VIEW
(limb extended)

Patient preparation: No special preparation is required.

Patient positioning: The patient is placed in ventral recumbency with the forelimb to be studied pulled as far cranially as possible and held by sandbags or tied to the table. The opposite forelimb can be left in a more natural position. This positioning does not place the humerus parallel to the tabletop.

X-ray beam direction: The vertically directed beam is angled distoproximally 10° to 20° in an effort to decrease geometric distortion.

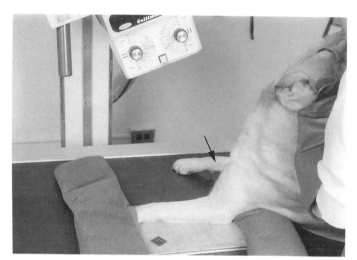

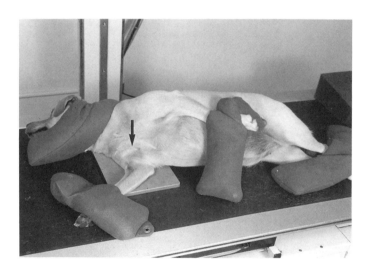

HUMERUS—CRANIOCAUDAL VIEW
(limb flexed)

Patient preparation: No special preparation is required.

Patient positioning: The patient is placed in dorsal recumbency with the forelimb to be studied flexed at the shoulder and pulled as far caudally as possible and tied to the table. The opposite forelimb is extended and either held or tied to the table. This positioning places the humerus more nearly parallel to the tabletop, however, there is a rather large object-film distance.

X-ray beam direction: The vertically directed beam is centered on the humerus.

HUMERUS—CAUDOCRANIAL VIEW
(horizontal beam)

Patient preparation: No special preparation is required.

Patient positioning: The patient is placed in lateral recumbency with the affected limb uppermost and the cassette positioned against the cranial aspect of the forelimb. The limb rests on a large sponge and is extended. The opposite forelimb can be left in a more natural position on the dependent side.

X-ray beam direction: The x-ray tube is positioned caudally and the horizontally directed beam is directed perpendicular to the cassette face.

Comments: It may not be possible to place the cassette far enough proximally to be able to study the humeral head and shoulder joint.

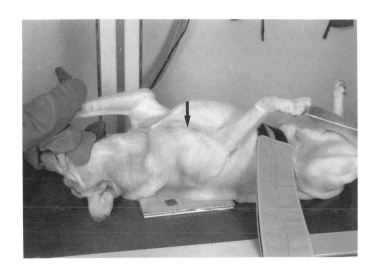

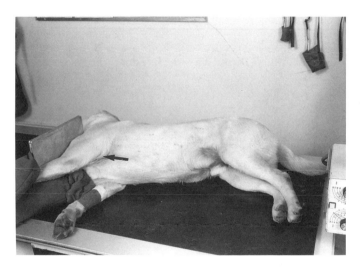

E. ELBOW JOINT

ELBOW JOINT—LATERAL VIEW (extended)

Patient preparation: No special preparation is required.

Patient positioning: Place the patient in lateral recumbency with the affected limb next to the tabletop. Forcefully pull the limb downward and cranially and position the limb so that the elbow joint is in a 120° extended position. Use sandbags to hold the limb in position. Arch the head and neck dorsally using sandbags to hold the position. Pull the unaffected leg caudally and hold it with sandbags or tie to the tabletop. Sandbags can be used to hold the pelvic limbs.

X-ray beam direction: The vertically directed x-ray beam is centered on the elbow joint.

Comments: If the lateral view of the elbow joint is made with the limb in partial extension of a specific angle, it is relatively easy to repeat that positioning on subsequent studies. With the elbow joint positioned in full extension, rotation of the limb into a position of supination is common and this alters the way the bones are seen on the radiograph.

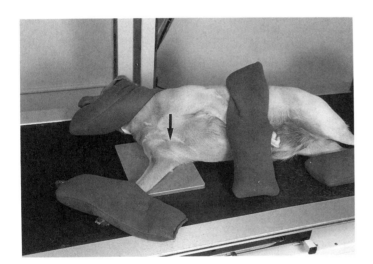

ELBOW JOINT—LATERAL VIEW (flexed)

Patient preparation: No special preparation is required.

Patient positioning: Place the patient in lateral recumbency with the affected leg next to the tabletop. Position the limb so that the elbow joint is in 90° flexion. Use sandbags to hold the limb in position. Arch the head and neck dorsally using sandbags to hold the position. Pull the unaffected leg caudally and hold it with sandbags or tie to the tabletop. Sandbags can be used to hold the pelvic limbs.

X-ray beam direction: The vertically directed x-ray beam is centered on the elbow joint.

Comments: If the lateral flexed view of the elbow joint is made with the limb flexed at 90°, evaluation of the anconeal process of the ulna is possible. It is relatively easy to repeat this positioning on subsequent studies.

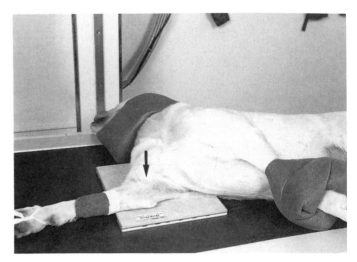

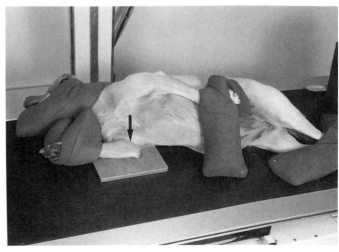

ELBOW JOINT—CRANIOCAUDAL VIEW
(vertical beam)

Patient preparation: No special preparation is required.

Patient positioning: The patient is placed in sternal recumbency with the forelimb to be studied pulled as far cranially as possible and held by sandbags or tied to the table. The opposite forelimb can be left in a neutral position. Hyperextend the dog's neck and pull the head laterally toward the unaffected limb so that it is not within the primary beam. This positioning places the radius and ulna parallel to the tabletop but the humerus remains at an angle to the tabletop.

X-ray beam direction: The vertically directed beam is angled distoproximally 10° to 20° in an effort to display the joint surfaces better.

ELBOW JOINT—CRANIOCAUDAL VIEW
(horizontal beam)

Patient preparation: No special preparation is required.

Patient positioning: The patient is placed in lateral recumbency with the forelimb to be studied uppermost, placed on a large sponge, pulled as far cranially as possible, and held by sandbags or tied to the table. The dependent forelimb can be left in a neutral position. Partially hyperextend the dog's neck to remove it from the x-ray beam. Rest the cassette in a vertical position next to the caudal aspect of the forelimb. Extend the limb forcing it into complete extension using the elbow joint as a fulcrum. Place the x-ray tube cranially. This positioning places the radius and ulna parallel to the cassette.

X-ray beam direction: The craniocaudally directed horizontal beam is perpendicular to the cassette.

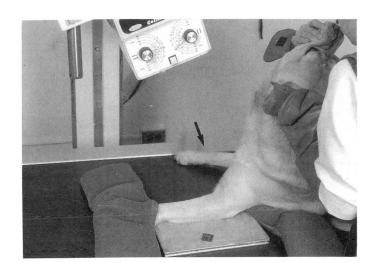

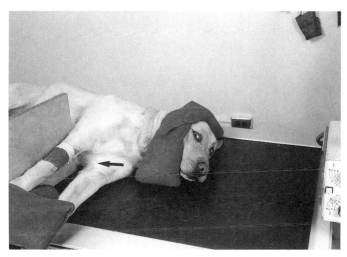

ELBOW JOINT—CAUDOCRANIAL VIEW
(horizontal beam)

Patient preparation: No special preparation is required.

Patient positioning: The patient is placed in lateral recumbency with the forelimb to be studied uppermost, placed on a large sponge, pulled as far cranially as possible, and held by sandbags or tied to the table. The dependent forelimb can be left in a neutral position. Partially hyperextend the dog's neck to permit placement of the cassette in a vertical position adjacent to the cranial aspect of the forelimb. Extend the limb forcing it into complete extension. Place the x-ray tube caudally. This positioning places the radius and ulna parallel to the cassette.

X-ray beam direction: The caudocranially directed horizontal beam is perpendicular to the cassette.

ELBOW JOINT—OBLIQUE VIEWS
(vertical beam)

Patient preparation: No special preparation is required.

Patient positioning: The patient is placed in sternal recumbency with the forelimb to be studied pulled as far cranially as possible and held by sandbags or tied to the table. Rotate the patient approximately 30° laterally for the lateral oblique and 30° for the medial oblique. The dog's head can be positioned laterally toward the unaffected limb so that it is not within the primary beam for both oblique views. The opposite forelimb can be left in a neutral position.

X-ray beam direction: The vertically directed beam is perpendicular to the tabletop for the oblique views.

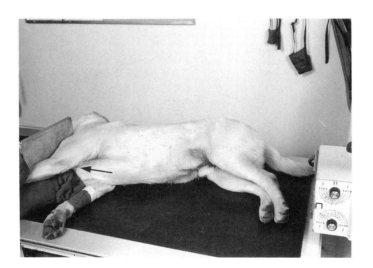

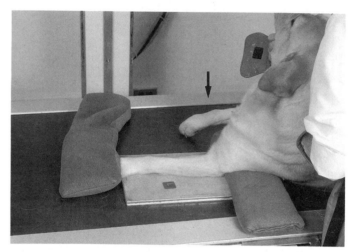

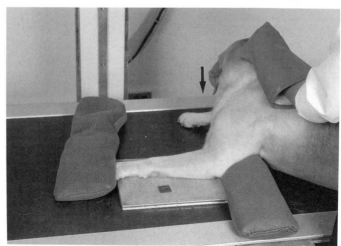

F. RADIUS AND ULNA (Antebrachium)
RADIUS AND ULNA—LATERAL VIEW

Patient preparation: No special preparation is required.

Patient positioning: Place the patient in lateral recumbency with the affected leg next to the tabletop. Forcefully extend the limb and hold it with sandbags or tied to the table. Slightly flex the carpus to avoid supination of the limb. Pull the unaffected leg caudally and hold it with sandbags or tie to the tabletop. Use sandbags to hold the head in a slightly extended position.

X-ray beam direction: The vertically directed x-ray beam is centered on the midshaft of the radius and ulna.

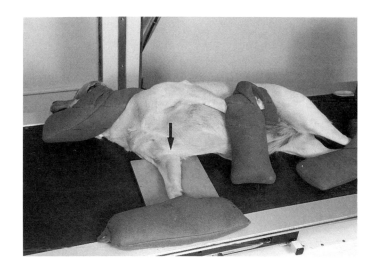

RADIUS AND ULNA—CRANIOCAUDAL VIEW

Patient preparation: No special preparation is required.

Patient positioning: The patient is placed in sternal recumbency with the forelimb to be studied pulled as far cranially as possible and held by sandbags or tied to the table. A sandbag can be placed just behind the elbow. The opposite forelimb can be left in a neutral position. The head is displaced laterally toward the unaffected limb.

X-ray beam direction: The vertically directed beam is centered on the midshaft of the radius and ulna.

Comments: It is also possible to make this study with a horizontally directed x-ray beam. Position the patient with the affected limb uppermost and resting on a large sponge. The cassette is placed against either the caudal or cranial aspect of the limb and the x-ray tube positioned in front or behind the limb with the x-ray beam directed at the midshaft of the radius and ulna.

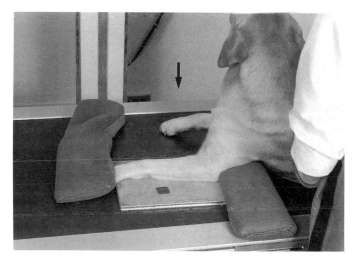

G. CARPUS-METACARPUS-DIGITS (Foot)
FOOT—LATERAL VIEW

Patient preparation: No special preparation is required.

Patient positioning: Place the patient in lateral recumbency with the affected leg next to the tabletop. Forcefully extend the limb cranially and position it through the use of sandbags placed on the proximal portion of the limb. Use a wooden paddle or plastic spoon to assist in positioning. Pull the unaffected leg caudally and hold it with sandbags or tie to the tabletop. Slightly flex the carpus so that you avoid supinating the limb.

X-ray beam direction: The vertically directed x-ray beam is centered on the carpal bones.

FOOT—LATERAL VIEW (hyperflexed)

Patient preparation: No special preparation is required.

Patient positioning: Place the patient in lateral recumbency with the affected leg next to the tabletop. Extend the limb cranially and position it through the use of sandbags placed on the proximal portion of the limb. Use a wooden paddle or plastic spoon to achieve a hyperflexed position. Pull the unaffected leg caudally and hold it with sandbags or tie to the tabletop. Use sandbags to position the head and neck.

X-ray beam direction: The vertically directed x-ray beam is centered on the carpal bones.

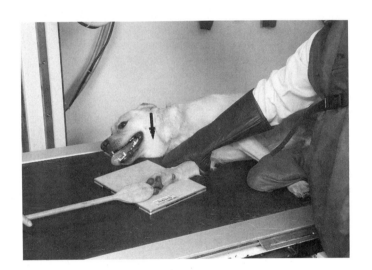

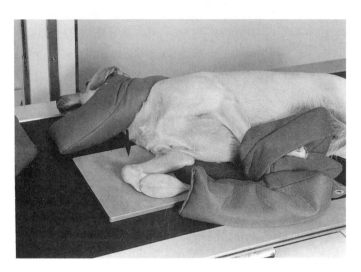

FOOT—LATERAL VIEW (hyperextended)

Patient preparation: No special preparation is required.

Patient positioning: Place the patient in lateral recumbency with the affected leg next to the tabletop. Extend the limb cranially and position it through the use of sandbags placed on the proximal portion of the limb. Use a wooden paddle or plastic spoon to achieve a hyperextended position. Pull the unaffected leg caudally and hold it with sandbags or tie to the tabletop.

X-ray beam direction: The vertically directed x-ray beam is centered on the carpal bones.

FOOT—DORSOPALMAR VIEW

Patient preparation: No special preparation is required.

Patient positioning: The patient is placed in sternal recumbency with the forelimb to be studied held as far cranially as possible with sandbags placed over the proximal portion of the limb. The opposite forelimb can be left in a neutral position. The head is displaced laterally toward the unaffected limb or placed in a hyperextended position.

X-ray beam direction: The vertically directed beam is centered on the carpal region.

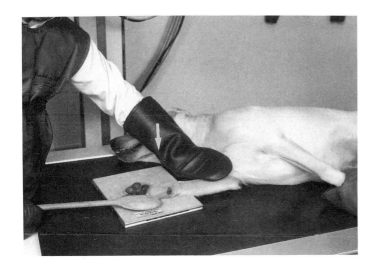

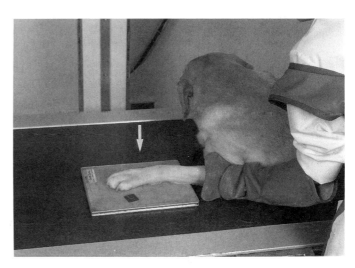

FOOT—DORSOPALMAR VIEW (obliques)

Patient preparation: No special preparation is required.

Patient positioning: The patient is placed in sternal recumbency with the forelimb to be studied held as far cranially as possible with the limb held or positioned by sandbags placed over the proximal portion of the limb. The opposite forelimb can be left in a natural position. The head is displaced laterally toward the unaffected limb or placed in a hyperextended position. Rotate the body medially and laterally with the limb in this position to obtain internal and external oblique views.

X-ray beam direction: The vertically directed beam is centered on the carpal region.

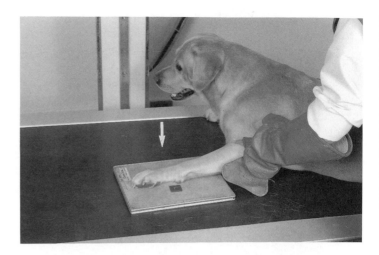

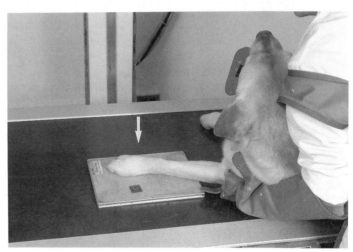

8. RADIOGRAPHY OF THE PELVIC LIMB

A. INTRODUCTION

The lateral views of the pelvic limb are relatively easy to make. The craniocaudal views of the proximal portion of the limb are difficult to obtain because of the problem of positioning the bones parallel to the tabletop. For this reason some bones are better studied using a caudocranial view. Oblique views of the tarsus, metatarsus, and digits can be made with relative ease and are helpful in radiographic diagnosis (Table 8-1). Many of the views are made in patients that are showing lameness or pain, however, usually sedation or anesthesia is not required. Most studies are made with tabletop technique without a grid except in examinations of large breeds. Often a comparable view of the opposite limb is helpful in diagnosis, especially if the growth plates have not closed. If the study is proximal on the limb, the lateral view of the opposite limb is the most easy comparison study to make. If the lesion if thought to be more distal, the craniocaudal or dorsoplantar/ plantarodorsal view is the most easy comparison study to make. No special preparation of the limb is necessary for the studies except to clean the haircoat.

A survey view of the limb can be made rather easily and can be of use in evaluation of a skeletally immature patient. Usually the study is made using a lateral beam and includes the stifle joint distally. These studies are usually made in a young dog suspected of having developmental bone or joint disease.

Table 8-1
PROTOCOL FOR RADIOGRAPHY OF THE PELVIC LIMB

FEMUR
Routine views
    lateral
    craniocaudal
Optional views
    caudocranial (vertical beam)
    caudocranial (horizontal beam)

STIFLE JOINT
Routine views
    lateral
    caudocranial
Optional views
    flexed lateral
    skyline patella
    caudocranial (horizontal beam)

TIBIA
Routine views
    lateral
    caudocranial
Optional views
    caudocranial (horizontal beam)

TARSAL JOINT
Routine views
    lateral
    plantarodorsal
Optional views
    plantarodorsal internal oblique (supination)
    plantarodorsal external oblique (pronation)

METATARSUS AND DIGITS
Routine views
    lateral
    plantarodorsal
Optional views
    plantarodorsal, internal oblique (supination)
    plantarodorsal, external oblique (pronation)

B. FEMUR

FEMUR—LATERAL VIEW

Patient preparation: Remove dirt and debris from the hair coat.

Patient positioning: Place the patient in lateral recumbency with the affected leg down. Extend the limb and hold it in position with sandbags or tied to the tabletop. Flex the opposite unaffected limb and remove it from the x-ray beam by abducting the limb and pulling it laterally. It may be possible to use sandbags to hold it in position or tie it to the tube stand. Sandbags are used to position the head and forelimbs.

X-ray beam direction: The vertically directed beam is centered on the midshaft of the femur.

Comments: The beam may be angled distoproximally to include the proximal femur if the upper limb cannot be completely removed from the x-ray beam.

FEMUR—CRANIOCAUDAL VIEW
(vertical beam)

Patient preparation: No special preparation.

Patient positioning: Place the patient in dorsal recumbency. Use a trough to support the abdomen or use a compression band. Extend the affected limb as far as possible caudally and hold it in a position similar to that used for a ventrodorsal views of the pelvis. Tie the affected pelvic limb to the tabletop or use sandbags to hold it in position. Because of the necessity of obtaining complete extension, it may be required to handhold the foot especially in a large dog. The body is slightly rotated so the pelvis on the affected side is higher so that the somewhat normally externally rotated limb is more perfectly positioned. Tie the forelimbs to the tabletop or use sandbags to hold them.

X-ray beam direction: The vertically directed x-ray beam is centered on the midshaft of the femur.

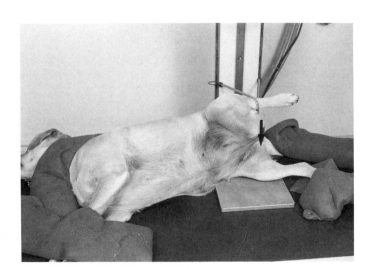

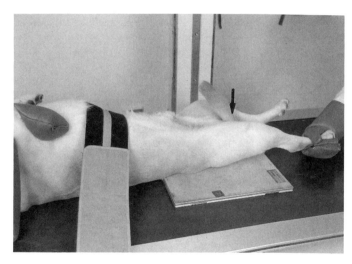

FEMUR—CAUDOCRANIAL VIEW
(horizontal beam)

Patient preparation: No special preparation.

Patient positioning: Place the patient in lateral recumbency with the affected limb uppermost supported on a sponge. Support the abdomen with sandbags or use a compression band. Place a cassette vertically against the cranial surface of the limb. Extend the affected limb, tying it to the tabletop or using sandbags to hold it in position. Because of the necessity of obtaining complete extension, it may be required to handhold the foot especially in a large dog. Tie the forelimbs to the tabletop or use sandbags to hold them. The x-ray tube is placed caudally.

X-ray beam direction: The horizontally directed x-ray beam is centered on the midshaft of the femur.

Comments: This positioning can also be used to obtain a caudocranial view of the stifle joint using a horizontal beam. It is also possible to obtain maximum flexion placing the femur next to the abdomen—the cassette is positioned next to the dog's back. The horizontal x-ray beam is directed in a caudocranial direction.

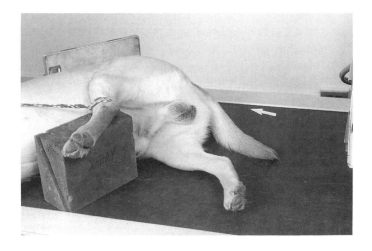

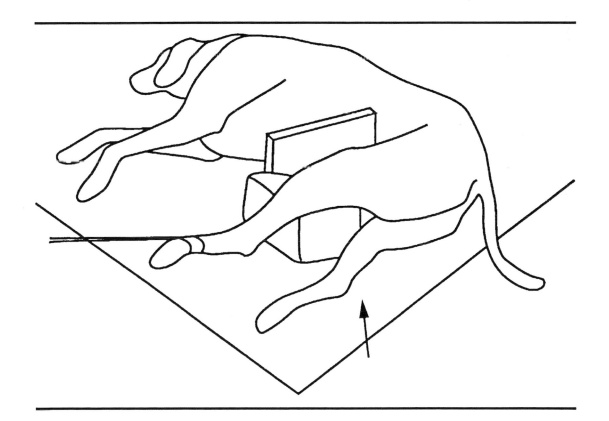

161

C. STIFLE JOINT
STIFLE JOINT—LATERAL VIEW

Patient preparation: Remove dirt and debris from the hair coat.

Patient positioning: Place the patient in lateral recumbency with the affected leg down. Extend the limb and hold it in position with sandbags or tied to the tabletop. Flex the opposite unaffected limb and remove it from the x-ray beam by abducting the limb and pulling it laterally. It may be possible to use sandbags to hold it in position or tie it to the tube stand. Sandbags are used to position the head and forelimbs.

X-ray beam direction: The vertically directed beam is centered on the stifle joint.

Comments: By always using the same degree of flexion of the stifle joint for the lateral view, the patella remains in the same relationship with the trochlea of the distal femur on the radiograph.

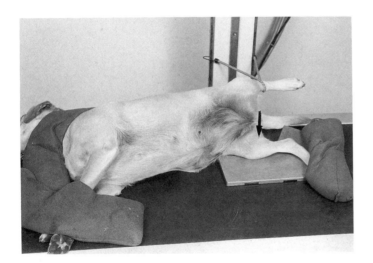

STIFLE JOINT—CAUDOCRANIAL VIEW
Patient preparation: No special preparation.

Patient positioning: Place the patient in ventral recumbency. Use a trough to support the thorax and a compression band or sandbags to position the body. Extend both limbs as far as possible caudally. Tie the affected pelvic limb to the tabletop or use sandbags to hold it in position. Because of the necessity of obtaining complete extension, it may be required to handhold the foot especially in a large dog. Place a sponge under the unaffected pelvic limb slightly rotating the pelvis so the unaffected limb is higher. This positions the somewhat externally rotated affected pelvic limb better. Tie the forelimbs to the tabletop or use sandbags to hold them.

X-ray beam direction: The vertically directed x-ray beam is centered on the stifle joint.

Comments: To be in good position, the affected limb must rest on the patella. This may be uncomfortable and a positioning sometimes rather difficult to accomplish. It may be possible to position a small sponge beneath the patella to relieve the pain.

It is possible to angle the beam distoproximally 10° to 20° and obtain a more prominent "tunnel" view of the distal femur.

It is possible to make a caudocranial view with the affected limb uppermost using a horizontally directed beam by positioning a cassette against the cranial surface of the affected limb and using the stifle joint as a fulcrum to obtain full extension. The x-ray tube is positioned caudally.

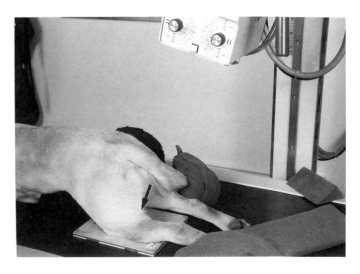

PATELLA—PROXIMODISTAL (skyline) VIEW

Patient preparation: No special preparation.

Patient positioning: Place the patient in ventral recumbency using a trough to support the thorax and compression band or sandbags to stabilize the body. Completely flex the pelvic limb to be studied and hold it in position lateral to the caudal abdomen with the foot flexed and placed beneath the limb to provide for some elevation of the patella. Let the unaffected pelvic limb flex partially and position itself laterally. Rotate the pelvis toward the affected limb so the femur to be studied is perpendicular to the tabletop and the unaffected side is elevated. Position a sandbag or sponge under the nonaffected limb to maintain this pelvic rotation. Use sandbags or tie the forelimbs to the tabletop.

X-ray beam direction: The vertically directed x-ray beam is centered on the patella.

Comments: To be in good position, the affected limb must rest on the tibia. This may be uncomfortable and a small sponge may be placed beneath the patella to relieve the pain.

It is possible to angle the beam craniocaudally 10° and obtain a greater skyline view of the patella. The exact beam angle may be estimated by palpating the patella as it fits against the trochlea.

The radiographic technique is decreased markedly for this view because of the decrease in tissue thickness.

The skyline view of the patella can also be made with the patient in lateral recumbency with the affected limb uppermost and resting on a sponge. Completely flex the limb. Place the cassette against the cranial surface of the upper limb. Use a horizontally directed beam with the x-ray tube positioned caudally.

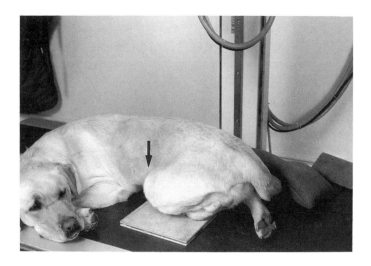

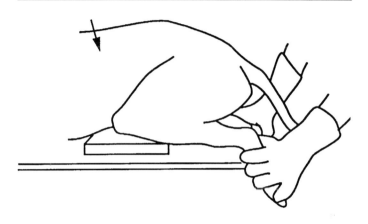

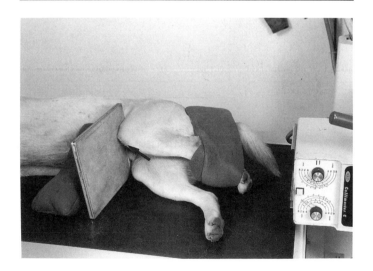

D. TIBIA

TIBIA—LATERAL VIEW

Patient preparation: Remove dirt and debris from the hair coat.

Patient positioning: Place the patient in lateral recumbency with the affected leg down. Extend the limb fully and hold the limb with sandbags or tie it to the tabletop. Place a sponge under the tarsus to elevate it and avoid obliquity of the limb. The opposite unaffected limb is removed from the x-ray beam by abducting the limb and pulling it laterally. It may be held with sandbags or tied to the tube stand. The forelimbs and head may be held using sandbags.

X-ray beam direction: The vertically directed beam is centered on the midshaft of the tibia.

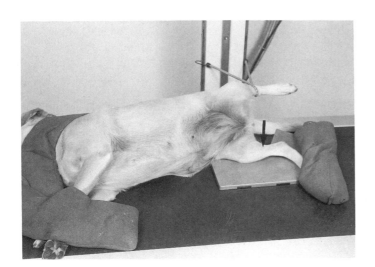

TIBIA—CAUDOCRANIAL VIEW (vertical beam)

Patient preparation: No special preparation.

Patient positioning: Place the patient in ventral recumbency. Use a trough to support the thorax and a compression band or sandbags to position the body. Extend both limbs as far as possible caudally. Tie the affected pelvic limb to the tabletop or use sandbags to hold it in position. Because of the necessity of obtaining complete extension, it may be required to handhold the foot especially in a large dog. The body is slightly rotated so the unaffected leg is higher so that the somewhat externally rotated limb to be studied is more perfectly positioned. Place a sponge beneath the unaffected pelvic limb to achieve this obliquity. Tie the forelimbs to the tabletop or use sandbags to hold them.

X-ray beam direction: The vertically directed x-ray beam is centered on the midshaft of the tibia.

Comment: This positioning is much more comfortable since the weight of the dog is not on the patella because it has shifted proximally.

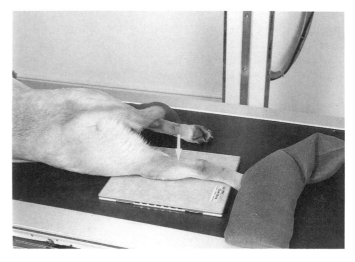

TIBIA—CAUDOCRANIAL VIEW
(horizontal beam)

Patient preparation: No special preparation.

Patient positioning: Place the patient in lateral recumbency with the affected limb uppermost and placed on a sponge. Use a compression band or sandbags to position the body. Extend the affected pelvic limb as far as possible and tie it to the tabletop or use sandbags to hold it in position. Because of the necessity of obtaining maximum traction, it may be required to handhold the foot especially in a large dog. Tie the forelimbs to the tabletop or use sandbags to hold them. The x-ray tube is caudal to the limb.

X-ray beam direction: The horizontally directed x-ray beam is centered on the midshaft of the tibia.

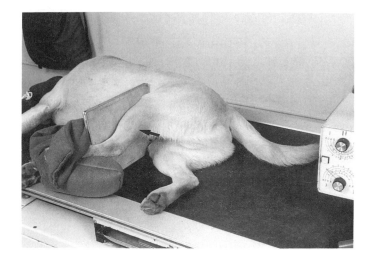

E. TARSUS-METATARSUS-DIGITS (Foot)

FOOT—LATERAL VIEW

Patient preparation: Remove dirt and debris from the hair coat.

Patient positioning: Place the patient in lateral recumbency with the affected leg down and the tarsal joint at a 90° angle of flexion. Hold the limb with sandbags positioned proximally or use a paddle to assist in positioning the foot. The opposite unaffected limb is removed from the x-ray beam by abducting the limb and pulling it laterally or by simply extending the limb.

X-ray beam direction: The vertically directed beam is centered on the foot.

FOOT—PLANTARODORSAL VIEW

Patient preparation: No special preparation.

Patient positioning: Place the patient in ventral recumbency with the body within a trough. Use a compression band or sandbags if necessary. Position the affected pelvic limb as far caudally as is possible. Place sandbags on the limb proximally or tie the limb to the tabletop to maintain the extended position. Rotate the patient's body by elevating the pelvis on the unaffected side. Position a sponge beneath the unaffected pelvic limb to maintain this position.

X-ray beam direction: The vertically directed x-ray beam is centered on the foot.

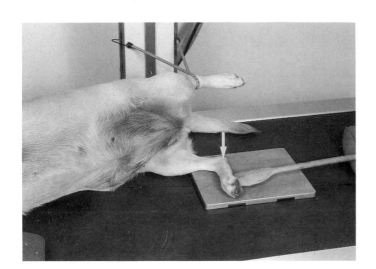

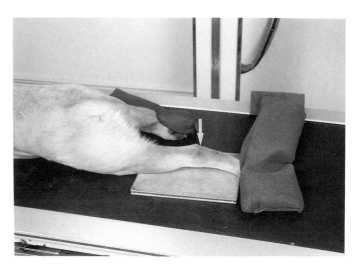

FOOT—PLANTARODORSAL VIEW
(oblique views)

Patient preparation: No special preparation.

Patient positioning: Place the patient in ventral recumbency with the body within a trough. Use a compression band or sandbags if necessary. Position the affected pelvic limb as far caudally as is possible. Place sandbags on the limb proximally or tie the limb to the tabletop to maintain the extended position. Rotate the patient's body additionally by further elevating the pelvis on the unaffected side for the medial oblique view. Position a larger sponge beneath the unaffected pelvic limb to maintain this oblique position. No rotation of the pelvis is required for the lateral oblique view since the limb is in an oblique position naturally.

X-ray beam direction: The vertically directed x-ray beam is centered on the foot.

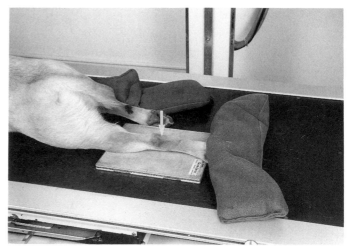

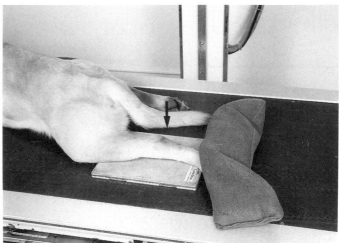

REFERENCES

Bur ke RL Corwin LA and Zimmerman D. Use of a medified occipital view for radiographic examination of the skull. Vet Med/SAC. April 1978 pages 460-3.

den Toom OI Miyabayashi T and Morgan JP. Application of positional radiographic techniques in the dog and cat. Part 1 -Thorax. Cal Vet. 5:19-22, 1983.

Grandage J. The radiology of the dog's diaphragm. J sm Anim Pract 15:1-7, 1974.

Grandage J. Some effects of posture on the radiographic appearance of the kidneys of the dog. J Am Vet Med Assoc 166:165-6, 1975.

Hare WCD. Radiographic anatomy of the canine skull. J Am Vet Med Assoc. 133:149-57, 1958.

Kus SP and Morgan JP. Radiography of the canine head. Vet Rad 26:196-202, 1985.

Miyabayashi T denToom OI and Morgan JP. Application of positional radiographic techniques in the dog. Part II - Abdomen, Cal Vet 6:15-21, 1983.

Miyabayashi T denToom OI and Morgan JP. Application of positional radiographic techniques in the dog and cat. Part III-Skeleton, Cal Vet 7:11-5, 1983.

Myer W. Radiography review: Pleural effusion. Vet Rad 19:75-9, 1978.

Reuhl WW and Thrall DE. The effect of dorsal versus ventral recumbency on the radiographic appearance of the canine thorax. Vet Rad 22:10-6, 1981.

Silverman S and Suter PF. Influence of inspiration and espiration on canine thoracic radiographs. J Am Vet Med Assoc 166:502-10, 1975.

Smith RN. The normal and radiological anatomy of the hip joint of the dog. J sm Anim Pract. 4:1-9, 1962.

Spencer CP Ackerman and Burt JK. The canine lateral thoracic radiograph. Vet Rad 22:262-6, 1981.

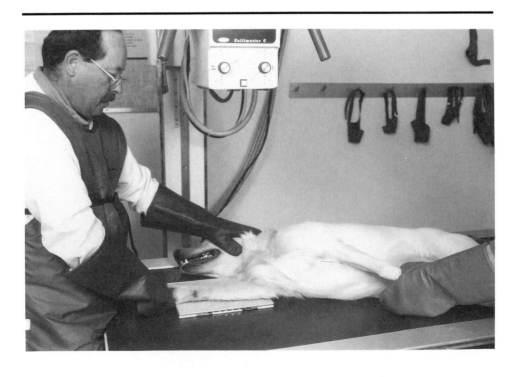

SECTION C

RADIOGRAPHY OF THE CAT

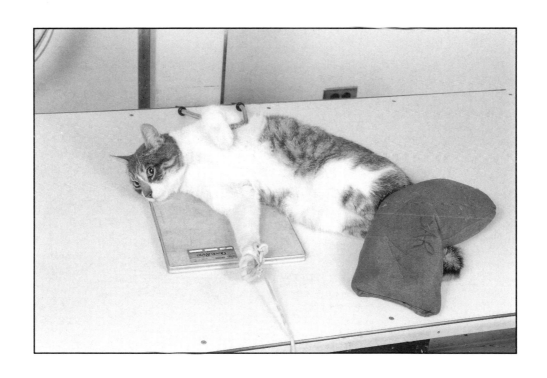

1. INTRODUCTION

Radiography of the cat is similar in many respects to that of the dog, but much easier because of the smaller size of the patient, and therefore the relative easy in positioning the patient for study. Because of the similarity in size of the patients, determination of the correct technique often does not require as careful a measurement and the technique can be obtained directly from the technique chart. There is an additional advantage in radiography of cats in that the difference in tissue density between the thorax and abdomen is minimal, meaning that the entire body can be radiographed using only one machine setting. This makes the concept of "whole body" survey very workable in radiography of the cat. The skeletal structures can even be evaluated on the whole body study. However, it is suggested that following evaluation of the survey film, "coned-down" views be made of areas of special interest so that better evaluation of the suspect lesion can be made.

Because of the small size of the patient, it is tempting to use manual restraint because of the relative ease. If the beam is well collimated, the technician can remain outside of the primary beam even while holding the patient. However, it is safer to use chemical restraint on the patient so that no technicians need to be within the room during the exposure. Sandbags, compression bands, positioning troughs, sponges, as well as tie-down ropes, tape, and gauze are all available for use in positioning the sedated, anesthetized, or awake patient. As in most things, a compromise can usually be reached in which there can be use of some positioning devices so that only one technician must remain within the room during the examination of a severely injured or diseased cat and that technician can be positioned at a greater distance from the x-ray beam. It is expected that radiation safety practices, such as beam collimation, use fast film-screen system, and lead aprons and gloves be used in all examinations

Two views are required for almost all radiographic examinations and are preferably made at right angles to each other. Beam direction is described by terms that indicate the entrance and exit of the x-ray beam. Thus, a dorsoventral beam enters dorsally and exits ventrally. Identification markers are required for each radiograph and contain the name of the patient, owner's name, date of examination, and name of the clinic. Right and left markers are needed. Because of the small size of the patient, frequently both views are made on the same film.

Most floor-to-ceiling tube stands accommodate an x-ray tube that is appropriate for use with cats and a capability of 100 mA and 100 kVp is sufficient for radiography of cats. Focal-film distances need to be standardized at 40" (100 cm) prior to development of the technique chart. Most studies are made in a tabletop mode. Grids can be positioned in undertable trays but are only used in studies of the thorax, abdomen, and spine in very large cats. Non-screen film can be used to study the thin extremities, increasing the detail of the study and helping to compensate for the small size of the bones. High detail screen-film systems can be used as well for radiography of extremities.

Non-screen film can also be used in studies of the teeth.

Because of the similarity in appearance of the breeds of cats, it is much easier to learn the radiographic anatomy making film evaluation easier.

Special procedures in cats are performed in much the same way as they are in the dog with some specific differences. These are discussed in greater detail in the section on special procedures.

INDICATIONS

Trauma is one of the most common reasons for radiography of the cat and the "whole body" survey film is often used. Because of the high frequency of lymphoma or lymphosarcoma and cardiomyopathy, studies of the thorax are commonly performed. Indications for abdominal radiography are similar to those found in the dog. Cats do not have the developmental dysplasias within the bones and joints that lead to lameness, therefore, most causes of studies of the limbs are trauma induced.

CONTRAINDICATIONS

There are probably no reasons why radiography should not be used in diagnosis of disease in the cat. Even in the most ill or fractious patient, it is possible to position the patient for lateral views of the whole body. It should be remembered that cats often do not clearly show a severity of clinical signs that is in proportion to the severity of the disease. In patients with pulmonary, mediastinal, or pleural lesions, the stress of a radiographic examination plus ventrodorsal positioning may cause compression of the remaining functional lung fields and rather sudden death from anoxia.

PROTOCOL

The protocol of radiographic studies is similar to that used for the dog, except that so much more of the body of the cat can be included in each view. This has the advantage in not requiring as many radiographs, but has the disadvantage in that the x-ray beam is often not centered on an area of interest. It is for this reason that additional coned-down views are of great value.

Patient preparation is essentially the same for all studies and consists in cleaning and drying the hair coat because wet hair and debris cause confusing artifacts on the radiographs. Because the hair coat in the cat is so thick, it is possible for matted hair to make rather prominent shadows on the radiograph. Leashes and collars are removed prior to radiography to avoid radiographic artifacts. Remove bandages, splints, casts, or tape when possible prior to radiography since they all influence the manner of exposure of the film and create some type of film artifact.

2. THORACIC RADIOGRAPHY

INTRODUCTION

Radiology remains a most important diagnostic test in the investigation of thoracic diseases especially in the cat. Radiology usually reveals more specific information than physical examination and can be performed relatively cheaply, quickly, and safely, providing rapid results on which to base the next set of decisions. Radiographs reproduce the character of the patient's body on film and can be examined both at the time of the original examination as well as being available for review at another time. The good contrast provided by the air in the lungs opens up a window to the thoracic organs on non-contrast radiographs to an extent not possible with the abdominal radiographic study. In addition, radiographic examinations provide a temporal dimension that permits evaluation of changes as you observe the progression of a disease. The trachea and lungs, pleural space, heart and great vessels, esophagus, lymph notes, diaphragm, and ribs, sternum, and spine can all be examined.

INDICATIONS

Indications for thoracic radiography in the cat include suspect pneumonia, pleural disease, cardiomyopathy, and thoracic cavity tumors. Thoracic radiography often provides an indication of what other clinical examination or test should be performed next. Some general indications for thoracic radiography are listed (Table 2-1).

PROTOCOL

Thoracic studies usually consist of a single lateral view and a dorsoventral view. Studies made especially to evaluate the heart consist of a right lateral and dorsoventral view to obtain the most correct evaluation of the heart shadow. Views using small size cassettes usually include both thoracic inlet and diaphragm. With certain clinical signs, it is desirable to use a larger cassette and include the larynx and cervical trachea within the study. Medium kVp settings (70 to 90 kVp) provide a long scale of radiographic contrast and are recommended. In the patient with dyspnea, it is necessary to use the shortest time of exposure possible, hopefully, this is 1/60 or 1/120 second (Table 2-2).

Positioning for thoracic studies is relatively easy. Extension of the forelimbs is easy and removes the muscle mass of the forelimbs from over the precardiac lung field. Attempt to superimpose the sternum and spine in the dorsoventral or ventrodorsal views. The use of an esophageal swallow of barium sulfate suspension prior to exposure provides information useful in the diagnosis of mediastinal disease characterized by displacement of the esophagus.

Table 2-1
GENERAL INDICATIONS FOR THORACIC RADIOGRAPHY

1. suspect lower respiratory disease (acute or chronic)
2. recurrent non-responsive respiratory disease
3. presence of cough
4. presence of dyspnea
5. suspect feline asthma
6. known or suspected thoracic trauma,
7. known or suspected non-cardiogenic edema
    —electrical shock
    —near-drowning
    —head trauma
    —near-asphyxiation
8. preanesthesia study because of
    —patient's older age
    —post-trauma status
    —presence of associated respiratory disease
    —presence of associated cardiac disease
    —presence of malignant disease
9. evaluation for pulmonary metastases
10. postoperative study in the event of respiratory complications
11. suspect cardiac disease, either congenital or acquired
12. suspect swallowing dysfunction
13. survey examination in an older patient without specific clinical signs

Table 2-2
PROTOCOL FOR THORACIC RADIOGRAPHY

Routine views
  lateral
  dorsoventral
Additional views
  opposite lateral
  ventrodorsal
  pulmonary metastasis—both lateral views
  mediasinal mass—increase exposure by 10 kVp
  pleural fluid—increase exposure by 10 kVp

VIEWS
THORAX—LATERAL VIEW

Patient preparation: None is required except to clean the hair coat and remove a collar.

Patient positioning: Place the cat in either right or left lateral recumbency. Selection of laterality is dictated by ease of handling the patient, comfort of the patient, and location of lesion. Pull the forelimbs together and extend them cranially and pull the pelvic limbs caudally. Avoid placing the head and neck in a hyperextended position because of the effect on tracheal position and diameter. It is best to use sandbags for positioning of the limbs, however, they can be tied to the table.

X-ray beam direction: The vertically directed beam is centered on the heart at the 5th intercostal space.

Comments: Make the exposure at or near full inspiration.

A lateral view of the thorax may be a part of a "whole body" survey.

THORAX—DORSOVENTRAL VIEW

Patient preparation: None is required except to clean the hair coat and remove a collar.

Patient positioning: Place the cat in sternal recumbency with the spine superimposed over the sternum. Pull the forelimbs cranially with the elbows lateral to the thoracic inlet. Position the pelvic limbs in a relaxed manner. Use ropes to tie the feet to the table if possible. Use a trough or sandbags to help in positioning the abdomen if the patient is large or difficult to position.

X-ray beam direction: The vertically directed beam is centered on the midthoracic spine.

Comments: Make the exposure near full inspiration.

A ventrodorsal view of the thorax may be made with the cat in dorsal recumbency, however, that positioning usually causes the patient to be uncomfortable and it is not recommended.

A dorsoventral view of the thorax may be part of a "whole-body" survey.

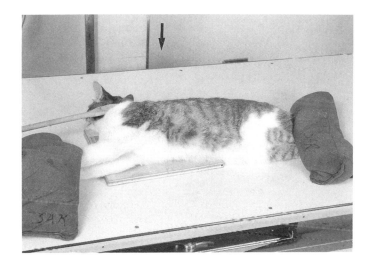

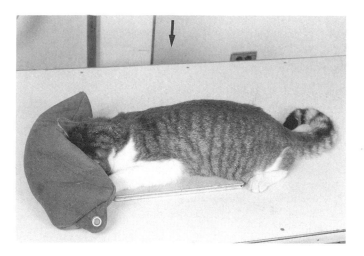

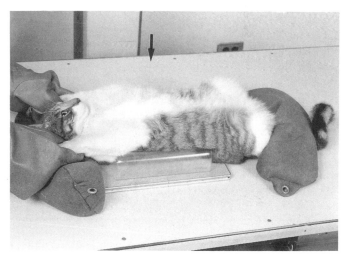

3. ABDOMINAL RADIOGRAPHY

INTRODUCTION

Abdominal radiography in the cat is frequently a part of a "whole-body" survey study. Because of the amount of abdominal fat, the urinary and gastro-intestinal systems are easier to visualize than in the dog. The routine abdominal study may be followed by a special radiographic study of the gastrointestinal or urinary system using contrast agents.

INDICATIONS

Since the study is a form of a survey study, the indications for examination are widespread and relate to the body systems that can be evaluated (Table 3-1). Any signs of anorexia, vomiting, or diarrhea suggest gastrointestinal disease, while problems of hematuria, dysuria, or crystalluria suggest urinary disease. A painful abdomen may relate to peritoneal disease, trauma to the abdominal wall, or a spinal injury.

PROTOCOL

Because of the presence of abdominal fat, ingesta or feces do not cause the problems in interpretation as they do in the dog. The rapid gastric emptying and rapid small bowel transit empties the stomach and small bowel so they contain little ingesta. The cat swallows only minimal amount of air so the presence of air within the stomach and small bowel does not cause a problem in interpretation of the radiographs. Because of these reasons, most cats can be examined radiographically without preparation.

Include the diaphragm and pelvic region on both views. The patient can be positioned in either right or left lateral recumbency for the lateral projection. The ventrodorsal view is preferred over the dorsoventral view for routine studies of the abdomen since positioning of the cat for this view can usually be more easily controlled in dorsal recumbency. The dorsoventral view may be used, however, if patients cannot tolerate dorsal recumbency because of respiratory distress or because of pelvic injury (Table 3-2).

The kVp scale selected should be in the medium range (70 to 80 kVp) since this provides a scale of contrast that is most diagnostic. Exposure times should be as brief as possible, but patient motion is not a usual problem. The beam is centered in the mid-portion of the abdomen at a point just caudal to the last rib.

Certain special techniques can be used to increase the value of the abdominal study. These include the use of: (1) a compression paddle that shifts overlying abdominal organs and permits better visualization of those beneath, (2) ingestion of a small amount of barium sulfate suspension or CO_2 spanules into the stomach to increase the contrast between cranial abdominal organs, or (3) injection of a small amount of barium sulfate suspension or air per rectum to permit evaluation of the caudal abdominal organs.

Table 3-1
INDICATIONS FOR
ABDOMINAL RADIOGRAPHY

---

those suggesting gastrointestinal disease
    anorexia
    vomiting
    diarrhea
    known ingestion of foreign body
    melana
    dyschezia
those suggesting urinary disease
    hematuria
    pyuria
    dysuria
    stranguria
    frequent urination
post trauma
findings on physical examination
    palpation of abdominal mass
    abdominal tenderness or pain
    tense abdominal wall
suspect malignancy

Table 3-2
PROTOCOL FOR ABDOMINAL
RADIOGRAPHY

Routine views
    right lateral
    ventrodorsal
Optional views
    left lateral
    compression paddle views
    dorsoventral

VIEWS

ABDOMEN—LATERAL VIEW

Patient preparation: No particular preparation is required except to clean the hair coat.

Patient positioning: Most commonly the lateral view is made with the cat in right lateral recumbency. The forelimbs can be positioned cranially being held by sandbags while the pelvic limbs need to be extended slightly and are held by hand or by sandbags or are tied to the table.

X-ray beam direction: The vertically directed x-ray beam is centered on the middle of the abdomen just caudal to the last ribs.

Comment: A lateral view of the abdomen may be a part of a "whole-body" study.

ABDOMEN—VENTRODORSAL VIEW

Patient preparation: No particular preparation is required except to clean the hair coat.

Patient positioning: The forelimbs and the pelvic limbs are extended and held in position by sandbags or by hand.

X-ray beam direction: The vertically directed central beam is centered on the middle of the abdomen just caudal to the last ribs.

Comment: A similar view of the abdomen may be made in sternal recumbency using a dorsoventral view, however, the rear limbs are difficult to position and the abdomen is usually obliques so this technique is not recommended.

A ventrodorsal view of the abdomen may be a part of a "whole-body" study.

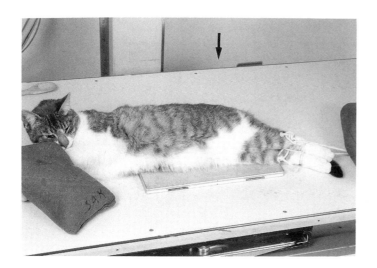

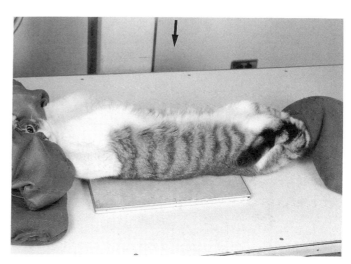

4. RADIOGRAPHY OF THE HEAD

INTRODUCTION

The head of the cat is much more spherical than in the dog and radiography is somewhat like radiographing a ball, thus making positioning more difficult. A decision needs to be made at the time of radiography of the purpose of the study and the need for sedation or anesthesia. It is possible to divide the studies of the head into the following: (1) survey study, (2) nasal cavity and sinuses, (3) maxilla and maxillary teeth, (4) mandible and mandibular teeth, (5) temporomandibular joints, and (6) tympanic bullae and odontoid process.

INDICATIONS

The indications for radiography of the head include: (1) trauma usually resulting from being hit by a car or falling a great distance or (2) lesions within the nasal cavity due to inflammation or tumors.

PROTOCOL

A survey study consisting of lateral and dorsoventral views can be made on an awake patient. However, anesthesia or sedation is needed if special views are to be accomplished. Consideration needs to be given to the location of the endotracheal tube and the tongue at the time of exposure. Both the tube and the tongue may create dense soft tissue shadows that confuse interpretation of the nasal cavity and should be located so that they are removed from the field of interest (Table 4-1).

Studies of the teeth are a special problem because the difficulty in positioning of the head and placement of the film to obtain the most diagnostic lateral views. Non-screen dental film in an intra-oral position is used in some practices to assist in solving these problems.

Table 4-1
PROTOCOL FOR HEAD

Routine views
  lateral
  dorsoventral
Optional views
  opposite lateral
  lateral obliques
  ventrodorsal
  frontal
  basilar for tympanic bullae or odontoid process
  open-mouth ventrodorsal (extraoral film placement)
  ventrodorsal with intraoral film placement
  dorsoventral of maxillary incisors with intraoral film
    placement
  ventrodorsal of mandibular incisors with intraoral film
    placement
  lateral oblique for temporomandibular joints

VIEWS

HEAD—LATERAL VIEW

Patient preparation: No special preparation is needed other than cleaning the haircoat and removal of a collar.

Patient positioning: Place the patient with the affected side next to the cassette unless the injury is of a nature that prevents this positioning. Place a foam wedge under the mandible and nose to elevate the nose so that it is parallel to the tabletop and the body of the mandible is superimposed. A line drawn through the medial canthus of the eyes should be perpendicular to the tabletop. The endotracheal tube may remain in position if the cat is anesthetized. The forelimbs are drawn back and held by sandbags or tied to the table. It is possible to use a wooden spoon or paddle to help position the head.

X-ray beam direction: The vertically directed beam is perpendicular to the tabletop and centered at a point on the zygomatic arch midway between the eye and the ear.

HEAD—DORSOVENTRAL VIEW

Patient preparation: No special preparation is required other than cleaning the haircoat and removal of a collar.

Patient positioning: Place the patient in sternal recumbency. The body of the mandible makes positioning for this study relatively easy since it rests evenly on the tabletop. Hold the head in position by putting pressure on the dorsum of the neck through use of a sandbag or through use of a gloved hand.

X-ray beam direction: The vertically directed beam is perpendicular to the tabletop and centered between the eyes.

Comments: It is possible, but difficult, in an awake patient to make a ventrodorsal view of the head with the patient in dorsal recumbency. Use a sponge to elevate the nose slightly and tape stretched across the mandible to hold the head in position. The forelimbs can be positioned lateral to the chest cavity and held by sandbags or tied or extended and held lateral to the head. The vertically directed beam is perpendicular to the tabletop and centered between the two parts of the mandible. There are only rare circumstances that require ventrodorsal positioning.

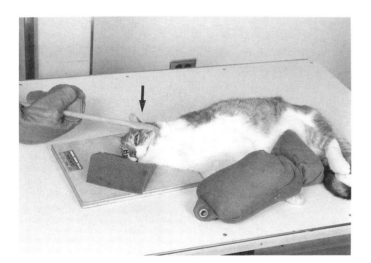

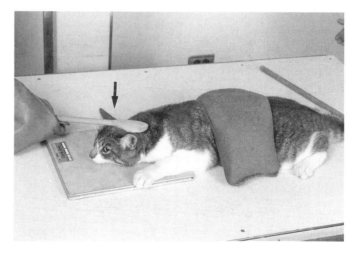

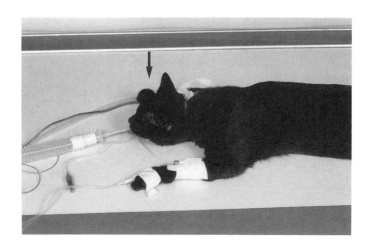

HEAD—FRONTAL VIEW

Patient preparation: No special preparation is required other than cleaning the haircoat and removing a collar.

Patient positioning: Place the anesthetized or sedated patient in dorsal recumbency with the head positioned with the nose pointing upward. Use gauze to hold the head in position. The forelimbs are positioned lateral to the chest cavity and can be held by sandbags or tied to the table.

X-ray beam direction: The vertically directed beam is perpendicular to the tabletop and centered between the eyes. If the skull is positioned correctly, the beam is parallel to the bridge of the nose.

Comments: The kVp is decreased for this study because of the decrease in thickness of the tissue. Therefore, the remainder of the radiograph of the head is greatly underexposed.

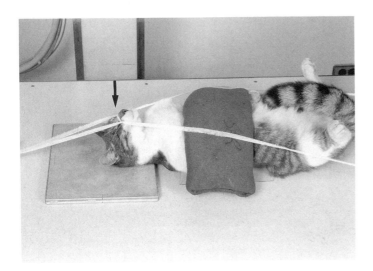

HEAD—BASILAR VIEW

Patient preparation: No special preparation is required other than cleaning the haircoat and removing a collar.

Patient positioning: Place the anesthetized or heavily sedated patient in dorsal recumbency with the head positioned with the mouth closed and the nose pointing upward. Place a gauze strip around the nose and pull caudally so the hard palate is angled approximately 45° to the table top. To stabilize the head, attach the gauze to a sandbag near the cat's hind feet or to the end of the table. Position the head so the vertically directed beam is centered between the eyes. Avoid any lateral angulation of the head. The forelimbs are best positioned lateral to the thorax and held by sandbags. Allow the pelvic limbs to be in a neutral position.

X-ray beam direction: The vertically directed beam is perpendicular to the table top and centered between the eyes.

Comment: Use the exposure settings used for the other routine views of the head. This study permits evaluation of the occipital bone, foramen magnum, atlanto-occipital articulation, tympanic bullae, and odontoid process. The positioning used for this view in the cat is in contrast to the positioning with the mouth open that would be used in the dog.

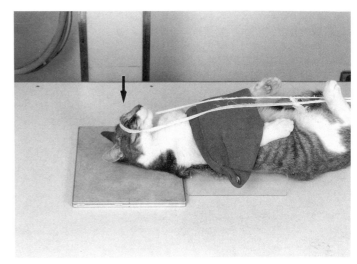

HEAD—OPEN MOUTH VENTRODORSAL VIEW (with extraoral film placement)

Patient preparation: No special preparation other than cleaning the haircoat and removing a collar.

Patient positioning: Place the anesthesized or sedated patient in dorsal recumbency with the nose elevated slightly by placement of a foam wedge beneath the nose and the tabletop so the hard palate is parallel with the tabletop. The mouth is opened as widely as possible with gauze placed around the lower canine teeth. Include the tongue within the gauze so that it does not cause an artifact on the radiograph. The nose is held in position by tape or gauze fastened to the tabletop. Place sandbags lateral to the head to achieve a degree of stabilization. The forelimbs are positioned lateral to the chest cavity and can be held by sandbags.

X-ray beam direction: The vertically directed beam is angled between 20° and 30° to the tabletop in a rostrocaudal direction.

Comment: Decrease the kVp technique used for the routine views of the skull since only the nasal tissue is to be penetrated.

HEAD—CLOSED MOUTH DORSOVENTRAL VIEW (with intraoral film placement)

Patient preparation: No special preparation is required other than cleaning the haircoat and removing a collar.

Patient positioning: Place the anesthetized patient in sternal recumbency with a sponge elevating the mandible. The non-screen film is placed into the mouth and the mouth closed on the film. Place a sandbag over the neck for positioning. The endotracheal tube is removed for this view. The forelimbs are positioned lateral to the thorax and can be held by sandbags or tied to the table.

X-ray beam direction: The vertically directed beam is perpendicular to the tabletop for the routine view. Angle the beam at a rostrocaudal angle to the film between 10° and 15° to better evaluate the upper incisor region and also obtain a view of the more caudal portion of the nasal region.

Comment: Decrease the kVp technique used for the routine views of the skull since only the nasal tissue is to be penetrated.

Position the film carefully since the teeth may penetrate the film envelope causing a focal exposure of the film.

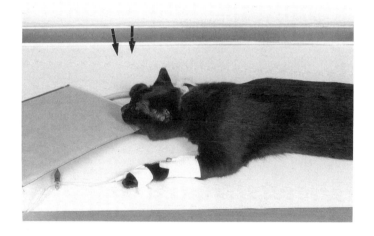

HEAD—LATERAL VIEW FOR TEMPOROMANDIBULAR JOINTS

Patient preparation: No special preparation other than cleaning the haircoat and removing a collar.

Patient positioning: Place the anesthesized or sedated patient in lateral recumbency with the joint to be studied dependent. Elevate the nose using a wedge shaped sponge. In addition, rotate the head 10° so that the joint to be studied is positioned ventrally. The mouth is held partially open by a gauze roll used as a speculum. Place a sandbag over the neck to assist in positioning. The endotracheal tube can be removed for this view. The forelimbs are positioned lateral to the thorax and can be held by sandbags or tied to the table.

X-ray beam direction: The vertically directed beam is centered just below the eye and is perpendicular to the tabletop.

Comments: Use the kVp technique used for the routine views of the skull since it is necessary to penetrate the heavy portion of the calvarium

Usually this view is made of both joints so they can be compared.

The tympanic bullae are also identified on this oblique lateral view to good advantage.

HEAD—OBLIQUE VIEW FOR THE UPPER DENTAL ARCADE

Patient preparation: No special preparation is required other than cleaning the haircoat and removing a collar.

Patient positioning: Place the anesthetized patient in lateral recumbency with the affected side positioned next to the cassette. Open the mouth using a gauze roll as a speculum to separate the dental arcades. Place a foam wedge under the mandible to elevate the nose and rotate the head. The degree of obliquity should be between 30° and 45°. The endotracheal tube may remain in position if the cat is anesthetized. The forelimbs are held in position with sandbags or are tied to the table.

X-ray beam direction: The vertically directed beam is perpendicular to the tabletop and centered on the open-mouth at the 2th premolar.

Comments: You can use gauze strips fastened on the canine teeth to open the mouth. This study also provides evaluation of the bony lesions of the upper maxilla. Usually this view is used bilaterally and both upper dental arcades are radiographed.

This view may be thought of as a ventrodorsal oblique while the study for the lower dental arcade is more of a dorsoventral oblique.

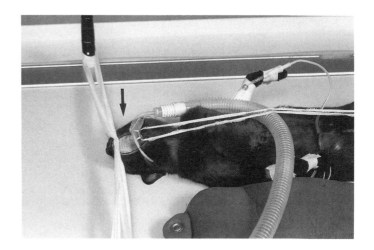

HEAD—OBLIQUE VIEW FOR THE LOWER DENTAL ARCADE

Patient preparation: No special preparation is required other than cleaning the haircoat and removing a collar.

Patient positioning: Place the anesthetized or sedated patient in lateral recumbency with the dental arcade to be studied on the dependent side. Open the mouth widely using a speculum of some type. Place a sponge under the nose to elevate the maxilla and rotate the head. Obtain an angle of approximately 30° to 45°. The forelimbs are positioned lateral to the thorax and can be held by sandbags or tied to the table.

X-ray beam direction: The vertically directed beam is perpendicular to the tabletop and centered on the open-mouth at the 2nd lower premolar tooth.

Comments: Usually oblique views of both lower dental arcades are made.

A roll of gauze or tape may be used as a speculum since a metal mouth speculum is undesirable because of its opacity. It is possible to use gauze strips fastened to the canine teeth to hold the mouth in an open position.

This study also provides evaluation of the bony lesions of the mandible.

This view may be thought of as a dorsoventral oblique while the study for the upper dental arcade is more of a ventrodrosal oblique.

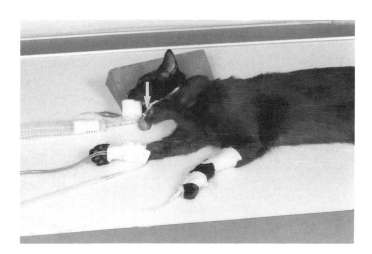

5. RADIOGRAPHY OF THE SPINE

INTRODUCTION

Studies of the spine are often included in the "whole-body" survey. It is important to remember to make "coned-down" views of areas of interest.

INDICATIONS

Most patients requiring spinal radiography have suffered acute spinal injury and present with paresis or paralysis that is partial or complete. The patient should be sedated or anesthetized and be carefully handled.

CONTRAINDICATIONS

There are no contraindications for spinal radiography. Even if the patient cannot be perfectly positioned because it cannot be sedated or anesthetized, it is possible to position the patient carefully and make both views for a survey type study of the spine.

PROTOCOL

The survey studies are made on a single large cassette. It may be of additional value to use small cassettes and include several views of the spine so that the intervertebral disc spaces are parallel to the central beam and can be more accurately evaluated.

Dynamic radiography of the spine is rarely used in the cat but is possible to make hyperextended and hyperflexed views in the cervical and lumbosacral regions (Table 5-1).

Table 5-1
PROTOCOL FOR RADIOGRAPHY OF THE SPINE

Routine views
  lateral
  ventrodorsal
Optional views
  opposite lateral
  ventrodorsal oblique
  dorsoventral
  stress

VIEWS
SPINE—LATERAL VIEW

Patient preparation: None is required except for cleaning the haircoat and removing a collar.

Patient positioning: Place the patient in lateral recumbency. Use sponges under the sternum if necessary to achieve lateral positioning. The forelimbs and pelvic limbs are extended and held with sandbags or tied to the table.

X-ray beam direction: The vertically directed beam is perpendicular to the tabletop and centered on T 6-7 or the area of interest.

Comments: Coned-down views can be made as desired.

SPINE—VENTRODORSAL VIEW

Patient preparation: None is required except for cleaning the haircoat.

Patient positioning: Place the patient in dorsal recumbency using a trough or placing sandbags lateral to the body. The forelimbs are pulled cranially and held by sandbags or by hand while the pelvic limbs are pulled in a caudal position.

X-ray beam direction: The vertically directed beam is centered on T 6-7 or the area of interest.

Comment: The spine can be rotated 20° from the ventrodorsal position and oblique views made.

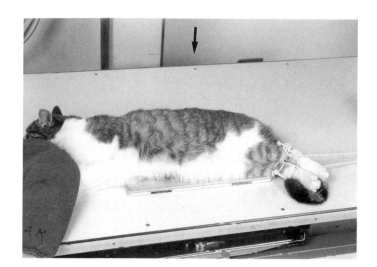

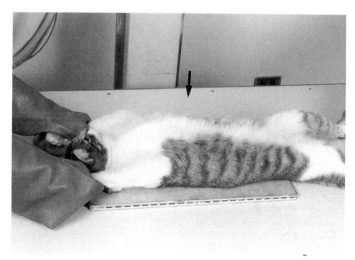

6. RADIOGRAPHY OF THE PELVIS AND HIP JOINTS

INTRODUCTION

Radiography of the pelvis is common because of frequent trauma that involved both the pelvic bones and the hip joints. Usually the trauma patient can be radiographed without sedation or anesthesia (Table 6-1).

Table 6-1
PROTOCOL FOR RADIOGRAPHY OF THE PELVIS AND HIP JOINTS

Routine views of the pelvis
    lateral
    ventrodorsal with limbs extended
    ventrodorsal with limbs in flexed position
Routine views of the hip joints
    lateral hip joint
    lateral pelvis
    ventrodorsal with limbs in flexed position

VIEWS

PELVIS—LATERAL VIEW

Patient preparation: The only preparation required is to clean the hair coat since this is often a film made following trauma.

Patient positioning: The cat is placed in lateral recumbency with the affected side next to the tabletop. The pelvic limbs are placed in a neutral position in a "scissored" position with the down limb flexed cranial and the upper limb extended caudally and are held or positioned with sandbags or tied to the table. Notice the position of the tail especially if it is long. The forelimbs are either held or positioned by sandbags.

X-ray beam direction: The vertically directed beam is centered on the hip joint.

PELVIS—VENTRODORSAL VIEW
(with limbs extended)

Patient preparation: Nothing is required other than cleaning the hair coat.

Patient positioning: The cat is placed in dorsal recumbency using a trough for positioning. The pelvic limbs are in an extended position and can be tied to the table or held. Place the pelvic limbs in internal rotation so the patellas are on or near the midline. The forelimbs are extended forward and held or positioned by sandbags.

X-ray beam direction: The vertically directed beam is centered on the hip joints.

Comments: If the view is made following trauma, perfect positioning may not be obtainable. It is most important to position both limbs in the same manner even if the positioning of the limbs is not perfect.

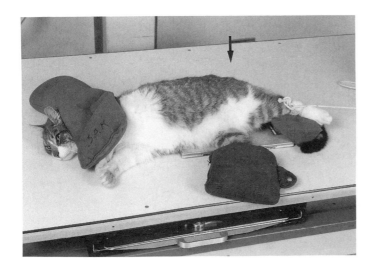

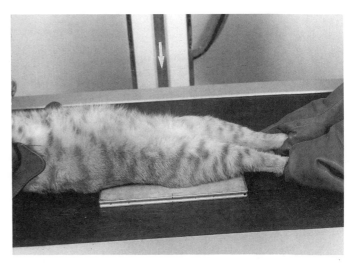

PELVIS—VENTRODORSAL VIEW
(with limbs flexed—frogleg view)

Patient preparation: Clean the hair coat.

Patient positioning: The cat is placed in dorsal recumbency placing the body in a trough to assist in positioning. The pelvic limbs are held lateral to the pelvis forcing the limbs into a tight flexed position. It is possible to use sandbags over each foot to hold the pelvic limbs in position. The forelimbs are extended forward and held or positioned by sandbags.

X-ray beam direction: The vertically directed beam is centered on the hip joints.

Comments: This view is used to obtain a study of the pelvis, especially of the hip joints, following trauma in which there is great pain associated with extension of one of the limbs. Position both pelvic limbs equally so that a comparison can be easily made on the radiograph.

PELVIS—LATERAL VIEW OF THE HIP JOINT

Patient preparation: No special preparation is required.

Patient positioning: Place the cat in lateral recumbency with the limb to be studied next to the table using sandbags to hold the limb in position or tying it to the table. Place a sponge beneath the sternum to rotate the body slightly. Abduct the unaffected leg and remove it from the field of view by tying it to the tube-stand or by use of sandbags. Use sandbags to stabilize the forelimbs.

X-ray beam direction: The vertically directed beam is centered on the dependent hip joint which is easier to project because of the rotated body.

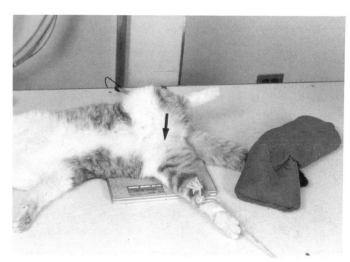

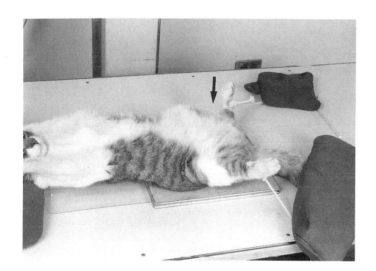

7. RADIOGRAPHY OF THE FORELIMB

INTRODUCTION

The lateral view of the forelimb is relatively easy to make with the patient in lateral recumbency. The position of sandbags may be altered because of the region of interest and the location of the vertically directed central x-ray beam is changed. The craniocaudal and dorsopalmar views are easier in the cat because of the ease in fully extending the limb. Oblique views are not often used, but may be of value in examination of the elbow, carpus, metacarpus, and digits. All studies are made with tabletop technique without a grid. Often a lateral view of the opposite limb is made as a comparison view and is helpful in diagnosis, especially when the growth plates have not closed (Table 7-1). Remember that growth plates close at an older age in the cat than in the dog.

Table 7-1
PROTOCOL FOR RADIOGRAPHY OF THE FORELIMB

Routine views
    lateral
    craniocaudal (dorsopalmar)
Optional views
    craniocaudal (dorsopalmar) in internal rotation
    craniocaudal (dorsopalmar) in external rotation
    caudocranial with horizontal beam
    stress views of the foot
        hyperextension
        hyperflexion

VIEWS

FORELIMB—LATERAL VIEW

Patient preparation: Remove dirt and debris from the hair coat.

Patient positioning: Place the patient in lateral recumbency with the affected leg down. Extend the limb cranially and place traction on the limb. The opposite unaffected limb is removed from the x-ray beam by flexing the limb and pulling it caudally

X-ray beam direction: The vertically directed beam is centered on the region of interest.

Comments: This view permits good evaluation of the entire limb. A shifting of the mechanism of restraint is needed when examining the distal portion of the limb.

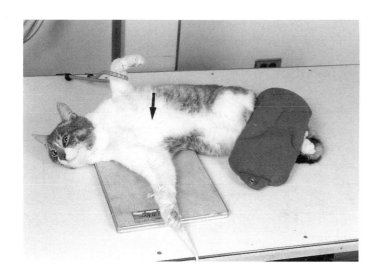

FORELIMB—CRANIOCAUDAL VIEW

Patient preparation: No special preparation is required.

Patient positioning: The patient is placed in ventral recumbency with the forelimb to be studied pulled as far cranially as possible and held or positioned by sandbags or tied to the table. The opposite forelimb can be left in a neutral position. This positioning does not place the humerus parallel to the tabletop.

X-ray beam direction: The vertically directed beam is centered on the region of interest. If the proximal portion of the limb is to be studied, the x-ray beam may be angled craniocaudally 10° to 20° in an effort to decrease geometric distortion.

Comments: This view permits good evaluation of the entire limb. A shifting of the mechanism of restraint is needed when examining the distal portion of the limb.

It is also possible, but more difficult, to position the patient in dorsal recumbency with the forelimb pulled caudally so the humerus is lateral to the thoracic cavity. A vertically directed beam is used with that positioning.

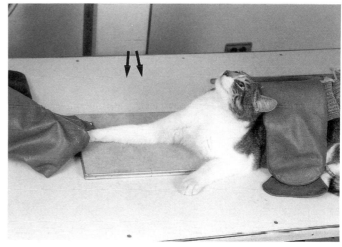

FORELIMB—CAUDOCRANIAL VIEW
(horizontal beam)

Patient preparation: This study is usually performed on a severely traumatized patient when other more conventional patient positioning cannot be accomplished easily.

Patient positioning: The patient is placed in lateral recumbency with the affected limb uppermost resting on a large sponge with the cassette positioned against the cranial aspect of the forelimb. Extend the limb as much as possible using a line tied to the foot. The opposite forelimb can be left in a neutral position on the dependent side.

X-ray beam direction: The x-ray tube is positioned caudally and the horizontally directed beam is directed perpendicular to the cassette face at the point of interest.

Comments: It may not be possible to place the cassette far enough proximally to be able to study the humeral head and shoulder joint.

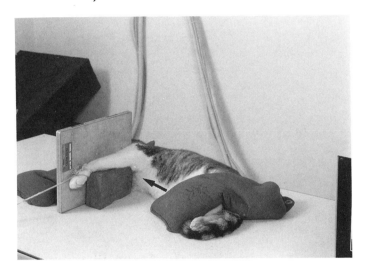

FORELIMB—OBLIQUE VIEWS

Patient preparation: No special preparation is required.

Patient positioning: The patient is placed in sternal recumbency with the forelimb to be studied pulled as far cranially as possible and held or positioned by sandbags or tied to the table. Rotate the patient approximately 30° laterally for the lateral oblique and 30° for the medial oblique. The cat's head is positioned laterally toward the unaffected limb so that it is not within the primary beam for either oblique views. The opposite forelimb is left in a neutral position.

X-ray beam direction: The vertically directed beam is perpendicular to the tabletop for the oblique views.

CARPUS-METACARPUS-DIGITS— LATERAL VIEW

Patient preparation: No special preparation is required.

Patient positioning: Place the patient in lateral recumbency with the affected foot next to the tabletop. Forcefully extend the limb cranially and restrain it through the use of sandbags placed on the proximal portion of the limb. Use a wooden paddle or plastic spoon to assist in positioning the foot. Pull the unaffected leg caudally and hold it with sandbags or tie it. Slightly flex the carpus so that you avoid supination of the limb.

X-ray beam direction: The vertically directed x-ray beam is centered on the carpal bones.

CARPUS-METACARPUS-DIGITS— LATERAL VIEW (hyperflexed)

Patient preparation: No special preparation is required.

Patient positioning: Place the patient in lateral recumbency with the affected leg next to the tabletop. Forcefully extend the limb cranially and restrain it through the use of sandbags placed on the proximal portion of the limb. Use a wooden paddle or plastic spoon to achieve a hyperflexed position of the foot. Pull the unaffected leg caudally and hold it with sandbags or tie to the tabletop. Use sandbags to position the head.

X-ray beam direction: The vertically directed x-ray beam is centered on the carpal bones.

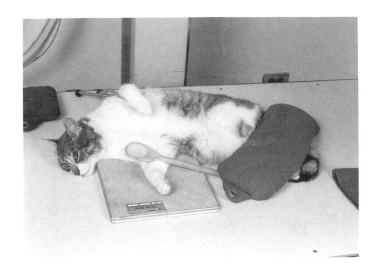 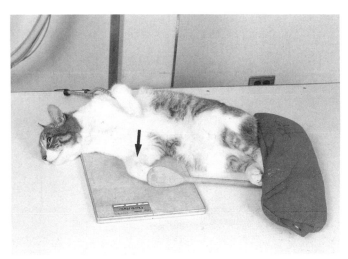

CARPUS-METACARPUS-DIGITS— LATERAL VIEW (hyperextended)

Patient preparation: No special preparation is required.

Patient positioning: Place the patient in lateral recumbency with the affected limb next to the tabletop. Forcefully extend the limb cranially and restrain it through the use of sandbags placed on the proximal portion of the limb. Use a wooden paddle or plastic spoon to achieve a hyperextended position of the foot. Pull the unaffected leg caudally and hold it with sandbags or tie to the table.

X-ray beam direction: The vertically directed x-ray beam is centered on the carpal bones.

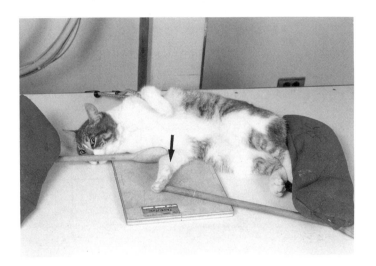

CARPUS-METACARPUS-DIGITS— DORSOPALMAR VIEW

Patient preparation: No special preparation is required.

Patient positioning: Place the patient in ventral recumbency with the affected limb extended using a rope or gauze. Restrain the limb through the use of sandbags placed in the more proximal portion of the limb. Use a wooden spoon or plastic paddle to achieve positioning.

X-Ray beam direction: The vertically directed x-ray beam is centered on the foot.

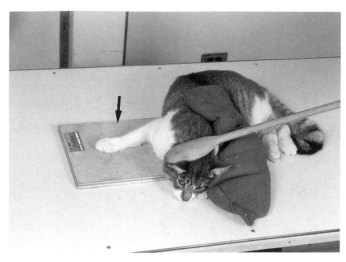

8. RADIOGRAPHY OF THE PELVIC LIMB

INTRODUCTION

The lateral view of the pelvic limb is relatively easy to make and the entire limb can be obtained on a single view. The craniocaudal view is made with the patient in dorsal recumbency with the limb extended caudally. Oblique views of the tarsus, metatarsus, and digits may be helpful (Table 8-1). Often a lateral view of the opposite limb can serve as a comparison view and is helpful in diagnosis, especially if the growth plates have not closed.

Table 8-1
PROTOCOL FOR RADIOGRAPHY OF THE PELVIC LIMB

Routine views
  lateral
  craniocaudal (vertical beam with patient in dorsal recumbency)
  caudocranial (vertical beam with patient in ventral recumbency)
Optional views
  caudocranial (horizontal beam)
  craniocaudal in internal oblique
  craniocaudal in external oblique
  caudocranial in internal oblique
  caudocranial in external oblique

VIEWS

PELVIC LIMB—LATERAL VIEW

Patient preparation: Remove dirt and debris from the hair coat.

Patient positioning: Place the patient in lateral recumbency with the affected limb down. Extend the limb and hold it in position or use sandbags or tie it to the tabletop. Flex the opposite unaffected limb and remove it from the x-ray beam by abducting the limb and pulling it laterally or remove it by placing it into extension or flexion. Hold the unaffected limb or use sandbags to hold it in position or tie it to the tube stand. Sandbags are used to position the forelimbs.

X-ray beam direction: The vertically directed beam is centered on the point of interest.

Comments: Shifting of the restraint devices is required to examine the distal part of the limb.

PELVIC LIMB—CRANIOCAUDAL VIEW (vertical beam)

Patient preparation: No special preparation.

Patient positioning: Place the patient in dorsal recumbency and extend the pelvic limbs as far caudally as possible and hold them in a position by tying them or using sandbags. This is the same position used for making a ventrodorsal view of the pelvis.

X-ray beam direction: The vertically directed x-ray beam is centered on the region of interest.

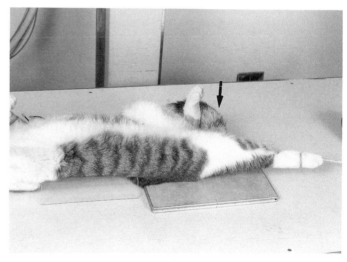

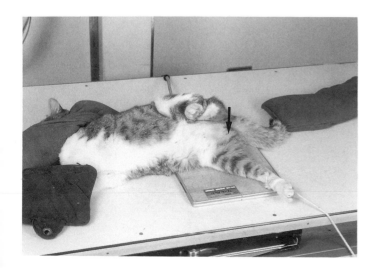

PELVIC LIMB—CAUDOCRANIAL VIEW
(horizontal beam)

Patient preparation: No special preparation.

Patient positioning: Place the cat in lateral recumbency with the affected limb uppermost supported on a sponge. Place a cassette vertically against the cranial surface of the limb. Extend the affected limb and hold it in position or tie the affected pelvic limb to the tabletop or use sandbags to hold it. Use sandbags to restrain the forelimbs.

X-ray beam direction: The x-ray tube is placed caudally and the horizontally directed x-ray beam is centered on the point of interest.

Comments: Shifting of the restraint devices is required to examine the distal part of the limb.

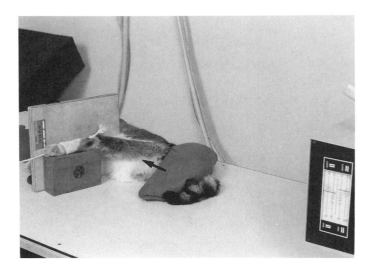

PELVIC LIMB—CAUDOCRANIAL VIEW
(vertical beam)

Patient preparation: No special preparation.

Patient positioning: Place the patient in ventral recumbency and extend both pelvic limbs as far as possible caudally. Hold the pelvic limbs or tie them to the tabletop or use sandbags to hold them. Tie the forelimbs to the tabletop or use sandbags to hold them.

X-ray beam direction: The vertically directed x-ray beam is centered on the more distal portion of the limb to be studied.

Comments: It is possible to angle the beam caudocranially 10° to 20° and obtain a greater "tunnel" view of the distal femur.

Shifting of the restraint devices may be required to examine the distal part of the limb.

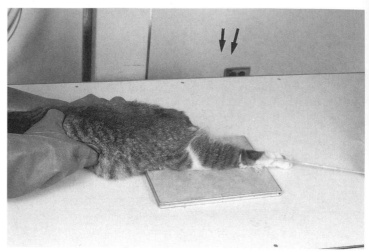

TARSUS-METATARSUS-DIGITS—LATERAL VIEW

Patient preparation: Remove dirt and debris from the hair coat.

Patient positioning: Place the cat in lateral recumbency with the affected leg down and the tarsal joint at a 90° angle of flexion. Hold the limb or use sandbags positioned proximally. The opposite unaffected limb is removed from the x-ray beam by abducting the limb and pulling it laterally or by simply extending the limb.

X-ray beam direction: The vertically directed beam is centered on the tarsal joints.

TARSUS-METATARSUS-DIGITS—PLANTARODORSAL VIEW

Patient preparation: No special preparation.

Patient positioning: Place the patient in ventral recumbency and position the affected pelvic limb as far caudally as is possible. Hold the limb proximally or place sandbags on the limb proximally to maintain the extended position.

X-ray beam direction: The vertically directed x-ray beam is centered on the tarsal joints.

Comments: By rotating the patient medially or laterally 30°, oblique views of the foot can be made.

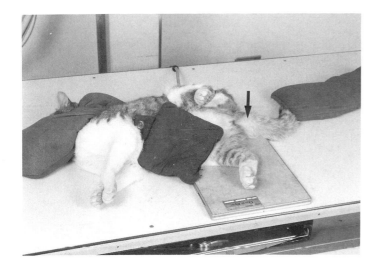

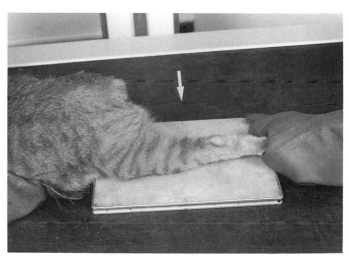

REFERENCES

Carlisle CH and Thrall DE. A comparison of normal feline thoracic radiographs made in dorsal versus ventral recumbency. Vet Rad 23:3-9, 1982.

den Toom OI Miyabayashi T and Morgan JP. Application of positional radiographic techniques in the dog and cat Part 1 Thorax. Cal Vet 5:19-22, 1983.

Hare WCD. Radiographic anatomy of the feline skull. J Am Vet Med Assoc 134:349-56, 1959.

Miyabayashi T denToom OI and Morgan JP. Application of positional radiographic techniques in the dog and cat. Part III—Skeleton. Cal Vet 7:11-5, 1983.

Sis RF and Getty R. Normal radiographic anatomy of the cat. Vet Med/SAC May 1968 pages 475-92.

SECTION D

SPECIAL RADIOGRAPHIC PROCEDURES IN THE DOG AND CAT

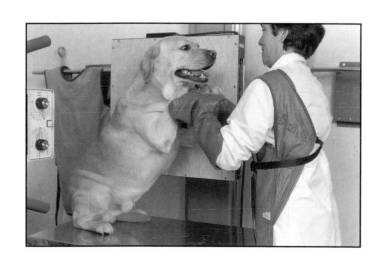
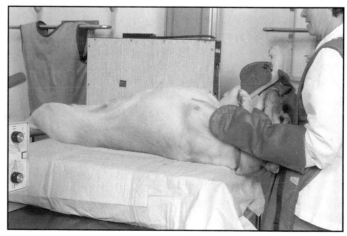

1. INTRODUCTION

Special radiographic procedures are used to make available additional information than can be obtained from a routine radiographic examination. Most procedures utilize either negative or positive contrast agents that enhance the contrast between body organs and therefore enhance radiographic contrast. Other procedures may be more simple and utilize only special positioning of the patient to improve visualization of an organ or lesion. Patient preparation is important in the conduct of these special procedures. In all studies, the use of preliminary non-contrast radiographs is important to establish a data base from which to evaluate the contrast study and the special procedure should never replace or precede the survey study.

Definition

Any radiographic study that requires some special positioning of the patient or x-ray beam or use of a negative or positive contrast agent can be considered as a special radiographic procedure. Another more general definition might include those radiographic studies that are in addition to any that are included within a routine examination. The special studies are easily divided into those that are morphological in character and those that are functional. Morphological studies are used to: (1) identify an organ's normal or abnormal size, shape, position, or contour, (2) provide information concerning the mucosal surface of a viscus or its luminal contents, (3) evaluate the character of the wall of a hollow viscus for a mural lesion, or (4) determine the presence of some extra-mural lesion. Functional studies provide assessment of organ function, often transit time of the contrast meal, and are usually more detailed and require a longer time to perform.

Indications

It is important to recognize that the special study provides information necessary to: (1) make a diagnosis, (2) further evaluate the character of a suspected lesion, or (3) determine an appropriate method of treatment in patients in which this information is not available from a non-contrast or survey radiographic study. In some patients, the special study may be used to determine the size and location of a lesion that enables a surgical procedure to be conducted with greater efficiency.

Contraindications

As in any diagnostic procedure, there are contraindications that are specific for the examination to be performed. These are considered in the description of the specific studies. A consideration prior to use of any of the studies deals with the fact that they generally require special positioning of the patient, and the use of additional radiographic views that are often made in a progressive manner over a period of minutes or even hours. The procedure entails the use of technical assistance for some period of time to provide the required positioning and may be an indication that the study is contraindicated because

of the financial cost to the owner. Hopefully, this financial consideration is balanced against the potential value of the special procedure to provide information that can be used in diagnosis or treatment.

Prior to performing the special procedure it should be determined: (1) if the patient is a good anesthetic risk should anesthesia be required, (2) if the patient can tolerate the withholding of food prior to the study if this should be required, (3) if the time required to perform the diagnostic study might be better used in performing other diagnostic techniques, (4) if enough information is already available to take the patient directly to surgery, and (5) whether surgical treatment can be safely postponed while the radiographic study is being performed.

Patient Preparation

The patient being considered for a routine non-contrast radiographic study may only need to have its hair coat cleaned, however, the same patient being prepared for a special procedure may require much more elaborate preparation.

Contrast Medium

Barium sulfate is the contrast medium most commonly used for studies of the gastrointestinal tract. Iodinated products are available for parenteral use for study of the urinary system. Myelography requires a special nonionic iodinated product because of the sensitivity of the meninges. Air is used as a contrast agent alone or mixed with the positive contrast agents. Iodinated contrast agents used for urographic studies are injected intravenously while barium sulfate suspensions may be administered orally or rectally.

Equipment

General equipment to perform a special procedure consists of some method of placing it within the body organ to be evaluated. This may be intravenous, per os, per rectum, or in a retrograde manner into the urethra, vagina, or sinus tract. Other more specific items required for a study are described in detail below.

Technique

The technique used for each of the special procedures is different and presented in detail in the following pages. A point of important consideration, however, applies to all of the studies. That is, the special radiographic procedures must be performed in a systematic manner using a predetermined technique of administration of the contrast agent or positioning of the patient. Standardization of the technique minimizes the complications and prevents failures when performing these procedures. The amount of contrast agent administered need be noted, and the sequence of radiographic exposures noted indicating the time the radiographs are made. Having made the point of the importance of standardization of the study, it is important to add that the special studies should be modified wherever necessary to meet the needs of the particular patient being studied.

2. GASTROINTESTINAL SPECIAL PROCEDURES IN THE DOG AND CAT

A. INTRODUCTION

Radiographic examination of the gastrointestinal tract remains a valuable technique in veterinary medicine and has progressed considerably from the early use of rubber bags full of lead that were swallowed by unsuspecting patients prior to radiography. While this technique was successful radiographically, it was somewhat toxic to the patient if the bag ruptured during the study. While ultrasound has assumed a valuable role in examination of the urinary system, diagnostic radiology is still a most successful method of evaluation of the esophagus, stomach, small bowel, and large bowel. Endoscopy also adds information relative to diagnosis of esophageal, gastric, and colonic lesions, however, there are limitations for that technique.

Indications

The usual indications for study of the gastrointestinal tract (excluding the esophagus) include; (1) vomiting, (2) diarrhea, (3) constipation, (4) hematochezia, (5) melana, (6) abdominal mass, (7) abdominal pain, (8) historical knowledge of foreign body ingestion, or (9) following abdominal trauma. The radiographic studies are used to detect alterations in: (1) structure or morphology or (2) function that includes time of transport of the contrast meal. While there are many reports of the radiographic appearance of mucosal disease, it should be understood that the techniques described do not easily permit dilatation of a hollow viscus and thus the organ cannot be expanded to enable complete evaluation of the mucosa. It is recommended that the studies should be used only for detection of intraluminal lesions, mass mural lesions, and extramural lesions.

The indications for study of the esophagus are usually related to an inability of a patient to successfully swallow and are most often used to evaluate a suspect foreign body. Extramural masses may also cause difficulty in swallowing and can be evaluated with an esophageal study.

Contraindications

Contraindications for these studies are related to the presence of a fluid-filled distended esophagus, stomach, or bowel in which there is a lack of motility. The use of barium sulfate suspension in a chronically obstructed patient with a mechanical ileus in which the stomach or bowel loops have become atonic and distended with fluid usually adds little information. Patients with an ileus due to torsion or necrosis due to loss of blood supply or with a paralytic ileus due to trauma or peritonitis are not good candidates for contrast studies. The addition of positive-contrast agent in these patients usually does little except create some very persistent white shadows to the radiograph that remain because of the atonic character of the gut and the tendency for the contrast agent to mix slowly with the watery contents.

Contrast Agents

Barium sulfate remains the most commonly used contrast agent for study of the gastrointestinal tract and is available in a liquid, powder, or paste form. The liquid form is available in containers from a size of 280ml to 1900ml bottles (Fig. 2-1). It has a particle size that is controlled but it does settles under the influence of gravity. The descriptive term, micronized, indicates a particle size range that has made flocculation, or the agglomeration of the particles, no longer the problem that it was in the past. Suspending agents used today also help to prevent flocculation and sedimentation. It is recommended that the suspension be shaken well prior to using. Barium sulfate is not hypertonic and does not increase the amount of intraluminal fluid. Perhaps, the only disadvantage of barium sulfate is the slow transit time through the small bowel. Use of the suspension chilled for the upper gastrointestinal studies provides a more rapid transit from the stomach into the small bowel. For use in lower gastrointestinal studies it is more comfortable should the suspension be administered between room and body temperature. Fears of inspisation within the large bowel have not been supported in clinical practice. Even with perforation of a hollow viscus, the mediastinal or peritoneal response is minimal and probably of little additional clinical significance to the already present inflammatory response.

It should be appreciated that barium sulfate powder or liquid suspensions are not produced in a sterile manner. If a container is opened, it is possible that contamination from patient-personnel contact may probable result. Preparation of barium sulfate suspension should not be performed in a dirty sink area. The reservoir-type of container for the barium sulfate enemas and the enema tubes are easily contaminated and it difficult to clean them thoroughly. Syringes used for

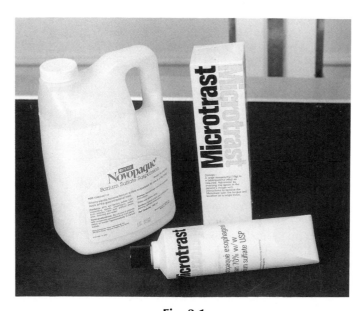

Fig. 2-1
FORMS OF BARIUM SULFATE
This commonly used contrast medium is available in a suspension form or a much thicker past formulation.

oral or rectal administration of barium sulfate suspension need to be thoroughly cleaned and sterilized prior to reuse.

The concentration of the barium mixture varies relative to its intended use from 30% to 60% (w/w). A suspension can be diluted with water using 1 part of 60% barium sulfate suspension and 4 parts water creating a 12% concentration (w/w). Barium sulfate can be obtained in a cream or paste form that is 70% w/w (Fig. 2-1).

Previously touted iodinated water-soluble agents, such as Gastrografin, are osmotically active and actually dangerous to use in the patient that is dehydrated or has severe electrolyte imbalance. The renal excretion of iodine can be used to detect the crossing of mucosal surfaces by the water-soluble organic iodine preparation. It has been suggested that resulting hypermotility was due in addition to the potentiation of cholinergic stimuli through the release of serotonin.

The production of nonionic iodinated products, such as metrizamide, makes them readily available today for successful use in radiographic evaluation of the gastrointestinal tract. Minimal fluid is drawn into the bowel lumen with resulting minimal dilution of the contrast agent. Little change in hematocrit is noticed. A mild cathartic effect occurs that is beneficial since the transit time for the contrast meal is increased. Their high cost unfortunately makes them of little practical use except with small patients (Williams et al, 1993).

Technique

The studies of the gastrointestinal tract are much more easily performed using the technique of fluoroscopy, since the visualization of passage of the contrast meal converts the study into a functional study instead of one of static images that demonstrate only a morphological picture. The more active the function, such as passage of a bolus through the esophagus, the more the lack of fluoroscopy is felt.

Certain techniques partially compensate for the lack of fluoroscopic equipment. Some of these include the use of oblique projections. Segments of the digestive system may be obscured by other overlying organs. The organ in question may be orientated so that it is not well visualized in the standard VD or lateral projection, but can be seen on an oblique view. The use of right and left lateral projections can be used to control and shift the position of the contrast medium and intraluminal gas. This can be used advantageously to evaluate an organ in question, particularly the stomach. Abdominal compression moves the organ of interest to a location that provides for better visualization, or shifts overlying organs so that they do not superimpose the area of interest. Compression also decreases tissue thickness therefore enhancing radiographic contrast by decreasing secondary radiation that fogs the film. The sequence of radiographic exposures provides additional information of a functional nature that can be used to better understand a suspected lesion. As in any special procedure, following a specific protocol is necessary to fully evaluate the organ in question.

Problems

The most commonly encountered errors noted in gastrointestinal studies are the use of an insufficient amount of contrast medium that results in a failure in distention of the organ in question and markedly alters gastric emptying time and small bowel transit time suggesting a partially obstructing lesion. Another serious problem in radiographic diagnosis results from the mixing of the contrast agent with digestive tract contents with resulting filling defects within the contrast column frequently misdiagnosed as luminal foreign bodies or mural masses. The contrast agent may fail to coat the mucosal surface equally, resulting in a compromised radiograph that prohibits accurate evaluation of the mucosal surface of the gut wall. While the mixture of barium sulfate suspension with bowel contents compromises a morphological study, it may be possible to use this mixture to measure gastric emptying or small bowel transit time.

REFERENCES

Allan GS Rendano VT Quick CB et al. Gastrografin as a gastrointestinal contrast medium in the cat. J Am Vet Rad Soc 20:110, 1979.

Allan GS Wentworth RA Rendano VT Meumier PC and Marmor M. The renal excretion of iodine following oral administration of gastrografin to domestic cats. Invest Rad 15: 47, 1980.

Amberg JR and Unger JD. Contamination of barium sulfate suspension. Radiology 97: 182, 1970.

Johansen JG. Assessment of a non-ionic contrast medium (Amipaque) in the gastrointestinal tract. Invest Rad 13:523, 1978.

Rubin DL Carroll BA and Snow HD. The harmful effects of aqueous contrast agents on the gastrointestinal tract: A study of mechanism and means of counteraction. Invest Rad 16:50, 1981.

Williams J Biller DS Myer CW Miyabayashi T and Leveille R. Use of iohexal as gastrointestinal contrast agent in three dogs, five cats, and one bird. J Am Vet Med Assoc 203:624-7, 1993.

B. ESOPHAGOGRAPHY IN THE DOG AND CAT

Definition

Esophagography is the radiographic study that may permit evaluation of both esophageal function and morphology (Fig. 2-2). The study is best performed under fluoroscopic examination, however, much can be learned from a sequential series of static radiographs. Understanding the limitations of the study along with the advantages is important, especially when forced to use a series of radiographs rather than fluoroscopy. Esophagography can be performed using a barium sulfate suspension to evaluate function or can be performed with air or a double-contrast study using barium sulfate and air to evaluate morphology. Use of barium sulfate suspension mixed with food permits determination of the degree of esophageal distensibility. It is important to tailor the study to the unique nature of the individual patient. The technique is performed in a similar manner in the dog as in the cat. Plan the study in conjunction with esophagoscopy realizing that there is some retention of the contrast agent on the mucosal surface. The addition of a barium sulfate suspension to a chronically fluid-filled esophagus severely compromises esophagoscopy.

Usually two radiographic views are satisfactory to perform the examination and the right lateral and dorsoventral view are used most commonly. However, it is possible to use left lateral and ventrodorsal views instead of, or in conjunction with, the first mentioned views.

Indications

Regurgitation of undigested food immediately after swallowing is a frequent indication for an esophageal study and may be associated with gagging or retching. A history of dysphagia or salivation or a history of swallowing a foreign body are also indications for obtaining an esophagram. Often the study is performed to evaluate the location of the esophagus relative to suspected extramural cervical, mediastinal, or pulmonary masses. Examination of the survey non-contrast radiographs assists in determining how the esophagram should be performed.

Specific indications include: (1) regurgitation of undigested food, (2) acute gagging or retching, (3) dysphagia, (4) excessive salivation, (5) change in attitude of eating and/or drinking. Suspect lesions include: (1) esophageal wall mass lesion, (2) esophagitis due to gastroesophageal reflux, regurgitation, or vomiting, (3) esophageal wall diverticula, (4) esophageal wall tear or rupture, (5) persistent vascular ring anomaly, (6) mediastinal mass causing esophageal displacement, (7) gastro-esophageal herniation or invagination, or (8) esophageal foreign body.

Contraindications

A patient who has dysphagia may aspirate the contrast medium at the time of administration. Small amounts of barium sulfate aspirated into the lungs usually have no serious consequences unless it is superimposed on severe acute or chronic lung disease. Even then, the radiographic appearance of the barium sulfate suspension within the lungs is more frightening than are the clinical consequences.

A dilated, fluid-filled, or food-filled esophagus usually has sufficient contrast within it to preclude the necessity for a barium sulfate study. If the cause of the mega-esophagus needs to be evaluated, attempt to empty the esophagus before performing the double-contrast study as described below.

If the esophagram includes the use of barium sulfate impregnated kibble, evaluation of a subsequent gastrogram is compromised. If only liquid barium sulfate is used, the gastrography can follow without problem.

The study can be performed in the cat in a similar manner as in the dog except for the use of smaller amounts of contrast agent.

Contrast Medium

Several forms of barium sulfate suspension, from a thin liquid to a thick cream or paste, may be used. Usually, a radiographic sequence begins with liquid contrast agent (30% w/w) and these films are evaluated prior to proceeding with the study. The use of thicker, more viscous, agents (70% w/w) or the use of a barium sulfate suspension (30% w/w) mixed with solid food may follow determining the distensibility of the esophagus during the act of swallowing. A double-contrast study may be used to further evaluate a mural lesion.

Equipment

1. 30 or 50 cc syringe
2. stomach tube
3. oral speculum
4. barium sulfate liquid or paste
5. kibble

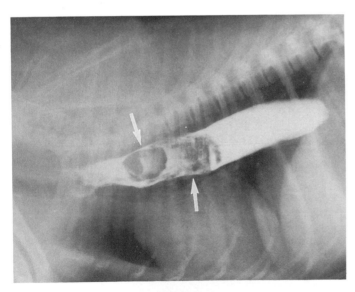

Fig. 2-2
ESOPHOGRAM
A lateral thoracic radiograph of a dog made after administration of a barium sulfate suspension. The dilated esophagus is filled with the positive-contrast agent and outlines two large filling defects (arrows) caused by foreign bodies (meat).

Technique—Liquid barium sulfate suspension

The technique using <u>liquid barium sulfate suspension</u> described below confirms the patency of the esophagus, esophageal location, and can provide functional evidence that the patient can pass a liquid bolus into the stomach.

1. place the patient on the radiographic table in a comfortable position
2. obtain precontrast radiographic studies of the cervical region and thorax
3. empty a fluid-filled distended esophagus, if possible
4. administer barium sulfate suspension (30% w/w) into the buccal pouch and close the mouth awaiting the patient to swallow the liquid
5. position the patient in lateral recumbency and make serial radiographs that include the oral pharynx cranially and the stomach caudally
6. administer additional barium sulfate suspension into the buccal pouch and close the mouth awaiting the patient to swallow the liquid
7. position the patient in ventral recumbency and make radiographs that include the oral pharynx cranially to the stomach caudally
8. repeat administration of the liquid contrast agent until diagnostic radiographs demonstrate coating of the esophageal mucosa throughout
9. paper towels placed on the tabletop or a towel tied around the patient's neck can be used to absorb contrast agent that is spilled from the patients mouth
10. in the event an esophageal lesion is suspected by passage of a esophageal tube or scope, it may be helpful to pass a tube to the level of the suspected lesion and make the injection of the barium sulfate suspension at that site—make the radiographs following injection—understand that this is not a complete study of the esophagus

Technique—Barium sulfate soaked kibble

The technique using <u>barium sulfate soaked kibble</u> described below confirms the ability of the patient to swallow and pass a more solid bolus through the esophagus and into the stomach. This functional study confirms that the esophagus is able to distend and permit passage of a large bulky mass of food and permits radiographic diagnosis of partially obstructive esophageal disease that might have been missed on the study using liquid barium sulfate suspension. The study using kibble also evaluates esophageal function as the bolus passes into the stomach.

1. place the patient on the radiographic table in a comfortable position
2. obtain precontrast radiographic studies of the cervical region and thorax
3. perform an esophageal study using liquid barium sulfate suspension (30% w/w) (as described above)
4. place barium soaked kibble into the buccal pouch and close the mouth awaiting the patient to swallow the bolus (use either 30% w/w or 60% w/w)
5. position the patient in lateral recumbency and make radiographs that include the oral pharynx cranially to the stomach caudally
6. place additional barium soaked kibble into the buccal pouch and close the mouth awaiting the patient to swallow the bolus
7. position the patient in ventral recumbency and make radiographs that include the oral pharynx cranially to the stomach caudally
8. repeat administration of barium soaked kibble until diagnostic radiographs are obtained
9. paper towels placed on the tabletop or a towel tied around the patient's neck can be used to absorb contrast agent that is spilled from the patients mouth

Technique—Double-contrast technique

The <u>double-contrast technique</u> described below evaluates for morphologic abnormalities within the esophagus where determination of esophageal function is not of concern. Mucosal abnormality, intraluminal foreign bodies, or partial stricture or stenosis can be well evaluated using this technique. Usually the patient is sedated or anesthetized for this procedure, however, it can be performed with some degree of success on an awake patient. The technique is usually performed following gastrography on the sedated or anesthetized patient when the stomach tube is pulled back into the esophagus. The patient may have already experienced some gastro-esophageal reflux so all that is needed is to inject air. The technique is uncommonly performed, but is most inform-ative when done correctly.

1. place the patient on the radiographic table in a comfortable position
2. obtain precontrast radiographic studies of the cervical region and thorax
3. perform an esophageal study using liquid barium sulfate suspension (30% w/w) (as described above)
4. using an oral speculum as required, pass a stomach tube into the esophagus avoiding forceful attempts to pass the tube through an area of partial ob-struction
5. if possible, make a radiograph to confirm the position of the stomach tube (you may wish to reposition the tip of the tube depending on the specific portion of the esophagus to be studied)
6. attach a syringe and inject 3 to 5 cc (small dog or cat) or 8 to 10 cc (large dog) of barium sulfate suspension (use either 30% w/w or 60% w/w) OR use barium sulfate suspension in the esophagus as a result of gastroesophageal reflux
7. attach the air-filled syringe to the tube
8. position the patient in lateral recumbency, inject 20 to 30 cc (small dog or cat) or 40 to 50 cc (large dog) of air, and make a single radiograph of the thorax immediately after completing the injection
9. re-attach the air-filled syringe to the tube
10. position the patient in sternal recumbency, inject a similar amount of air and make a single radiograph of the thorax immediately after completing the injection

Comments

It is possible to use additional mixtures to evaluate deglutition in the patient. The barium sulfate suspension may be mixed with infant cereal mix to obtain an intermediary consistency. If required, the barium sulfate suspension can be made thinner by diluting it with equal parts of water. It is possible to make a study using the technique described above using only air.

Aspirated barium sulfate is well tolerated in the healthy lung and even fairly large volumes are cleared from the airways within 24 hours.

REFERENCES

Brawner WR and Bartels JE. Contrast radiography of the digestive tract—indications, techniques and complica-tions. Vet Clin North Am 13:599, 1983.

Kneller SK and Lewis R. Contrast radiography of the normal cat esophagus. JAAHA 9:50, 1973.

Morgan JP. Normal radiographic anatomy of the gastro-intestinal tract of the dog. Scientific Proceedings AVMA 101st Annual meeting Vol 155, 1964.

Root CR and Morgan JP. Contrast radiography of the upper gastrointestinal tract in the dog. J sm Anim Pract 10:279, 1969.

C. GASTROGRAPHY IN THE DOG AND CAT

Definition

The radiographic study of the stomach including the proximal portion of the duodenal loop is referred to as gastrography. The contrast agent is administered orally and radiographs are made with the patient in various positions. The study can be performed as a: (1) positive-contrast study, (2) negative-contrast study, and (3) double-contrast study.

The study can be designed either to evaluate the morphology of the stomach or gastric function. A morphologic study examines the character and location of the gastric wall or gastric contents looking for an: (1) extramural lesion, (2) mural lesion, or (3) intraluminal lesion. A functional study examines gastric motility and pyloric function and is most often evaluated by determination of the time of onset of gastric emptying and the time of complete gastric emptying. These times depend directly on the size of the test meal and the nature of the meal, liquid or solid. The liquid phase of the meal should begin to enter the small intestine immediately following administration, however, the patient may need to be returned to a quiet environment before gastric emptying commences. A decision must be made as to the purpose of the study, since a functional study is performed differently from a morphologic study (Table 2-1). In certain cases, one type of study can be followed by the other, but often this cannot be done. A study to determine morphology can be performed on a sedated or anesthetized patient, however, the functional study is best performed on a patient who has not received any medication.

Fixation of a small area of the stomach to the abdominal wall of dogs or establishment of a gastric fistula was reported to shorten gastric emptying time significantly (Jefferson et al 1963).

In most patients, gastroscopy cannot immediately follow the radiographic study.

Indications

Clinical signs that suggest use of a gastrography, however the study is performed, include: (1) vomition, (2) hematemesis, (3) cranial abdominal pain, (4) anorexia, (5) melena, or (6) cranial abdominal mass lesion. Specific morphologic lesions include: (1) intraluminal gastric foreign body, (2) gastric mural lesion, (3) gastric mucosal lesion, (4) diaphragmatic hernia with gastric displacement, (5) gastric dilatation, and (6) gastric displacement due to adjacent cranial abdominal mass lesion. Specific functional lesions include the determination of gastric emptying that might indicate a pyloric outflow dysfunction (Table 2-2).

Table 2-1
GASTROGRAPHY IN THE DOG AND CAT

Information desired	Technique of gastrography
determine size, shape, and/or position	negative gastrography positive gastrography
determine extramural lesion	negative gastrography positive gastrography
determine mural lesion	double-contrast gastrography negative gastrography
determine intraluminal mass	double-contrast gastrography negative gastrography
determine gastric emptying time	positive gastrography using liquid and kibble

Table 2-2
COMPLETE GASTRIC EMPTYING TIMES (APPROXIMATE)

	Dog adult	Dog immature	Cat adult
full liquid meal	2 hr (0.5-3)	1 hr (1-1.5)	0.5 hr (0.25-1)
full intact kibble meal	8 hr (6-10)	5 hr (4-6)	
full ground kibble meal	7 hr (5-9)		
half ground kibble meal	5 hr (4-5.5)		

Contraindications

1. Usually the study can be performed in some manner in every patient, however, determination of gastric emptying time should begin early in the day so that the study does not need to continue into the evening.
2. Usually the patient is anorectic or vomiting and the stomach is empty prior to gastrography. This permits performing either a morphological or functional study without special preparation. If the study is to be morphological in nature, the stomach must be empty prior to administration of the contrast meal. If the study is functional in character, the fluid-filled stomach should be at least partially emptied prior to administration of the contrast meal.
3. While some describe the use of gastrography in evaluation of patients with gastric dilatation/volvulus syndrome, the addition of contrast agent into a fluid-filled distended stomach usually offers little additional information and frequently may be complicating. The degree of gastric distention and rotation can be determined from non-contrast radiographs made using several different body positionings.
4. Use of gastrography that requires gastric distention is not suggested immediately following gastric surgery or deep biopsy.
5. If the survey radiographs show the stomach to be filled with ingesta, consider delaying the study.

Contrast Medium

Several forms of barium sulfate suspension are available ranging from 30% w/w to 60% w/w. It is recommended to consider diluting the more concentrated agents. Double-contrast studies may be performed with the higher concentrations and may be used to further evaluate a mural lesion.

Equipment

1. barium sulfate suspension (30% w/w or 60% w/w)
2. gastric tube
3. oral speculum
4. 50 cc syringe

POSITIVE-CONTRAST GASTROGRAPHY AS A FUNCTIONAL STUDY IN THE DOG

Specific Indications

As a functional study, the primary indication is to determine gastric emptying time.

Technique to determine function using a liquid contrast agent

1. make a routine noncontrast abdominal radiographic study
2. either using the buccal pouch and a syringe or a gastric tube, administer barium sulfate suspension (diluted to 30% if necessary) using the following dosages: (1) 8 to 10 cc/kgbw in small-sized dogs less than 10 kg, (2) 5 to 8 cc/kgbw in medium-sized dogs between 10 and 40 kg, and (3) 3 to 5 cc/kgbw in large dogs more than 40 kg. The dosage may be slightly modified if esophagography has been performed prior to gastrography.
3. make dorsoventral, ventrodorsal, right lateral, and left lateral radiographs centering on the cranial abdomen immediately following administration of the contrast agent (0-time films)
4. make ventrodorsal and left lateral radiographs centering on the cranial abdomen 30 minutes following administration of the contrast agent (30-minute films)
5. make ventrodorsal and left lateral radiographs centering on the cranial abdomen 60 minutes following administration of the contrast agent (60-minute films)

Comments

After determining that gastric emptying of the liquid contrast agent is progressing in a normal manner through filling of the proximal portion of the small intestine within 30 minutes to 1 hour, proceed with the second portion of the study. The study can be converted into a double-contrast morphologic study following partial emptying of the stomach through the administration of air.

Technique to determine function using a solid contrast meal

1. using the buccal pouch, administer kibble mixed with barium sulfate suspension using the following dosages: 8 g/kg of intact kibble plus 5 to 7 ml/kg of the barium sulfate suspension (30%w/w or 60%w/w)
2. make dorsoventral and right lateral radiographs centering on the cranial abdomen following administration of the kibble mixed with contrast agent (0-time films)
3. make dorsoventral and right lateral radiographs centering on the cranial abdomen 3 hours following administration of the kibble mixed with contrast agent (3-hour films)
4. make dorsoventral and right lateral radiographs centering on the cranial abdomen 5 hours following administration of the kibble mixed with contrast agent (5-hour films)
5. make additional radiographs until stomach is empty

POSITIVE-CONTRAST GASTROGRAPHY AS A MORPHOLOGIC STUDY IN THE DOG

Specific Indications

The positive-contrast study is good to evaluate gastric size, shape, and location in examination of an extramural gastric lesion. The study is not good to evaluate a mural gastric lesion or an intraluminal gastric lesion.

Technique

1. make a routine noncontrast abdominal radiographic study
2. either using the buccal pouch or a gastric tube, administer barium sulfate suspension (30% w/w or 60% w/w) using the following dosages: (1) 8 to 10 cc/kgbw in small-sized dogs less than 10 kg, (2) 5 to 8 cc/kgbw in medium-sized dogs between 10 and 40 kg, and (3) 3 to 5 cc/kgbw in large dogs more than 40 kg. The dosage may be slightly modified if esophogography has been performed prior to gastrography.
3. make dorsoventral, ventrodorsal, right lateral, and left lateral radiographs centering on the cranial abdomen immediately following administration of the contrast agent (0-time films) (this provides information on gastric location or extramural gastric lesion and the study may be terminated)
4. make ventrodorsal and left lateral radiographs centering on the cranial abdomen 30 minutes following administration of the contrast agent (30-minute films)
5. make ventrodorsal and left lateral radiographs centering on the cranial abdomen 60 minutes following administration of the contrast agent (60-minute films)
6. make ventrodorsal and left lateral radiographs centering on the cranial abdomen 180 minutes following administration of the contrast agent (3-hour films) (by this time the stomach has emptied adequately so that any intraluminal lesion is coated and visible)

Comments

If a gastric lesion is not identified, the study can be continued as double-contrast gastrography following the administration of air following emptying of some of the positive-contrast agent from the stomach. The study can also be continues as a small-bowel follow-through study since the amount of contrast agent administered orally insures that both gastric emptying and small bowel transit times observed can be evaluated.

DOUBLE-CONTRAST GASTROGRAPHY AS A MORPHOLOGIC STUDY IN THE DOG

Specific Indications

Double-contrast gastrography provides coating of the stomach wall and permits determination of the gastric location or extramural gastric lesion In addition, because of your ability to "see through" the stomach it is possible to determine mural gastric lesions and intraluminal gastric lesions.

Technique

1. the study is more easily performed on a sedated or anesthetized patient.
2. make a routine noncontrast abdominal radiographic study
3. using a gastric tube, administer barium sulfate suspension (30% w/w) using the following dosages: (1) 10 cc in small-sized dogs less than 10 kg, (2) 20 cc in medium-sized dogs between 10 and 40 kg, and (3) 30 cc in large dogs more than 40 kg
4. attach the air-filled syringe and inject air using the following dosages: (1) 50 to 100 cc in small-sized dogs less than 10 kg, (2) 100 to 200 cc in medium-sized dogs between 10 and 40 kg, and (3) 200 to 300 cc in large dogs (inject until the stomach is distended)
5. withdraw the tip of the tube into the caudal esophagus
6. rotate the patient carefully
7. make dorsoventral, ventrodorsal, right lateral, and left lateral radiographs centering on the cranial abdomen immediately following administration of the air
8. if necessary inject additional air since air can be lost by regurgitation or into the small bowel
9. make dorsoventral, ventrodorsal, right lateral, and left lateral radiographs centering on the cranial abdomen immediately following additional administration of the air

Comments

It is difficult to determine the exact volume of air to inject since not all of the air remains within the stomach, some is regurgitated immediately and some passes into the small bowel. Therefore, it is important to rely on resistance to injection of air and palpation of the distended stomach.

If a gastric lesion is not identified, the study can be continued as a positive-contrast study of the stomach or the study can be continued as a double-contrast morphologic small-bowel study with the distended small bowel easily evaluated.

If tubing the patient is not practical, it is possible to orally administer CO_2-producing tablets or spanules. These act immediately and radiographs made within 30 to 90 seconds after administration show the stomach to be greatly distended with gas (Fig. 2-3).

NEGATIVE-CONTRAST GASTROGRAPHY AS A MORPHOLOGIC STUDY IN THE DOG

Specific Indications

Using air or gas to distend the stomach permits evaluation of gastric location or the presence of an extramural gastric lesion. Because of the negative contrast agent, it is possible to evaluate a gastric mural lesion or an intraluminal gastric lesion.

Technique

1. the study is more easily performed on a sedated or anesthetized patient.
2. make a routine noncontrast abdominal radiographic study
3. pass an orogastric tube
4. attach the air-filled syringe to the gastric tube and inject air using the following dosages: (1) 50 to 100 cc in small-sized dogs less than 10 kg, (2) 100 to 200 cc in medium-sized dogs between 10 and 40 kg, and (3) 200 to 300 cc in large dogs
5. withdraw the tip of the tube into the caudal esophagus
6. make dorsoventral, ventrodorsal, right lateral, and left lateral radiographs centering on the cranial abdomen immediately following administration of the air
7. if necessary inject additional air since air can be lost by regurgitation or into the small bowel
8. make dorsoventral, ventrodorsal, right lateral, and left lateral radiographs centering on the cranial abdomen immediately following additional administration of the air

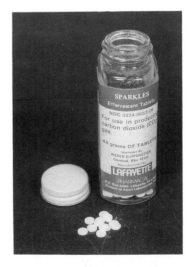

Fig. 2-3
EFFERVESCENT TABLETS
These small spanules produce CO_2 when swallowed and are of value in creation of negative-contrast and double-contrast radiographic studies.

Comments

It is difficult to determine the exact volume of air to inject since not all of the air remains within the stomach, some is regurgitated immediately and some passes into the small bowel. Therefore, it is important to rely on resistance to injection of air and palpation of the distended stomach.

If a gastric lesion is not identified, the study can be continued as a double-contrast morphologic small-bowel study with the distended small bowel easily evaluated.

It is also possible to generate sufficient gas through the introduction of CO_2 spanules that release the gas on contact with the acid environment of the stomach (Fig. 2-3).

POSITIVE-CONTRAST GASTROGRAPHY AS A FUNCTIONAL OR MORPHOLOGICAL STUDY IN THE CAT

Specific Indications

The use of a positive-contrast study permits evaluation of gastric size, shape, and location that might indicate an extramural gastric lesion (Fig. 2-4). Evaluation of a mural gastric lesion or an intraluminal gastric lesion is more difficult because of the density of the contrast agent. The study can also be used to determine gastric emptying.

Technique

1. make a routine noncontrast abdominal radiographic study
2. pass an orogastric tube
3. administer barium sulfate suspension (30% w/w or 60% w/w) using the dosage of 12 to 16 cc/kgbw
4. make dorsoventral, ventrodorsal, right lateral, and left lateral radiographs centering on the cranial abdomen immediately following administration of the contrast agent (0-time films) (this provides information on gastric location or extramural gastric lesion and the study may be terminated)
5. make ventrodorsal and left lateral radiographs centering on the cranial abdomen 15 minutes following administration of the contrast agent (15-minute films)
6. make ventrodorsal and left lateral radiographs centering on the cranial abdomen 30 minutes following administration of the contrast agent (30-minute films)

Comments

If a gastric lesion is not identified, the study can be continued as a small-bowel follow-through study. The amount of contrast agent administered orally insures that both gastric emptying and small bowel transit times observed can be evaluated. The study can also be converted into a double-contrast study by waiting for partial gastric emptying and administering air.

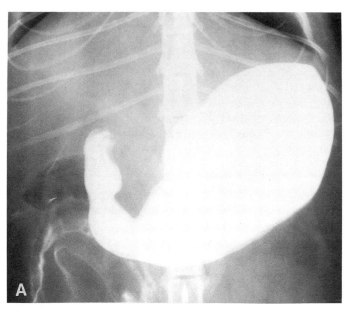

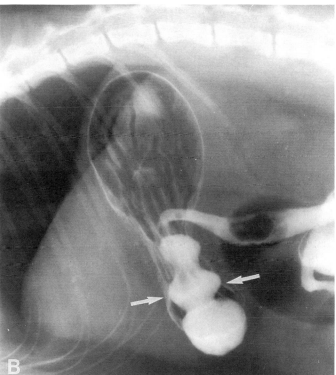

Fig. 2-4
GASTROGRAM
A ventrodorsal radiograph (A) of a cat following administration of barium sulfate suspension to perform positive-contrast gastrography. The stomach is distended and it can be understood how an intraluminal mass could be "hidden" in the contrast pool. A lateral radiograph (B) of the cranial abdomen of a cat following double-contrast gastrography. Infusion of a small amount of barium sulfate suspension was followed by infusion of a large quantity of air. The cat is in right lateral recumbency and the heavier barium sulfate suspension outlines the pyloric antrum (arrows) and the duodenum.

DOUBLE-CONTRAST GASTROGRAPHY AS A MORPHOLOGIC STUDY IN THE CAT

Specific Indications

Use of double contrast technique permits visualization of the size, shape and location of the stomach in the evaluation of a mural or extramural gastric lesion (Fig. 2-4). In addition, because you can see "into the stomach" it is possible to evaluate a mural gastric lesion or an intraluminal gastric lesion.

Technique

1. the study is more easily performed on a sedated or anesthetized patient
2. make a routine noncontrast abdominal radiographic study
3. using a gastric tube, administer 3 to 5 cc of barium sulfate suspension (30% w/w)
4. attach the air-filled syringe and inject air using the dosage of 30 to 50 cc
5. withdraw the tip of the tube into the caudal esophagus
6. rotate the patient carefully
7. make dorsoventral, ventrodorsal, right lateral, and left lateral radiographs centering on the cranial abdomen immediately following administration of the air
8. if necessary, inject additional air since air can be lost by regurgitation or into the small bowel
9. make dorsoventral, ventrodorsal, right lateral, and left lateral radiographs centering on the cranial abdomen immediately following additional administration of the air

Comments

It is difficult to determine the exact volume of air to inject since not all of the air remains within the stomach, some is regurgitated immediately and some passes into the small bowel. Therefore, it is important to rely on resistance to injection of air and palpation of the distended stomach.

If a gastric lesion is not identified, the study can be continued as a double-contrast morphologic small-bowel study with the distended small bowel easily evaluated.

NEGATIVE-CONTRAST GASTROGRAPHY AS A MORPHOLOGIC STUDY IN THE CAT

Specific Indications

The study permits evaluation of gastric size, shape, or location in the determination of an extramural gastric lesion. Because of the negative-contrast agent it is possible to evaluate mural gastric lesions or an intraluminal gastric lesion.

Technique

1. the study is more easily performed on a sedated or anesthetized patient.
2. make a routine noncontrast abdominal radiographic study
3. pass an orogastric tube
4. attach the air-filled syringe to the gastric tube and inject air using dosage of 30 to 50 cc
5. withdraw the tip of the tube into the caudal esophagus
6. make dorsoventral, ventrodorsal, right lateral, and left lateral radiographs centering on the cranial abdomen immediately following administration of the air
7. if necessary inject additional air since air can be lost by regurgitation or into the small bowel
8. make dorsoventral, ventrodorsal, right lateral, and left lateral radiographs centering on the cranial abdomen immediately following additional administration of the air

Comments

It is difficult to determine the exact volume of air to inject since not all of the air remains within the stomach, some is regurgitated immediately and some passes into the small bowel. Therefore, it is important to rely on resistance to injection of air and palpation of the distended stomach.

If a gastric lesion is not identified, the study can be continued as a negative-contrast morphologic small-bowel study with the distended small bowel easily evaluated.

REFERENCES

Burns J and Fox SM. The use of a barium meal to evaluate total gastric emptying time in the dog. Vet Rad 27:169-72, 1986.

Dyce KM Merlen RHA and Wadsworth FJ. Radiological studies of the gastro-intestinal tract of the dog. Brit Vet J 110:83-87, 1954.

Evans SM and Biery DN. Double contrast gastrography in the cat: Technique and normal radiographic appearance. Vet Rad 24:3-5, 1983.

Evans SM and Laufer I. Double contrast gastrography in the normal dog. Vet. Rad 22:2-9, 1981.

Evans SM. Double versus single contrast gastrography in the dog and cat. Vet Rad 24:6-10, 1983.

Gelfand DW and Hachiya J. The double-contrast examination of the stomach using gas-producing granules and tablets. Radiology 93:1381-2, 1969.

Gomez JA. The gastrointestinal contrast study. Vet Clin of NA 4:805-42, 1974.

Grandage J. Radiological appearance of stomach gas in the dog. Aust Vet J 50:529-32, 1974.

Happe RP van den Brom WE and van der Gaag I. Duodenogastric reflux in the dog, a clinicopathological study. Res Vet Sci 33:280-6, 1982.

Hornof WJ Koblik PD Strombeck DR Morgan JP and Hansen G. Scintigraphic evaluation of solid-phase gastric emptying in the dog. Vet Radiol 30:242-8, 1989.

Jefferson NC Kuroyanagi Y and Necheles H. Mechanical factors affecting gastric emptying. Am J Surg 106:464-6, 1963.

Leonardi L. Combined pneumogastography (using contrast media) in the radiological examination of small animals. Clinica Veterinaria 100:67-76, 1977.

Miyabayashi T and Morgan JP. Gastric emptying in the normal dog. A contrast radiographic technique. Vet Rad 25:187-91, 1984.

Miyabayashi T and Morgan JP. Upper gastrointestinal examinations: a radiographic study of clinically normal beagle puppies. J sm Anim Pract 32: 83-8, 1991.

Morgan JP. Normal radiographic anatomy of the gastrointestinal tract of the dog. AVMA Scientific Proceedings 101st annual meeting, p155, 1964.

Morgan JP. The upper gastrointestinal examination in the cat: Normal radiographic appearance using positive contrast medium. Vet Rad 22:159-69, 1981.

Morgan JP. The upper gastrointestinal tract in the cat: A protocol for contrast radiography. JAVRS 18:134-7, 1977.

Root CR and Morgan JP. Contrast radiography of the upper gastrointestinal tract in the dog. J. small Anim Pract 10: 79-286, 1969.

Rosenquist CJ Carrigg JW Regal A-MY and Kohatsu S. Electrical, contractile, and radiographic studies of the stomach after proximal gastric vagotomy. Am J Surg 134:338-342, 1977.

Thrall DE. Contrast radiography of the canine and feline stomach and small bowel; Indictions, method, and roentgen signs. Biweekly Sn An Vet Med Update Series 11:2-11,1978.

Thrall DE. Technique for radiographic examination of the canine and feline. in "Veterinary Gastroenterology" edited by Neil V Anderson p 61, Lea & Febiger Philadelphia 1980.

Van Liere EJ and Crisler G. Normal emptying time of the stomach of the dog. Proc Soc Exp Biol and Med 31:85-7, 1931.

Zontine WJ. Effect of chemical restraint drugs on the passage of barium sulfate through the stomach and duodenum of dogs. J Am Vet Med Assoc 162:878-84, 1973.

D. SMALL INTESTINAL SPECIAL RADIOGRAPHIC STUDY IN THE DOG AND CAT

Definition

Previously, the radiographic study of the stomach and small intestine was referred to as an upper gastrointestinal examination (UGI). This implied that a contrast agent administered orally could be followed through the stomach and small intestine, into the large intestine, and accurate radiographic evaluation of these organs could be made. However, the filling of the small intestine is dependent on the volume of contrast agent administered and on gastric emptying assuming that the contrast agent is administered orally or through an orogastric tube. Since gastric emptying cannot be regulated, the contrast meal that enters the small bowel cannot be controlled and distention of the bowel loops cannot be guaranteed. Actually, the small bowel radiographic study has little morphologic value and only minimal function value in proving that the contrast meal passed through the gastrointestinal tract. If the study is intended to be functional, the time of passage of the head of the meal into the colon, and the time of passage of the entire meal into the colon may both be of value.

The first part of the small bowel and the terminal ileum may be reached by endoscopy, however, the mesenteric small intestine cannot be easily evaluated by endoscopy and remains in the purview of radiographic examination.

The study can be performed with barium sulfate suspension (Fig. 2-5). The volume of the contrast agent administered is important to insure rapid gastric emptying. If you use one of the newer nonionic water-soluble contrast agents, the small intestinal transit time may be slightly increased because osmotic activity of the contrast agent pulls minimal water into the intestinal lumen increasing the volume.

Patient preparation is probably not necessary if it is to be a morphologic study to determine partial or complete obstruction, since the gastrointestinal tract is probably empty from the resulting vomiting and/or diarrhea. The study is not recommended to evaluate mucosal disease, but if it is used in this manner, the patient should be off feed for 24 hours offering an empty gastrointestinal tract for the special radiographic study. Evaluation of transit time of the contrast meal can be determined with relative accuracy.

Indications

Clinical signs are usually associated with vomiting, regurgitation, or anorexia supported by suggestive findings of obstructive ileus as seen on the noncontrast radiographs. Specific indications for the study include: (1) a suspicion of mechanical ileus (obstructive ileus), (2) the need to determine the size, shape, and position of the small bowel, (3) a suspicion of an intraluminal linear foreign body, (4) a determination of transit time through the small bowel (Table 2-3), and (5) a determination of the small bowel emptying time (Table 2-4). Specific lesions include an: (1) intraluminal foreign body, (2) bowel wall tumors, (3) bowel wall rupture, (4) bowel torsion, and (5) intussusception.

Contraindications

Study of the small bowel has its greatest value in proving the presence of a mechanical ileus (obstructive ileus) within the small bowel. The fallacy in listing this indication lies in the fact that the non-contrast radiographic studies of the abdomen usually have such prominent changes associated with the obstruction that the use of a special contrast study is not warranted because of the delay in surgical intervention and because of the additional expense. In the event of a partial obstructive lesion, the bowel is patent and the non-contrast findings are much less prominent. In a patient of this type, the contrast study may be extremely helpful in reaching a diagnosis.

Specific contraindications are: (1) suspect gastric distention and/or torsion, (2) known bowel perforation, (3) prior use of tranquilizer or other drug that affects bowel transit time, (4) suspect chronic obstructive bowel disease, and (5) suspect paralytic ileus, bowel torsion, or bowel volvulus.

Techniques

There are descriptions of the use of anticholinergic drugs as an aid to radiographic studies of the small bowel. Propantheline bromide (Pro-Banthine) is widely used as an antispasmodic and blocks neural impulses at autonomic ganglia and at parasympathetic effector sites in tissue by interfering with acetylcholine which normally conducts impulses across cell walls. Important effects on organ systems include diminished tone and mobility of smooth muscle in the alimentary tract which would otherwise aid in the evaluation of contrast studies of the bowel. The delaying effects of this drug on small bowel transit times in cats have been reported (Noonan and Margulis, 1970).

Frequently, the terminal ileum is involved with disease. This is a common site for intussusception and for disease related with the ileocecocolic lymph nodes. Retrograde ileography is a valuable technique for the evaluation of this region. The procedure necessitates reflux of barium sulfate suspension, with or without air, into the terminal ileum. This can be accomplished with the administration of an excessive amount of liquid or air into the colon. The passage of contrast agent through the ileocolic valve can be assisted through the use of glucagon. Studies of this type are much easier performed under fluoroscopic guidance.

This study can be transformed into a double-contrast study through the oral administration of an effervescent agent that generates CO_2. These small spanules are administered by placing them into the buccal pouch and closing the patients mouth. Radiographs must be made within 1 minute following swallowing of the spanules since the gas produced either is belched from the stomach or passes into the small bowel quickly. Additional spanules can be administered to achieve a greater effect in producing the double-contrast study (Fig. 2-5).

Equipment

1. barium sulfate suspension or nonionic contrast agent such as Isovue or Iohexal
2. 50-cc syringe
3. speculum
4. orogastric tube

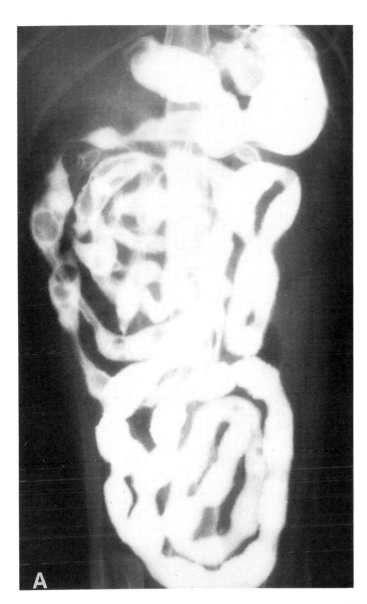

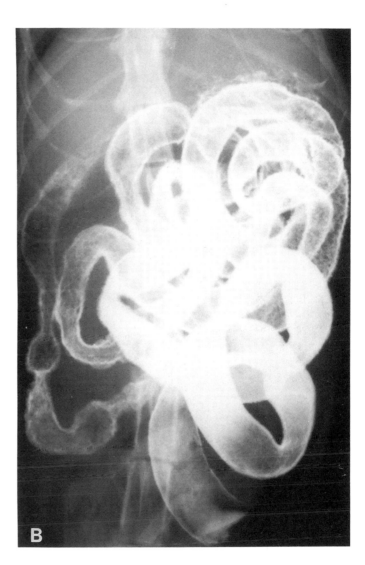

Fig. 2-5
SMALL INTESTINAL RADIOGRAPHY
Ventrodorsal radiographs of two cats were made after a positive contrast study (A) and a double-contrast study (B). Notice the difference in appearance of the barium sulfate suspension filled bowel loops when compared with those in which the barium sulfate suspension coats the bowel walls and the loops are distended by air.

Table 2-3
SMALL INTESTINAL TRANSIT TIMES (APPROXIMATE)

	Dog adult	Dog immature	Cat adult
full barium meal	1 hr (0.5-2)	1.5 (1-2)	0.75hr (0.5-1)
full intact kibble meal	1-5 (1-2)		
full ground kibble meal			

Table 2-4
SMALL INTESTINAL EMPTYING TIMES (APPROXIMATE)

	Dog adult	immature	Cat adult	immature
full liquid meal	3.5hr (3-5)			
full intact kibble meal				
full ground kibble meal				

SMALL INTESTINAL RADIOGRAPHY IN THE DOG

Technique
1. make noncontrast survey radiographic study of the abdomen
2. if the stomach, small bowel, or colon are filled with ingesta or feces, consider the appropriateness of the study in the evaluation of a mechanical ileus, also the difficulty created in evaluation of the radiograph if the study is to be functional in character
3. administer barium sulfate suspension (20% w/w or 30%w/w) according to the following schedule, 8 to 10 cc/kgbw in small dogs that are less than 10 kg, 5 to 8 cc/kgbw in medium sized dogs that are between 10 to 40 kg, and 3 to 5 cc/kgbw in large sized dogs that are greater than 40 kg
4. make ventrodorsal and right lateral studies of the abdomen at 1 hour, 3 hours, and 5 hours and later as appropriate

Comments
The study described can be functional to determine passage of the contrast meal or morphologic to determine gross abnormality such as is seen in an intraluminal linear foreign body.

It is possible to orally administer an effervescent agent to generate CO_2 gas after the head of the barium meal has entered the colon. The patient is positioned in left lateral recumbency so that the gas that is generated can enter the duodenum and small bowel. A good double-contrast study of the small intestine can be obtained in over one-half of the patients.

SMALL INTESTINAL RADIOGRAPHY IN THE CAT

Technique
1. make noncontrast survey radiographic study of the abdomen
2. if the stomach, small bowel, or colon are filled with ingesta or feces consider the appropriateness of the study in the evaluation of a mechanical ileus and the difficulty created in evaluation of the radiograph if the study is to be functional
3. administer barium sulfate suspension (20% w/w or 30% w/w) according to the following schedule, 12 to 16 cc/kgbw
4. make ventrodorsal and right lateral studies of the abdomen at 5, 30, and 60 minutes and later as appropriate

Comments
The study described can be functional to determine passage of the contrast meal or morphologic to determine gross abnormality such as is seen in an intraluminal linear foreign body.

It is possible to orally administer an effervescent agent to generate CO_2 gas after the head of the barium meal has entered the colon. The patient is positioned in left lateral recumbency so that the gas enters the duodenum and small bowel. A good double-contrast image of the small intestine can be obtained in over one-half of the patients.

SMALL INTESTINAL RADIOGRAPHY USING NON-IONIC AGENTS IN THE DOG AND CAT

Problems exist with the use of barium sulfate suspension for the study of gastrointestinal systems in the puppy or kitten if there is a suspected perforation or if intestinal surgery is contemplated. The newer non-ionic, nearly isotonic agents provide excellent visualization of the gastrointestinal system with no dilutional problems. Transit times are rapidly increased (Williams, et al 1993). Apparently there is no need for fear following aspiration of contrast containing vomitus since studies performed on baby piglets showed that following aspiration of diluted nonionic agents there were no acute clinical or radiologic abnormalities and only mild, self limiting persistent infiltrates in the lungs up to four days after aspiration (Isdale et al, 1987).

RETROGRADE ILEOGRAPHY IN THE DOG AND CAT

The terminal ileum can be evaluated following retrograde colonic administration of contrast media. Since this is an important region anatomically and is poorly evaluated by other radiographic techniques, retrograde filling using either barium sulfate suspension alone or a combination of barium sulfate and air can be used to great advantage. The administration of glucagon facilitates the retrograde flow.

Indications for a study of this type include any disease causing enlargement of the ileocecocolic lymph nodes or any type of intussusception at the ileocecocolic region

Contraindications

Any factors that prevent the patient from being sedated or anesthetized.

Equipment

1. some method to instill the barium sulfate solution into the colon by gravity flow and then change to instill air rectally through a catheter that has some type of retention tip.

Technique

1. it is best to have the patient sedated or anesthetized for the study
2. perform a retrograde barium sulfate study of the colon in a conventional manner
3. continue instillation of liquid contrast agent using not more than a 30" container height above the table
4. make a single radiograph of the abdomen and evaluate the level of flow of the barium sulfate
5. continue or stop instillation as required
6. make additional radiographs

OR

1. perform the retrograde barium sulfate study of the colon in a conventional manner
2. drain the barium sulfate suspension by dropping the bag to the floor
3. attach a syringe or air hose to the catheter and instill air
4. make a single radiograph of the abdomen and evaluate the level of flow of the double-contrast pattern
5. continue or stop instillation of air as required
6. make additional radiographs

Comments

It is also possible to perform this technique as a double-contrast study following a small bowel follow-through study in which air is administered per rectum after the orally administered barium sulfate has passed to the right side of the colon.

The amount of air to inject is difficult to predict because of the inability to determine how much air passes in a retrograde direction through the ileocecal valve and because of the difficulty in determining how much air has escaped rectally. It is best to palpate the abdomen and to estimate the amount of air within the colon.

REFERENCES

Cohen MD Weber TR and Grosfeld JL. Bowel perforation in the newborn: Diagnosis with metrizamide. Radiology 150:65, 1984.

Ferrucci JTJr and Benedict KT. Anticholinergic-aided study of the gastrointestinal tract. Rad Clinics of NA 9:23, 1971.

Gomez JA. The gastrointestinal contrast study. Vet Clin of NA 4:805, 1974.

Grandage J. The radiological appearance of stomach gas in the dog. Aust Vet J 50:529, 1974.

Isdale JM Leibowitz B Austin JC Wright PG and Schmaman A. Blood gas pH and pulmonary response to the inhalation of low osmolar contrast media iopamidol and ioxaglate. Invest Radiol 22:908, 1987.

Johansen JG. Assessment of a non-ionic contrast medium (Amipaque) in the gastrointestinal tract. Invest Radiol 13:523, 1978.

Kuhns LR and Kanellitsas C. Use of isotonic water-soluble contrast agents for gastrointestinal examinations in infants. Radiology 144;411, 1982.

Maglinte DDT Lappas JC Kelvin FM Rex D and Chernish SM. Small bowel radiography: How, when, and why? Radiology 163:297, 1987.

McAlister WH and Margulis AR. Small bowel transit time of barium sulfate preparation and iodine contrast media in dogs. Am J Roentgenol 91:814, 1964.

Miyabayashi T and Morgan JP. Upper gastrointestinal examinations: a radiographic study of clinically normal beagle puppies. J sm Anim Pract 32:83-8, 1991.

Miyabayashi T Morgan JP Atilola MAO and Muhumuza L. Small intestinal empyting time in normal beagle dogs: A contrast radiographic study. Vet Rad 27:164-8, 1986.

Monsein LH Halpert RD Harris ED and Feczko PJ. Retrograde Ileography:Value of Glucagon. Radiology 161:558, 1986.

Morgan JP. Protocol for contrast radiography of the upper gastrointestinal tract in the cat. J Am Vet Rad Soc 18:134, 1977.

Morgan JP. The upper gastrointestinal examination in the cat: Normal radiographic appearance using positive-contrast medium. Vet Rad 22:159, 1981.

Noonan CD and Margulis AR. Small bowel transit time of water soluble iodinated contrast medium and barium sulfate in cats with simulated surgical acute abdomen. Am J Roentgen 110:334, 1970.

Root CR and Morgan JP. Contrast radiography of the upper gastrointestinal tract in the dog. J sm An Pract 10:279, 1964.

Thrall DE and Leininger JR. Irregular intestinal mucosal margination in the dog; Normal or abnormal? J sm An Pract 17:305, 1976.

Thrall DE. Contrast radiography of the canine and feline stomach and small bowel; Indictions, method, and roentgen signs. Biweekly Sn An Vet Med Update Series 11:2, 1978.

Williams J Biller DS Myer CW Miyabayashi T and Leveille R. Use of iohexal as gastrointestinal contrast agent in three dogs, five cats, and one bird. J Am Vet Med Assoc 203:624-7, 1993.

Wolvekamp WThC. Enteroclysis and reflux examination; two new radiographic techniques for investigation of the small intestine in the dog. Proc Voorjaarsdagen, Netherlands Small Anim Vet Asoc 1978; pp14.

Zontine WJ. Effect of chemical restraint drugs on the passage of barium sulfate through the stomach and duodenum of dogs. J Am Vet Med Assoc 162:878, 1973.

E. LARGE INTESTINAL SPECIAL RADIOGRAPHIC STUDY IN THE DOG AND CAT

Definition

Radiographic examination of the cecum, colon, and rectum with retrograde administration of contrast medium can be performed as: (1) a positive-contrast study, (2) a negative-contrast study (pneumocolon), or (3) a double-contrast study. Studies performed following the oral administration of positive-contrast media do not distend the large intestine and are complicated by the mixture of the contrast media with colonic contents and, therefore, are not considered adequate for a large intestinal study except for demonstrating anatomic location and providing minimal information relative to function.

These studies of the large intestine are generally morphologic in character and can evaluate extramural masses, mural, or mucosal lesions, and intraluminal lesions. Since mucosal lesions are more accurately studied using endoscopy, the lesions studied radiographically are usually larger mass lesions.

Radiographic evaluation of the large intestine is often combined with fiber-optic endoscopy if the descending colon or rectum are thought to be involved. However, disease in the region of the ileocecocolic valves, ascending and transverse colon may be better studied using a radiographic technique.

Indications

Major indications for study of the large intestine are: (1) abnormal defecation characterized by excessive mucus or bright red blood coating the stool, (2) pencilling of the stool due to stricture, or (3) pain or difficulty during defecation (tenesmus or dyschezia). Other indications are a need to determine the position of the colon because of a suspected caudal abdominal or pelvic mass, or to ascertain whether gas-filled loops of bowel are the result of small bowel ileus or are a part of a normal large bowel. These radiographic studies cannot evaluate minimal mucosal disease but are, instead, used to determine the presence of larger morphologic changes. Diarrhea, while a common clinical problem, is probably not a good indication for a special radiographic study of the colon. Specific lesions to evaluate include: (1) colonic wall tumor, (2) extramural mass causing displacement of the colon, (3) ileocolic intussusception, (4) cecal inversion, (5) colonic wall rupture, or (6) ileocecocolic mass lesions.

Contraindications

Contraindications include: (1) suspected perforation of the colonic wall in which situation there is the possibility of further peritoneal contamination, (2) previous colonic biopsy (determine nature of biopsy) that might have weakened the colonic wall and made it susceptible to rupture, (3) fecal contents that create filling-defects and make evaluation of the mucosal surface difficult, and (4) soapy-water enemas that create an acute colitis.

Experimental studies showed that a superficial biopsy of the rectum or colon in pigs that included tissues superficial to the muscularis propria could be performed with small colonoscopic forceps (rectal suction biopsy cannula) and was a safe procedure and no waiting period was necessary before performing a barium enema study. However, biopsy of the colon or rectum with proctoscopic forceps including the muscularis propria appeared to have a greater potential for perforation and a waiting period between biopsy and barium enema study was recommended (Harned et al, 1982).

Contrast Agent

A barium sulfate suspension (10% w/w or 20% w/w) is usually used. It may be necessary to dilute the concentration of the barium sulfate suspension you have available to decrease the density. Nonionic iodinated contrast agents can be used for colonic studies, however, they are much more expensive. Any agent that is to be placed within the colon should be brought to body temperature prior to injection.

Equipment

1. a Bardex catheter, which is an enema tube with an inflatable cuff to hold it in position within the rectum, or a Foley catheter with an inflating bulb—the tip of the catheter can be cut off to avoid producing colonic spasticity if the tip of the catheter contacts the colonic wall
2. some type of contrast agent reservoir—an enema bag, enema can, or commercial enema set or may only be a 50 cc syringe (Fig. 2-6)
3. lubricant
4. compression paddle

Comments

Preparation of the colon for examination varies depending on the luminal contents and the purpose of the examination. Since mucosal disease is poorly studied radiographically, there is little value in "washing" the colonic wall with a cleansing enema. The colon may be empty due to the patient's disease or can be adequately prepared by stimulating defecation with a "low" water enema.

Discussion of the method of preparation of the colon prior to a radiographic study has probably created an environment in which the study is currently underutilized. Another problem has been the idea that the colon must be distended with contrast agent to obtain a satisfactory radiographic study and this has been threatening because of the resulting problems following expulsion of the barium tip from the rectum at a time the colon is full. By achieving a partial cleansing of the colon and by partially filling the colon with contrast agent, it is possible to make a satisfactory study using the barium sulfate suspension and/or air. The study is definitely easier to perform in the sedated or anesthetized patient.

LARGE INTESTINAL STUDY USING POSITIVE-CONTRAST TECHNIQUE IN THE DOG

The technique to be used is determined by the information desired. If there is a need to determine the character of a suspected lesion within the large intestine a larger amount of positive-contrast agent is required than if the large intestine is simply to be located radiographically. A 50 cc syringe or bulb syringe can be used to inject a minimal amount of contrast agent or a more complicated injection scheme is required if the entire colon is to be distended. Placement of the hand on the abdomen is a good technique to estimate the level of filling of the colon.

Technique

1. consider sedating or anesthetizing the patient prior to performing this study
2. use a low enema to stimulate defecation—the colon need not be "washed" clean
3. make a survey radiographic study of the abdomen
4. dilute the barium sulfate suspension until it has a concentration of 10% w/w to 20% w/w
5. insert catheter rectally and inflate bulb
6. infuse the contrast medium with a minimal pressure of the syringe or a minimal gravity pressure by positioning the reservoir only slightly above the tabletop—stop infusion if there is resistance to flow of the contrast agent
7. the volume infused is dependent on the purpose of the study—to fill the large intestine and permit its location use 10 cc in a small dog, 30 cc in a medium sized dog, and 60 cc in a large dog—to only fill the rectum and permit its evaluation and location use 10 to 20 cc
8. make ventrodorsal and both right and left lateral radiographs
9. determine the need for administration of additional contrast medium after evaluation of the radiographs
10. remove the catheter from the rectum in an appropriate location, preferably near a floor drain

LARGE INTESTINAL STUDY USING DOUBLE-CONTRAST TECHNIQUE IN THE DOG

The need for this technique is determined by a suspected lesion within the large intestine. It can also be used to determine the location of the large intestine. A 50 cc syringe or bulb syringe can be used to inject a minimal amount of positive-contrast agent with a second syringe used to inject air.

Technique

1. consider sedating or anesthetizing the patient prior to performing this study
2. use a low enema to stimulate defecation—the colon need not be "washed" clean
3. make a survey radiographic study of the abdomen
4. dilute the barium sulfate suspension until it is 10% w/w to 20% w/w concentration
5. insert the syringe tip or bulb syringe into the rectum
6. infuse 5 to 10 cc of barium sulfate suspension
7. place a new syringe tip into the rectum
8. inject 50 to 200 cc of air
9. remove the syringe tip
10. make ventrodorsal and both right and left lateral radiographs
11. determine the need to repeat the study upon evaluation of the radiographs
12. remove the patient to an appropriate location for defecation, preferably near a floor drain

Comments

A per-rectal pneumocolon examination can be used to obtain a double-contrast image of the terminal ileum and right-sided colon by insufflating air through a small catheter inserted into the rectum at the time an orally ingested barium sulfate suspension meal reaches the right colon. The examination is indicated if a view of the ileocecal region is required or the patient is unable to tolerate a conventional barium enema study (Kressel et al, 1982).

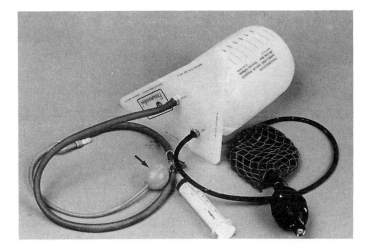

Fig. 2-6
LARGE BOWEL RADIOGRAPHY
Use of a contrast agent reservoir, tubing, Bardex catheter (arrow), and pressure bulb make large bowel radiographic studies easier. The reservoir can be rotated so that liquid (barium sulfate suspension) flows through the tubing or so that air flows through the tubing. The reservoir can also be lowered to floor level and be used as a container into which the liquid can drain after completion of the study.

LARGE INTESTINAL STUDY USING NEGATIVE-CONTRAST TECHNIQUE (PNEUMOCOLON) IN THE DOG

Use of this technique is determined by the need to evaluate a suspected lesion within the large intestine or by the need to know the location of the large intestine within the abdomen (Fig. 2-7). A 50-cc syringe or bulb syringe can be used to inject the air. Preparation of the patient is much less rigid and in an emergency situation, no preparation is required.

Technique

1. use a low enema to stimulate defecation or perform the examination without preparation
2. make a survey radiographic study of the abdomen
3. place the syringe tip or bulb syringe into the rectum
5. infuse 60 to 100 cc of air
6. make ventrodorsal and both right and left lateral radiographs
7. determine the need to repeat the study upon evaluation of the radiographs
8. remove the patient to an appropriate location for defecation

Comments

The amount of air injected can be decreased if distention of the entire colon is not required. Often the amount of air within the colon is difficult to ascertain until radiographs are made.

LARGE INTESTINAL STUDY USING POSITIVE-CONTRAST TECHNIQUE IN THE CAT

The technique to be used is determined by the information desired. If there is a need to determined the character of a suspected lesion within the large intestine a larger amount of contrast agent is required than if the large intestine is simply to be located radiographically. A 50 cc syringe or bulb syringe can be used to inject the contrast agent. Placement of the hand on the abdomen is a good technique to estimate the level of filling of the colon.

Technique

1. consider sedating or anesthetizing the patient prior to performing this study
2. use a low enema to stimulate defecation—the colon need not be "washed" clean
3. make a survey radiographic study of the abdomen
4. dilute the barium sulfate suspension until it is 10% w/w to 20% w/w concentration
5. insert a syringe tip or bulb syringe rectally
6. infuse the contrast medium using minimal pressure on the syringe (a total of 10 cc partially fills the large intestine and permits its location while 10 to 20 cc fills the colon)
7. make ventrodorsal and both right and left lateral radiographs
8. determine the need for additional contrast medium upon evaluation of the radiographs
9. remove the catheter from the rectum in an appropriate location, preferably near a floor drain

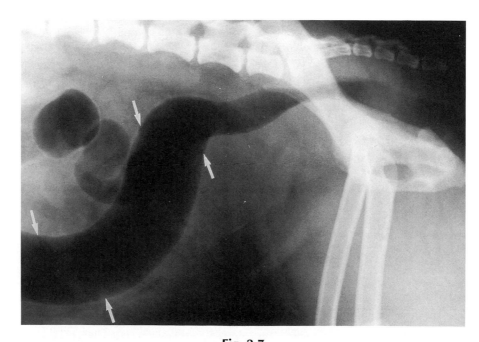

Fig. 2-7
PNEUMOCOLON
A lateral radiograph of the pelvic region in a dog following the administration of air per rectum. The air filled colon (arrows) is well outlined by the study.

LARGE INTESTINAL STUDY USING DOUBLE-CONTRAST TECHNIQUE IN THE CAT

The technique is used to evaluate a suspected lesion within the large intestine or to simply locate the large intestine anatomically. A 50 cc syringe or bulb syringe can be used to inject the contrast agent and the air.

Technique

1. consider sedating or anesthetizing the patient prior to performing this study
2. use a low enema to stimulate defecation—the colon need not be "washed" clean
3. make a survey radiographic study of the abdomen
4. dilute the barium sulfate suspension until it is 10% w/w to 20% w/w concentration
5. place the syringe tip or bulb syringe into the rectum
6. infuse 2 to 3 cc of barium sulfate suspension
7. place a new syringe tip into the rectum
8. inject 25 to 50 cc of air
9. remove the syringe tip
10. make ventrodorsal and both right and left lateral radiographs
11. determine the need to repeat the study upon evaluation of the radiographs
12. remove the patient to an appropriate location for defecation (near a floor drain)

Comments

A per-rectal pneumocolon examination can be used to obtain a double-contrast image of the terminal ileum and right colon by insufflating air through a small catheter inserted into the rectum at the time orally ingested barium sulfate meal reaches the right colon. The examination is indicated if a view of the ileocecal region is required or the patient is unable to tolerate a conventional barium enema study (Kressel et al, 1982).

LARGE INTESTINAL STUDY USING NEGATIVE-CONTRAST TECHNIQUE (PNEUMOCOLON) IN THE CAT

The use of the technique is determined by the need to evaluate a suspected colonic lesion or by the need to simply located the position of the large intestine. A 50 cc syringe or bulb syringe can be used to inject the air. Preparation of the patient is much less rigid and in an emergency situation, no preparation is required.

Technique

1. use a low enema to stimulate defecation or perform the examination without preparation
2. make a survey radiographic study of the abdomen
3. place the syringe tip or bulb syringe into the rectum
4. infuse 20 to 30 cc of air
5. make ventrodorsal and both right and left lateral radiographs
6. determine the need to repeat the study upon evaluation of the radiographs
7. remove the patient to an appropriate location for defecation

Comments

The amount of air injected can be decreased if distention of the entire colon is not required. It may be difficult to determine the amount of air within the colon until the first radiographs are made.

REFERENCES

Gomez JA. The gastrointestinal contrast study. Vet Clin North Amer 4:805,1974.

Harned RK Consigny PM Cooper NB Williams SM and Woltjen AJ. Barium enema examination following biopsy of the rectum or colon. Radiology 145:11, 1982.

Kressel HY Evers KA Glick SN Laufer I and Herlinger H. The peroral pneumocolon examination. Radiology 144:414, 1982.

Nyland TG and Ackerman N. Pneumocolon: A diagnostic aid in abdominal radiography. J Am Vet Rad Soc 19:203,1978.

Walters JW. Radiography of the canine colon using different contrast agents. J Am Vet Med Assoc 156:423,1970.

3. UROGRAPHY IN THE DOG AND CAT

A. INTRODUCTION

Definition

Urographic studies include those that provide a method of radiographic evaluation of the kidneys, ureters, urinary bladder, prostate gland, and urethera. The examinations are generally morphological in character, but may be functional. They can be performed in several ways and the specific information desired determines how the examination is to be performed. In general, the studies can be made following intravenous injection of the contrast agent or following the retrograde injection of the contrast agent into the urethra or urinary bladder. While the intravenous study must utilize a positive-contrast agent prepared for parenteral injection, the retrograde study can be made using a positive, negative, or double-contrast technique. Studies in the dog and cat are performed in the same manner.

Evaluation of non-contrast survey abdominal radiographs is important especially in the detection of radiopaque calculi within the urinary system. The nature of the contents of the over-lying bowel loops greatly influences the detection of small calculi and preparation of the bowel for radiographic examination by taking the patient off food or through the administration of enemas may be required. Also, focal abdominal compression studies are helpful in displacing overlying bowel shadows.

A generalized abdominal compression can be utilized in certain patients in which an intravenous urogram is to be performed in an effort to permit better visualization of the renal collecting system. The purpose of abdominal compression is to delay drainage of the contrast agent from the renal collecting systems and thus permit their better evaluation on the radiograph. This goal is reached by compressing the urinary bladder so that the intraluminal pressure increases and prevents drainage from the kidneys through the ureters. The best abdominal compression can be obtained through the use of elastic bandages encircling the prepelvic abdomen. A flat piece of radiolucent sponge on the central abdomen increases the effectiveness of the compression. Commercially available compression devices are available. Some of these include an inflatable bladder that produces inwardly directed compression. Some x-ray tables are equipped with a compression band that tightens mechanically with a ratchet device. Use of these devices require that the patient remain immobilized on the table and are thus not always appropriate for use with all patients especially those that are awake. Use of abdominal compression may be inappropriate in the presence of a suspected caudal abdominal mass. Abdominal compression in the cat is relatively easy because of the small size of the patient although placement of the band caudal to the urinary bladder without obtaining any compression of the bladder is common.

Indications

While the information gained from the radiographic studies may be helpful in diagnosis of renal disease, the studies rarely provide qualitative information about renal function and do not evaluate the reserve renal capacity. Visualization of the contrast agent within the kidneys implies patent renal arteries. Evaluation of sequential radiographs made following an intravenous pyelogram can serve as a rough indicator of renal function by permitting you to make a comparison between the two kidneys of the volume and rate of excretion of the contrast agent. Movement of the contrast-laden urine is expected through the ureters and into the urinary bladder. Morphologic information is limited to the determination of the size, shape and location of the structures within the urinary system. Disruption of the renal collecting systems is indicative of a mass lesion that maybe cystic or solid in character while irregularity in the diverticula or pelvis of the collective system usually indicates chronic inflammatory disease. A filling defect within the contrast pool in the pelvis or within the urinary bladder is often indicative of the presence of a calculus while a mural lesion originating from the bladder wall is usually due to a tumor.

Indications for urography may relate to the detection of an abdominal mass and the desire to determine if the mass is associated with a kidney or if the mass is a part of the urinary bladder or the prostate gland. Determination of the intactness of the urinary system following trauma is a frequent indication for urography since the studies can detect rupture of kidney, ureter, bladder, or urethra. Displacement of organs within the urinary system may follow trauma and be associated with organ herniation. Site of insertion of the distal end of the ureter can be determined with special urographic studies and determination of the possibility of ectopic location in the bladder, urethra, or vagina can be made.

Specific indications for urographic studies include those related to urination and include: (1) hematuria, (2) pyuria, (3) dysuria, (4) straining, and (5) frequency.

The advent of ultrasound has provided a safer and more accurate method for evaluation of the kidneys and prostate gland and provides for ultrasound guided biopsy. This has markedly reduced the use of urography in the study of urinary disease, however, there remain specific indications for urography and also many instances where the combination of urography and ultrasonography provides the greatest amount of information.

Contraindications

Renal failure is not a contraindication for urography, but suggests that the quality of the intravenous study will be compromised because of the delay in excretion of contrast agent through the kidneys. Therefore, elevated blood urinary nitrogen or creatinine levels do not predict the failure of intravenous urographic studies. If these levels are abnormally high, it may be possible to enhance the intravenous study by maintaining abdominal compression for a longer period of time waiting for accumulation of the contrast agent within the renal pelvis or by injecting a higher than usual volume of the contrast agent.

Because of renal disease, the opacification of the renal collecting system may be delayed and not as easily evaluated on the radiograph and much of the contrast agent cycles through the highly-vascularized liver, spleen, and bowel waiting for excretion by the kidneys.

In the event of suspected abdominal trauma or in the presence of an abdominal mass or in patients with severe dyspnea, it is recommended that abdominal compression not be used.

A single case of acute renal failure associated with intravenous contrast medium administration has been reported in a female dog with possible hermaphroditism that was otherwise normal. Acute renal failure developed 10 hours after administration of 2.2 ml/kgbw of Hypaque M 75%. The dog recovered after 4 days following aggressive fluid therapy, furosemide therapy, dopamine hydrochloride, and cimetidine (Ihle and Kostolich, 1991).

Equipment

The type of equipment required varies with the technique used. Either the contrast agent is injected intravenously or in a retrograde manner through a catheter. Different types of catheters may be used with some requiring a retension bulb. A timing device is positioned on the edge of the radiograph and records the length of time between intravenous injection and filming. Towels are required to keep the table and patient clean of any contrast agent that has spilled.

Contrast Agent

Conventional agents for urography are positive-contrast, water-soluble, ionic products with high osmolarity containing organic iodine (Z=53). They contain 141 to 400 mg of iodine/ml and are rapidly cleared from the circulation and are excreted by the kidneys. All are sodium or meglumine salts (Table 3-1). The toxicity is related to high osmolarity, presence of sodium ion, and hypersensitivity reactions. Nausea and vomiting sometimes occur, but this response is transient. Severe reactions are rare, however, anaphylactoid-like reactions do occur.

In addition, lower-osmolar, water-soluble, nonionic monomers such as iohexol (Omnipaque), iopamidol (Isovue), or metrizamide (Amipaque) as well as a low osmolar ionic monoacid dimer such as ioxaglate sodium meglumine (Hexabrix) are available. These low-osmolar agents are more expensive than ionic contrast media. Their safety as measured in man following intravenous application indicates that the nonionic contrast agents have a lower frequency of adverse drug reactions than are noted with the usage of ionic contrast media. Room air is obviously the cheapest contrast agent available and it or CO_2 or N_2O can be used in negative studies or in double contrast studies performed in a retrograde manner.

Technique

The techniques to be used in urography vary widely according to the study performed and are explained in detail below. The dosage of contrast media when injected intravenously is usually between 200 to 400 mg of iodide/kgbw (approximately 1cc/lbbw or 2cc/kgbw up to a maximum dosage of 90cc).

Table 3-1
UROGRAPHIC AGENTS AVAILABLE FOR USE IN ANIMALS

Contrast Medium	Generic Name	Manufacturer	Mg Iodide/ml
Conray	meglumine iothalamate	Mallinckrodt	282
Conray-400	sodium iothalamate	Mallinckrodt	400
Hypaque-50	sodium diatrizoate	Winthrop	300
Hypaque meglumine, 60%	meglumine diatrizoate	Winthrop	282
Hypaque, 25%	sodium diatrizoate	Winthrop	150
Hypaque-DIU, 30%	meglumine diatrizoate	Winthrop	141
Renovist	meglumine diatrizoate and sodium diatrizoate	Squibb	370
Renografin-76	meglumine diatrizoate and sodium diatrizoate	Squibb	370
Renografin-60	meglumine diatrizoate and sodium diatrizoate	Squibb	288

REFERENCES

Ihle SL and Kostolich M. Acute renal failure associated with contrast medium administration in a dog. J Am Vet Med Assoc 199:899-901, 1991.

Katayama H Yamaguchi K Kozuka T Takashima T Seez P and Matsuura K. Adverse reactions to ionic and nonionic contrast media. Radiology 175:621-8, 1990.

Thrall DE and Finco DR. Canine excretory urography: Is quality a function of BUN? JAAHA12:446-50, 1976.

Wilcox J Evill CA Sage MR and Benness GT. Urographic excretion studies with nonionic contrast agents, iopamidol vs iothalamate. Invest Rad 18:207-10, 1983.

B. INTRAVENOUS UROGRAPHY (Pyelography) IN THE DOG AND CAT

Definition

A radiographic study performed following the intravenous injection of an iodinated agent that is excreted through the kidneys, passes through the ureters into the urinary bladder, and can be seen radiographically because of the radiodensity of the iodine (Fig. 3-1). The character of the study may be altered according to specific clinical findings or according to specific findings as the study develops.

Indications

The study is performed primarily to determine the size, shape, location, and integrity of the kidneys as well as the size, shape, and appearance of the collecting systems. Extrarenal, parenchymal lesions, and filling defects within the renal collecting systems are visualized. In determining the morphology of the kidneys, renal function is partially determined as well. In addition, it is possible to determine the size, shape, and location of the ureters and determine something of ureteral peristaltic activity as well as possible leakage of the contrast agent into the retroperitoneal space. Blockage of the flow of contrast laden urine through the ureters can be determined. Another use of intravenous urography is to achieve filling of the urinary bladder when a retrograde cystogram cannot be performed

Specific indications include: (1) hematuria, (2) dysuria, (3) pyruria, (4) straining at urination, and (5) frequency of urination.

Contraindications

The quality of the study is compromised if the patient is in renal failure. The nature of the technique may need to be modified because of conditions that preclude the use of abdominal compression. Dehydration can result in kidney damage (acute tubular necrosis) and rehydration prior to excretory urography should be used to avoid this complication.

Equipment

1. indwelling intravenous catheter
2. syringe
3. system for abdominal compression
4. marker to identify time of film exposure (Fig. 3-2)

Contrast Agent

1. positive-contrast organic iodide agent recommended for parenteral injection (Table 3-1).

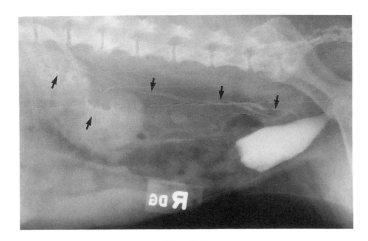

Fig. 3-1
INTRAVENOUS UROGRAM
A lateral radiograph of a dog made after intravenous injection of an iodinated contrast agent. The renal collecting systems (arrows), ureters (arrows) and urinary bladder are outlined by the positive-contrast agent. Notice the film marker with the initials of the technician.

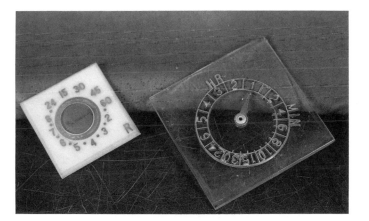

Fig. 3-2
TIME MARKERS
The time of the radiographic exposure following the intravenous injection or oral administration of a contrast agent can be recorded on the radiographs using a marker with "minutes" and "hours" indicated.

Technique (Table 3-2)

1. obtain non-contrast abdominal studies that include kidneys, ureters, and bladder
2. position the indwelling venous catheter
3. inject the contrast medium over 2 minutes using the following dosage: 2 ml/kgbw (maximum of 90 ml in a dog and 15 ml in a cat)
4. make a ventrodorsal radiograph at 5 minutes—if both kidneys are functioning as evidenced by visualization of contrast agent within both renal collecting systems apply abdominal compression
5. make the next ventrodorsal radiograph at 10 minutes
6. if both collecting systems are filled with contrast agent, remove the abdominal compression
7. allow the contrast-laden urine to drain into the urinary bladder and make the next ventrodorsal and lateral radiograph at 15 minutes
8. if the urinary bladder fills, make oblique and lateral radiographs of the bladder

Comments

1. the dosage in the cat can be lowered to 1ml/kgbw and still produce a diagnostic urogram
2. the patient may become nauseated and vomit if the intravenous injection is made quickly
3. if both renal collecting systems are not visualized on the first study, make an additional ventrodorsal radiograph at 15 minutes without compression—if the collecting systems are not visualized on the 15 minutes radiograph, make an additional ventrodorsal radiograph at 60 minutes—this last film probably provides all the information you can gain from the study and the study can be terminated
4. if both kidneys are noted to function but the compression study does not show good distention of the renal collecting systems, leave the compression on and make an additional ventrodorsal radiograph 15 minutes later
5. if post-compression radiographs show the contrast-laden urine to remain in the renal collecting systems and visualization of the ureters is less than expected, suspect a blockage to flow and make another series of radiographs 15 minutes later
6. if the study is primarily to evaluate the ureters, the rate of contrast medium injection can be slower and the filming sequence delayed.
7. do not use abdominal compression on a ureteral study
8. intravenous use of glucagon has been described as a technique to prevent ureteral peristalsis and cause better filling of both renal collecting systems and ureters with the effect lasting for 16 to 22 minutes
9. fluid restriction prior to excretory urogaraphy has been suggested to improve the quality of intravenous urography but may be contraindicated because of the resulting dehydration and is reported to be ineffectual in improving the urogram
10. urothelial cells obtained from the pelvicalyceal system of patients following intravenous urography may show changes induced by contrast material that would affect the interpretation of urine cytology
11. bacterial growth from urine following urography is inhibited by a diatrizoate concentration suggesting that samples for culture should be taken prior to intravenous urography
12. the fifth position in the aromatic ring of certain urographic agents determines whether the molecule is lipophilic and excreted through the liver or hydrophilic and excreted through the kidneys while certain agents pass in either direction, thus, it is possible to have the intravenous contrast agent visualized in both the liver and bowel as well as in the kidneys

Table 3-2
SUMMARY FOR PERFORMING INTRAVENOUS UROGRAPHY

Time	Procedure	Radiographic views
prior to injection	non-contrast radiographs	VD and lateral
0 time	injection of contrast agent	—
5 minutes	—	VD
(if excretion is noted bilaterally)	apply abdominal compression	—
10 minutes	—	VD
(if collecting systems are distended)	remove abdominal compression	—
15 minutes	—	VD and lateral
—	reposition patient for bladder study	Obliques and lateral

REFERENCES

Ackerman N. Intravenous pyelography. J Am An Hosp Assoc 10:277-80, 1974.

Bartels JE. Feline intravenous urography. J Am An Hosp Assoc 9:349-353, 1973.

Bock J Heilbron DC Hoeft A Korb H and Hellige G. No pulmonary edema or congestion after central venous injection of conventional and newer contrast media in dogs. Invest Rad 23:836-41, 1988.

Borthwick R and Robbie B. Large volume urography in the cat. J small Anim Pract 12:579-83, 1971.

Borthwick R and Robbie B. Urography in the dog by an intravenous transfusion technique J small Anim Pract 10:465-70, 1969.

Dure-Smith P. Fluid restriction before excretory urography. Radiology 118:487-9, 1976.

Feeney DA Barber DL Culver DH Prasse KW Thrall DE and Lewis, RE. Canine excretory urogram: Correlation with base-line measurements. Am J Vet Res 41:279-83, 1980.

Feeney DA Johnston GR Osborne CA and Tomlinson MJ. Maximum-distention retrograde urethrocystography in healthy male dogs: Occurrence and radiographic appearance of urethroprostatic reflux. Am J Vet Res 45:948-52, 1984.

Feeney DA Johnston GR Osborne CA and Tomlinson MJ. Maximum-distention retrograde urethrocystography in healthy male dogs: Occurrence of vesicoureteral reflux. Am J Vet Res 45:953-4, 1984.

Feeney DA Osborne CA and Jessen CR. Effect of multiple excretory urograms on glomerular filtration of normal dogs: A preliminary report. Am J Vet Res 41:960-63, 1980.

Feeney DA Osborne CA and Jessen CR. Effect of radiographic contrast media on results of urinalysis with emphasis on alteration in specific gravity. J Am Vet Med Assoc 176;1378-81, 1980.

Feeney DA Thrall DE Barber DL Culver DH and Lewis RE. Normal canine excretory urogram: Effects of dose, time, and individual dog variation. Am J Vet Res 40:1596-1604, 1979.

Hillman BJ Ovitt TW and Doering JW. Improved pyeloureteral visualization using glucagon during experimental intravenous urography. Invest Rad 15:313-7, 1980.

Hillman BJ Ovitt TW and Doering JW. Intravenous glucagon as an alternative to abdominal compression: Experimental urograms in dogs. Abstract Invest Rad 15:419, 1980.

Lord PF Scott RC and Chan KF. Intravenous urography for evaluation of renal diseases in small animals. J Am An Hosp Assoc 10:139-51, 1974.

McClennan BL Oertel YC Malmgren RA and Mendoza M. The effect of water soluble contrast material on urine cytology. Acta Cytologica 22:230-3, 1978.

Olsson O. Excretion of sodium metrizoate through the liver during urography. Acta Rad Diag 11:85-90, 1971.

Ruby AL Ling GV and Ackerman N. Effect of sodium diatrizoate on urinary bacteria. Vet Radiol 24:222-5, 1983.

Thrall DE and Finco DR. Canine excretory urography: Is quality a function of BUN. J Am An Hosp Assoc 12:446-450, 1976.

C. CYSTOGRAPHY IN THE DOG AND CAT

Definition

Cystography is a radiographic study performed to evaluate the urinary bladder for extramural, mural, or intraluminal lesions. These lesions may be primary within the urinary bladder or may originate from an adjacent organ with the effect on the bladder being secondary. The cystogram may be performed: (1) following the intravenous injection of an iodinated agent that is excreted through the kidneys and fills the bladder or (2) following retrograde injection of the positive-contrast agent, air, or be a combination (double-contrast study).

Indications

Cystography should be considered when the clinical signs suggest the origin of the disease process is in the urinary bladder or if the urinary bladder is involved secondarily by an adjacent disease process. The cause of abnormal urine which does not respond to medical treatment such as hematuria, crystalluria, or bacteriuria can be studied with cystography. Abnormal urination such as dysuria, straining to urinate, frequency, or urinary incontinence are additional indications. Following the detection of urinary bladder calculi, cystography can provide additional information as to associated bladder wall disease. The study may determine the size, shape, location, and integrity of the urinary bladder wall as well as to determine extramural, mural, and intraluminal bladder lesions. The integrity of the vesicoureteral valves can be estimated. Bladder location can be determined in patients in which the bladder may by herniated.

Specific indications include:

1. congenital anomaly such as a persistent urachus
2. non-opaque or small calculi
3. inflammatory bladder wall disease
4. bladder wall tumor
5. bladder wall rupture
6. bladder wall diverticula
7. extrensic bladder mass
8. determination of bladder location
9. assistance in evaluation of prostatic disease
10. assistance in location of ureterovesicle junction

Contraindications

At one time, the presence of blood clots within the urinary bladder was suggested to be a complicating factor and their removal was suggested. Repeated flushing of the urinary bladder with sterile water was suggested. Additional experience has shown that the filling defects that are created by the blood clots can be differentiated radiographically from those caused by more clinically significant mural lesions and the additional effort to remove the clots is not necessary and often not rewarding.

Following trauma or chronic bladder wall or urethral disease, the catheter tip should be positioned carefully so that it is not placed into a damaged ureteral or bladder wall with the possibility of air embolisation or bladder wall rupture. Fatal air embolization has been reported as a complication of pneumocystography in both cats and dogs. Venous air embolism is characterized by primary respiratory failure. An air trap is formed in the right ventricular outflow tract and constitutes an obstructive mechanism to the flow of blood into the lungs. The air trap can be displaced by appropriate positioning. The patient reported had had active hemorrhage within the bladder mucosa and it was assumed that air entered the low pressure venous system via bleeding capillaries. Positioning the patient in left lateral recumbency decreases the opportunity for the emboli reaching the lungs. Either CO_2 or N_2O are 20 times more soluble in serum than air or oxygen and there use is to be recommended.

Technique

The study is described in a similar manner for both sexes of the dog and cat. Differences exist, for example, the compression technique is much more satisfactorily performed in the cat because of the smaller size, however, the principles remain the same.

The study is tailored to provide the specific information required considering the clinical signs and patient history. A trauma patient may need to be handled more carefully and the selection of the technique be more limited than it would be in a patient with chronic hematuria. If urinary calculi are suspected, the entire urinary tract should be evaluated radiographically, while hematuria associated with pelvic trauma may necessitate only a retrograde cystogram to evaluate for possible urinary bladder or urethral rupture. Full distention of the bladder is not required if the study is to evaluate integrity of the bladder wall, however, full distention using a double-contrast technique is often needed to identify a small mural lesion. Often the study is combined with a study of the urethra, especially in the male dog.

The degree of filling of the urinary bladder in a retrograde manner may be influenced by anesthesia with the depth of anesthesia often inversely proportional to the degree of filling. If the level of anesthesia is light, abdominal straining may result in voiding of urine especially with the presence of inflammatory disease within the bladder wall.

Retrograde studies should be performed in as aseptic a manner as is possible using sterile catheters. In the male dog, the penis can be rather easily expressed from the sheath and swabbed with alcohol prior to aseptic catherization. In the male cat, the penis is swabbed with alcohol and an open ended tomcat catheter is introduced approximately 2 cm into the distal urethra. In the female dog, a speculum assists in performing the catheterization under direct visualization using a sterile otoscope speculum. In the female cat, an open-ended tomcat catheter can be introduced into the urethral orifice. While urethrography is commonly and easily performed in the male dog, the same technique is much more difficult and less rewarding in the female dog or in the cat.

Often the intravenous technique is used to study the urinary bladder in the cat, especially in the traumatized female, because of the greater ease in performing an intravenous injection as compared with urethral catheterization. In other trauma patients, a urethral catheter may have been positioned prior to radiography to obtain urine, in which case the retrograde study is easily accomplished.

Extravasation of contrast media into the bladder wall or intra or extra peritoneally may be noted in association with cystography. The intramural extravasation is usually self limiting and does not require surgical intervention. Leakage of contrast agent outside the bladder may be due to: (1) rupture of the bladder wall that may be the result of weakness due to previous bladder wall disease, (2) rupture of a normal bladder wall through the use of an excessive amount of contrast media or through the improper positioning of a rigid catheter, or (3) leakage through a traumatic tear. Each patient should be evaluated prior to the study and a determination made of the status of the bladder. During the infusion, the bladder should be palpated so as to avoid overdistention.

Routinely, the radiographic projections used to study the bladder are lateral views and oblique views made 30 degrees from the ventrodorsal positioning. The oblique projections avoid superimposing the bladder neck over the pelvis or the shadows cast by the colon and rectum. Also, if urethrography is performed, it is helpful in the male dog to not superimpose the portions of the urethra. With negative-contrast or double-contrast cystography, both lateral views should be made since it is possible for the shifting air bubble to delinate a lesion on one lateral view to a better advantage.

Catheter tip positioning should be determined by measuring the length required prior to positioning the catheter. Radiography may be necessary to positively determine the location of the catheter tip. Catheter kinking or knotting within the urethra or within the bladder may occur during studies of the bladder. The exact nature of the problem can be evaluated by filling the catheter with either air or a positive-contrast agent. Manipulation of the catheter may resolve the problem, otherwise, surgical relief may be required.

Urine samples for bacteriologic studies should be obtained prior to the infusion of contrast media since most agents contain bacteriostatic substances. Infusion of a suitable antibiotic solution is warranted after the catheterization procedure if the patient is not on systemic antiobiotic therapy.

Leakage of urine around or through the catheter may occur during the procedure. Since the urine contains contrast media, it needs to be cleaned from the table, cassette, and patient, to minimize the radiographic artifacts that are produced on the radiograph.

Comments

1. the quality of the study can be improve by withholding food for 24 hours prior to the study so that the small bowel is empty
2. a low enema may be required to empty the colon of fecal material
3. the non-contrast survey radiographic study includes the entire abdomen to enable evaluation of the entire urinary system
4. the non-contrast survey radiographic study determines proper preparation of the patient, correct radiographic exposure, and the presence of artifacts due to wet hair coat or foreign material on the skin
5. avoid use of a stiff urinary catheter because of possible injury to the urethera or bladder mucosa
6. the use of lidocaine solution without epinephrine further decreases the possibility of spasm and helps to insure that complete bladder distention can be obtained
7. vesicoureteral reflux and urethroprostatic reflux occurs frequently in mature healthy dogs undergoing maximum distention urethrocystography

POSITIVE CYSTOGRAPHY SECONDARY TO INTRAVENOUS UROGRAPHY IN THE DOG AND CAT

Definition

Toward the end of an intravenous urogram, the contrast agent accumulates within the urinary bladder and provides an opportunity for positive cystography. The bladder is distended to varying degrees depending on bladder filling prior to the intravenous injection of contrast agent. Because the urogram usually takes 20 to 30 minutes to perform, it is possible that the patient urinates prior to maximum bladder filling. This is particularly noted in a patient in which a cystitis or other disease makes complete distention of the bladder uncomfortable. Because of the mixing of the contrast-laden urine with the residual urine in the bladder, the contrast is decreased.

Equipment

1. needle and syringe required for intravenous injection

Contrast Agent

1. positive-contrast organic iodide agent recommended for parenteral injection

---

Technique

1. obtain non-contrast abdominal studies that include the urinary bladder
2. position the indwelling venous catheter
3. inject the contrast medium over 2 minutes using the following dosage: 2 ml/kgbw with a maximum of 90 ml in the dog, 1 ml/kgbw with a maximum of 15 ml in the cat
4. 15 to 30 minutes following injection, make oblique and lateral radiographs of the bladder

---

Comments

1. the study is more easily and more quickly performed if the patient is anesthetized
2. it is assumed that the intravenous study is selected because the patient cannot be easily catheterized
3. if the patient can be catheterized, the study is more quickly performed in a retrograde manner
4. move the contrast pool through use of a paddle to make evaluation of the bladder more complete
5. extravasation of positive-contrast agent into the extraperitoneal soft tissues or into the peritoneal cavity is well tolerated

RETROGRADE POSITIVE CYSTOGRAPHY IN THE DOG AND CAT

Definition

Retrograde positive cystography is a study in which the urinary bladder is filled through a catheter with a contrast agent similar to that used to perform the intravenous urogram (Fig. 3-3). This is the best technique to evaluate the character of the bladder wall in a trauma patient or to locate the bladder following trauma or herniation. It is of value in determining the character of caudal abdominal masses in the absence of ultrasound. The degree of patient preparation and bladder distention is dependent on the level of information desired.

Equipment

1. sterile male or female urinary catheter
2. vaginal speculum or adapted otoscope for female dogs
3. flashlight or other light source
4. sterile lubricating jelly
5. 20 to 50 cc syringe
6. adapter for urethral catheter
7. 2% lidocaine jelly
8. 3-way valve
9. irrigation pan

Contrast Agent

1. positive-contrast organic iodide agent recommended for parenteral injection

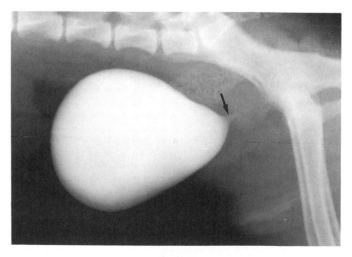

Fig. 3-3
RETROGRADE POSITIVE-CONTRAST CYSTOGRAM
A lateral radiograph of the caudal abdomen of a dog shows a distended urinary bladder filled with a positive-contrast agent. The bladder neck and a small portion of the urethra (arrow) can be identified. The feces within the rectum just dorsal to the prostate gland somewhat compromises the quality of the study.

Technique

1. the study is performed more easily if the female is anesthetized and the male is sedated
2. obtain non-contrast abdominal studies that include the urinary bladder
3. dilute the positive-contrast medium with two parts of sterile water
4. fill the catheter with sterile water prior to placement to prevent the introduction of air bubbles
5. place 2% lidocaine jelly on the tip of the catheter
6. catheterize the patient in lateral recumbency placing the catheter tip within the urinary bladder
7. withdraw as much urine from the bladder as possible
8. the volume of diluted contrast agent to be injected should be determined by constant palpation of the bladder at the time of injection rather than by strict adherence to published dosages—use the following dosages as guidelines—50 to 300 cc in dogs—35 cc in cats
9. make oblique and lateral radiographs of the bladder with the catheter tip in position immediately following the injection
10. if further distention of the bladder is required inject additional contrast agent
11. if an inflatable cuff is used within the urethra, it should not be inflated for a period beyond that needed for the injection and making the radiographs
12. remove catheter when appropriate
13. it may be preferred to flush the urinary bladder with a broad spectrum antibiotic solution before the catheter is removed or to place the patient on systemic antibiotics

Comments

1. determine the length of the catheter by measuring the required length on the outside of the patients body prior to positioning or make a radiograph to determine the location of the catheter tip as it is positioned
2. the character of the diseased bladder determines the degree of distensibility—a neurogenic bladder may hold 2 to 3 times the expected volume while a bladder with chronic cystitis may only hold a fraction of the expected volume before contrast begins to leak around the catheter
3. to help determine the volume of contrast agent to be infused, place your hand on the caudal abdomen and note the pressure within the bladder at the time of infusion—if the bladder becomes distended or if back-pressure on the syringe becomes great, stop the infusion
4. following positive-contrast cystography, it is possible to remove as much positive-contrast agent as possible and inject air to perform a double-contrast agent if desirable
5. compression through use of a paddle should be performed carefully and may move the contrast pool and make evaluation of the integrity of the bladder wall more complete
6. following positive-contrast cystography, it is possible to reposition the catheter tip into the urethra to perform a urethrogram—this is important since the positioning of the catheter tip within the bladder often produces a study that fails to detect injury to the bladder neck following trauma or the presence of a bladder neck tumor
7. ureteral reflux of positive-contrast agent may be a normal finding
8. if the contrast agent remains in the bladder for a relatively long period of time especially in patients with cystitis, the amount of iodine absorbed may be sufficient to produce an excretory urogram
9. to evaluate for a ruptured urinary bladder, the contrast agent may be used without dilution to enable better visualization of a small quantity of contrast agent within the peritoneal cavity
10. extravasation of a positive-contrast agent into the extraperitioneal soft tissues or into the peritoneal cavity is well tolerated

RETROGRADE NEGATIVE CYSTOGRAPHY IN THE DOG AND CAT

Definition

Retrograde negative cystography is a study performed by catheterization of the patient and filling of the urinary bladder with air or other gas. This study is performed only is specific clinical situations where it is used to identify the integrity of the bladder wall following trauma or to locate the bladder. Use of negative cystography usually requires use of a large quantity of air. The study fails to delineate mucosal lesions that would be more easily seen on a double-contrast study.

Equipment

1. vaginal speculum for female dogs or cats or adapted otoscope
2. flashlight or other light source
3. sterile lubricating jelly
4. 20 to 50 cc syringe
5. adapter for urethral catheter
6. 2% lidocaine jelly
7. 3-way valve
8. irrigation pan

Technique

1. obtain non-contrast abdominal studies that include the urinary bladder
2. place lidocaine jelly on the catheter tip
3. catheterize the patient in lateral recumbency placing the catheter tip within the urinary bladder
4. remove as much urine from the bladder as possible
5. inject air slowly using abdominal palpation to determine adequate distention of the bladder—use the following dosages as guidelines—50 to 300 cc in dogs—35 cc in cats
6. make both oblique and both lateral radiographs of the bladder with the catheter in position
7. inject additional air if further distention of the bladder is required
8. remove catheter when appropriate
9. it may be preferred to flush the urinary bladder with a broad spectrum antibiotic solution before the catheter is removed or to place the patient on systemic antibiotics

Comments

1. the study is more easily and more quickly performed if the patient is anesthesized
2. measure the length of the catheter against the outside of the patients body or make a radiograph to determine the location of the catheter tip
3. place your hand on the caudal abdomen and note the pressure within the bladder at the time of injection—stop injection if the bladder becomes distended or if back-pressure on the syringe becomes great
4. a neurogenic bladder may hold 2 to 3 times the expected volume of air while a bladder with chronic cystitis may only hold a fraction of the expected volume before air begins to leak around the catheter
5. leakage of air around the catheter may be undetected and the volume of air within the bladder may be impossible to estimate other than by abdominal palpation
6. it is possible to follow the injection of air with the injection of a positive-contrast agent and perform a double-contrast agent
7. If the catheter has an inflatable cuff it should not be inflated for a period beyond that needed for the injection and making the radiographs
8. ureteral reflux of air may be a normal finding
9. the kVp is reduced 4 to 6 in cats and small dogs and 10 to 15 in larger dogs because of the reduced tissue density

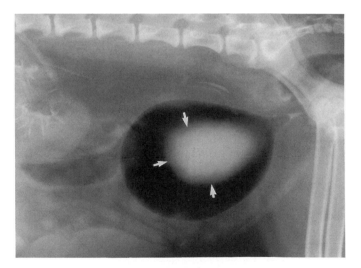

Fig. 3-4
DOUBLE-CONTRAST CYSTOGRAM
A lateral radiograph of the caudal abdomen of a dog shows a distended urinary bladder filled with air with a minimal coating on the bladder wall by a positive-contrast agent. The bladder neck and a small portion of the urethra can be identified. Notice the dense pool of positive contrast agent within the bladder (arrows). The double-contrast cystogram was made following an intravenous urogram.

RETROGRADE DOUBLE-CONTRAST CYSTOGRAPHY IN THE DOG AND CAT

Definition

Double-contrast cystography performed in a retrograde manner is the best study to delineate mural or intraluminal disease of the urinary bladder and has become a popular form of bladder examination (Fig. 3-4). The double-contrast study may: (1) follow intravenous urography, (2) follow positive retrograde cystography, or (3) be injected as a separate study. To perform the study, catheterize the patient and remove as much urine as is possible and follow by the injection of a positive-contrast agent and air.

Equipment

1. vaginal speculum or adapted otoscope
2. flashlight or other light source
3. sterile lubricating jelly
4. 20 to 50 cc syringe
5. adapter for urethral catheter
6. 2% lidocaine jelly
7. 3-way valve
8. irrigation pan

Contrast Agent

1. positive-contrast organic iodide agent recommended for parenteral injection

Technique

1. obtain non-contrast abdominal studies that include the urinary bladder
2. place lidocaine jelly on the catheter tip
3. catheterize the patient in lateral recumbency placing the catheter tip within the urinary bladder
4. remove the contrast-laden urine from the urinary bladder through a catheter if the study follows an intravenous urogram or positive-contrast cystography OR remove undiluted urine if the study is performed as a separate study
5. inject the positive-contrast medium using the following dosages as guidelines—5 to 10 cc in a dog and 3 cc in a cat
6. rotate the patient to coat the mucosal surface and massage the bladder gently
7. remove as much of the contrast agent as possible
8. infuse air slowly through the catheter using bladder palpation to insure complete distention using a dosage of 50 to 300 cc in dogs and 35 cc in cats
9. reduce the kVp for the cystograms by 4 to 6 in cats and small dogs and 10 to 15 in larger dogs because of the reduced tissue density.
10. make both oblique and both lateral radiographs of the bladder with the catheter in position
11. if further distention of the bladder is required inject additional air
12. at the completion of the study remove the catheter

Comments

1. the study is more easily and more quickly performed if the patient is anesthetized
2. measure the length of the catheter against the outside of the patients body or make a radiograph to determine the location of the catheter tip
3. place your hand on the caudal abdomen and note the pressure within the bladder at the time of injection—stop injection if the bladder becomes distended or if back-pressure on the syringe becomes great
4. a neurogenic bladder may hold 2 to 3 times the expected volume while a bladder with chronic cystitis may only hold a fraction of the expected before air begins to leak around the catheter
5. more air may be needed to distend the bladder than the volume of fluid removed because the gas is compressible while the fluid is not.
6. iodinated organic agents can be diluted to a final concentration of 15% and decrease mucosal irritation.
7. extravasation of positive-contrast agent or air into the extraperitoneal soft tissues or into the peritoneal cavity is well tolerated
8. in the past, a diluted sodium iodide solution has been incorrectly recommended for retrograde cystography with a resulting acute hemorrhagic cystitis with epithelial ulceration and submucosal hemorrhage
9. if cystography is performed in conjunction with excretory urography, the study is more diagnostic if the bladder examination is performed prior to the excretory urography since the constant drainage of positive-contrast media opacified urine into the bladder compromises the double-contrast cystogram
10. if an inflatable cuff is used, it should not be inflated for a period beyond that needed for the injection and making the radiographs
11. ureteral reflux of either positive contrast, air, or a combination may be a normal finding
12. it may be preferred to flush the urinary bladder with a broad spectrum antibiotic solution before the catheter is removed or to put the patient on systemic antibiotics

CYSTOGRAPHY VIA CYSTOCENTESIS IN THE DOG AND CAT

Definition

Either positive or negative cystography can be performed following the injection of a positive contrast agent or air into the urinary bladder following adominal cystocentesis. Cystography may be done in this manner if urethral obstruction prevents catheterization. This technique may be more useful in cats than in dogs. This is an uncommon technique but it should be appreciated that it can be performed if necessary.

Equipment

1. 1" 22 ga needle in a cat and a 2" 22 ga needle in a dog
2. 20 to 50 cc syringe

Contrast Agent

1. positive-contrast organic iodide agent recommended for parenteral injection

Technique

1. manually palpate the urinary bladder and immobilize it with your fingers against the ventral or lateral abdominal wall
2. aseptically introduced the needle into the bladder through the midline abdominal wall
3. drain as much urine as possible from the bladder
4. infuse a diluted positive-contrast media or air creating minimal bladder distention
5. remove the needle
6. make lateral and oblique radiographs

Comments

1. anticipate minimal leakage of the positive-contrast agent or air into the peritoneal cavity
2. do not compress the bladder following injection because of possible leakage

REFERENCES

Ackerman N and Nyland TG. Cystography. Calif Vet p13-16, June 1978.

Ackerman N Wingfield WE and Corley EA. Fatal air embolism associated with pneumourethrography and pneumo-cystography in a dog. J Am Vet Med Assoc 160:1616-8, 1972.

Ackerman N. Radiology of Urogenital Diseases in Dogs and Cat, 2nd edition, ISU Press, Ames, 1991.

Breton L Pennock PW and Valli VE. The effects of hypaque 25% and sodium iodide10% in the canine urinary bladder. J Am Vet Rad Soc 19:116-24, 1978.

Buchanan JW. Kinked catheter: A compliation in pneumo-cystography. J Am Vet Rad Soc 8:54-6, 1967.

Currarino G Weinberg A and Putnam R. Resorption of contrast material from the bladder during cystoure-thrography causing an excretory urogram. Radiology 123:149-50, 1977.

Johnston GR Feeney DA and Osborne CA. Urethrography and cystography in cats Part 1. Techniques, normal radiographic anatomy, and artifacts. Continuing education 4:823-35, 1982.

Johnston GR Feeney DA and Osborne CA. Urethrography and cystography in cats Part 11. Abnormal radiographic anatomy and complications. Continuing education 4:931-46, 1982.

Johnston GR Stevens JB and Jessen CR. Complications of retrograde contrast urethrography in dogs and cats. Amer J Vet Res 44:1248, 1983.

Kizer KW and Goodman PC. Radiographic manifestations of venous air embolism. Radiology 144:35-9, 1982.

Oppenheimer MJ Durant TM and Lynch P. Body position in relation to venous air embolism and the associated cardiovascular-respiratory changes. Am J Med Sci 225:362-73, 1953.

Osborn CA and Jensen CR. Double-contrast cystography in the dog. J Am Vet Med Assoc 159:1400-04, 1971.

Park RD. Contrast studies of the lower urinary tract. Vet. Clinics of North Am 4:863, 1974.

Rhodes WH and Biery DN. Pneumocystography in the dog. J Am Vet Rad Soc 8:45-53, 1967.

Thayer GW Carrig CB and Evans AT. Fatal venous air embolism associated with pneumocystography in a cat. J Am Vet Med Assoc 176:643-5, 1980.

Zontine WJ and Andrews LK. Fatal air embolization as a complication of pneumocystography in two cats. J Am Vet Rad Soc 19:8-11, 1978.

D. UROGRAPHY FOR ECTOPIC URETERS IN THE DOG

Definition

Excretory urography used for diagnosing ureteral abnormalities such as ruptures, obstruction, or ectopic insertion into the urinary bladder, urethra or vagina is performed in a special way. With the urinary bladder filled with air, the positive-contrast filled ureters and their entrance into the bladder, urethra, or vagina are visible. The ureters can be filled following an intravenous urogram or they can be filled following a retrograde vaginourethrogram (see later). The study is best performed on sedated or anesthetized patients.

Indications

The principle indication is urinary incontinence that often is first noted in the young female patient.

Contraindications

A clinical problem that prevents sedation or anesathesia may prevent the study.

Equipment

Equipment is the same as that required for the intravenous urogram (or retrograde vagino-urethrogram).

Contrast Agent

1. positive-contrast organic iodide agent recommended for parenteral injection

Technique

1. patient preparation is important and enemas may be needed to remove all fecal material from the distal colon
2. make non-contrast abdominal radiographs including the pelvic region
3. pass a urinary catheter
4. remove all urine possible
5. infuse air causing distention of the bladder
6. expand the retention bulb of the catheter keeping the air within the bladder
7. make an intravenous injection of the positive-contrast agent using a dosage of 2 cc/kgbw
8. 10 minutes following the injection, make lateral and oblique ventrodorsal abdominal radiographs centering on the bladder neck
9. repeat the radiographs to insure location of the distal ureters

Comments

1. if air leaks out of the bladder during the study, additional volumes of air should be infused to maintain a distented bladder
2. if the insertion of the ureters cannot be clearly seen, minimal compression of the bladder with a spoon or paddle may reposition overlying structures

E. VAGINOGRAPHY (Vaginourethrogram) IN THE FEMALE DOG

Definition

Retrograde placement of either positive-contrast agent or negative-contrast agent within the vagina is called retrograde vaginography and may assist in evaluation of the location, size, and shape of this organ and provide for the detection of strictures or other intraluminal masses. Rectal or vaginal digital palpation or direct visualization of the vagina may be inadequate to fully evaluate an extramural, mural, or intraluminal lesion. Fistulous tracts originating from the vagina may also require further evaluation radiographically to determine the origin of the tract. The success of the study is based primarily on your ability to maintain the pool of contrast agent within the vagina during the examination.

Because of the technique often used, a vaginourethrogram is often produced. This results from the creation of a pressure within the vaginal vault that causes contrast agent to fill the urethra. In certain patients, this may be a most successful technique to perform urethrography. While this is a retrograde passage, there does not seem to be any untoward effects related to the production of uretheritis or cystitis. This may be due in part to the minimal bacteriostatic properties of the contrast agent. However, a course of antibiotic therapy is recommended.

Indications

The most common indication for performing the study is to evaluate the vaginal vault for stricture or other mass lesions that serve as a persistent cause of incomplete vaginal drainage and a resulting chronic vaginitis. It is also possible to use this study to evaluate urinary incontinence in the young female puppy that has often been present since birth. The study is performed to determine if the entrance of the ureters is abnormal and if an ectopic ureteral orifice is detected, where is its location and is the abnormality unilateral or bilateral.

Other indications include: (1) vaginal discharge, (2) dysuria, (3) physical vaginal abnormalities that prevent examination, (4) vaginal mass, (5) extra-vaginal mass, (6) fistulous tract, (7) congenital stricture, or (8) determination of ectopic ureteral orifice.

Contraindications

Some thought should be given to performing the examination in the presence of marked vaginitis since it is a retrograde study.

Equipment

1. large catheter with inflatable bulb (such as a Foley catheter)
2. 50 cc syringe
3. catheter adapter
4. tongue forceps
5. urinary catheter

Contrast Agent

1. positive-contrast organic iodide agent recommended for parenteral injection

Technique

1. anesthesia is recommended because of the discomfort to the patient
2. use low enemas to obtain emptying of the distal colon and rectum
3. catheterize the urinary bladder and drain all urine possible
4. remove the catheter
5. make both lateral and oblique ventrodorsal non-contrast radiographs of the pelvic region
6. fill the catheter with positive contrast agent to avoid filling defects due to air bubbles
7. place the catheter tip within the vagina and inflate the bulb
8. inject contrast agent using the following dosages—30 cc in a small dog, 45 cc in a medium sized dog, and 90 cc in a large dog—using the back pressure on the syringe to determine an adequate volume
9. make lateral and oblique ventrodorsal radiographs

Comments

Vaginography is often performed in conjunction with cystography and it may be helpful to perform a negative-contrast cystogram in conjunction with a positive-contrast vaginogram to more clearly outline the urethra or ureters. In the search for ectopic ureters, the study should be made with a persistent high injection pressure of the positive-contrast media. The volume of contrast medium required is less in spayed or incontinent bitches.

Contrast agent may by forced into the uterine horns creating a hysterogram, or this study can be performed by positioning the catheter tip through the cervical canal into the uterus and injecting a radiopaque contrast solution in that location. Because of the angle of the cervical canal, difficulty may be experienced in positioning the catheter into the uterine horns. With the advent of ultrasound, hysterography is not usually recommended, but there may be specific indications that warrant its use.

REFERENCES

Adams WM Biery DN and Millar HC. Pneumovaginography in the dog: A case report. J Am Vet Rad Soc 19:80-2, 1978.

Cobb LM and Archibald J. The radiographic appearance of certain pathological conditions of the canine uterus. J Am Vet Med Assoc 134:393-7; 1959.

Holt PE Gibbs C and Pearson H. Canine ectopic ureter: a review of twenty-nine cases. J small Anim Pract 23:195 1983.

Leveille R and Atilola MAO. Retrograde vaginocystography: A contrast study for evaluation of bitches with urinary incontinence. Comp Cont Ed 13:934-43, 1991.

F. URETHROGRAPHY IN THE DOG AND CAT

Definition

Urethrography is the radiographic technique most easily accomplished in a retrograde manner that permits evaluation of the urethra using a positive-contrast, negative-contrast, or possibly a double-contrast study. The study can also be performed by providing compression on a positive-contrast filled bladder causing a voiding urethrogram. It is also possible to fill the urethra in a retrograde manner during the performance of a vaginogram in the female dog. During the urethrogram in a male dog, it is possible to force contrast agent into the prostate gland and thus gain some information concerning that organ. The technique that is selected varies between the sexes and between the dog and cat.

Indications

Urethrography is indicated in the presence of apparent difficult in passing a stream of urine. This may be due to: (1) acute injury to the urethra, (2) obstruction with urinary calculi, (2) partial obstruction secondary to chronic injury following repeated urethritis or repeated catheterization, or (4) malignant disease. The study may be valuable to determine the cause of hematuria. The study can be used to evaluate the urethra post-operatively to insure patency and complete healing without fistulization.

Specific indications include: (1) urethral calculi, (2) luminal stenosis following chronic urethritis, (3) mucosal injury caused by tumor, urethritis, or post-surgical fibrosis, (4) mural disease due to tumor, urethritis, or rupture, and (5) prostatic disease (cystic prostate, prostatic abscessation) with communication with the urethra

Contraindications

The only contraindication may occur with the use of air as the contrast agent in the even of injury to the mucosa or placement of the catheter tip within the corpus cavernosum. Injected air may enter the venous system and may result in life threatening venous air embolisation.

Equipment

1. catheter preferably with inflatable bulb
2. sterile lubricating jelly
3. catheter adapter
4. syringe
5. positive-contrast agent
6. sterile saline solution
7. 2% lidocaine jelly
8. 2% lidocaine solution

Contrast Agent

1. positive-contrast organic iodide agent recommended for parenteral injection

Technique

Sedation or anesthesia may facilitate the conduction of the examination since there is some patient discomfort. Cleaning the descending colon and rectum improves the quality of the study in removing superimposed shadows due to the fecal material.

Either use the largest catheter possible or one with an inflatable cuff. The catheter should be filled with contrast media prior to insertion to avoid injection of air bubbles that can be incorrectly diagnosed as radiolucent calculi or other intraluminal filling defects.

Studies usually consist of lateral and oblique radiographs made at 30° from the ventrodorsal positioning. The lateral views are often made with the hindlimbs positioned cranially to permit visualization of the ischial portion of the urethra in the male dog. It may be helpful in some patients to make one lateral view with the hindlimbs pulled caudally and a second view with the hindlimbs pulled cranially.

Dilute an iodinated contrast agent with an equal amount of sterile water to achieve a solution with less opacity. It is also possible to use a small amount of positive-contrast agent and follow with an injection of air to obtain a double-contrast study. Air can be injected to perform a negative-contrast study.

Catheter kinking or knotting may occur during positioning of the catheter for studies of the urethra. The exact nature of the problem can be evaluated by filling the catheter with either air or positive-contrast. Manipulation of the catheter may resolve the problem, otherwise, surgical relief may be required.

URETHROGRAPHY IN THE MALE DOG

Urethrography in the male dog is relatively easy to perform because of the ease of catheter placement. The catheter tip is usually positioned in the penile urethra to permit evaluation of the entire urethra. Usually this study is performed after completion of a retrograde cystogram by simply repositioning the catheter tip (Fig. 3-5).

Vesicoureteral relux can be induced during retrograde urethrography or by manual compression of the urinary bladder in male and female dogs and in male and female cats. The duration of the digital pressure on the urinary bladder or the degree of distention of the urinary bladder increased the vesicoureteral reflux. Urethroprostatic reflex was observed in male dogs, but not in male cats.

Technique

1. make lateral and both ventrodorsal oblique non-contrast radiographs of the pelvic region insuring that the urethra is included
2. place lidocaine jelly on the tip of the catheter
3. fill the catheter with sterile water
4. pass the catheter in an aseptic manner
5. position the retention bulb within the distal portion of the penile urethra and inflate the catheter bulb
6. dilute the contrast agent to 1/2 or 1/4 concentration
7. attach the catheter to the syringe containing the diluted contrast material avoiding leaving any air within the catheter
8. inject 1/2 the diluted contrast agent (10 ml in a small male dog, 20 ml in a medium-sized male dog, 30 ml in a large male dog)
9. make a lateral radiograph
10. inject the remaining 1/2 of the diluted contrast agent
11. make a lateral radiograph to coincide with the completion of the injection
12. make the oblique exposures to coincide with the completion of additional injections

---

Comments

1. if the catheter does not have a retention bulb, select the largest catheter to limit leakage of the contrast agent placing a towel or surgical sponge under the dog to absorb the leaking contrast agent
2. if the catheter does not have a retention bulb, use some form of manual compression to prevent leakage of the contrast during injection
3. the location of the tip of the catheter may be varied dependent upon the portion of the urethra in which there is the greatest clinical interest
4. retrograde urethrography, especially in the presence of urinary bladder distention, has been reported to cause histologically detected lesions ranging from focal hemorrhagic cystitis
5. avoid the use of a mixture of positive-contrast agent with KY jelly since this has the possibility of creating filing defects within the contrast column that result in false positive diagnoses
6. the inflated catheter balloon should not be left inflated for a long period of time since inflation for 15 minutes duration in the distal part of the urethra of dogs and cats results in a mild reversible inflammatory reaction
7. it is possible to place pressure on the urinary bladder to start urination and perform a voiding urethrography—usually this is not done in a male dog because of the ease of performing the retrograde study

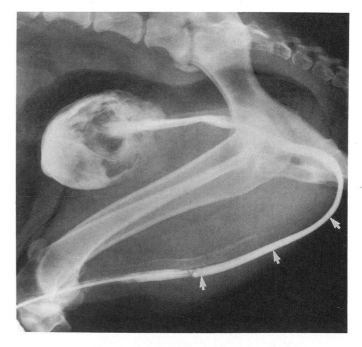

Fig. 3-5
POSITIVE CONTRAST URETHROGRAM
A lateral radiograph of the caudal abdomen of a dog shows the urethra (arrows) filled with positive contrast agent with some of the contrast agent flowing into the urinary bladder creating a "mixing" pattern. Notice the shadow cast by the urethral catheter within the penile urethra.

RETROGRADE URETHROGRAPHY FOR PROSTATIC URETHRA IN THE MALE DOG

The study is performed primarily to identify extravasation of contrast media within the diseased prostate gland. This type of pathologic change is best seen using positive-contrast media, but the study can also be performed with air. Since the contrast media tends to remain within the diseased prostate, there is not as much urgency in making the radiographs. The lateral projection is recommended because of the ease in positioning the patient. The oblique studies may be used to more completely visualize the prostate gland. This study is rarely performed because the character of the prostate gland is so well studied by ultrasound. This special study is performed essentially as described above except that the tip of the catheter is placed just distal to the prostatic urethra.

URETHROGRAPHY IN THE FEMALE DOG

Urethrography in the female dog can be performed by positioning a catheter tip within the urethra and making a retrograde infusion. However, the length of the urethra is so short that the catheter positioning makes it impossible to visualize more than a part of the urethra. It is, however, also possible to apply pressure to the bladder following filling through a positive cystogram and perform a voiding study. Gentle pressure is placed on the bladder with a paddle and a lateral radiograph is made at the time urine is noted at the urethral orifice. Place a towel under the patient to absorb the contrast-laden urine as it is voided. Usually only lateral radiographs are made. Performing the study in this manner is contraindicated in the presence of a badly disease bladder where rupture would be a possibility.

Technique

1. make lateral and both ventrodorsal oblique non-contrast radiographs of the pelvic region insuring that the urethra is included
2. place lidocaine jelly on the catheter tip
3. position the catheter in an aseptic manner
4. dilute the positive-contrast agent to 1/2 or 1/4 concentration
5. attach the catheter to the syringe containing the diluted contrast material using a catheter adapter
6. avoiding having air within the catheter
7. position the catheter in an aseptic manner positioning the retention bulb within the distal portion of the urethra
8. inflate the catheter bulb
9. inject the diluted contrast agent (4 ml in a small female dog, 8 ml in a medium-sized female dog, 12 ml in a large female dog)
10. make a lateral exposure to coincide with the completion of the injection
11. make the oblique exposures to coincide with the completion of additional injections

Comments

1. the inflated catheter balloon should not be left inflated for a long period of time since inflation for 15 minutes duration in the distal part of the urethra results in a mild reversible inflammatory reaction
2. if a double-contrast study is to be performed, inject a small amount of positive-contrast agent (2 ml) and follow this immediately with an injection of air

URETHROGRAPHY IN THE MALE AND FEMALE CAT

It is possible to perform the urethrogram in the cat by positioning a catheter within the urethra and making a retrograde infusion. However, the length of the urethra is so short that the catheter positioning makes it impossible to visualize more than a limited portion. It is, however, also possible to apply pressure to the bladder following filling through a positive cystogram and perform a voiding study. Gentle pressure is placed on the bladder with a paddle and a lateral radiograph made at the time urine is noted at the urethral orifice. Usually only lateral studies are made. Performing the study in this manner is contraindicated in the presence of a badly disease bladder where rupture would be a possibility.

REFERENCES

Ackerman N Wingfield WE and Corley EA. Fatal air embolism associated with pneumourethrography and pneumo-cystography in a dog. J Am Vet Med Assoc 160:1616-18, 1972.

Ackerman N. Prostatic reflux during positive-contrast retrograde urethrography in the dog. Vet Radiol 24:251-9, 1983.

Ackerman N. Urography-Technique. Calif Vet 33:6-9, 1979.

Ackerman N. Use of pediatric Foley catheter for positive-contrast retrograde urethrography. Mod Vet Pract 61:684-6, 1980.

Barsanti JA Crowell W Losonsky J and Talkington FD. Complications of bladder distention during rdtrograde urethrography. Am J Vet Res 42: 819-21, 1981.

Christie BA. Vesicoureteral reflux in dogs. J Am Vet Med Assoc 162:772-6, 1973.

Christie BA. Incidence and etiology of vesicoureteral reflux in apparanently normal dogs. Invest Urol 8:184-94, 1971.

Christie BA. Occurrence of vesicoureteral reflux and pyelonephritis in apparently normal dogs. Invest Urol 21:359-66, 1973.

Feeney DA Osborne CA and Johnston GR. Vesicoureteral reflex indiced by manual compression of the urinary bladder of dogs and cats. J Am Vet Med Assoc 182:795-7, 1983.

Johnston GR Feeney DA and Osborne CA. Urethrography and cystography in cats Part 1. Techniques, normal radiographic anatomy, and artifacts. Continuing Education 4:823-35, 1982.

Johnston GR Feeney DA and Osborne CA. Urethrography and cystography in cats Part 11. Abnormal radiographic anatomy and complications. Continuing Education 4:931-46, 1982.

Johnston GR Stevens JB and Jessen CR. Complications of retrograde contrast urethrography in dogs and cats. Amer J Vet Res 44:1248, 1983.

Johnston GR Stevens JB Jessen CR and Osborne CA. Effects of prolonged distention of retention catheters on the urethra of dogs and cats. Am J Vet Res 44:223-8, 1983.

Johnston GR Stevens JB Jessen CR et al. Complications of retrograde contrast contrast urethrography in dogs and cats. Am J Vet Res 44; 1248, 1983.

Kipnis RM. Vesicoureteral reflux in a cat. J Am Vet Med Assoc 167:288-92, 1975.

Lenaghan D and Cussen LJ. Vesicoureteral reflux in pups. Invest Urol 5:449;61, 1968.

Park RD. Contrast studies of the lower urinary tract. Vet Clin North Am 4:863-8, 1974.

Ticer JW Spencer CP and Ackerman N. Positive contrast retrograde urethography: a useful procedure for evaluating urethral disorders in the dog. Vet Radiol 21:2-11, 1980.

Zontine WJ. The urethra. Mod Vet Pract 56:411-5, 1975.

4. NEUROLOGICAL PROCEDURES IN THE DOG AND CAT

A. MYELOGRAPHY IN THE DOG AND CAT

Definition

Myelography, without further qualification, describes the placement of a radio-opaque contrast agent into the subarachnoid apace either through injection in the cisterna magna or in the lumbar region (Fig. 4-1). The radiographic assessment of the lumbosacral nerves is probably more correctly referred to as radiculography while the evaluation of the spinal cord is myelography. The description of the technique and equipment required is divided by the site of injection and by the species to be studied.

Indications

Myelography assists in the localization and characterization of the cause of a suspected transverse spinal myelopathy. Non-contrast studies often cannot identify the cause of the myelopathy or the location of the lesion and the final diagnosis relies entirely on the myelogram. In other patients, the lesion can be identified by physical examination or by non-contrast radiography and the myelogram is used to gain additional information about the size of the lesion or the extent of cord compression. In certain cases, the myelogram is used to determine location of several lesions, especially protruded intervertebral discs, and to determine which lesion is causing the currently observed clinical signs.

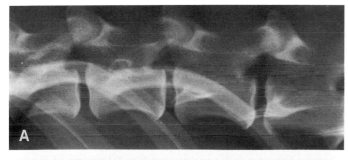

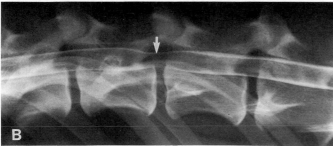

Fig. 4-1
MYELOGRAM
Lateral radiographs of the thoraco-lumbar spine of a dog made before (A) and after (B) the injection of contrast agent. Notice the deflection of the dorsal column of contrast agent (arrow) that represents extra-dural masses at T13-L1.

The myelogram also proves that a suspect lesion determined clinically or on non-contrast radiographs may not be the cause of the neurologic signs present at the time of examination. With the visualization of the lesion myelographically comes the possibility to determine whether the lesion is to be treated surgically or medically.

The specific indications for myelography include a patient with paresis, paralysis, proprioceptive or sensory deficit, or spinal pain thought to be due to a transverse myelopathy.

Contrast Agent

Newer contrast agents are available that are water-soluble, contain additional iodine atoms to improve the density of the fluid, are nonionic, have improved osmolality, and have varying viscosity. They are triiodinated benzoic-acid derivatives with either a glucosamine moiety or hydrophilic side chains added to increase water solubility. Agents that can be used include: (1) iopamidol (Isovue), E.R.Squibb & Sons Company, Princeton, NJ 08540 and (Niopam) or (Solutrast), Bracco Industria Chimica, Milan, Italy—available in 200 mgI/ml in 20 ml vials and in 300 mgI/ml in 15 ml vials, (2) metrizamide (Amipaque), Winthrop-Breon Laboratories, New York NY 10016 and Nyegaard & Company, Oslo, Norway—available as 170 mgI/ml or 300 mgI/ml, (3) iohexol (Omnipaque), Winthrop-Breon Laboratories, New York NY 10016 and Nyegaard & Company, Oslo, Norway—available in 180 mgI/ml in 10 and 20 ml vial and in 240 mgI/ml in 10, 100, and 200 ml vial, or (4) iotrolan, Schering AG, Berlin and Berlex Laboratories, Wayne, NJ—available as 300 mgI/ml.

Most myelographic agents are sensitive to light and therefore should be protected from exposure. Most are hypertonic relative to plasma or cerebrospinal fluid.

Contraindications

1. anything that prevents performing general anesthesia
2. presence of significant local or systemic infection, especially myelitis or meningitis especially as indicated by examination of the CFS
3. presence of sepsis of the overlying skin, subcutis, and muscle that would make placement of a needle into the spinal canal inappropriate
4. use of phenothiazine derivatives in the anesthetic regimen
5. intrathecal administration of corticosteroids along with the myelographic agent
6. recent myelography within 5 days (an interval of 48 hours is probably sufficient prior to a repeat myelogram)
7. dehydration, since the frequency of side effects and complications from aqueous myelography is increased due to delayed elimination of contrast medium from the subarachnoid space

Comments

The recommended contrast agents are Iopamidol 200 mg I/ml or Iohexol 180 mgI/ml or 240 mgI/ml.

Flexion and extension of the cervical and lumbosacral spine may aid diagnosis by moving the cord and contrast filled subarachnoid columns dorsally and ventrally and exaggerate the appearance of an extradural mass. In addition, those spinal movements may influence the character of a dorsal disc protrusion by forcing annulus into the spinal canal or decreasing the amount of protrusion. This movement of the disc results is an increased or decreased compression of the subarachnoid columns and/or spinal cord.

Lateral movements are used to a lesser degree, but may cause the contrast-filled subarachnoid columns to move against an extradural mass making it more prominent.

Oblique views of the spine often demonstrate the effect of the extradural mass on the contrast columns when the mass is located dorsal and lateral or ventral and lateral.

Cerebrospinal fluid analysis in the dog has been reported to be influenced by the effect of metrizamide myelography with an increase in the percentage of neutrophils and a pleocytosis. Increase in total protein concentration and erythrocyte numbers and a decrease in the percentage of small nomonuclear cells were attributed to repeated intracisternal puncture.

Removal of the myelographic agent has been reported to decrease the number of seizures (Widner et al, 1990). This involves an additional placement of a needle, but may be practice to consider especially when associated with cisternal injection.

MYELOGRAPHY BY INJECTION AT THE CISTERNA MAGNA IN THE DOG

Injection at the cisterna magna may be easier to perform for many than lumbar injection. The difficulty with the examination performed in this manner is that there is no method of insuring that the contrast column will flow caudally into the lumbar area. Thus, a thoracolumbar lesion may not be clearly identified or at best, only the cranial aspect of the lesion may be detected.

Equipment

1. 20 ga spinal needle with a flat bevel usually 2" to 4" in length
2. 10 cc syringe (2)
3. sponges or sandbags to assist in positioning the head
4. contrast agent using a dosage of 0.45 cc/kgbw to outline the entire spine and 0.30 cc/kgbw to study the cervical spine
5. test tube to collect CSF

Technique

1. the patient needs to be under general anesthesia to avoid injury to the spinal cord by the needle tip through body movement
2. obtain a series of lateral and ventrodorsal non-contrast radiographs of the entire spine
3. aseptically prepare the region just caudal to the external occipital protruberance (approximately 4" square—10 cm square)
4. position the patient in lateral recumbency using sponges to insure a perfect lateral position (positioning dependent on whether you are right or left handed)
5. position the head in maximum ventral flexion using sandbags or sponges so that the midline of the neck and the midline of the head are parallel to the tabletop
6. position an assistant in a comfortable manner in front of the dog holding the head in a flexed position using both hands in a cupped position resting on the tabletop
7. position of the head is controlled by the individual who positions the needle
8. with the patient's head to your left, determine the location of the needle site to be within the center of a triangle created by placing the thumb and tip of the second finger of your right hand on the lateral processes of C1 and the tip of the first finger on the external occipital protuberance
9. insure that the needle site in on the midline
10. check to insure that the patient is perfectly lateral and maintain the needle in a horizontal plane as it is advanced

11. rest your left hand on the patient's head with the thumb and first finger holding the shaft of the needle (never move this hand during the procedure and never release your hold on the needle)
12. with the right hand advance the needle in steps removing the stylet at the end of each step to continuously monitor the position of the needle tip
13. as the needle passes through the dura you experience a subtle "pop"
14. on removing the stylet, CSF flows from the needle hub and can be collected for examination
15. permit a volume of CSF to flow at least equal to the volume of contrast agent you intend to inject
16. attach the syringe to the hub of the spinal needle and inject the total volume over a 3 to 4 minute period (use 0.45 cc/kgbw)
17. remove the needle (this releases your assistant from holding the head)
18. make a lateral radiograph of the cervical spine to confirm the location of the contrast pool and determine the level of flow
19. it may be necessary to raise the patients head to assist in the flow of the contrast pool caudally
20. rotate the patient to insure equal mixing of the contrast agent with the CSF
21. complete the series of lateral and ventrodorsal radiographs
22. keep the patient under general anesthesia for an hour after the study to lessen the frequency of post-myelographic convulsions

Comments

Some prefer to position the patient in sternal recumbency with the head flexed for a cisternal puncture. This still requires that an assistant carefully position the head during needle placement, but has the advantage of making it easier to define the midline for needle placement.

Lateral positioning can be reversed from that described above for a person preferring to position the needle with their left hand.

Obviously, the placement of a needle tip into the cisterna magna is with some risk since malpositioning laterally results in puncture of the vertebral sinuses and the resulting bleeding. Malpositioning cranially can result in placement of the tip into the hind brain causing respiratory collapse and death. Slight movement of the needle tip during positioning can lead to laceration of the spinal cord or medulla with disastrous results.

With correct positioning of the needle and accurate injection, the most common problem using a cisternal site for injection is that the contrast column does not flow caudally permitting full visualization of the lesion. This can be partially controlled by positioning the patient with the head up either during injection or following removal of the spinal needle. The problem is exacerbated by your inability to avoid the flow of contrast agent into the head. This results in an insufficient volume of contrast agent in the subarachnoid space around the spinal cord. If positioning the patient does not correct this problem, a lumbar injection may be necessary. Unfortunately, the spinal needle must be withdrawn prior to radiography. This means that it is impossible to inject additional contrast agent as determined radiographically without placement of another spinal needle.

In the event of post-myelographic convulsions, intravenous diazepam (Valium, Roche) is recommended in therapeutic doses, with intravenous barbiturates recommended if the diazepam is not effective.

MYELOGRAPHY BY INJECTION IN THE LUMBAR REGION IN THE DOG

Placement of the needle for injection in the lumbar region requires more skill than placement in the cervical region, but is much safer than a cisternal injection (Fig. 4-2). If the injection is accurate, you have a better chance for evaluation of the entire spinal cord. A minor difficulty with the examination performed in this manner is that the anatomical sites used to assist in the positioning of the needle may be more sometimes difficult to locate especially if the dog has congenital lumbosacral vertebral segments. Examination of the non-contrast lateral radiograph of the spine assist in solving this problem.

Equipment
1. 20 or 22 ga spinal needle with a flat bevel usually 2" to 4" in length
2. 10 cc syringe (2)
3. sponges or sandbags to assist in positioning the patient
4. contrast agent using a dosage of 0.3 cc/kgbw to study the thoracolumbar region and a dosage of 0.45 cc/kgbw to study the entire spinal cord
5. glass collection tube for CSF

Technique
1. the patient needs to be under general anesthesia to avoid injury to the spinal cord by movement of the needle tip during body movement
2. obtain a series of lateral and ventrodorsal non-contrast radiographs of the entire spine
3. aseptically prepare the region over the lumbar region centered on L5-6 level (approximately 4" square—10 cm square)
4. position the patient in lateral recumbency using sandbags or sponges to insure a perfect lateral position
5. it may be helpful to flex the pelvic limbs so the feet are along the dog's abdomen and hold them in position with sandbags
6. palpate the tips of the spinous processes locating the L5-6 interspace (evaluate the non-contrast radiographs to ensure there are no congenital anomalies to interfere with the needle location)
7. determine the location of the needle site just caudal and lateral to the cranial edge of the spinous process of L6
8. advance the tip of the needle at a slight cranial angle and angled toward the midline so that the tip of the needle falls into the interarcuate space between L5-6
9. the needle is almost parallel to the table but slightly angled toward the midline
10. during needle placement repeatedly insure that the patient is positioned perfectly lateral
11. continue to advance the needle tip waiting for the "pop" that you experience as the needle tip passes through the dura
12. a muscle twitch, leg extension, or movement of the tail is often noted as the needle tip passes through the meninges and cord
13. it is difficult to position the tip of the needle in the dorsal subarachnoid space and usually the tip passes through the cord into the ventral subarachnoid space
14. make a lateral radiograph at any time during placement of the needle to more accurately locate the needle tip
15. on removing the stylet, CSF may flow from the needle hub and can be collected for examination
16. permit a volume of CSF to flow at least equal to the volume of contrast agent you intend to inject
17. attach the syringe to the hub of the spinal needle and inject the total volume over a 5 minute period
18. replace the stylet
19. make a lateral radiograph of the lumbar spine to confirm the location of the contrast columns and determine the cranial extent of the flow
20. it may be necessary to inject additional contrast agent or lower the patients head to assist in the flow of the contrast pool cranially
21. when the radiographs show adequate filling of the subarachnoid space remove the needle
22. rotate the patient to insure equal mixing of the contrast agent with the CSF
23. complete the series of lateral and ventrodorsal radiographs
24. keep the patient under general anesthesia for an hour after the study to lessen the frequency of post-myelographic convulsions

Comments

Some prefer to have the patient positioned in sternal recumbency because they have a better feeling during needle placement. The disadvantage is that the patient cannot safely be moved to lateral recumbency for radiography to determine needle tip location. The radiographs made in sternal recumbency can only determine placement of the needle tip relative to the midline and not the depth of the needle tip. Dorsoventral radiographs made following injection are more difficult to evaluate to determine the level and extent of subarachnoid filling.

The volume of contrast agent should be based on the volume of CSF, however, it is based on body weight which may not be accurate. Therefore, note the nature of the patient in an effort to adjust the volume lower in an obese patient or higher in a very thin patient.

The placement of a needle tip into the lumbar spine usually can be performed safely. Malpositioning of the tip laterally results in puncture of the venous sinuses and creation of a bloody tap that compromised interpretation of the CSF.

Do not inject contrast agent in the presence of a bloody tap since the mixture of blood and contrast agent within the subarachnoid space is highly irritative.

Frequently there is no reverse flow of CSF through the needle following a lumbar tap even though the bevel is in the correct position. This may be due to the meninges forming a flap that covers the bevel preventing back-flow of CSF. In this situation, make a trial injection of <0.5 cc of contrast agent and make a radiograph. Adjust the needle tip as needed before proceeding with the rest of the injection.

The most common problem in lumbar myelography results in the injection of contrast agent into the epidural space and/or into the venous sinuses. This is usually due to the large size of the needle bevel and the small size of the subarachnoid space with the length of the bevel extending beyond the subarachnoid space. The contrast agent flows freely into the epidural space if several attempts have been made at needle placement leaving multiple holes within the meninges.

Filling of the venous sinuses usually does not extend cranial to the thoracolumbar junction, however, the filling in the lumbar area compromises your ability to study the subarachnoid spaces in that location.

Extradural contrast media severely compromises your diagnostic ability and usually produces a non-diagnostic myelogram. With loss of the contrast media into the epidural space, the most common problem is that the remaining contrast medium that forms the subarachnoid columns is not of sufficient quantity to flow cranially permitting full visualization of the cord. This problem can be partially alleviated by positioning the patient with head down and by injecting additional contrast agent. In the event that complete subarachnoid filling cannot be achieved or interpretation is compromised by epidural contrast agent, it may be necessary to consider a cisternal injection.

In the event of post-myelographic convulsions, intravenous diazepam (Valium, Roche) is recommended in therapeutic doses, with intravenous barbiturates recommended if the diazepam is not effective.

The person wanting to place the needle with their left hand would reverse the positioning described above.

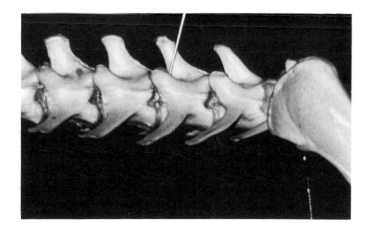 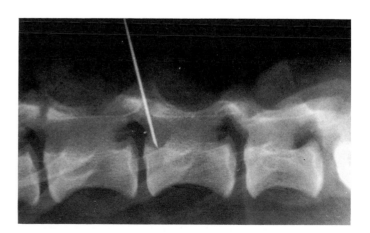

Fig. 4-2
NEEDLE PLACEMENT FOR MYELOGRAPHY
A photograph of the lateral aspect of the lumbar vertebrae shows the needle correctly positioned for lumbar myelography. The radiograph shows successful placement of the needle, but using a slightly different angle.

MYELOGRAPHY BY INJECTION AT THE CISTERNA MAGNA IN THE CAT

Injection at the cisterna magna is easier for many than lumbar injection especially in the smaller sized cat. The difficulty with the examination performed in this manner is that there is no method of insuring that the contrast column will flow caudally into the lumbar area. Thus, a thoracolumbar lesion may not be identified or at best, only the cranial aspect of the lesion.

Equipment

1. 22 ga spinal needle with a flat bevel—1 1/2" length
2. 5 cc syringe (2)
3. sponges or sandbags to assist in positioning the head
4. contrast agent using a dosage of 0.3 cc/kgbw for cervical study, 0.45 cc/kgbw for cervicothoracic study, and 0.5 cc/kgbw for complete spinal study
5. a cassette tunnel or tabletop that angles
6. glass collection tubes for CSF

Technique

1. the patient needs to be under general anesthesia
2. obtain a series of non-contrast radiographs of the entire spine
3. aseptically prepare the region just caudal to the external occipital protuberance (approximately 2" square—5 cm square)
4. position the patient in lateral recumbency with the head elevated 10° using sponges to insure a perfect lateral position
5. position the head using sandbags or sponges
6. position an assistant in a comfortable manner in front of the cat holding the head in a flexed position using both hands
7. the individual who places the needle controls the position of the head
8. determine the location of the needle site in the center of a triangle created by placing the thumb and second fingertip of the right hand on the lateral processes of C1 and the tip of the first finger on the external occipital protuberance
9. insure that the needle site in on the midline
10. check to insure that the patient is perfectly lateral and maintain the needle in a horizontal plane as it is advanced
11. rest your left hand on the patients head with the thumb and first finger holding the shaft of the needle (never move this hand during the procedure and never release your hold on the needle)
12. with the right hand start to advance the needle removing the stylet to monitor position of the needle tip
13. as the needle passes through the dura you experience a subtle "pop"
14. on removing the stylet, CSF flows from the needle hub and can be collected for examination
15. permit a volume of CSF to flow at least equal to the volume of contrast agent you intend to inject
16. attach the syringe to the hub of the spinal needle and inject the total volume over a 3 minute period
17. replace the stylet and remove the needle (this releases your assistant from holding the head)
18. make a lateral radiograph of the cervical spine to confirm the location of the contrast pool and determine the level of flow
19. to assist in the flow of the contrast pool caudally, it may be necessary to raise the patients head by tilting the table between 30° and 45° from horizontal
20. rotate the patient to insure mixing of the contrast agent and the CSF
21. complete the series of lateral and ventrodorsal radiographs
22. keep the patient under general anesthesia for an hour after the study to lessen the frequency of post-myelographic convulsions

Comments

Some prefer to position the patient in sternal recumbency with the head flexed while performing the cisternal puncture. This still requires that an assistant carefully position the head during needle placement, but has the advantage of more clearly defining the midline.

Obviously, the placement of a needle tip into the cisterna magna is with some risk since malpositioning laterally results in puncture of the vertebral sinuses and the resulting bleeding. Malpositioning the needle cranially can result in placement of the tip into the hind brain causing respiratory collapse and death.

With correct positioning of the needle and accurate injection, the most common problem using a cisternal site for injection is that the contrast column does not flow caudally permitting full visualization of the lesion as seen radiographically. The problem is exacerbated by your inability to avoid the flow of contrast agent into the head, resulting is an insufficient volume of contrast agent in the subarachnoid space around the spinal cord. This leads to the assumption that stoppage of the contrast column within the spinal canal indicates a space occupying lesion. This possible error can be controlled by positioning the patient with head up. If positioning the patient does not correct this problem, a lumbar injection may be necessary.

For the person wishing to make the needle placement with their left hand, the directions given above should be reversed.

In the event of post-myelographic convulsions intravenous diazepam (Valium, Roche) is recommended in therapeutic doses, with intravenous barbiturates recommended if the diazepam is not effective.

MYELOGRAPHY BY INJECTION IN THE LUMBAR REGION IN THE CAT

Placement of the needle for injection in the lumbar region of the cat is easier than in the dog and much safer than a cisternal injection. The anatomical site is much easier to palpate than in the dog. If the injection is accurate, you have a good chance of evaluation of the entire spinal cord.

Equipment

1. 22 ga spinal needle with a flat bevel usually 1 1/2" in length
2. 5 cc syringe (2)
3. sponges or sandbags to assist in positioning the patient
4. contrast agent using a dosage of 0.3 cc/kgbw to study the lumbar spine, 0.45 cc/kgbw to study the thoracolumbar spine and 0.6 cc/kgbw to study the entire spinal cord
5. cassette tunnel or tabletop that can be angled
6. glass collection tubes for CSF

Technique

1. the patient needs to be under general anesthesia
2. obtain a series of lateral and ventrodorsal non-contrast radiographs of the entire spine
3. aseptically prepare the lumbar region centered on L5-6 (approximately 2" square—5 cm square)
4. position the patient in lateral recumbency using sponges to insure a perfect lateral position noting whether you are right or left handed
5. it may be helpful to flex the pelvic limbs and hold them in position with sandbags
6. palpate the tips of the spinous processes locating the L5-6 interspace (evaluate the non-contrast radiographs to ensure there are no congenital anomalies to confuse the needle location)
7. determine the location of the needle site just caudal and lateral to the cranial edge of the spinous process of L6
8. advance the tip of the needle so that the needle is at a slight cranial angle and angled toward the midline so that the tip of the needle falls into the interarcuate space between L5-6
9. the needle is almost parallel to the table but slightly angled toward the midline
10. during needle placement repeatedly insure that the patient is positioned perfectly lateral
11. continue to advance the needle tip waiting for the "pop" that you experience as the needle tip passes through the dura
12. a twitch, leg extension, or movement of the tail may be noted as the needle tip passes through the meninges or cord
13. it is difficult to position the tip of the needle in the dorsal subarachnoid space and usually the tip is passed through the cord into the ventral subarachnoid space

14. make a lateral radiograph at any time during placement of the needle to more accurately locate the needle tip
15. on removing the stylet, CSF may flow from the needle hub and can be collected for examination
16. permit a volume of CSF to flow at least equal to the volume of contrast agent you intend to inject
17. attach the syringe to the hub of the spinal needle and inject 0.5 cc of contrast agent
18. replace the stylet
19. make a lateral radiograph of the lumbar spine to confirm the location of the columns of contrast media
20. attach the syringe to the hub of the spinal needle and inject the total volume over a 3 minute period
21. replace the stylet
22. make a lateral radiograph of the lumbar spine to reconfirm the location of the contrast columns and determine the cranial extent of the flow
23. it may be necessary to inject additional contrast agent or lower the patients head to assist in the flow of the contrast pool cranially
24. when the radiographs show adequate filling of the subarachnoid space remove the needle,
25. rotate the patient to insure equal mixing of the contrast columns
26. complete the series of lateral radiographs
27. make the ventrodorsal radiographs
28. keep the patient under general anesthesia for an hour after the study to lessen the frequency of post-myelographic convulsions

Comments

Some prefer to have the patient positioned in sternal recumbency because they have a better feeling during needle placement. The disadvantage is that any radiographs made during needle placement cannot indicate the level of the needle tip and the radiographs made following injection prior to the removal of the needle are more difficult to evaluate to determine the level of subarachnoid filling. It is not safe to move the patient with the needle in position.

The volume of contrast agent should be based on the volume of CSF, however, it is based on body weight which may not be accurate. Therefore, note the nature of the patient in an effort to adjust the volume lower in an obese patient or higher in a very thin patient.

The placement of a needle tip into the lumbar spine usually can be performed safely. Malpositioning of the tip laterally results in puncture of the venous sinuses and creation of a bloody tap that compromises interpretation of the CSF. Epidural leakage of contrast agent is common in lumbar injections, probably because of the small size of the subarachnoid space and the large size of the needle bevel or because of multiple attempts at needle placement resulting in leakage through the holes within the meninges.

Frequently there is no reverse flow of CSF through the needle even though the bevel is in the correct position. This may be due to the meninges forming a flap that covers the bevel preventing back-flow of CSF. In this situation, make a trial injection of < 0.5 cc of contrast agent and make a radiograph. Adjust the needle tip as needed before proceeding with the rest of the injection.

The most common problem results in the injection of contrast agent into the epidural space and/or into the venous sinuses. This is usually due to the large size of the needle bevel and the small size of the subarachnoid space.

With loss of the contrast media into the epidural space, the remaining subarachnoid contrast column is not large enough to permitting full visualization of the cord. This can be partially controlled by positioning the patient with head down or by injecting additional contrast agent. In the event that subarachnoid filling cannot be achieved or interpretation is compromised by epidural contrast agent, it may be necessary to consider a cisternal injection.

If the person wishes to make the needle placement with their left hand, the description above should be reversed.

In the event of post-myelographic convulsions, intravenous diazepam (Valium, Roche) is recommended in therapeutic doses, with intravenous barbiturates recommended if the diazepam is not effective.

REFERENCES

TECHNIQUE AND MEDIA

Adams WM and Stowater JL. Complications of metrizamide myelography in the dog; a summary of 107 clinical case histories. Vet Radiol 22:27-34, 1981.

Allan GS and Wood AKA. Iohexol for contrast radiology of the vertebral canal in dogs and cats. IVRA meeting Sydney 1988.

Allan GS and Wood AKA. Iohexol myelography in the dog. Vet Radiol 29:78-82, 1988.

Bartels JE and Braund KG. Experimental arachnoid fibrosis produced by metrizamide in the dog. Vet Radiol 21:78-81, 1980.

Bartels JE Braund KG and Redding RW. An experimental evaluation of a non-ionic agent amipaque (Metrizamide) as a neuroradiologic medium in the dog. J Amer Vet Rad Soc 18:117-23, 1977.

Boring G. Transmedullary myelography. J Am Vet Radiol Soc. 18:3, 1977.

Carakostas MC Gossett KA Watters JW and MacWilliams PS. Effects of metrizamide myelography on cerebro-spinal fluid analysis in the dog. Vet Radiol 24:267-70, 1983.

Cox FH and Jakovljevic S. The use of iopamidol for myelography in dogs: a study of twenty-seven cases. J small Anim Pract 27:159-65, 1986.

Davis EM Glickman LT Rendano VT and Short CE. Seizures in dogs following metrizamide myelography. J Am Anim Hosp Assoc 17:642-8, 1981.

Dennis R and Herrtage ME. Low osmolar contrast media. Vet Radiol 30:2-12, 1989.

Funquist B. Thoraco-lumbar myelography with water-soluble contrast medium in dogs I. Technique of myelography; side effects and complications. J small Anim Pract 3:53-66, 1962.

Gray PR Indriere RJ and Lowrie CT. Use of pentobarbital sodium to reduce seizures in dogs after cervical myelography with metrizamide. J Am Vet Med Assoc 190:1422-4, 1987.

Gray PR Indriere RJ Lipert AC et al. The influence of anesthetic regimen on the frequency of seizures after cervical myelography in the dog. J Am Vet Med Assoc 190:527-30, 1987.

Gray PR Lowrie CT and Wetmore LA. Effect of intravenous administration of dextrose or lactated Ringer's solution on seizure development in dogs after cervical myelography with metrizamide. Am J Vet Res 48:1600-2, 1987.

Haughton VM and Ho KC. Arachnoid response to contrast media: a comparison of iophendylate and metrizamide in experimental animals. Radiology 143:699-702, 1982.

Haughton VM Ho KC and Lipman BT. Experimental study of arachnoiditis from iohexol, an investigational nonionic aqueous contrast medium. AJR 3:375-7, 1982.

Johnson GC Fuciu DM Fenner WR and Krakowka L. Transient leakage across the blood-cerebrospinal fluid barrier after intrathecal metrizamide administration to dogs. Am J Vet Res 46:1303-8, 1985.

Lang J. Flexion-extension myelography of the canine cauda equina. Vet Radiol 29:242, 1988.

Lord PF and Olsson S-E. Myelography with metrizamide in the dog. J Am Vet Rad Soc 17:42-49, 1976.

Pasaoglu A Gok A and Patrioglu TE. An experimental evaluation of response to contrast media pantopaque, iopamidol and iohexol in the subarachnoid space. Invest Radiol 23:762-6, 1988.

Puglisi TA Green RW Hall CL Read WK Green RA Tangner CH Mann FA and Robson HP. Comparison of metrizamide and iohexol for cisternal myelographic examination of dogs. Am J Vet Res 47:1863-9, 1986.

Reidesel DH. The relationship between premedication and postmyelographic seizure activity. Cal Vet 8:23-4, 1980.

Sovak M Ranganathan R and Hammer B. Early experience with iotrol, a nonionic dimer for intrathecal use. Invest Radiol 19:139, 1984.

Spencer CP Chrisman CL Mayhew IG and Kaude JV. Neurotoxicologic effects of the nonionic contrast agent iopamidol on the leptomeninges of the dog. Am J Vet Res 43:1958-62, 1982.

Stowater JL and Kneller SK. Clinical evaluation of metrizamide as a myelographic agent in the dog. J Am Vet Med Assoc 175: 191-5, 1979.

Stowater JL Menhusen MJ and Gendreau CL. Canine myelography with skiodan. VMSAC 1207-1214, September 1976.

Tamas PM Walker MA Paddleford RR et al. Prevention of postmetrizamide myelographic seizures in dogs, using 5% dextrose solution. J Am Vet Med Assoc 188:710-2,1986.

Thrall DW Lewis RE Walker MA Kneller SK and Losondky JM. The basis for dosing water soluble myelographic medium for lumbar administration: Body weight or crown rump length. J Am Vet Radiol Soc 16:130-2, 1975.

Tilmant L Ackerman N and Spencer CP. Mechanical aspects of subarachnoid space puncture in the dog. Vet Radiol 25:227-32, 1984.

van Bree H van Rijssen B and van Ham L. Comparison of nonionic contrast agents iohexol and iotrolan for cisternal myelography in dogs. Am J Vet Res 52:926-33, 1991.

Wheeler SJ and Davies JV. Iohexol myelography in the dog and cat: A series of one hundred cases, and a comparison with metrizamide and iopamidol. J small Anim Pract 26:247-56, 1985.

Widmer WR and Blevins WE. Veterinary Myelography: A review of contrast media, adverse effects, and technique. J Am Anim Hosp Assoc 27:163-77, 1991.

Widmer WR Blevins WE Cantwell HD Cook JR and DeNicola DB. A comparison of iopamidol and metrizamide for cervical myelography in dogs. Vet Radiol 29:108-15, 1988.

Widmer WR Blevins WE Cantwell HD Cook JR and DeNicola DB. Effects of postmyelographic removal of metrizamide in dogs. Vet Radiol 31:2-10, 1990.

Widmer WR Blevins WE Jakovljevic S Teclaw RF Han CM and Hurd CD. Iohexol and iopamidol myelography in the dog: A clinical trial comparing adverse effects and myelographic quality. Vet Rad & Ultrasound 33:327-33, 1992.

Widner WR Blevins Cantwell HD et al. Effects of postmyelographic removal of metrizamide in dogs. Vet Radiol 31:2-10,1990.

Widner WR. Iohexol and iopamidol: New contrast media for veterinary myelography. J Am Vet Med Assoc 194:1714-16, 1989.

Wilcox J Evill CA and Sage MR. Rate of clearance of intrathecal iopamidol in the dog. Neuroradiology 28:359-61, 1986.

Wood AKW. Iohexol and iopamidol: new nonionic contrast media for myelography in dogs. Comp Cont Ed Pract Vet 10:32-6, 1988.

CAT

Hilal SK Dauth GW Burger LC and Gilman S. Effect of isotonic contrast agents on spinal reflexes in the cat. Radiology 122:149-55, 1977.

Luttgen J Braund WR Brawner WR and Vandevelde M. A retrospective study of twenty nine spinal cord tumors in the dog and cat. J small Anim Pract, 21:213-26, 1980.

Murphie A Prescott R and Eubank K. Myelography in the cat. Mod Vet Pract 63:893-5, 1982.

Northington JW. Metrizamide myelography in five dogs and two cats with spinal cord neoplasia. Vet Radiol 21: 149-53, 1980.

Pardo AD and Morgan JP. Myelography in the cat. A comparison of cisternal versus lumbar puncture, Using metrizamide. Vet Radiol 29:89-95, 1988.

Skalpe IO. Myelography with metrizamide, meglumine iothalamate and meglumine iocarmate: an experimental investigation in cats. Acta Radiol (Suppl) 1973:35-57, 1973.

Wheeler SJ and Davies JV. Iohexol myelography in the dog and cat: A series of one hundred cases, and a comparison with metrizamide and iopamidol. J small Anim Pract 26:247-56, 1985.

Wheeler SJ Clayton Jones DG and Wright JA. Myelography in the cat. J small Anim Pract 26:143-52, 1985.

DOG

Adams WM. Myelography. Vet Clin North Am 12:295-311, 1982.

Lewis DD and Hosgood G. Complications associated with the use of iohexol for myelography of the cervical vertebral column in dogs: 66 cases (1988-1990). J Am Vet Med Assoc 200:1381-84, 1992.

Luttgen J Braund WR Brawner WR and Vandevelde M. A retrospective study of twenty nine spinal cord tumors in the dog and cat. J Small Anim Pract, 21:213-26, 1980.

Morgan JP Suter PF and Holliday TA: Myelography in the dog: with water soluble contrast medium. Acta Radiol Suppl. 319: 217-30, 1972.

Northington JW Biery DN and Glickman LT: Intrathecal dextrose to prevent seizures after metrizamide myelography in dogs. Invest Radiol 17:282-3, 1982.

Northington JW. Metrizamide myelography in five dogs and two cats with spinal cord neoplasia. Vet Radiol 21: 149-53, 1980.

Suter PF Morgan JP Holliday TA and O'Brien TR: Myelography in the dog: diagnosis of tumors of the spinal cord and vertebrae. Vet Radiol 12:29-44, 1971.

Ticer JW and Brown SG. Water-soluble myelography in canine intervertebral disk protrusion. J Am Vet Radiol Soc 15:3-9, 1974.

Webbon PM and Woolley GE. Contrast radiography of the spine of the dog. 21:247-.

Wood ADW Farrow BRH and Fairburn AJ. Cervical myelography in dogs using iohexol. Acta Radiol (Diag) 26:767-70, 1988.

Wright JA and Clayton Jones DG. Metrizamide myelography in sixty-eight dogs. J small Anim Pract 22:415-35, 1981.

Wright JA. Metrizamide myelography in 68 dogs. J small Anim Pract 22:415-36, 1981.

B. DISCOGRAPHY IN THE DOG

Definition

Discography is the outlining of the central portion of the intervertebral disc by injecting radiopaque contrast media into the disc permitting evaluation of the size and shape of the central cavity within the disc and the determination of the amount of and direction of nuclear herniation or annular rupture (Fig. 4-3). It is the only method other than MRI available for demonstrating degenerative change in a disc which has not protruded nuclear material. Discography is usually performed in a disc with an intact annulus fibrosus and thus the contrast pool is retained within the disc. However, discography can be performed on a disc in which the annulus fibrosus is ruptured with the contrast medium seen to leak outside of the disc. Discography is most commonly performed to evaluate the lumbosacral disc in patients with signs of cauda equina syndrome because the needle can be placed with accuracy because of the available anatomic landmarks. Discography can be performed within the cervical or lumbar region but the location of the needle tip needs to be controlled by making repeated radiographs, unless fluoroscopy is available.

Because of the proximity of the subarachnoid space, the contrast agent used must be safe for myelography were it to be accidentally injected into the subarachnoid space.

Indications

Discography permits evaluation of the extent of discal degeneration and resulting disc protrusions. The technique could be used to evaluate discal tears although the lesions associated with that type of disc disease are more accurately evaluated with subarachnoid myelography. Discography is performed after the neurologic and non-contrast radiographic studies have confirmed that there is a suspect spinal lesion that can be further studied by knowing the degree of discal protrusion that cannot be evaluated as easily by subarachnoid myelography. It is for this reason that the lumbosacral disc is so often selected for study by discography.

Discography has the definite limitation in not being able to show the intradural structures or the configuration of the bony canal, and therefore should be combined with either epidurography or subarachnoid myelography.

Contrast Agent

Newer contrast agents are available that are water-soluble, contain additional iodine atoms to improve the density of the fluid, are nonionic, have improved osmolality, and have varying viscosity. Agents that can be used include: (1) iopamidol (Isovue, Squibb) available as Isovue-M 200 with 200 mg organically bound iodine per mL or Isovue-M 300 with 300 mg organically bound iodine per mL, (2) metrizamide (Amipaque, Winthrop-Breon, Nyegaard, Oslo) available with 170 mg organically bound iodine per mL or 300 mg organically bound iodine per mL, (3) iohexol (Omnipaque, Winthrop-Breon, Nyegaard,Oslo) available with 180 mg organically bound iodine per mL , and (4) ioxaglate sodium-meglumine (Hexabrix, Mallinckrodt) available with 320 mg organically bound iodine per mL.

Contraindications

1. any condition that would prevent use of general anesthesia
2. discospondylitis at the site to be injected
3. presence of sepsis of the overlying skin, subcutis, and muscle that would make placement of a needle into the spinal canal inappropriate
4. use of phenothiazine derivatives in the anesthetic regimen

Equipment

1. positive-contrast agent—any of the newer low osmolality contrast agents such as Ioxaglate sodium-meglumine (hexabrix), Isovue (iopamidol), Omnipaque (iohexol), or Amipaque (metrizamide)
2. short bevel spinal needle, 18, 20, or 22 ga with a length required to reach the lumbosacral disc
3. 10 cc syringe

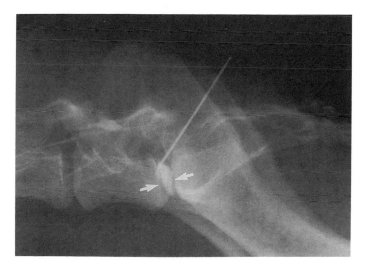

Fig. 4-3
DISCOGRAM
A lateral radiograph of the lumbosacral region in a dog showing a needle tip placed within the nuclear portion of the lumbosacral disc. Positive-contrast agent has been injected filling the degenerative cavity within the disc (arrows).

Technique for lumbosacral discography

1. make a survey radiographic study of the lumbosacral region and study the anatomy noting especially congenital anomalies or degenerative changes that would affect placement of the needle
2. place the anesthetized patient in lateral recumbency and aseptically prepare the lumbosacral region
3. with the patient's head to your left, palpate the lumbosacral region by placing the tips of the thumb and second finger of the left hand on the ilial wings and the tip of the first finger falls into the lumbosacral depression—another method of location the lumbosacral depression is to palpate the tips of the spinous processes recognizing that the process of L7 is much shorter than L6
4. place the tip of the needle on the midline over the lumbosacral space and pass the needle horizontally—there is a "pop" as the needle tip passes through the interarcuate ligament into the spinal canal and passage of the needle into the disc is signaled by a feeling of increased resistance to needle advancement
5. make a lateral radiograph to confirm the location of the needle tip
6. remove the stylet from the needle and attach the syringe
7. begin the injection expecting resistance because of the location of the needle tip within the disc—move the needle ventrally and then dorsally "looking" for the cavity within the diseased disc that permits the injection to be made without any resistance
8. inject 1cc of contrast agent, remove the syringe, replace the stylet and make a lateral radiograph
9. evaluate the radiograph for the location of the contrast agent
10. if the test radiograph shows satisfactory discal filling, complete the injection until no more contrast agent can be injected (up to 5cc in a severely degenerated disc in a large patient)
11. remove the needle
12. make the following radiographs (**minimum)
    a. lateral—neutral position**
    b. lateral—hyperflexion of the pelvic limbs
    c. lateral—hyperextension of the pelvic limbs
13. position the patient in sternal recumbency
14. make a dorsoventral radiograph
15. the contrast pool remains within the disc without absorption for over 30 minutes providing ample time for repeated radiographic studies

Problems

1. if difficulty is experienced in placement of the needle—examine the survey radiography to determine if a congenital lesion or degenerative changes influences placement of the needle
2. if injection of the contrast agent is not possible—re-examine the needle placement noting if the needle tip is against the caudal end plate of L7 vertebral body and therefore cannot be placed within the nuclear portion of the disc—further advancement of the needle cannot be made in this position—a new needle direction may be necessary striving for a more vertical placement—also examine the dorsoventral or ventrodorsal radiograph to determine needle position is on the midline
3. if injection of the contrast agent is difficult—slightly shift the needle tip ventrally or dorsally since it may be within the cranial or ventral portion of the annulus fibrosus of the lumbosacral disc—this change in needle tip position can be made with the syringe in position and pressure placed on the plunger as you "search" for the cavity—injection becomes very easy when the tip moves into the discal cavity—unfortunately injection also becomes very easy with the tip moves into the spinal canal as well
4. flow of CFS when stylet is first removed from the needle—reposition tip further ventrally so that it is not within the subarachnoid space
5. radiograph shows contrast in the epidural space, subarachnoid space, or within vertebral sinuses—this may occur following injection with the needle tip in the spinal canal but usually doesn't affect a subsequently performed discogram—reposition the needle tip into the disc
6. contrast agent injected into the muscle dorsal to the spinal canal—wait 30 minutes for absorption of the contrast agent and reposition the needle tip for a second attempt at a discogram

Comments

The patient can be positioned in sternal recumbency for placement of the needle. The patient then needs to be placed into lateral recumbency following placement of the needle to make a lateral radiograph since the dorsoventral radiograph does not permit determination of the location of the needle tip as does the lateral radiograph.

The needle tip can be correctly place within the center of a healthy disc and not be able to make an injection of contrast medium because of the absence of a cavity that is secondary to disc degeneration.

Lumbosacral epidurography can follow discography by simply retracting the needle tip into the epidural space and making another injection of contrast agent.

Discograms can be made of discs other than at the lumbosacral junction but this requires entrance of the needle laterally. The presence of prominent anatomic landmarks assists in needle positioning. However, the location of the needle tip can only controlled by multiple radiographs or by fluoroscopy which is time consuming and a technique not recommended.

Discography is often performed prior to chemonucleolysis.

REFERENCES

Garrick JG and Sullivan CR: Long-term effects of diskography in dogs. Minn. Med. 53:849, 1970.

Garrick JG and Sullivan CR: A technique of performing diskography in dogs. Mayo Clin Proceed 39:270, 1964.

Morgan JP and Bailey CS. Cauda equina syndrome in the dog: radiographic evaluation. J small Anim Pract 31:69, 1990.

Sisson AF LeCouteur RA Ingram JT Park RD and Child G. Diagnosis of cauda equina abnormalities by using electromyography, discography, and epidurography in dogs. J Vet Int Med 6:253, 1992.

Hathcock JT Pechman RD Dillon AR Knecht CD and Braund KG. Comparison of three radiographic contrast procedures in the evaluation of the canine lumbosacral spinal canal. Vet Radiol 29:4, 1988.

C. LUMBOSACRAL EPIDUROGRAPHY IN THE DOG

Definition

Positive contrast agent may be injected into the spinal canal in an extradural location so that it surrounds the spinal cord and meninges and may outline an extradural mass or show a constricting lesion (Fig. 4-4). It is also possible to identify the spinal nerves within the spinal canal. It is particularly of value within the lumbosacral region to demonstrate dorsal disc protrusion. This area is difficult to study with subarachnoid myelography because of the tapering of the caudal arachnoid sac and the elevation of the contrast columns. In some dogs, the subarachnoid columns terminate cranial to the lumbosacral junction.

Epidurography has its greatest limitation because of the fact that the epidural space is not clearly defined and the contrast agent can freely drain out of the intervertebral foramina and therefore prevent complete filling of the epidural space. Because of the proximity of the subarachnoid space, the contrast agent used must be safe for myelography were it to accidentally injected into the subarachnoid space.

Indications

A suspect spinal lesion that requires further localization and definition that is located by neurologic examination or non-contrast radiographs to be within the lumbosacral region and therefore cannot be clearly evaluated by subarachnoid myelography.

Contraindications

1. anything that prevents performing general anesthesia
2. presence of sepsis of the overlying skin, subcutis, and muscle that would make placement of a needle into the spinal canal inappropriate
3. use of phenothiazine derivatives in the anesthetic regimen

Contrast Agent

Newer contrast agents are available that are water-soluble, contain additional iodine atoms to improve the density of the fluid, are nonionic, have improved osmolality, and have varying viscosity. Agents that can be used include: (1) iopamidol (Isovue, Squibb) available as Isovue-M 200 with 200 mg organically bound iodine per mL or Isovue-M 300 with 300 mg organically bound iodine per mL, (2) metrizamide (Amipaque, Winthrop-Breon, Nyegaard, Oslo) available with 170 mg organically bound iodine per mL or with 300 mg organically bound iodine per mL, (3) iohexol (Omnipaque, Winthrop-Breon, Nyegaard, Oslo) available with 180 mg organically bound iodine per mL, and (4) ioxaglate sodium-meglumine (Hexabrix, Mallinckrodt) available as 320 mg organically bound iodine per mL.

Equipment

1. positive-contrast agent—any of the newer low osmolality contrast agents such as Ioxaglate sodium-meglumine (hexabrix), Isovue (iopamidol), Omnipaque (iohexol), or Amipaque (metrizamide)
2. short bevel spinal needle, 18, 20, or 22 ga with a length required to reach the spinal canal
3. 10 cc syringe

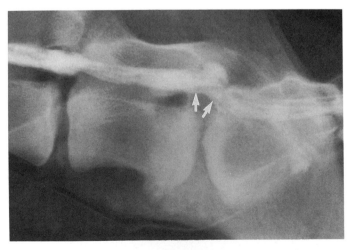

Fig. 4-4
EPIDUROGRAM
A lateral radiograph of the lumbosacral region in a dog showing the positive-contrast agent within the epidural space. Notice how the flow is displaced dorsally (arrows) at the site of the lumbosacral disc indicating dorsal herniation of that disc.

Technique

1. make a survey radiographic study of the lumbosacral region and study the anatomy noting especially any congenital anomalies that would affect placement of the needle
2. place the anesthetized patient in sternal recumbency and surgically prepare the lumbosacral region
3. with the patient's head to your left, palpate the lumbosacral region by placing the tips of the thumb and second finger of the left hand on the ilial wings and the tip of the first finger falls into the lumbosacral depression—another method of location the lumbosacral depression is to palpate the tips of the spinous processes recognizing that the process of L7 is much shorter than L6
4. place the tip of the needle on the midline over the lumbosacral space and pass the needle vertically into the spinal canal
5. remove the stylet from the needle and attach the syringe
6. begin the injection noting any resistance to injection since injection within the spinal canal should be without any resistance
7. inject 2cc of contrast agent, remove the syringe, replace the stylet and make a dorsoventral radiograph
8. evaluate the radiograph for the distribution of the contrast agent
9. if the test radiograph shows satisfactory epidural filling, complete the injection making a determination of the quantity needed by evaluation of the radiograph
10. remove the needle
11. make a dorsoventral radiograph
12. position the patient in lateral recumbency
13. make the following radiography (*minimum)
    a. lateral—neutral position*
    b. lateral—hyperflexion of the pelvic limbs
    c. lateral—hyperextension of the pelvic limbs

Problems

1. determination of the volume of contrast agent to inject is difficult since the epidural space is not well defined—the contrast agent drains dependently and also flows cranially or caudally—therefore, the dosage needed to outline a lesion varies with the patient and the lessions to be studied
2. difficulty in placement of the needle—examine the survey radiography to determine if a congenital lesion or degenerative changes prevents the placement of the needle—re-examine the proposed needle placement
3. difficult to inject—slightly retract needle tip since it may be within the dorsal annulus of the lumbosacral disc
4. flow of CFS when stylet is first removed from the needle—reposition tip so that it is not within the subarachnoid space
5. radiograph shows contrast in the epidural space, subarachnoid space, or within vertebral sinuses—this may occur and the contrast will clear from the subarachnoid space and vertebral sinuses within 15 minutes
6. contrast agent does not pool in the region of interest—elevate or depress patients body to encourage flow of the contrast pool in the direction desired
7. contrast agent injected into a degenerated lumbosacral disc—the injection may have been easy if the disc is severely degenerated—this does not compromise the epidurogram—withdraw the tip of the needle and make the injection in the epidural space
8. contrast agent is injected into the muscle dorsal to the spinal canal even though there was some resistance to the injection—wait 30 minutes for absorption of the contrast agent and reposition the needle for a second epidurogram

Comments

Placement of 20 or 22 gauge spinal needle 3.8cm (1.5 inch) can be made through the interarcuate ligament at the sacrococcygeal junction or between the first and fifth coccygeal vertebrae with resulting flow of the contrast pool cranial to the level of the lumbosacral junction. The flow of contrast agent is difficult to control.

Epidurography can also be performed with the patient in lateral recumbency although the contrast agent tends to flow dependently out of the LS intervertebral foramen.

Epidurography is often preformed following discography using the same needle and only repositioning the tip dorsally.

It is possible to perform lumbosacral epidurography by placement of a small catheter through a spinal needle with the tip placed into the spinal canal between the first caudal segments. This technique permits adjusting the catheter tip and controlling the placement of the contrast medium. The problem is the additional time and skill required for placement of the needle and catheter.

REFERENCES

Bromage PR Bramwell RSB Catachlove RFH Belanger G and Pearce CGA. Peridurography with metrizamide: Animal and human studies. Radiology 128:123-6, 1978.

Feeney DA and Wise M. Epidurography in the normal dog: Technic and radiographic findings. Vet Radiol 22:35, 1981.

Hathcock JT Pechman RD Dillon AR Knecht CD and Braund KG. Comparison of three radiographic contrast procedures in the evaluation of the canine lumbosacral spinal canal. Vet Radiol 29:4, 1988.

Kido DK Schoene W Baker RA and Rumbaugh CL: Metrizamide epidurography in dogs. Radiology 128:119-22, 1978.

Klide AM Steinberg SA and Pond MJ. Epiduralograms in the dog: the uses and advantages of the diagnostic procedure. J Am Vet Radiol Soc 8:39-43, 1967.

Morgan JP and Bailey CS. Cauda equina syndrome in the dog: radiographic evaluation. J small Anim Pract 31: 69, 1990.

Selcer BA Chambers JN Schwensen K and Mahaffey MB. Epidurography as a diagnostic aid in canine lumbosacral compressive disease: 47 cases (1981-1986) Vet Comp Orthop Trauma 1:97, 1988.

Sisson AF LeCouteur RA Ingram JT Park RD and Child G. Diagnosis of cauda equina abnormalities by using electromyography, discography, and epidurography in dogs. J Vet Int Med 6:253, 1992.

5. ARTHROGRAPHY IN THE DOG

Definition

Arthrography is a special radiographic technique used to evaluate the character of an extremital joint. The study is best described in the shoulder (Fig. 5-1) and stifle joint of the dog. Theoretically the study can be performed in any joint in any species. The study can be performed following the: (1) injection of air, (2) an iodine-containing positive-contrast agent, or (3) a mixture of air and positive-contrast agent referred to as a double-contrast technique.

The effective capacity of the joint and the capsular compliance determines: (1) the volume of contrast agent that can be injected and (2) the intra-articular pressure generated during injection. In the normal patient, a biphasic pressure vs. volume curve is seen with a relatively small rise in pressure in the initial filling phase followed by greatly increasing pressure as the maximum volume is reached. In the presence of a full thickness tear, the pressure vs. volume curve remains relatively flat with only a minimal rise in intra-articular pressure during the injection because of the leakage of fluid. In the presence of a partial thickness tear, there is a normal biphasic appearance of the curse followed by rapid extravasation of contrast agent from the joint and an immediate decrease in intra-articular pressure. In the event of adhesive capsulitis, there is an increased intra-articular pressure at all volumes with a greater than normal increase in the slope of the pressure vs. volume curve throughout the injection.

Indications

Arthrography is used to evaluate: (1) any alteration in morphology of the surface of articular cartilage, (2) the integrity of the joint capsule, (3) abnormal joint laxity, (4) the character of intra-articular ligaments or tendons, (5) the character of menisci, (6) the character of a connecting synovial sheath, or (7) the presence of a communicating bursae or abscess cavity. As a result of the arthrogram, the site and nature of a surgical exploration may be more clearly determined.

Contraindications

Any infectious process in the over-lying soft tissues is a contraindication since a needle needs to be passed percutaneously into the joint. Injection of a positive-contrast agent in the presence of an infectious arthritis or synovitis causes the joint to become more acutely inflamed. The injection of a positive-contrast agent into an inflamed, but non-infectious, joint in not contraindicated, but, causes that process to become much more acute. Arthrography is limited only by the volume of the joint with the larger volume providing contrast for better visualization of the structures, thus, a joint with a low-volume would not be as well studied.

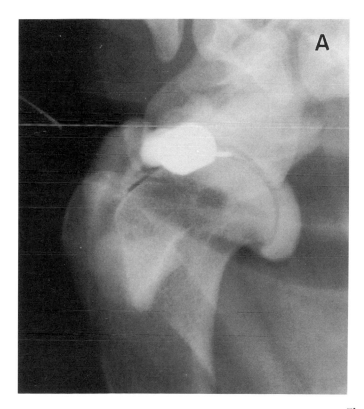 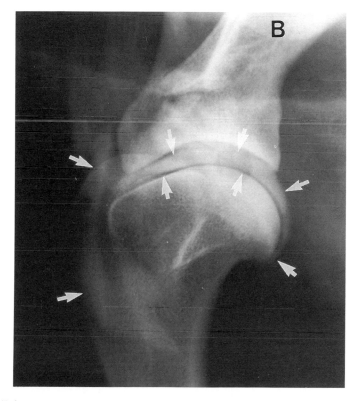

Fig. 5-1
POSITIVE CONTRAST ARTHROGRAM
Lateral radiographs of the shoulder joint of a dog following injection of the contrast agent. The needle is seen is position (A) along with the early portion of the injection. The complete filling of the joint (B) along with filling of the bicepetal tendon sheath was accomplished (arrows).

Equipment

1. positive-contrast agent—any of the newer low osmolality contrast agents such as Hexabrix (loxaglate sodium-meglumine), Isovue (iopamidol), Omnipaque (iohexol), Iotrol (Schering AG), or Amipaque (metrizamide).
2. short bevel spinal needle, 20 or 22 ga with a length required to reach the joint
3. 10 cc syringes (2)
4. collection tube for synovial fluid

Technique

1. survey radiographs are made of the joint to be studied (often the contralateral joint is radiographed as well)
2. aseptically prepare the site of injection
3. place the needle tip into the joint
4. control the location of the needle radiographically
5. remove the needle stylet and withdraw all synovial fluid possible
6. control the injection of contrast agent by finger pressure and/or predetermined volume
7. determine the amount of contrast agent injected by making a post-injection radiograph
8. if the amount of contrast is adequate, remove the needle, massage the needle tract, and gently manipulate the joint to insure uniform filling
9. make the appropriate radiographic views
10. submit the synovial fluid for analysis
11. time available to perform the radiographic study is dependent on contrast agent to be used:
    air—no limit
    positive-contrast agent—15 minutes
    double-contrast technique—15 minutes

REFERENCES

Guerra J Resnick D Haghighi P Sovak M and Cone R. Investigation of a new arthrographic contrast agent: Iotrol. Invest Radiol 19:228, 1983.

Johansen JG and Berner A. Arthrography with Amipaque (metrizamide) and other contrast media. A roentgenographic and histologic evaluation in rabbits. Invest Radiol 11:534, 1976.

Resnik CS Fronek J Frey C Gershuni D and Resnick D. Invest Radiol 19:45, 1984.

A. POSITIVE-CONTRAST SHOULDER (Scapulohumeral) ARTHROGRAPHY IN THE DOG

Definition

Injection of a positive-contrast agent into the shoulder joint clearly outlines the boundaries of the joint on the resulting radiographs (Fig. 5-1).

Indications

Originally shoulder joint arthrography was suggested to evaluate the presence of a defect within the articular cartilage (osteochondrosis). Currently, the technique is used more often to evaluate change within the bicipital tendon sheath, joint capsular tear, and excessive joint laxity.

Contraindications

(as described above)

Equipment

(as described above)
1. use a 3 in (7.5cm) needle

Technique

1. lateral and caudo-cranial survey radiographs are made of the shoulder joint to be studied (often the contralateral shoulder joint is radiographed as well)
2. aseptically prepare the site of injection
3. prepare contrast agent—dilute to 1/2 or 1/4 concentration in a small dog or to 1/2 in a large dog
4. estimate the amount of contrast agent to be injected—3cc in a 10 kgbw dog and 6cc in a dog over 25 kgbw
5. place the dog in lateral recumbency with the leg to be studied uppermost
6. adduct the limb at the shoulder joint (this opens the lateral aspect of the joint space more widely)
7. palpate the acromion process and place the needle tip through the skin just distal to the process in a smaller patient and 1cm distal to the process in a larger patient
8. pass the needle vertically into the joint—a slight "pop" is felt as the needle tip passes through the joint capsule
9. remove the needle stylet—the flow of synovial fluid indicates the correct placement of the needle tip— if you are unable to withdraw synovial fluid, control the needle location radiographically and reposition
10. withdraw all synovial fluid possible and save for analysis
11. slowly inject the contrast agent controlling the injection through the use of finger pressure on the syringe—when the joint is adequately distended, the intra-articular pressure increases enough to cause the syringe to refill with contrast agent following removal of your hand from the plunger
12. make a lateral radiograph to determine the amount of contrast injected before removing the needle
13. if the amount of contrast agent injected is adequate, remove the needle, massage the needle tract, and gently manipulate the joint to insure uniform filling
14. reposition the patient in the opposite lateral recumbency so that the affected limb is next to the tabletop
15. make the following radiographic views (*minimal view)
    a. lateral—limb in neutral position*
    b. lateral—limb in extended position
    c. lateral—limb in flexed position
    d. lateral—limb in external rotation
    e. lateral—limb in internal rotation
    f. lateral—limb with maximum tension
16. reposition the patient in dorsal recumbency and make a caudo-cranial radiograph with the limb in extended position

Problems

1. periarticular injection—the contrast agent is injected laterally but is absorbed in sufficient quantity so that the study can be reattempted within 15 to 20 minutes
2. bloody tap—reposition the needle and attempt to inject—you can proceed with the injection of the contrast agent in the face of a bloody tap
3. unable to inject contrast agent easily—the tip is outside the joint and the needle should be repositioned for an attempt to reinject
4. unable to inject contrast agent easily—it is possible that a joint with chronic synovitis may have a thickened and fibrotic capsule and cannot dilate
5. extravasation of contrast agent into extracapsular tissues due to injection of too much contrast agent— capsular "tears" or "separations" are common and have no clinical significance—extracapsular contrast absorbs rather quickly and another radiograph can be attempted 15 minutes later

Comments

Shoulder arthrography can be performed using air as a negative-contrast agent, however, the positive-contrast technique is strongly recommended as it provides more diagnostic radiographs. Double contrast arthrography is not recommended because of the problem of "foaming" with air bubble formation as the air and liquid contrast agent mix.

REFERENCES

Blevins WE. Arthrography of the canine shoulder: radiographic and histologic observations. Abs 3rd International IVRA Conference 1973.

Farrow CS. Application of shoulder arthrography: a case report. Vet Med Sm Anim Clin 69:266, 1974.

LaHue TR Brown SG Roush JC and Ticer JW. Entrapment of joint mice in the bicipital tendon sheath as a sequela to osteochondritis dissecans of the proximal humerus in dogs: A report of six cases. J Am Anim Hosp Assoc 24:99, 1988.

Muhumuza L Morgan JP Miyabayashi T and Atilola AO. Positive-contrast Arthrography. A study of the humeral joints in normal beagle dogs. Vet Radiol 29:157, 1988.

Person MW. Arthroscopy of the canine shoulder joint. Compend Contin Educ Pract Vet 8:537, 1986.

Rivers B Wallace L and Johnston GR. Biceps tenosynovitis in the dog: Radiographic and sonographic findings. V.C.O.T. 55:51, 1992.

Story E. Prognostic value of arthrography in canine shoulder osteochondrosis (osteochondritis) dissecans. Vet Clin North Am 8:301, 1978.

Suter PF and Carb AV. Shoulder arthrography in dogs—Radiographic anatomy and clinical application. J small Anim Pract 10:407, 1969.

van Bree H Van Rijssen B Peremans K and Peremans J. A comparison of diatrizoate and ioxaglate for positive contrast shoulder arthrography in dogs. Vet Radiol 32:291-6, 1991.

van Bree H Van Ryssen B and Desmidt M. Osteochondrosis lesions of the canine shoulder: Correlation of positive-contrast arthrography and arthroscopy. Vet Radiol and Ultrasound, 33:342-7, 1992.

van Bree H Verhaeghe B and Maenhout D. Positive contrast arthrography of the dog's shoulder with meglumine-sodium diatrizote. J Vet Med 36A:421, 1989.

van Bree H. Epinephrine enhanced positive-contrast shoulder arthrography in the dog. J Vet Med 36A:687, 1989.

van Bree H. Evaluation of the prognostic value of positive-contrast shoulder arthrography for bilateral osteochondrosis lesions in dogs. Am J Vet Res 7:1121, 1990.

van Bree H. The accuracy of positive-contrast shoulder arthrography in the evaluation of osteochondrosis lesions in dogs: A comparison with arthrotomy. J Am Vet Med Assoc 1991.

B. POSITIVE-CONTRAST STIFLE JOINT (Femorotibial) ARTHROGRAPHY IN THE DOG

Definition

Injection of a positive-contrast agent into the stifle joint clearly outlines the boundaries of the joint on the resulting radiographs.

Indications

Stifle joint arthrography in the dog has been suggested for the detection of: (1) tearing or rupture of the cruciate ligaments, (2) meniscal injury or tears, (3) joint capsule tears, or (4) the presence of a defect within the articular cartilage (osteochondrosis). The technique has never gained high clinical popularity.

Contraindications

(as described above)

Equipment

(as described above)
1. use a 1 in (2.5cm) needle

Technique

1. lateral and caudo-cranial survey radiographs are made of the stifle joint to be studied (often the contralateral stifle joint is studied as well)
2. prepare contrast agent dilute to 1/2 to 1/4 concentration in a small patient or to 1/2 in a large dog
3. estimate the amount of contrast agent to be injected—3cc in a 10 kgbw dog and 4cc in a dog over 25 kgbw
4. place the dog in lateral recumbency with the leg to be studied uppermost
5. aseptically prepare the site of injection medial to the patellar ligament
6. palpate the patellar ligament and apply digital pressure to the caudal aspect of the joint capsule causing a cranial bulging of the capsule facilitating placement of the needle tip
7. place the needle tip through the skin just medial to the ligament distal to the patella
8. pass the needle vertically into the joint—a slight "pop" is felt as the needle tip passes through the joint capsule
9. remove the needle stylet and withdraw synovial fluid indicating the correct placement of the needle tip—if you are unable to withdraw synovial fluid, control the needle location radiographically and reposition the needle
10. withdraw all synovial fluid possible and save for analysis
11. control the injection of contrast agent by finger pressure on the syringe—when the joint is filled adequately, the syringe refills following removal of your hand from the plunger
12. radiographically control the amount of contrast agent injected before removing the needle by making a lateral radiograph
13. if the amount of contrast medium appears adequate, remove the needle
14. massage the needle tract, and gently manipulate the joint to insure uniform filling
15. turn the patient so that the affected limb is next to the tabletop and make the following radiographic views (*minimal view)
    a. lateral—limb in neutral position*
    b. lateral—limb in extended position
    c. lateral—limb in flexed position
16. position the patient in sternal recumbency and extend the limb for a caudo-cranial radiograph

Problems

1. periarticular injection—the contrast agent absorbs quickly so that the study can be repeated within 15 to 20 minutes
2. injection of contrast agent into the patellar fat pat due to incorrect positioning of the needle tip is a common problem—it is best to delay a second injection for several hours because of the delayed absorption of the contrast agent from the fat
3. bloody tap—reposition the needle and attempt another injection
4. unable to inject contrast agent easily—reposition the needle and attempt to reinject

Comments

Stifle arthrography can be performed using air as a negative-contrast agent, however, the positive-contrast technique is strongly recommended as providing more diagnostic radiographs. Double-contrast arthrography is not recommended because of the problem of "foaming" with air bubble formation as the air and liquid contrast agent mix.

REFERENCES

Attiola MAO Pennock PW and Sumner-Smith G. Evaluation of analytical grade of metrizamide for canine stifle arthrography. J Am Vet Med Assoc 185:436, 1984.

Attiola MAO Lumsden JH Hulland TJ and Pennock PW. Intra-articular tissue response to analytical grade metrizamide in dogs. Am J Vet Res 45:2651, 1984.

van Gestel M A. Diagnostic accuracy of stifle arthroscopy in the dog. J Am Anim Hosp Assoc 21:757, 1985.

6. PERITONEOGRAPHY (Pneumoperitoneography, Celiography, Herniography) IN THE DOG AND CAT

Definition

Peritoneography is the placement of an appropriate gas (air, N_2O, CO_2) or iodinated contrast agent into the peritoneal cavity and the making of multiple positional radiographic views many of which are made with a horizontal x-ray beam. A positive-contrast study is used most commonly for evaluation of diaphragmatic integrity since it entails injection of a lower volume of contrast agent and a positive-contrast agent can be more easily seen than air or a gas if it were to flow through the diaphragmatic tear into the thoracic cavity.

Pneumoperitoneography is used commonly to evaluate an abdominal mass but is rarely used today because of the availability of ultrasound. The descriptive terms used to describe this technique provide additional information concerning the contrast agent to be used and the purpose of the examination, however, the principles are similar.

CO_2 or N_2O can be provided commercially in pressurized cylinders and are preferred to air as the contrast medium due to their more rapid absorption from the abdominal cavity and also the lower probability of causing a gas embolus. It is necessary to have a reducer valve between the compressed gas tank and the patient in order to fill syringes with the gas rather than injecting gas directly from the tank into the abdominal cavity. The use of the reducing valve prevents accidental overdistention of the abdomen.

Indications

Peritoneography is used for evaluation of: (1) traumatic diaphragmatic hernia, (2) congenital diaphragmatic/pericardial hernia, (3) large cranially located abdominal mass, (3) pre-pelvic or pelvic mass lesion. The study is used less frequently because of the ease of performing ultrasound examination in studying some of these lesions.

Contraindications

1. any inflammatory process such as peritonitis or pancreatitis that would be disseminated by the distention of the abdomen
2. abdominal fluid such as might be associated with mesenteric carcinomatosis, peritoneal hemorrhage, or peritoneal effusion because of the compromise of contrast between abdominal organs
3. distention of a portion of the gastrointestinal tract (stomach, small bowel, large bowel) that prevents free movement of the contrast agent
4. full urinary bladder because of the possibility of injection into the bladder

Contrast Agent

1. air, N_2O, or CO_2 can be used for pneumoperitoneography
2. any sterile positive-contrast agent used for parenteral injection can be used for positive peritoneography

Equipment

1. x-ray machine must have the capacity for horizontal radiography to take full advantage of the technique
2. plastic intravenous catheter of 20 -22 ga with stylet
3. lidocaine (2%) for local anesthesia or other drugs for sedation or general anesthesia
4. 50 cc syringe
5. 3 way valve

A. PNEUMOPERITONEOGRAPHY IN THE DOG AND CAT

Technique

1. withhold food for 24 hours prior to the examination to empty the gastrointestinal tract (an anorectic or vomiting patient may not require this preparation)
2. make ventrodorsal and lateral survey radiographs of the abdomen to evaluate level of patient preparation
3. sedation or general anesthetic makes the examination easier to perform
4. aseptic preparation of an injection site on the midline between the umbilicus and the pubis
5. place the plastic catheter and stylet through the abdominal wall into the peritoneal cavity
6. withdraw the inner stylet
7. attach a syringe and aspirate to test the location of the catheter tip to avoid being within a blood vessel, bowel loop, or abdominal organ
8. make a test injection of 3 to 5cc of a positive-contrast agent to insure the catheter tip is not within a blood vessel, bowel loop, or abdominal organ
9. make a lateral radiograph if there is a question concerning catheter tip location (this can be made during injection)
10. make a test injection of 10 cc sterile saline solution and attempt aspiration to further insure correct location of the catheter tip
11. inject air until the abdominal wall is moderately distended and a bongo drum sound is produced on abdominal percussion
12. observe the character of breathing and the color of the mucous membranes during the injection and be prepared to terminate the injection if problems are noted
13. remove the catheter and massage the injection site
14. reducing the kVp setting by 10 because of the reduction in tissue density
15. make the following radiographic views as determined by the character of the suspect lesion (*minimal views)
    1. recumbent right and left lateral views with vertical beam*
    2. recumbent dorsoventral and ventrodorsal views with vertical beam*
    3. erect lateral view with horizontal beam
    4. erect ventrodorsal (dorsoventral) view with horizontal beam
    5. lateral view with horizontal beam made with the patient erect with pelvic limbs elevated
    6. ventrodorsal view with horizontal beam made with the patient erect with pelvic limbs elevated
    7. lateral view with horizontal beam with the patient in sternal recumbency
    8. lateral view with horizontal beam with the patient in dorsal recumbency
    9. lateral view with a horizontal beam with the patient in lateral recumbency with affected side up

Problems

1. resistance to injection indicates that the catheter tip is not positioned correctly—plastic cannula is bent—catheter tip is resting against an abdominal organ—catheter tip is embedded within an abdominal structure—catheter tip is extra-abdominal
2. increase in the patient's respiratory rate as gas is being infused due to cranial displacement of the diaphragm resulting from increase in the abdominal contents that decreases pulmonary tidal volume
3. patient becomes severely dyspneic during injection of gas suggesting diaphragmatic hernia—stop the injection and radiograph to confirm the cause of the dyspnea—thoracocentesis may be required
4. subcutaneous air is common because of leakage and causes little problem in radiographic diagnosis of the pneumoperitoneum
5. cardiovascular abnormality may be due to venous or arterial air embolization and may be evident on cardiac auscultation

Comments

It is not necessary to remove the air or gas following the study.

B. POSITIVE-CONTRAST PERITONEOGRAPHY (Celiography) IN THE DOG AND CAT

Techniques
1. withhold food for 24 hours prior to the examination to empty the gastrointestinal tract (an anorectic or vomiting patient may not require this preparation)
2. make ventrodorsal and lateral survey radiographs of the abdomen to evaluate level of patient preparation
3. sedation or general anesthetic makes the examination easier to perform
4. aseptic preparation of an injection site on the midline between the umbilicus and the pubis
5. place the plastic catheter and stylet through the abdominal wall into the peritoneal cavity
6. withdraw the inner stylet
7. attach a syringe and aspirate to test the location of the catheter tip to avoid being within a blood vessel, bowel loop, or abdominal organ
8. make a test injection of 3 to 5 cc of positive-contrast agent to insure the catheter tip is not within a blood vessel, bowel loop, or abdominal organ
9. make a lateral radiograph if there is a question concerning catheter tip location (this can be made during injection)
10. make a test injection of 10cc sterile saline solution and attempt aspiration to further insure correct location of the catheter tip
11. inject 20 to 30ml of the positive-contrast agent
12. rotate the patient in an effort to move the contrast agent throughout the abdomen
13. make the following radiographic views as determined by suspect lesion (*minimal views)
    1. recumbent right and left lateral views with vertical beam*
    2. recumbent dorsoventral and ventrodorsal views with vertical beam*
    3. erect lateral view with horizontal beam
    4. erect ventrodorsal (dorsoventral) view with horizontal beam
    5. lateral view with horizontal beam made with the patient erect with pelvic limbs elevated
    6. ventrodorsal view with horizontal beam made with the patient erect with pelvic limbs elevated

Problems
1. resistance to injection indicates that the catheter tip is not positioned correctly—plastic cannula is bent—catheter tip is resting against an abdominal organ—catheter tip is embedded within an abdominal structure—catheter tip is extra-abdominal
2. subcutaneous location of the catheter tip—a more frequent problem in the cat
3. a greater amount of positive-contrast agent is needed if the study is performed in the presence of peritoneal effusion

Comments
1. use of newer nonionic positive-contrast agents with lower osmolality such as the nonionic myelographic agents are more expensive but highly recommended

REFERENCES

Andrew E Dahlstrøm K Sveen K and Renaa T. Amipaque® (Metrizamide) in vascular use and use in body cavities: A survey of the initial clinical trials. Invest Rad 16:455-65, 1981.

Carlson WD. Pneumoperitoneum in the dog. J Am Vet Med Assoc 130:245-51, 1957.

Ferron RF. Low-cost, pocket-sized CO_2 dispenser for medical use. J Am Vet Radiol Soc 17;18-9, 1976.

Margulis AR Burhenne HJ and Rambo ON. Evaluation of celiography in rats. Radiology 82:290-5, 1964.

Margulis AR Cook GB Tucker GL and Saltzstein SL. Celiography with iothalamic acid. Am J Roent 90:723-6, 1963.

Morgan JP. Celiography with iothalamic acid. J Am Vet Med Assoc 145:1095-9, 1964.

Rendano VT. Positive contrast peritoneography: An aid in the radiographic diagnosis of diaphragmatic hernia. J Am Vet Radiol Soc 20:67-72, 1979.

Silverman S and Morgan JP. Pneumoperitoneography in nonhuman primates. J Am Vet Med Assoc 167:622-7, 1975.

Stickle RL. Positive-contrast celiography (peritoneography) for the diagnosis of diaphragmatic hernia in dogs and cats. J Am Vet Med Assoc 185:295-8, 1984.

7. FISTULOGRAPHY AND SINUS TRACK INJECTIONS IN THE DOG AND CAT

Definition

Puncture wounds often create an injury in which the depth of the wound is important to determine. A chronic drainage may be associated with a lesion deep within the tissues. The character, depth, and origin of fistulous tracks and sinus cavities in either case can be determined by injecting positive- or negative-contrast medium and documenting the passage of the contrast medium radiographically. Because of the variability of the tracks, it is difficult to specifically describe the procedure.

Indications

A special radiographic procedure may be of value in examining a chronic draining wound or track of un-determined origin that is nonresponsive to therapy and surgical exploration is considered. It may be important to know the depth of an acute injury or the possible presence of a foreign body assumed to be associated with a puncture wound.

Contraindications

Chronic draining wound or track on the thorax or abdomen or in a location where subcutaneous pocketing of the contrast agent is probable. This usually limits the study to examination of lesions on the limbs or head.

Contrast Agent

Any iodinated contrast agent that can be used parentially can be used. Air can be used as a negative-contrast agent and a double contrast technique can be performed using both air and a positive-contrast agent.

In some patients it may be appropriate to use a rigid metallic probe or catheter to determine the depth of the track.

Equipment

1. catheter selection is dependent on the injury and the location and depth of the track—catheters may be rigid or flexible and may be radiopaque or radiolucent
2. 10 or 20cc syringe
3. type of connector to attach syringe to the catheter

Technique

1. survey radiographs of the region to examine for radiopaque foreign bodies, gas within the sinus track, or bony changes that might suggest the origin of the track
2. clean the skin and hair in the region to be studied to remove any material that would make a shadow on the radiograph that could be confused with a foreign body
3. introduce the catheter as deeply as possible—predict the location of the catheter and determine the positioning of the patient so that the contrast agent remains within the track and does not drain from the track following injection
4. inject the positive-contrast agent—reposition the catheter—inject additional contrast agent—make a radiographic exposure while the catheter remains in position
5. evaluate the radiograph to determine the extent of the track and decide the value of additional injection
6. consider the injection of air to better outline the track especially if the positive-contrast agent does not appear to completely outline the track
7. remove the catheter and reposition the patient for the orthogonal view

Comments

1. positive-contrast agent may drain over the skin surface after injection and the resulting radiograph may only show a large radiodense puddle—wash away the contrast agent and try to occlude the track openings using digital pressure and gauze pads or padded hemostats
2. failure to visualize the tracks because they are not open may require the use of more force in positioning of the catheter tip
3. failure to visualize the tracks because the contrast agent is draining out of the track can be helped by the injection of air and performing of a double-contrast study
4. contrast pooling in the subcutaneous spaces usually makes it impossible to see the sinus tracks and results in a technically unsatisfactory study
5. radiopaque markers can be placed on the patient's skin or needles inserted into the tissue to aid in the documentation of the track's course

8. BRONCHOGRAPHY IN THE DOG AND CAT

Definition

Bronchography is a radiographic procedure which renders the otherwise poorly visualized tracheobronchial tree radiographically visible through the administration of a radiopaque medium that coats the bronchial mucosa. It is performed by coating the wall of the airways with the radiopaque material and evaluating the resulting radiographic image. It appears to have been investigated in dogs and cats and reported safe; however, few clinical reports have been written in recent years. This is probably because of the increased use of bronchoscopy.

The study is obviously more easily performed if the catheter tip can be positioned under fluoroscopic control and this is another reason for the technique not being used often in practice.

Indications

Any tracheobronchial lesion that causes coughing or dyspnea and is due to a lesion in the intraluminal, mural, or extramural space. Specific lesions include: (1) intraluminal foreign bodies, (2) bronchial dilatation (bronchiectasis), (3) bronchial stenosis (tumor), (4) malpositioned bronchi (lung torsion), (5) parasites, and (6) bronchial wall granulomas.

Contrast Agents

Barium sulfate is the safest of all bronchographic media available because of its inertness. There is no danger of anaphylaxis or iodism, it does not cause fibrosis, and there are few reports of acute physiologic responses. 50% w/v propyliodone (aqueous) can also be used for bronchography. Other agents such as metrizamide powder have been used.

Contraindications

Since bronchography entails the infusion of an aqueous substance into the airways, the presence of severe lung disease might be a contraindication. Most techniques describe the use of general anesthesia which makes the technique not practical for many clinical patients with pulmonary disease.

Equipment

1. some type of catheter of a length that reaches into the main stem bronchi
2. technique for anesthesia
3. contrast agent
   Dionosil, 50% w/v propyliodone (aqueous)
   barium sulfate suspension (sterile)

Technique

1. anesthetize the patient
2. pass a polyethylene catheter into the cervical trachea
3. inject 10 to 20 ml of the contrast agent
4. make lateral and ventrodorsal radiographs
5. continue positioning of the catheter as desired
6. make additional radiographs

Comments

The volume of contrast agent to inject is dependent on the purpose for the study. The more proximal is the lesion and the more limited to one lobe, the less contrast agent is needed.

REFERENCES

Bishop EJ Medway W and Archibald J. Radiological methods of investigating the thorax of small animals, including a technic for bronchography. North Am Vet 36:477-83, 1955.

Cantwell HD and Blevins WE. Metrizamide insufflation bronchography: A new diagnostic approach. Vet Radiol 22:184-9, 1981.

Clarke KW and Webbon PM. The influence of anesthesia on bronchography in dogs J small Anim Pract 18:333-40, 1977.

Douglass SW and Hall LW. Bronchography in the dog. Vet Rec 72:901-3, 1959.

Douglass SW. The interpretation of canine bronchograms. J Am Vet Radiol Soc 15:18-22, 1974.

Dyce KM. Experimental bronchography of the dog. Brit Vet J 111:319-23, 1955.

Edmunds LH Jr Graf PD Sagel SS and Greenspan RH. Radiographic observations of clearance of tantalum and barium sulfate particles from airways. Invest Rad 5:131-41, 1970.

Hersman R Kleine LJ and Gilmore CE. A clinical evaluation of propyliodone bronchography. J Am Vet Radiol Soc 13:27-35, 1972.

Llamas R Ortiz J Perez AR and Baum GL. Experimental bronchography by tantalum insufflation. Dis Chest 56:75-7, 1069.

Meyer W Burt JK and Davis GW. A comparative study of propyliodone and barium bronchography in the dog. J Am Vet Radiol Soc 15:44-55, 1974.

Nelson SW Christoforidis AJ and Pratt PC. Further experience with barium sulfate as a bronchographic contrast medium. Am J Roent 92: 595-614, 1964.

Shook CD and Felson B. Inhalation bronchography. Chest 58:333-7, 1970.

Walker M and Goble D. Barium sulfate bronchography in horses. Vet Radiol 21:85-90, 1980.

Webbon PM and Clarke KW. Bronchography in normal dogs. J small Anim Pract 18:327-32, 1977.

9. PLEUROGRAPHY IN THE DOG AND CAT

Definition

Pleurography is the radiographic technique of placing either radiopaque contrast media or air/gas into the pleural space. The study evaluates the pleural cavity and thus determines the size, shape, and position of the lung lobes, the size, shape, and position of the mediastinum, and the character of the chest wall and diaphragm. The study is usually performed with a positive-contrast agent, but air or gas could be used.

Indications

The study is performed to evaluate a suspected mediastinal mass. Evaluation of pulmonary adhesions or other pleuropulmonary lesions is difficult, but can be attempted. Chest wall masses are most easily identified because of the absence of overlying shadows. The evaluation of diaphragmatic continuity can be performed be placing contrast agent on either side of the diaphragm. Size, shape and position of the lung lobes is a frequent indication, but the filling of the pleural space is not always uniform and evaluation of the lung lobes may be difficult.

Contraindications

The presence of a large amount of pleural fluid makes it impossible for the contrast agent to move freely and outline the intrathoracic organs. The presence of any infectious process within the pleural space is a contraindication since the movement of the contrast agent and positioning of the patient would probably assist in the spread of the infection. Any contraindication to sedating or anesthezing the patient may make it more difficult to perform the examination safely.

Contrast Agent

Any parenteral iodinated contrast agent used for urography is satisfactory, as are the nonionic products prepared for myelography. Any contrast agent recommended for angiography, are satisfactory, however, they are more irritating than the newer myelographic agents. Air or gas can be used in some patients, however, the contrast between the air and the lung surface may be difficult to detect on the radiograph.

Equipment

1. intracath 22 ga 2 inches
2. 50cc syringe

Technique for positive-contrast pleurography

1. use general anesthesia or sedate the patient
2. shave and surgically prepare a 2" (5cm) square area either at the third intracostal space ventrally or at the seventh intracostal space ventrally
3. insert the intracatheter and withdraw the needle
4. mix the positive-contrast agent with Lidocaine hydrochloride at the rate 1 ml to 10 ml of contrast agent
5. inject 1.0cc/kgbw of the contrast agent—use 0.5cc/kgbw in small dogs and cats and 1.5cc/kgbw in larger dogs
6. rotate the patient to insure equal distribution of the contrast agent
7. make right and left lateral and dorsoventral and ventrodorsal radiographic studies using a vertical x-ray beam
8. make radiographic studies using a horizontal x-ray beam as might be indicated recognizing that the contrast agent will migrate to the dependent portion of the thoracic cavity

Technique for pneumopleurography

1. use general anesthesia or sedate the patient
2. shave and surgically prepare a 2" (5cm) square area either at the third intracostal space ventrally or at the seventh intracostal space ventrally
3. insert the intracatheter and withdraw the needle
4. inject room air at the rate of 50cc for a small dog or cat, 100cc for a medium sized dog, and 200cc for a large dog.
5. make right and left lateral and dorsoventral and ventrodorsal radiographic studies using a vertical x-ray beam
6. make radiographic studies using a horizontal x-ray beam as might be indicated recognizing that the air or gas migrates to the superior portion of the thoracic cavity
4. observe the respiratory rate during the injection and stop if respiratory distress is observed

Comments

1. select the injection site based on the suspected location of the thoracic lesion using the caudal thoracic site if possible
2. avoid placement of the catheter near the caudal edge of a rib because of the presence of the intercostal arteries
3. if there is any resistance to injection, stop the injection and make a radiograph to evaluate the location of the catheter tip
4. observe the respiratory rate during the injection and stop if respiratory distress is observed
5. the mediastinum permits rapid penetration of fluids and air so that the pleural space on both sides of the thorax may be evaluated using a single injection site
6. if the mediastinum is intact, the amount of contrast injected may be excessive

REFERENCES

Bhargava AK Burt JK Rudy RL and Wilson GP. Diagnosis of mediastinal and heart base tumors in dogs using contrast pleurography. Am Vet Radiol Soc 11:56-64, 1970.

Bhargava AK Kentner DC Rudy RL and Burt JK. Contrast pleurography in rhesus monkeys (Macaca mulatta). Br Vet J 126:57-60, 1970.

Bhargava AK Rudy RL and Diesem CD. Radiographic anatomy of the pleura in dogs as visualized by contrast pleurography. Am Vet Radiol Soc 10:61-5, 1969.

Rudy RL Bhargava AK and Roenigk WJ. Contrast Pleurography: A new technic for the radiographic visualization of the pleura and its various reflections in dogs. Radiology 91:1034-6, 1968.

10. STRESS RADIOGRAPHY IN THE DOG AND CAT

Definition

Stress radiography may be defined as the application of a controlled force upon a joint in order to demonstrate an abnormal spatial relationship between two or more bones (Fig. 10-1). The abnormal motion to be evaluated may be congenital (absence of the odontoid process), traumatic (joint injury), or degenerative (cruciate ligament injury) in nature. The anatomical information obtained from the stress examination is often available on physical examination, however, the stress radiograph permits a permanent recording of the abnormality and a detailed studying of the corrective surgical technique that might be required. Certain basic maneuvers are possible, most of which are used to demonstrate joint instability. However, it is also possible to demonstrate instability at an acute or healing fracture site. Hyperextension and hyperflexion require use of a fulcrum of some type. Medial and lateral deviation also require the use of a fulcrum. Shear force can also be used to cause a joint instability. Rotary stress can be performed by simply twisting the limb while traction is performed by placing traction force on the limb. Stress studies of the vertebral column must be made with the knowledge that further injury to the spinal cord is possible. The radiographs can be made using: (1) weight-bearing stress on a standing patient with the radiograph made with a horizontal x-ray beam, (2) stress on a recumbent patient using a fulcrum to create the instability, or (3) rotary or traction force on a recumbent patient.

Indications

1. identify small avulsion or chip fracture fragments
2. determine the degree and nature of the instability present in an extremital joint injury
3. determine the degree and nature of spinal instability, particularly cervical and lumbosacral
4. determine the level of displacement of the condyloid process at the temporomandibular joint

Contraindications

1. stress radiography in the spine when further injury to the spinal cord or nerve roots is possible

Equipment

1. device such as a wooden spoon or plastic paddle to achieve the appropriate stress

Technique

1. make non-stress radiographs of the region of interest
2. position the patient appropriately for the stress views
3. generate the stress on the anatomical site of interest
4. make the radiographic exposure

REFERENCES

Farrow CS. Carpal sprain injury in the dog. J Vet Radiol Soc 18:38-43, 1977.

Farrow CS. Stress radiography: Applications in small animal practice. J Am Vet Med Assoc 181:777-84, 1982.

Miyabayashi T den Toom OI and Morgan JP. Application of positional radiographic techniques in the dog and cat: Part 111—Skeleton. Cal Vet 37:11-8, 1983.

Rijke AM Tegtmeyer CJ, Weiland DJ and McCue III FC. Stress examination of the cruciate ligaments: A radiologic Lachman test. Radiology 165:867-9, 1987.

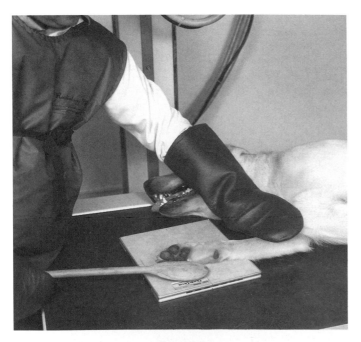

Fig. 10-1
STRESS RADIOGRAPHY
A photograph illustrates the positioning of a dog for stress radiography of the carpus. The paddle causes hyperextension of the antebrachiocarpal joint permitting evaluation of the abnormal laxity that might result from injury. The study uses a vertically directed x-ray beam.

11. HORIZONTAL BEAM RADIOGRAPHY IN THE DOG AND CAT

Definition

Standard radiographic evaluation includes two views of the area of interest that are usually made with a vertically directed x-ray beam. It is especially easy to position the patient for the lateral view, however, the opposite view (craniocaudal, dorsopalmar, dorsoplantar, or dorsoventral) may be more difficult to achieve. Since most patients are more comfortable when positioned in lateral recumbency, it may be possible to make the orthogonal view using a horizontal x-ray beam. In other patients, a radiograph made with a horizontal beam permits the evaluation of gas-capped fluid levels such as might be found an abscess or in a bowel loop that is obstructed. Horizontal radiography also is important in the identification of free pleural or peritoneal air in which the pocket of air is separated and easier to identify.

Horizontal beam radiography requires that the x-ray tube be easily lowered and rotated to be able to produce a usable horizontal beam. Some form of cassette holder is required that may range from a wall-mounted cassette holder (Fig. 11-1) to a sandbag braced against a cassette that stands vertically on the tabletop. If the object to be radiographed exceeds 13cm in thickness, it maybe necessary to have the cassette holder also hold a grid.

This technique can be used to advantage to make the following studies in the recumbent patient: caudocranial view of both limbs (Fig. 11-2), ventrodorsal view of the spine, ventrodorsal view of the thorax, ventrodorsal view of the abdomen, and a lateral view of the abdomen. Lateral view of the thorax can be made in the standing or erect patient.

Indications

The studies permit movement of air to improve radiographic evaluation of air normally or abnormally accumulated within an organ such as a: (1) pulmonary cystic lesion, (2) mediastinal air, (3) esophageal air, (4) gastric air to visualize pyloric lesion, (5) emphysematous cholecystitis, (6) emphysematous gallbladder wall, (7) abnormal gas collection within the urinary bladder, (8) emphysematous cystitis, and (9) gas-capped dilated intestinal loops (mechanical obstruction). Air may be free within a body cavity such as free pleural air or free peritoneal air.

The studies also permit the detection of movement of fluid within a body cavity to make visualization of a lesion easier, for example, moving pleural fluid to better see a thoracic wall lesion, a mediastinal mass, a pulmonary mass, or a diaphragmatic integrity. Moving abdominal fluid permits a better understanding of an abdominal wall lesion.

Horizontal radiography permits movement of fluid free within an organ such as a dilated esophagus or dilated fluid-filled small bowel loops to make visualization of a lesion easier.

The technique provides easier positioning in lateral recumbency for post-traumatic skeletal studies of the long bones or views of the spine suspected to be fractured.

Positioning for horizontal radiography permits movement within an organ of opaque material such as sand-like calculi within the urinary bladder or foreign bodies within the stomach.

Contraindications

1. in the presence of free pleural fluid, ventrodorsal positioning may cause dyspnea
2. in the presence of suspected cranial mediastinal mass, erect positioning may cause life-threatening dyspnea

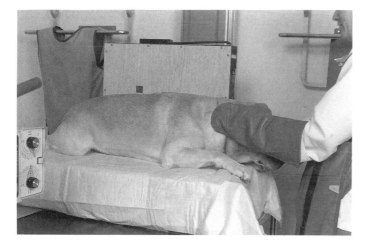
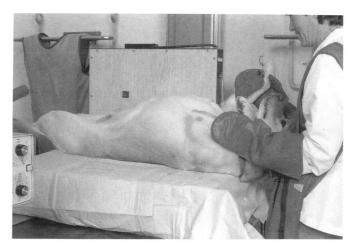

Fig. 11-1
HORIZONTAL BEAM RADIOGRAPHY
Photographs illustrate the position of a dog in sternal and dorsal recumbency for lateral thoracic radiograph using a horizontal x-ray beam.

Equipment

1. x-ray machine that permits repositioning of the tube
2. some form of cassette holder
3. sponges to elevate the patient above the tabletop so as to be able to center the x-ray beam

Technique

1. reposition the x-ray tube
2. position cassette and grid if necessary
3. position patient as required (may include elevation)
4. make radiographic exposure
5. make additional positional studies as required

Comments

If free air is suspected, wait 5 minutes to permit collection of the air dorsally before radiographic exposure.

REFERENCES

Beck KA. Caudocranial horizontal beam radiographic projection for evaluation of femoral fracture and osteotomy repair in dogs and cats. J Am Vet Med Assoc 198;1751-4, 1991.

den Toom OI Miyabayashi T and Morgan JP. Application of positional radiographic techniques in the dog and cat. Part 1—Thorax. Cal Vet 37:19-23, 1983.

Miyabayashi T den Toom OI and Morgan JP. Application of positional radiographic techniques in the dog and cat. Part 11—Abdomen. Cal Vet 37:15-21, 1983.

Miyabayashi T den Toom OI and Morgan JP. Application of positional radiographic techniques in the dog and cat. Part 111—Skeleton. Cal Vet, 37:11-8, 1983.

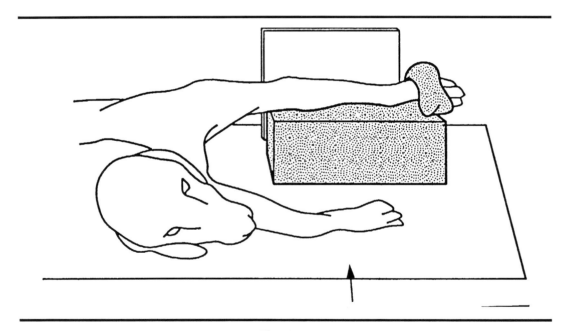

Fig. 11-2
HORIZONTAL BEAM RADIOGRAPHY
A drawing illustrates the use of a horizontally directed x-ray beam (arrow) in a study of the antebrachium of a dog.

12. ABDOMINAL COMPRESSION IN THE DOG AND CAT

Definition

Abdominal compression is a radiographic technique used to reduce the thickness of the anatomical part through the moving of an overlying organ in an effort to improve visualization of a suspect lesion. The study can be performed using a single paddle or spoon, or by wrapping the abdomen or using a compression band to decrease thickness. In addition to increasing visualization of an organ, reduction in the thickness of the abdomen proportionately reduces the amount of scatter radiation produced and thus improves the technical quality of the radiograph. It may be possible to compress the abdomen to the extent that use of a grid is not necessary and the radiographic technique can be decreased appreciably. The use of a compression device may be used to enhance a lateral view or may improve a ventrodorsal projection. Often the compression apparatus aids in the restraint of the patient and minimizes the risk of technical problems due to patient movement. The technique described is used in conjunction with use of a vertical x-ray beam.

Indications

Indications include the improvement of the visualization of an abdominal organ of interest by displacing an overlying organ to permit visualization of: (1) a kidney suspected of containing calculi, (2) the urinary bladder suspected of containing calculi, (3) an enlarged uterus superimposed between the rectum and urinary bladder, (4) a distended loop of small bowel suspected of being obstructed or containing a foreign body, (5) a tumor within an adrenal gland, (6) suspected peritoneal air by shifting it into a more visible location for easier visualization, (7) a gastric wall lesion through the shifting of air or fluid contents, (8) a space occupying lesion identified within the gastrointestinal tract as seen by the use of a positive-contrast agent, and (9) a space occupying lesion identified within the urinary bladder by the use of a positive-contrast agent.

The visualization of the spine may be improved by displacing gas or fecal-filled intestinal loops.

Contraindications

Contraindications include clinical situations where abdominal compression must be avoided, for example: (1) the presence of a large abdominal mass that might rupture (pyometra, splenic tumor), (2) the presence of a localized peritonitis that might be made generalized, (3) the presence of suspected pancreatic inflammation, (4) patients with severe respiratory distress, (5) patients with suspected diaphragmatic hernia, and (6) patients with generalized osteopenia where rib fractures might result.

Equipment

1. some type of compressive device, such as a wooden paddle or plastic (lucite) spoon, with reasonable rigidity that may incorporate an inflatable rubber bladder (Fig. 12-1)
2. compression band that attaches to the tabletop or wraps around the abdomen
3. wedge-shaped radiolucent sponge may be positioned beneath a compression band

Technique

1. make a routine radiographic study and detect a finding that requires further examination or fail to visualize an organ of particular clinical interest
2. place the compression device directly over the organ of interest so as to move overlying organs
3. alter radiographic technique either by decreasing kVp by 10 or decreasing the mAs to one-half
4. make the new radiographic study
5. consider repositioning the patient for a second study

REFERENCES

Carrig CB and Mostosky UV. The use of compression in abdominal radiography of the dog and cat. J Am Vet Radiol Soc 17:178-81, 1976.

Crowe J Sumner T and Ott D. Improved visualization of the lumbar spine and sacrum in pediatric patients by use of the pneumatic compression paddle. Radiology 128:812-4, 1978.

Miyabayashi T den Toom OI and Morgan JP. Application of positional radiographic techniques in the dog and cat. Cal Vet 37:15-21, 1983.

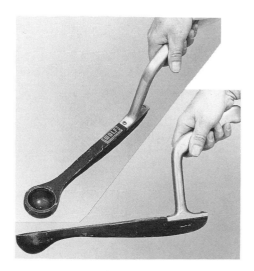

Fig. 12-1
COMPRESSION PADDLE
A photograph of a commercially produced cup-shaped paddle device used as a compression device in abdominal radiography.

13. MAGNIFICATION RADIOLOGY IN THE DOG AND CAT

Magnification in a radiographic study is based on how well the imaging system faithfully records the frequency characteristics of the object of interest. It is dependent on focal spot size and object film distance. Magnification radiography requires a small focal spot size that became available with the advent of high-speed rotating anodes and sizes of 0.3mm or smaller. Unfortunately, equipment of this type is expensive. Further developments included gird-controlled x-ray tubes with wire mesh surrounding the focusing cup of the cathode. With a negative charge on the grid there is reduction in the size of the electron beam and reduction of the resulting focal spot size. In this manner, the focal spot size can be reduced to 0.1mm or less but the tube is limited to its heat capacity. Therefore, it is necessary to increase the radiographic exposure through a longer exposure time due to the decreased mA and kVp setting.

A second method of magnification is optical enlargement of a high detail radiograph. This may be as good as magnification radiography but it requires time for the photographic enlargement while radiographic magnification is immediate.

REFERENCES

Abel MS. Advantages and limitation of the 0.3mm focal spot tube for magnification and other techniques. Radiology 66:747, 1956

Bookstein JJ and Voegeli E. A critical analysis of magnification radiography. Radiology 98:23, 1971.

Freedman PJ and Greenspan RH. Observations on magnification radiography. Radiology 92:549, 1969.

James AE Rao GU Gray CR Heller RM and Bush MR. Magnification in Veterinary Radiology. J Am Vet Radiol Soc 16:52-64, 1975

Rao GUV Clark RL and Gaylor BW. Radiography Magnification. Appl. Radiology 2:37, 1973.

SECTION E

RADIOGRAPHY OF THE HORSE

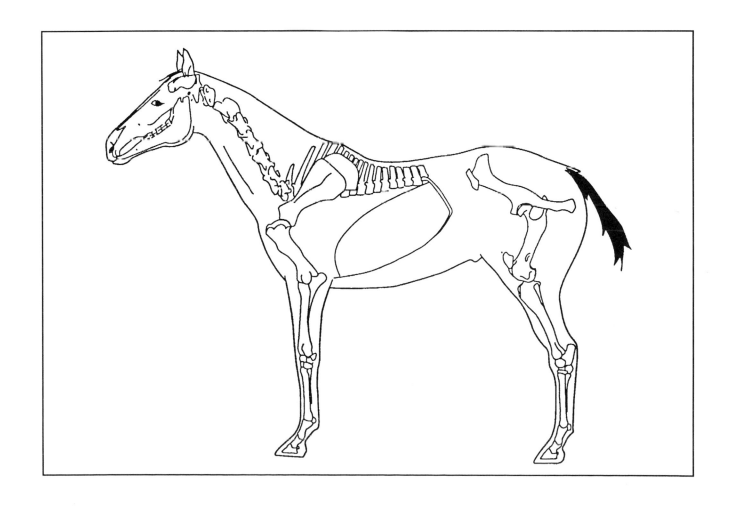

1. INTRODUCTION

Diagnostic radiography of the horse is different in form, function, and status as compared to radiography of other animals. In a practice in which a great deal of service is conducted on an ambulatory basis, examinations are often made on the ranch or farm utilizing a portable x-ray unit. Thus, the size of the x-ray machine has remained small and the scope of the radiographic examination has remained limited. The x-ray film is usually not processed at the time of exposure; therefore, it is not possible to make an immediate evaluation of the technical quality of the study and not possible to correct positioning or technique errors. In larger clinics that receive many of their patients on an in-patient basis, permanently installed x-ray equipment is larger, films are processed immediately and the limitations placed on examinations are fewer.

Radiographing a horse is a unique undertaking. The size of the horse, the fact that most examinations are made with the horse in a standing position, and the unpredictable disposition of the patient make radiography of the horse a truly challenging experience. Because of difficulties in positioning the horse for radiography, it is more common to move the x-ray tube and machine in an effort to re-direct the x-ray beam. Therefore, a mobile tubehead and movement of the patient are necessary to achieve satisfactory radiographs. Technically satisfactory machines must be positioned easily or they are of little practical value (Koblik and Toal, 1991). Many pieces of accessory equipment are indispensable for radiography of the horse's feet. Routine use of chemical restraint usually decreases patient movement and thus, the time required for a study resulting in higher quality radiographs.

The size and morphology of the bones and joints in the horse requires that oblique projections be made regularly in an effort to evaluate all of the surfaces of the bones. These views are included, along with the more conventional views, in describing what is required for a complete radiographic examination of each anatomical part.

EQUINE RADIOGRAPHIC TECHNIQUES

EQUINE RADIOGRAPHIC EQUIPMENT

Units for use in radiography of horses falls generally into three categories: (1) small portable x-ray units with minimal mA capabilities, (2) mobile x-ray units with high mA capabilities, and (3) ceiling- or wall-mounted x-ray units with high mA capabilities (Table 1-1). In the comparison of x-ray units, the maximum mA, kVp, and shortest exposure time are evaluated closely since they are a measure of the diagnostic capability of the unit.

Small Portable X-ray Units

These units typically weigh around 15 to 20 kg, have a stationary anode type x-ray tube, are easily transported to a ranch or farm, and are carried to the stall or paddock in which the patient is housed. The majority of these units have a capability of 10 to 20 mA and 80 to 90 kVp, and the shortest exposure times are usually a minimum of 1/25 second. It is possible to arrange a tube support system for these small units, but most are hand-held during exposures. A tripod-like device on wheels can be used, but it is difficult to position the device near the patient and there is a problem of safety to the machine, horses, and operator (Koblik and Toal, 1991).

While small portable units are popular because of their ease in transportation; they have definite limitations in diagnosis. Often they are used at a great distance from an electrical power source which compromises the electrical power available to the unit resulting in production of an underexposed radiograph. Because of the portable nature of the unit, all of the accessory equipment including lead aprons, lead gloves, and positioning devices must be carried to the site of the examination. While all portable units have collimators, light beam collimators are not commonly used. Since these exposures may be made in the open, the illuminated field is often not bright enough to make use of the collimator in identifying the field of exposure. These

---

Table 1-1
SUMMARY OF CHARACTERISTICS OF X-RAY MACHINES USED IN RADIOGRAPHY OF HORSES

Machine characteristics for a portable x-ray machine:
1. Stationary anode x-ray tube with 1.5 to 2.0 mm focal spot size
2. Capability of 0.05 to 0.1 second exposure
3. Capability of 10 to 20 mA
4. Capability of 75 to 90 kVp
5. Capability of 80 kVp setting at 1.5 mAs setting
6. Capability of readily positioning tube head
7. Method available to monitor incoming line voltage
8. Light-beam collimator, even though difficult to use
9. Hand switch (where permitted by law)
10. Minimal weight for easy transportation
11. Safe from potential electrical and radiation hazards
12. Examinations limited to limbs
13. Exposure consistency not good
14. Cost less than $5000

Machine characteristics of a large mobile or ceiling- or wall-mounted x-ray machine:
1. Rotating anode x-ray tube with 0.3 to 1.0 mm small focal spot size
2. Rotating anode x-ray tube with 1.0 to 2.0 mm large focal spot size
3. Capability of 1/120 to 1/60 second exposure
4. Capability of 100 to 500 mA
5. Capability of 100 to 120 kVp setting
6. Tube head permits easy and quiet vertical and horizontal adjustment of the x-ray beam
7. Tube head supported on a panographic arm or column
8. Capable of tube head being readily positioned
9. Method available to monitor and adjust the incoming line voltage
10. Light-beam collimator with device to determine focal-film distance easy to use
11. Switch mounted on tube head (where permitted by law)
12. Minimal operational noise
13. Cassette and grid holder easily positioned
14. Safe from potential electrical and radiation hazards.
15. Cost between $15,000 and $25,000
16. Unit mobility limited by size
17. Potential radiographic examinations limited only by tube head mobility
18. Exposure consistency high

portable x-ray units are limited in their use to examinations of the extremities from the carpus and tarsus distally, however, in immature patients, their use can be expanded to include studies more proximal on the limb.

Large Mobile X-ray Units

Another less commonly used type of x-ray unit is one that is mounted on wheels, has a rotating anode type of x-ray tube with a high-quality collimator and a large transformer, and can be moved within a clinic or hospital. Because of this type of mounting, relatively level, smooth surfaces are necessary upon which to move the unit. The units are capable of 100 to 300 mA, 100 to 120 kVp, and a timer with shortest exposures of 1/60 to 1/120 seconds.

The best use for this type of machine is found in a clinic or hospital that has need of both large and small animal radiographic capabilities. A mobile unit can be used: (1) in the area used for examination of lameness in horses, (2) in the surgery room for intra-operative studies, (3) to study a patient that cannot be moved from the back of a truck or trailer, (4) in a recovery stall for a post-operative study, and (5) over a stationary x-ray table for examination of smaller patients. It is this diversity of use that makes it a good solution for a large clinic that has need for a radiographic capability in examination of both large and small animals.

Ceiling Mounted X-ray Units

These large, permanently mounted x-ray units have a range of 100 to 1000 mA, 60 to 150 kVp, and exposure times as short as 1/60 to 1/120 second and use a rotating anode type of x-ray tube. The tube head support is ceiling-mounted and can be freely moved horizontally throughout the room and vertically from floor level to a height of 5 feet (2m) or more. This means that the tube head can be dropped to the floor level for a study of the horse's foot or can be raised quickly in the event of potential danger to the tube. It is best to have the exposure controls at the tube head so that the exposure can be made at the time of tube positioning.

PREPARATION OF THE HORSE

Preparation of the horse for radiography requires brushing or washing of the hair coat to remove obvious dirt, scruff, or any iodinated medicament that is present following wound treatment. If possible, any bandage, splint, or cast should be removed prior to examination. Keep a set of instruments available for use in preparing feet for radiography. Preparation of the foot is most important because of the prominent artifacts created by the uneven surface of the sole and the nature of the dirt and gravel that is packed in the sole. The shoe needs to be removed if possible and the foot cleaned and trimmed for the best radiographic study of the foot. Following this careful preparation, the sulci of the foot is packed with "Play-Doh" or another suitable material to eliminate the artifacts produced by those structures (Fig. 1-1).

Most people radiographing horses prefer to work with an animal free in an open room rather than using stocks. This decision is obviously based on the character of the patients. Use of a tranquilizer is highly recommended as safer for both the horse and you and results in the production of a technically better radiographic study. A twitch or ear-hold are other techniques used to control the horse, however, permission should be obtained from the owner prior to using either of these.

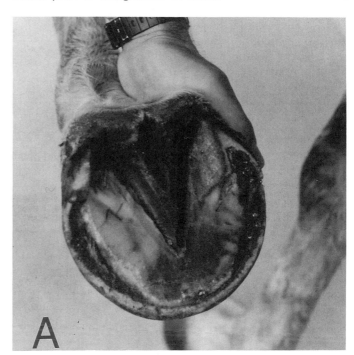

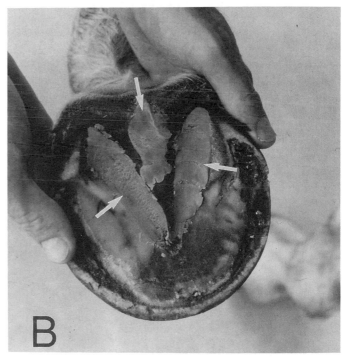

Fig. 1-1
PATIENT PREPARATION
Preparation of the foot must precede radiography for the navicular bone and third phalanx. After picking the sole clean, it is packed with a suitable material (arrows) to eliminate film artifacts.

Positioning Blocks and Cassette Holders

These accessories are necessary in radiographic examination of the horses feet if you intend to be able to consistently reproduce the positioning of the horse's foot, x-ray tube, and cassette. The blocks should be constructed with a slot so that they serve as a cassette holder as well. Positioning blocks have their greatest importance in radiography of the navicular bone and several types of blocks have been developed for that examination. Cassette tunnels are necessary in positioning of the foot and also provide protection for the cassette.

Cassette holders are important in ensuring that the film is positioned in a correct location and angle to the central beam and are held without motion enabling an assistant to move further from the primary x-ray beam. Most cassette holders are hand-held and may have an adjustable "leg" attached to provide greater stability to the cassette during the exposure and greater ease in movement (Fig. 1-2). The most commonly used holder is 8 x 10 inches but are available in 10 x 12 inch, 11 x 14 in, 7 x 17 in, or 14 x 17 in sizes. Holders can be constructed to have a provision for placement of a grid in addition to the cassette.

Use of X-ray Table

Examination of the patient can often be best performed on an x-ray table in which the cassette is placed within a tray beneath the patient. The tube head and cassette and grid are moved independently of the patient. Positioning of the cassette is easier and it is possible to develop a guidance system that ensures the central beam is centered on the cassette and the grid and is perpendicular to the surface of the grid. The tabletop can be made to shift laterally, making it easier to move or unload the patient.

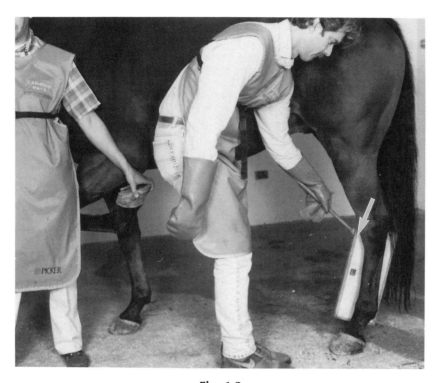

Fig. 1-2
CASSETTE HOLDERS
Different sizes of cassette holders (arrow) can be fabricated to match the various sizes of cassettes. They should be made with handles that are adjustable in position.

2. FOOT

Radiographic examinations of the distal extremities of the horse constitute the majority of radiographic examinations in the horse and include the: (1) proximal sesamoid bones, (2) fetlock joint, (3) navicular bone, and (4) distal phalanx. It is relatively easy to position for this group of examinations when they are performed on the forelimb, however, some difficulty is encountered in positioning of the tube and cassette when examining the hindlimb. Multiple radiographic views are used for the evaluation of these structures. The majority of the views, except the flexed and skyline views, are made in a weight-bearing manner. Positioning blocks and cassette holders are essential in obtaining standardized positioning.

Collimation of the primary x-ray beam keeps the x-ray field to a minimum and is a desirable goal. However, it should be kept in mind that the bones in the limb are aligned vertically making it easy to narrow the x-ray field laterally to the width of the bones examined and still keep the x-ray field as large as the cassette proximally and distally. This enables evaluation of as much of the skeletal structures as is possible.

It is important that radiographic artifacts not compromise the quality of this examination. The shoe should be pulled, the foot brushed and washed, hoof wall trimmed, the frog picked clean, and the sole and frog trimmed to remove debris. The sulcus should be packed on a study of the distal phalanx especially if a fracture in the area of the sulci is suspected. A wire placed along the dorsum of the hoof wall on the mid-sagittal plane permits evaluation of the normally parallel relationship between hoof wall and dorsum of the third phalanx.

DISTAL PHALANX
(Ungular Bone, Pedal Bone, Os Pedis, Third Phalanx, Coffin Bone)

A basic study of the distal phalanx consists of dorsopalmar (plantar), and lateral views. Oblique views are considered optional until a definite lesion is identified. The lateral projection is often used without other views for the single purpose of studying the relationship of the hoof wall to the dorsal border of the distal phalanx (Table 2-1). The hoof appears large, however, the density of both hoof wall and distal phalanx are less than anticipated. Thus, the radiographic techniques are not increased and in fact are less than those techniques used for other parts of the forelimb.

There are no consistently found separate ossification centers of the distal phalanx present at birth, however, it is possible to incorrectly diagnosis avulsed fragments from the extensor process as separate ossification centers. Fragmentation of the palmar processes appears as incomplete ossification but probably represents separated fracture fragments.

The markers for studies of the foot are not unique, but it is important that the lateral aspects of the radiograph be identified. In this manual, all markers are described as having been placed laterally.

Table 2-1
TECHNIQUE FOR RADIOGRAPHIC EVALUATION OF THE DISTAL PHALANX

Standard views
  dorsopalmar (plantar) 65°
  lateral (lateromedial)
Optional views
  single lateral (lateromedial) may be used for
    evaluation of the status of the distal phalanx
  obliques
  dorsopalmar (plantar) with x-ray beam parallel to the
    ground
Views of the opposite limb
  dorsopalmar (plantar) view of opposite limb if 6
    months of age or younger
Cassette size
  8 x 10 inches (18 x 24 cm)
Cassette tunnel
  use on the dorsopalmar (plantar) weight-bearing view
    to protect the cassette
Grid
  not required routinely but of value in examination of
    a thick foot
Markers
  lateral
  fore- or hindfoot
  right or left foot

DISTAL PHALANX—DORSOPALMAR (plantar) VIEW (65° dorsoproximal-palmarodistal)

Purpose of study—The number, size, and character of vascular channels can be noted. The size and shape of the crena, the large notch in the solar border, is often noted dorsally on the midline and may vary widely. The solar border extends medially and laterally to form the palmar processes or wings. The level of mineralization of the collateral cartilages (ungular cartilages) is dependent on the patients age, weight, and use. While mineralization of the collateral cartilages is not common in the lighter weight breeds, it is especially noticeable in heavier adult warm-blooded breeds.

Preparation of patient—There can be no compromise in the requirement to clean the hoof wall and sole, since, the presence of any dirt or rocks or roughening of the sole creates radiographic artifacts.

Foot Positioning—The cassette is placed within a tunnel and put on the ground in front of the horse. The foot to be examined is picked up and is placed near the center of the cassette tunnel with the toe near the forward edge of the tunnel. It is not necessary to lift the opposite forefoot, but with the unruly horse, the opposite foot can be lifted to force maximum weight-bearing on the cassette holder by the foot to be examined to insure there is no motion during the study.

Tube Positioning—The tube is positioned in front of the leg approximately 24 to 26 in (60 cm) off the ground and angled at approximately 65° so that the central x-ray beam strikes the middle of the hoof wall on the midline. The highly collimated beam is at a right angle to the hoof wall in a foot that is correctly trimmed (Fig. 2-1). In the patient with feet that are uncared for, the angle of intercept with the hoof wall changes as the toe lengthens. The x-ray beam is centered 1/2 to 1 in (1 to 2 cm) proximal to the coronary band.

Comments—It is possible to make this study with the shoe in place, however, a cassette tunnel should be used to avoid injury to the cassette.

The central beam can be directed parallel to the ground to better evaluate: (1) the character of the extensor process of the distal phalanx, (2) conformation of the foot and distal interphalangeal joint, (3) the quality of hoof care as indicated by differences in hoof wall length, and (4) the relationship of the foot to the surface of the ground (Fig. 2-2). This projection is recommended only as an additional view and is not recommended for the evaluation of disease within the distal phalanx because of the distortion of the shadows resulting from the x-ray beam being directed at an oblique angle with the axis of the bone (foot).

Radiographic Technique for Portable Unit (400 speed film-screen system)
- 80 kVp, 10 mA, 0.06 sec, 26 inches focal-film distance
- 80 kVp, 20 mA, 0.04 sec, 26 inches focal-film distance

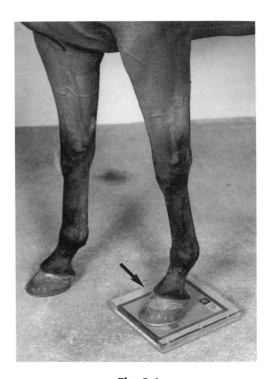

Fig. 2-1
Photograph of the positioning of the foot preparatory to making the dorsopalmar view of the distal phalanx. The direction of the central x-ray beam (arrow) is marked. It is helpful with some patients to lift the opposite forefoot. Use of a cassette tunnel is recommended.

DISTAL PHALANX—LATERAL VIEW
(lateromedial)

Purpose—The relationship and distance between the dorsal hoof wall and the dorsal border of the distal phalanx can be evaluated on this view as well as fractures of the extensor process of the third phalanx. The palmar processes are normally separated from the cartilages of the distal phalanx by a prominent parietal sulcus and may appear to be irregular with separate bony fragments.

Preparation—If this view is only used to study the relationship of the hoof wall-distal phalanx, cleanliness of the sole or trimming of the hoof is not as important. When this view is made as a part of a full examination of the distal phalanx, routine preparation is required.

Foot Positioning—The horse's foot is positioned on some form of block that may have a slot to hold the cassette in addition to elevating the foot sufficiently so that the x-ray beam is directed in a horizontal plane and is centered on the distal phalanx. The hoof is positioned toward the medial side of the block so that it is against the cassette as it is positioned in the slot or held in a holder (Fig. 2-3). This decreases object-film distance and limits the magnification of the foot on the film. Always confirm the positioning of the block relative to the horse's stance. Malpositioning the block to foot stance angle creates an obliqued projection of the distal phalanx relative to a horizontal beam making it is difficult to evaluate the relationship between the hoof wall and the dorsal (parietal) surface of the distal phalanx. It may be helpful to lift the opposite foot to insure full weight bearing on the foot to be examined to insure there is no motion during the exposure.

Tube Positioning—The tube head is positioned laterally with the x-ray beam parallel to the ground surface and the beam is centered on the hoof wall below the coronary band midway between the dorsal hoof wall and the bulbs of the heels. Visually superimpose the bulbs of the heels by drawing a line straight from the bulbs of the heel to the x-ray tube to avoid beam angulation cranially or caudally. The most common error occurs when positioning the x-ray tube cranially and angling the beam relative to the hoof. Evaluate the leg proximally and distally to avoid radiographing the foot with the leg abducted or adducted.

If the horse is non-weight bearing, the foot can be positioned forward and placed in a weight-bearing position on the tunnel and cassette. All studies of the distal phalanx in the pelvic limb are positioned forward as it is difficult to elevate the opposite limb and or get the horse to stand on the tunnel without placing the foot forward.

Radiographic Technique for Portable Unit (400 speed film-screen system)
- 80 kVp, 10 mA, 0.1 sec, 26 inches focal-film distance
- 80 kVp, 20 mA, 0.06 sec, 26 inches focal-film distance

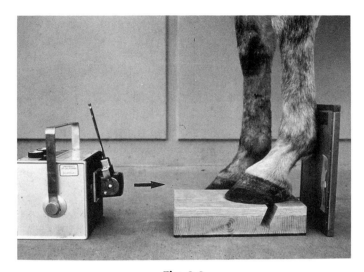

Fig. 2-2
Photograph shows the positioning of the foot used to obtain a special dorsopalmar angle of the foot using a horizontal x-ray beam. The direction of the central x-ray beam (arrow) is marked.

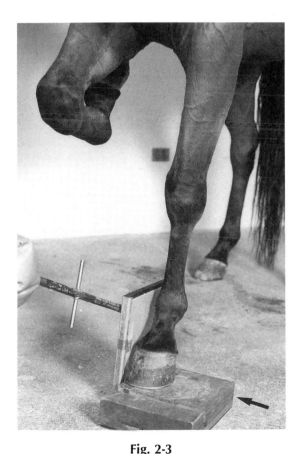

Fig. 2-3
Photograph shows the foot elevated on a block to obtain the lateromedial view for the distal phalanx. The opposite forefoot can be lifted to control motion during the exposure. Make certain that the assistant is not standing behind the cassette with their feet in the primary x-ray beam. The x-ray beam (arrow) is horizontal and centered just distal to the coronary band one half the distance between the dorsal wall and the heels.

DISTAL PHALANX—OBLIQUE VIEW
(65° dorsoproximolateral-palmarodistomedial or 65° dorsoproximomedial-palmarodistolateral)

Purpose—These special views assist in detection of non-displaced fractures in the quarters of the solar border and in the palmar or plantar processes of the distal phalanx.

Preparation—The studies have limited value unless the shoe is removed and the foot is well cleaned.

Foot Positioning—Place the cassette on the ground within the tunnel and position the foot on the tunnel with the foot off-center slightly toward the side to be studied (Fig. 2-4). Lift the opposite foot to insure weightbearing and an absence of motion.

Tube Positioning—The x-ray tube is positioned in front of the foot and to the medial or lateral side depending on which oblique view is being made. The beam is centered at an angle of 65° to the ground just below the coronary band in a plane 65° medial or lateral to the mid-sagittal plane (25° from a lateral projection).

Radiographic Technique for Portable Unit (400 speed film-screen system)
- 80 kVp, 10 mA, 0.1 sec, 26 inches focal-film distance
- 80 kVp, 20 mA, 0.06 sec, 26 inches focal-film distance

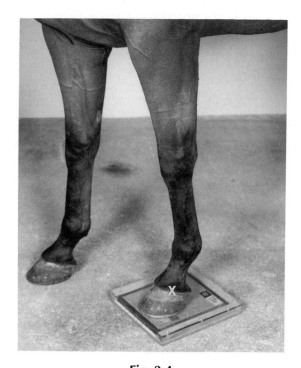

Fig. 2-4

Photograph showing the positioning of the foot used for the oblique view for the distal phalanx (dorsoproximolateral-palmarodistomedial). The foot is positioned on a cassette holder to provide protection for the cassette. The x-ray beam is angled 25° from lateral and is angled downward 65° from horizontal and centered (x) just distal to the coronary band one half the distance between the dorsal wall and the heels.

NAVICULAR BONE
(Distal Sesamoid Bone)

Radiography of the navicular bone is included in a soundness examination prior to purchase even in the absence of clinical signs. Therefore, it is most important that the radiographic study be of exceptional quality so that there is no opportunity that technical errors create radiographic shadows that may be misdiagnosed as a pathologic change or that prevent detection of abnormalities. Because of the small size of the navicular bone and its location, it is difficult to freely project the bone without having it superimposed over the adjacent middle and distal phalanges. Careful attention should be given to the proximodistal (flexor) study, since this is the only view in which most of the navicular bone is projected clearly without overlying bony shadows. The same possibility of an unencumbered projection applies to the lateral view, except in the presence of superimposed mineralization of the collateral ligaments of the distal phalanx, however it is less informative than the flexor view because of superimposition of bone tissue as the navicular bone is visualized 'on-end.'

A study of the navicular bone should not be attempted without first pulling the shoe and cleaning the foot using a brush and water as required. Trimming of the sole and hoof helps to remove tissue that creates unusual radio-graphic shadows. The sulci should be "opened-up" and trimmed sufficiently with a hoof knife to allow complete removal of debris with a hoof pick. This is done prior to packing the sulci with a material that has a density similar to the hoof wall (Fig.1-1), does not stick to the cassette or cassette holder, can be easily removed or cleaned from the sole after the examination, and does not cause the horse to slip when walking. We recommend a child's modeling compound called PLA-DOH (Rainbow Crafts, Cincinnati, Ohio 45202) because it has a uniform density that is equivalent to that of the hoof and may be easily packed into the sulci and other depressions in the sole. It is packed into the central as well as the lateral sulci of the frog and must stick to the sole and remain in position when the horse moves its foot during the examination. Pack the sulci so they are only 3/4 filled with the packing material to prevent it from sticking to the ground and pulling out when the horse moves. Also, gravel and dirt do not stick to the packing as easily when the sulci are not completely filled. Avoid trapping air in the packing material as it is pushed into the sulci since this creates prominent artifacts on the film. Between each view, repack the material with your thumb to insure that it remains deep within the sulci.

The dorsopalmar (plantar) views, made using two different angulations of the central beam, plus the lateral and the special flexor view complete the study. Oblique views that project the wings of the navicular bone free of overlying bony shadows can be made easily if necessary (Table 2-2).

The same radiographic technique is used for all of the studies except for the flexor view. In the flexor view, the technique is decreased because the focal-film distance is decreased and the amount and density of tissue that is penetrated by the primary beam is decreased. Identification required for study of the navicular bone includes: (1) right or left foot, (2) fore- or hindfoot, and (3) the lateral aspect of the foot.

Table 2-2
TECHNIQUE FOR RADIOGRAPHIC EVALUATION OF THE NAVICULAR BONE
(Distal Sesamoid Bone)

Standard views
  dorsopalmar (plantar) 45°
  dorsopalmar (plantar) 65°
  lateromedial
  proximodistal (flexor)
Optional views
  oblique
Views of the opposite limb
  degenerative changes of the navicular bone often involve both feet
  congenital anomalies often involve both feet
Cassette size
  small-sized cassettes (8 x 10 in, 18 x 24 cm) are satisfactory
Cassette holder
  special positioning blocks are necessary if using a horizontal beam (Oxspring positioning)
  cassette tunnel is necessary for weight-bearing studies
Grid
  not required but may be used, especially with a thick-footed horse
Collimation
  strict collimation required
  use of lead shield for dorsopalmar (plantar) views is recommended
Markers
  lateral
  right or left foot
  fore- or hindfoot

NAVICULAR BONE—
DORSOPALMAR (plantar) VIEW
(45° dorsoproximal-palmarodistal)

Purpose—The proximal border of the navicular bone is projected through the middle phalanx on this view permitting detection of new bone (enthesophytes) especially on the medial and lateral aspects of the proximal border.

Preparation—Preparation of the foot must be complete as described above.

Foot Positioning—The foot is either placed on a positioning block with the cassette in a slot in a near-vertical manner with the cassette against the bulbs of the heel (Fig. 2-5), or in a specially constructed positioning block with a slot that holds the cassette vertically. If the foot is placed in the special positioning blocks (Oxspring view), the cassette is positioned vertical to the ground and the x-ray beam is parallel to the ground making positioning of the hoof for these views more objective and thus easier for some people. However, these are not commonly used techniques in the United States.

Tube Positioning—The x-ray tube is positioned in front of the foot at a 45° angle to the ground with the x-ray beam within the mid-sagittal plane and centered just above the coronary band. It is important to notice the positioning of the foot, so that when the central beam is at a 45° angle to the ground, it is also at a 90° angle to the hoof wall.

Problems with the 45° dorsopalmar projection are often caused by the manner in which the hoof wall has been trimmed. If the heels are long, the foot axis is broken and the navicular bone is elevated changing its relationship with the middle and distal phalanges.

Radiographic Technique for Portable Unit (400 speed film-screen system)
- 80 kVp, 10 mA, 0.1 sec, 26 inches focal-film distance
- 80 kVp, 20 mA, 0.06 sec, 26 inches focal-film distance

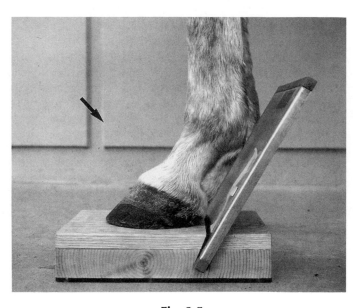

Fig. 2-5

Photograph of the positioning of the foot resting on a cassette holder with the cassette against the palmar aspect of the foot as would be used for making the 45° dorsopalmar study. The direction of the central beam is marked (arrow).

NAVICULAR BONE—
DORSOPALMAR (plantar) VIEW
(65° dorsoproximal-palmarodistal)

Purpose—This dorsopalmar view of the navicular bone creates a radiograph with apparent elevation of the navicular bone so that the distal border may be seen projected through the distal and palmar (plantar) portion of the middle phalanx.

Preparation—Must be complete as described above.

Foot Positioning—The foot is positioned on a cassette tunnel placed flat on the ground or floor (Fig. 2-6). If the foot is placed in the special positioning blocks (Oxspring view), the cassette is positioned vertical to the ground and the x-ray beam is parallel to the ground.

Tube Positioning—The x-ray tube is placed in front of the foot with the x-ray beam directed within the mid-sagittal plane. The beam is centered at a point 1 in (2.5 cm) proximal to the coronary band. If you are placing the foot on a cassette tunnel for this view, the central beam is directed at a 65° angle to the ground and is approximately 110° to the hoof wall. If special positioning blocks are used, the x-ray beam is directed parallel to the ground.

Major problems in obtaining this view of the navicular bone involve the angulation of the x-ray beam and the effect of improper trimming of the hoof wall on the rela-tionship between the hoof and the cassette.

> Radiographic Technique for Portable Unit (400 speed film-screen system)
> - 80 kVp, 10 mA, 0.12 sec, 26 inches focal-film distance
> - 80 kVp, 20 mA, 0.06-0.08 sec, 26 inches focal-film distance

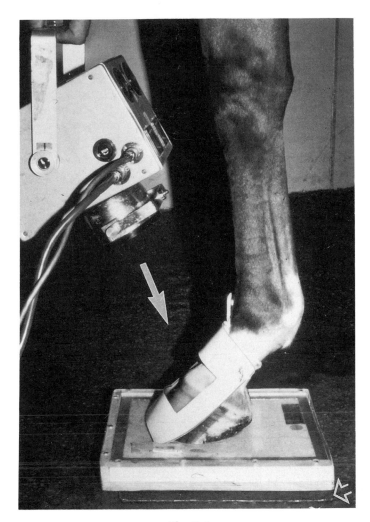

Fig. 2-6
Photograph of the positioning of the foot resting on a cassette holder as required for the 65° dorsopalmar view showing the use of a lead shield ("navicular mask") and a lead sheet under the cassette tunnel (hollow white arrow) that assist in limiting the amount of scatter radiation that can fog the radiograph in a study of the navicular bone. The direction of the x-ray beam (arrow) is shown.

NAVICULAR BONE—LATERAL VIEW
(lateromedial)

Purpose—This view assists in evaluation of change in the shape of the bone that is often associated with chronic degenerative changes of navicular disease.

Preparation—Preparation for this single view is not a special problem and involves only the washing or brushing of the hoof wall.

Tube Positioning—The foot is positioned on a wooden block that provides sufficient elevation so the x-ray beam can be directed in a horizontal plane. The x-ray tube is positioned lateral to the foot (Fig. 2-7). It is convenient if the positioning block has a slot to hold the cassette. It is also possible to position the cassette on the floor adjacent to the medial side of the positioning block.

Tube Positioning—The x-ray beam is directed to a point in the center of the coronary band above the bulbs of the heel.

Radiographic Technique for Portable Unit (400 speed film-screen system)
- 80 kVp, 10 mA, 0.12 sec, 24-26 inches focal-film distance
- 80 kVp, 20 mA, 0.06 sec, 24-26 inches focal-film distance

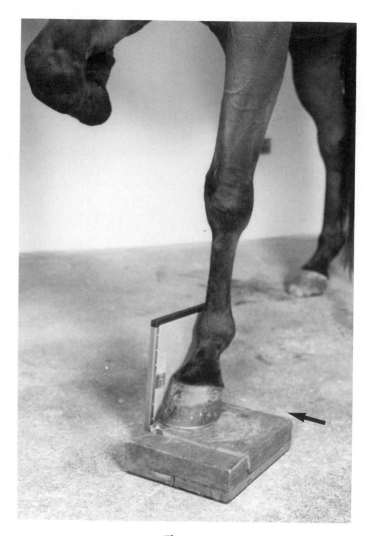

Fig. 2-7
Photograph of the positioning of the foot used for making the lateral view of the navicular bone. The foot is elevated on a positioning block and the central beam (arrow) is directed in a horizontal direction centered just below the coronary band.

NAVICULAR BONE—
PALMAROPROXIMAL-PALMARODISTAL VIEW
(flexor or skyline view)

This should be the first view made in the navicular series since the radiographic study is probably being performed just after the horse has received a nerve block as part of the physical examination. In the event of navicular disease, the local anesthetic makes it possible to pull the foot in a caudal direction required for the flexor view. After the effect of the anesthetic has worn off, it may be more painful for the foot to be positioned correctly for this important view.

Purpose—The width of the flexor cortex as it interfaces with the more lucent medullary cavity and the size and shape of the ridge on the flexor surface can be evaluated along with the character of the medullary cavity.

Preparation—Preparation includes the earlier described care given to cleaning the sole and sulci of the foot.

Foot Positioning—The cassette is placed on the ground within a protective tunnel and the foot is placed on the cassette (Fig. 2-8). If the forefoot is being examined, the foot should be placed as far back under the horse as is possible with the fetlock joint in an extended position. This positions the middle phalanx nearly vertical. If the hindfoot is to be examined, positioning the foot caudally is extremely difficult and can be hazardous to both x-ray equipment and radiographer. Therefore, you may have to be content with making this view of the hindfoot with the horse standing in a nearly normal manner.

Tube Positioning—In radiography of either fore- or hindfoot, the x-ray tube is positioned directly behind the distal-palmar (plantar) portion of the fetlock joint, and the focal-film distance is decreased to 18 to 20 inches (45 to 50 cm). The beam is directed along the palmar (plantar) surface of the digit within the mid-sagittal plane and is centered between the bulbs of the heel. The angle of the central beam is directed in the same plane as the flexor cortex. The field of exposure should be made as small as possible. The radiographic technique is altered because of the change in focal-film distance.

Radiographic Technique for Portable Unit (400 speed film-screen system)
- 80 kVp, 10 mA, 0.08 sec, 20 inches focal-film distance
- 80 kVp, 20 mA, 0.04 sec, 20 inches focal-film distance

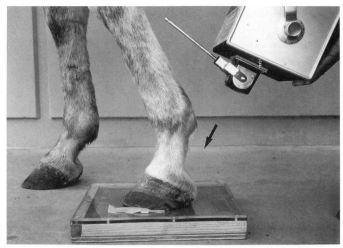

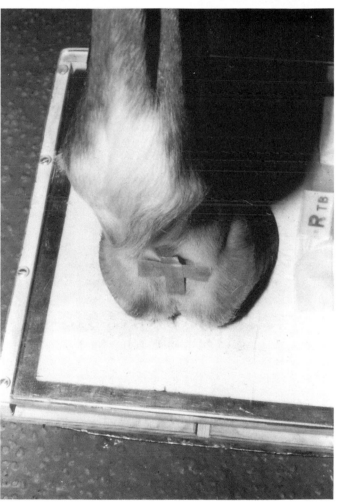

Fig. 2-8
Photographs shows the positioning of the foot used to obtain the flexor view of the navicular bone. The foot is positioned on a cassette tunnel to provide protection for the cassette and is drawn as far caudally as is possible. The x-ray beam (arrow) is angled cranially and is centered between the bulbs of the heels (x). Focal-film distance is decreased for this view.

NAVICULAR BONE—OBLIQUE VIEWS
(65° dorsoproximolateral-palmarodistomedial
or
65° dorsoproximomedial-palmarodistolateral)

Purpose—The oblique studies cause the wings to be projected in such a way that they are not superimposed over adjacent bones and permit more accurate evaluation of fractures in this part of the navicular bone.

Preparation—Preparation of the foot is the same as described above.

Foot Positioning—The cassette is placed on the ground, preferably within a cassette tunnel, and the foot is placed directly on the cassette with the angle to be projected closer to the edge of the cassette.

Tube Positioning—The x-ray tube is positioned in front of the foot and to the medial or lateral side depending on which oblique is being made. The beam is centered on the coronary band toward the side that is being examined. The x-ray beam is directed downward at an angle of 65° to the ground and is in a plane 65° medial or lateral from the mid-sagittal plane or 25° from a lateral position. This is the same positioning used for the oblique view of the third phalanx but with a heavier radiographic technique.

Radiographic Technique for Portable Unit (400 speed film-screen system)
- 80 kVp, 10 mA, 0.12 sec, 26 inches focal-film distance
- 80 kVp, 20 mA, 0.08 sec, 26 inches focal-film distance

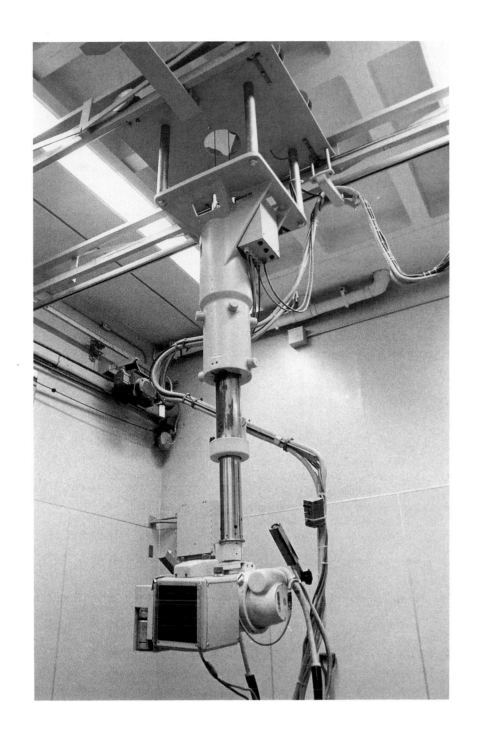

3. FORELIMB
PASTERN JOINT
(Proximal Interphalangeal Joint)

Studies of the phalangeal area include the proximal (os compedale) and middle (os coronale) phalanges and center on the proximal interphalangeal joint (pastern joint) but often include the metacarpophalangeal joint (fetlock joint) and distal interphalangeal joint (coffin joint) as well. The suspensory ligament, the common digital extensor tendon, the lateral digital extensor tendon, the proximal digital annular ligament, the distal digital annular ligament, the superficial digital flexor tendon, the short sesamoidean ligaments, the deep or cruciate sesamoidean ligaments, the middle or oblique sesamoidean ligament, the superficial or straight sesamoidean ligament, and the collateral ligaments all attach to these bones and enthesophyte production at the site of the attachments is often secondary to chronic injury.

This is a relatively easy study to perform, and errors in positioning are minimal and usually related to conformational problems in the patient. It is suggested that the foot be placed on a positioning block so that both interphalangeal joints can be seen on the radiograph.

Physes are present in the proximal ends of the proximal and middle phalanges and close between 6 to 9 months of age, and comparison views of the opposite limb are indicated in young foals. Comparison studies permit evaluation of physeal closure and avoid the erroneous diagnosis of developmental disease in normal patients.

Identification of the film requires marking right or left and fore- or hindfoot. The lateral aspect should be identified consistently by the use of one of these markers (Table 3-1).

Table 3-1
TECHNIQUE FOR RADIOGRAPHIC EVALUATION OF THE PASTERN (proximal interphalangeal) JOINT

Routine views
  dorsopalmar
  lateral

Optional views
  obliques

Views of the opposite limb
  required under 9-months of age

Cassette size
  small cassette (8 x 10 in, 18 x 24 cm)

Cassette holder
  required to decrease the incidence of radiation exposure

Grids
  not needed

Film markers
  lateral
  right or left foot
  fore- or hindfoot

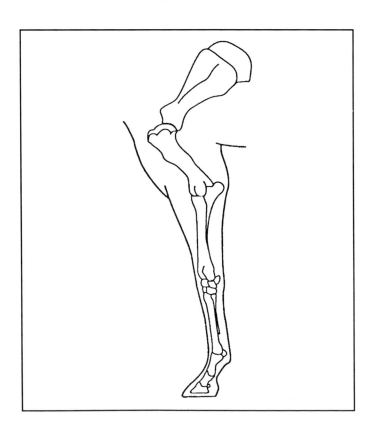

PASTERN JOINT—DORSOPALMAR VIEW
(45° dorsoproximal-palmarodistal)

Purpose—This view is a standard part of the study used to evaluate causes of forelimb lameness.

Preparation—No specific preparation of the digit is required except for brushing the hair coat.

Foot Positioning—The foot is positioned on the ground or on a positioning block with the cassette positioned close behind the digit and held in a cassette holder or in a slot in the positioning block (Fig. 3-1). The horse is weight bearing with the opposite forefoot elevated.

Tube Positioning—The x-ray tube is placed in front of the digit with the central beam directed within the midsagittal plane. The angle of the beam is dependent on the positioning of the foot, but is usually between 30° and 45° to the ground. Attempt to place the foot so the x-ray beam is perpendicular to the foot axis. The beam is centered on the proximal interphalangeal joint or a point of interest.

Radiographic Technique for portable unit (400 speed film-screen system)
- 80 kVp, 10 mA, 0.1 sec, 26 inches focal-film distance
- 80 kVp, 20 mA, 0.06 sec, 26 inches focal-film distance

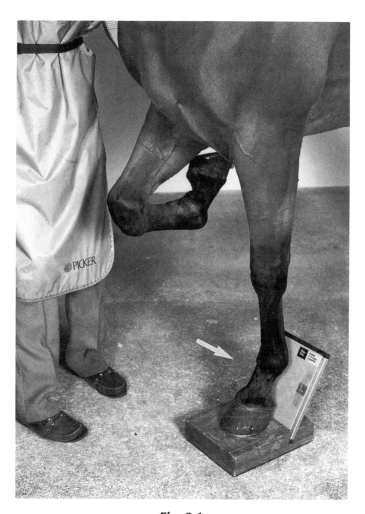

Fig. 3-1
Photograph of the positioning of the foot resting on a cassette holder with the cassette behind the foot for the dorsopalmar views of the pastern region. The central beam is identified (arrow). Note the use of the slot in the wooden positioning block in positioning the cassette thus alleviating the need for someone to hold the cassette.

PASTERN JOINT—LATERAL VIEW
(lateromedial)

Purpose—In addition to learning of the character of the bone and joints in the digit, the lateral view provides valuable information on the character of the foot axis.

Preparation—No special preparation is required except for brushing the hair coat.

Foot Positioning—The x-ray beam must be parallel to the ground as it is centered on the digit as the foot may need to be elevated by placing it on a wooden block (Fig. 3-2). View the foot from the front to ensure that medial or lateral angulation of the digit is not present. If there is a conformational problem, it may require subsequent angulation of the x-ray beam to insure that the digit is projected correctly.

Tube Positioning—The x-ray tube is positioned laterally and the beam is centered on the proximal interphalangeal joint or point of interest.

Radiographic Technique for Portable Unit (400 speed film-screen system)
- 80 kVp, 10 mA, 0.1 sec, 26 inches focal-film distance
- 80 kVp, 20 mA, 0.06 sec, 26 inches focal-film distance

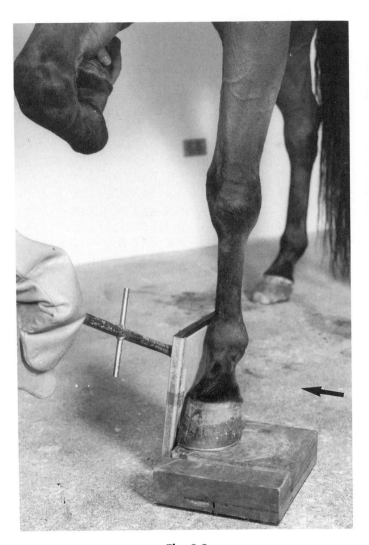

Fig. 3-2
Photograph of the positioning of the foot resting on a positioning block with the cassette against the medial aspect of the foot for the lateromedial view of the pastern region. The central beam is identified (arrow). Note the use of the cassette holder in positioning the cassette.

PASTERN JOINT—OBLIQUE VIEWS
(dorsoproximomedial-palmarodistolateral or dorsoproximolateral-palmarodistomedial)

Purpose—Oblique views are necessary to detect areas of new bone production that are located medially and laterally from the dorsal or palmar borders of the phalanges and to show periarticular new bone formation around the interphalangeal joints.

Preparation—No special preparation is required.

Foot Positioning—The foot is positioned in a similar manner as used for the dorsopalmar (plantar) view. The foot may be resting on the ground or on a wooden block.

Tube Positioning—The x-ray beam is angled downward at an angle of 45° to the ground so that the central beam is perpendicular to the foot axis and is centered on the proximal interphalangeal joint or point of interest (Figs. 3-3, 3-4). The tube is rotated 30° from the mid-sagittal plane medially or laterally and 60° from the lateral direction.

> Radiographic Technique for Portable Unit (400 speed film-screen system)
> • 80 kVp, 10 mA, 0.1 sec, 26 inches focal-film distance
> • 80 kVp, 20 mA, 0.06 sec, 26 inches focal-film distance

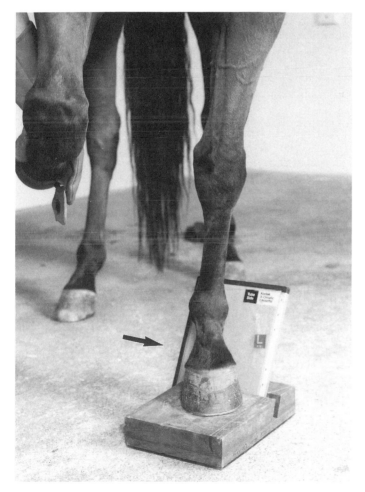

Fig. 3-3
Photograph of the positioning of the foot resting on a positioning block with the cassette behind the foot prior to making the dorsomedioproximal-palmarolaterodistal oblique view of the pastern region. The central beam is identified (arrow). Note the use of the slot in the wooden positioning block in positioning the cassette thus alleviating the need for someone to hold the cassette.

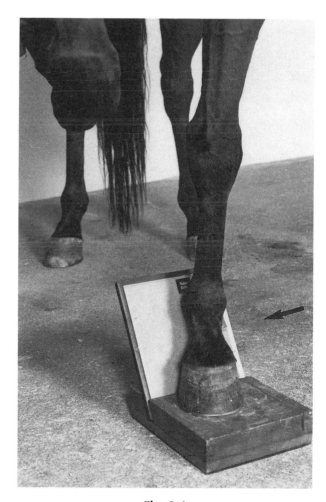

Fig. 3-4
Photograph of the positioning of the foot resting on a positioning block with the cassette behind the foot prior to making the dorsolateroproximal-palmaromediodistal oblique view of the pastern region. The central beam is identified (arrow). Note the use of the slot in the wooden positioning block in positioning the cassette thus alleviating the need for someone to hold the cassette.

FETLOCK JOINT AND
(Metacarpo-metatarso-phalangeal joint)
and PROXIMAL SESAMOID BONES

Radiographic examination of the metacarpo-phalangeal or metatarsophalangeal joints permits evaluation of: (1) the character of the articular surfaces of these bones, (2) the width of the joint spaces, (3) the nature of the subchondral bone, and (4) the presence of periarticular new bone. The study also includes the proximal sesamoid bones that appear as paired triangular shaped bones located palmar (plantar) to the fetlock joint. They play an integral part in the structure and function of the suspensory apparatus, as well as of the fetlock joint. Their cartilaginous surfaces articulate with the palmar (plantar) aspect of the distal articular surface of the third metacarpal (tarsal) bone. They position the superficial and deep flexor tendons away from the center of rotation of the fetlock joint increasing the force these tendons can exert on the fetlock joint and give stabilization to the angulation of these flexor tendons which pass between their axial and abaxial borders.

The ligaments that attach to the proximal sesamoid bones include: (1) deep or cruciate, (2) middle or oblique, (3) superficial or straight, (4) intersesamoidean, and (5) collateral. All of these have the possibility of having their attachments to the sesamoid bones torn with resulting enthesophyte formation. While clinical signs related to joint disease may be different from those associated with the proximal sesamoid bones, the radiographic examination is essentially the same for both anatomical structures with several noted exceptions. The distal tips of the second and fourth metacarpal (metatarsal) bones are usually seen on the radiographs of the fetlock region.

The radiographic views commonly used to examine this region include: (1) dorsopalmar, (2) lateral extended, (3) lateral flexed, and (4) oblique views. The 125° dorso-palmar view of the distal metacarpal (tarsal) bone and flexor studies of the proximal sesamoid bones are additional views. Angles for the dorsopalmar, lateral, and oblique views are illustrated (Fig. 3-5). Radiographic technique uses a standard focal-film distance dependent on the x-ray unit, except for a decreased distance for the flexor studies.

Preparation of the patient is relatively easy requiring only brushing of the ankle. Film identification requires indicating whether the limb is right or left and fore- or hind. Although the difference in appearance of the proximal sesamoid bones permits identification of medial or lateral sides, it is still helpful to mark these sides (Table 3-2). The studies are usually made weight bearing except for the flexed lateral and the 125° dorsopalmar view.

The distal physis of the third metacarpal (metatarsal) bone closes between 6 and 12 months while the proximal physis of the first phalanx closes between 6 and 9 months. The proximal sesamoid bones each form from a single ossification center. Growth plates in the hindlimbs close at a slightly older age than in the forelimbs.

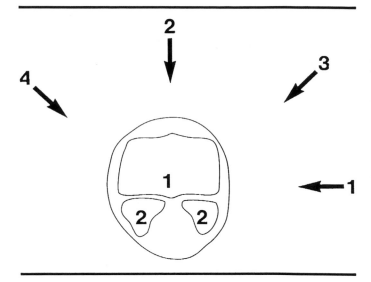

Fig. 3-5
Cross sectional drawing of the distal metacarpal (tarsal) bone (1) and the proximal sesamoid bones (2) showing x-ray beam direction for: (1) lateral (lateromedial), (2) dorsopalmar, (3) medial (dorsolateral-palmaromedial) oblique, and (4) lateral (dorsomedial-palmarolateral) oblique views.

Table 3-2
TECHNIQUE FOR RADIOGRAPHIC EVALUATION OF THE FETLOCK
(Metacarpo-metatarso-phalangeal) JOINT
AND THE PROXIMAL SESAMOID BONES

Standard views
  dorsopalmar
  lateromedial, extended
  lateromedial, flexed
  obliques
Optional views
  dorsopalmar made with a horizontal beam
  125° dorsopalmar distal metacarpal (tarsal) bone
  proximodistal (flexor) studies of the proximal sesamoid bones
  distal third metacarpal (tarsal) bone, extensor view or skyline view
Studies of opposite limb
  under the age of 12 months
Cassette size
  small cassette (8 x 10 in, 18 x 24 cm)
Cassette holders
  use separately or built into positioning block
Grid
  not necessary
Film markers
  lateral
  right or left limb
  fore- or hindlimb

FETLOCK JOINT—DORSOPALMAR (plantar) VIEW (45° dorsoproximal-palmarodistal)

Purpose—Both fetlock joint and the proximal sesamoid bones are seen on this view and the technique may be altered slightly if greater penetration is required to visualize the proximal sesamoid bones. The medial sesamoid bone appears as a full triangle while the lateral sesamoid bone has a shorter rounded apex.

Preparation—Only brushing of the ankle is required.

Foot Positioning—The foot is placed on the ground with the cassette positioned against the palmar (plantar) surface (Fig. 3-6) or on a positioning block with the horse fully weight-bearing. If motion of the foot is a problem, the opposite foot can be elevated. Recognize the potential for an artifactually produced alteration in width of the joint space due to altered weight-bearing. This degree of joint narrowing that commonly occurs at the lateral portion of the fetlock joint can be misinterpreted as disease.

Tube Positioning—The x-ray tube is placed in front of the foot and the cassette is held in contact with the digit. The x-ray beam is directed in the mid-sagittal plane at a right angle to the foot axis and centered at the fetlock joint. The angle with the ground depends on the position of the foot but is usually less than 45° from horizontal (greater than 45° from vertical).

Some radiographers prefer to have the cassette vertical and use a horizontal x-ray beam centered on the fetlock joint that results in projection of the distal palmar aspect of the articular surface of the metacarpal (tarsal) bone. This is not a recommended technique since it results in an oblique projection of the proximal phalanx, but it may be helpful as a second dorsopalmar view.

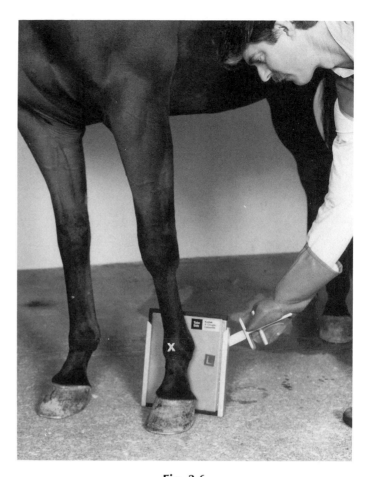

Fig. 3-6
Photograph of the positioning of the foot on the ground prior to making the dorsopalmar view of the fetlock joint. The point of centering of the central beam (X) is marked.

Radiographic Technique for Portable Unit (400 speed film-screen system)
- 80 kVp, 10 mA, 0.1 sec, 26 inches focal-film distance
- 80 kVp, 20 mA, 0.06 sec, 26 inches focal-film distance

FETLOCK JOINT—DORSOPALMAR (plantar) VIEW (dorsodistal-palmarproximal)

Purpose—Lesions on the palmar (plantar) surface of the distal metacarpal (tarsal) bone can be evaluated by this view. Because of the unique positioning of the horse's foot that is required, special consideration should be given to radiation safety.

Preparation—Care must be used in positioning the assistant for this study and strict collimation of the beam is required, since it is relatively easy for the assistant to be near the primary x-ray beam.

Foot Positioning—The foot is elevated by holding it in your hand or positioning it on a wooden block. The cassette is held in a short handled cassette holder that is placed against the palmar (plantar) surface of the joint (Fig. 3-7).

Tube Positioning—The x-ray tube is positioned in front of the limb and the cassette positioned against the palmar (plantar surface). Determination of the angle of the x-ray beam is made easier by relating it to the long axis of the metacarpal (metatarsal) bone. The angle of the x-ray beam is usually near parallel to the ground and it is centered on the fetlock joint.

This view can also be made in a palmarodorsal (plantarodorsal) direction. The foot is placed on the ground, the x-ray tube is positioned behind the foot, and the central beam is directed proximopalmar-distodorsal at an angle of 110° toward the ground. The cassette is positioned in a vertical manner just in front of the foot.

Radiographic Technique for Portable Unit (400 speed film-screen system)
- 80 kVp, 10 mA, 0.16 sec, 26 inches focal-film distance
- 80 kVp, 20 mA, 0.08 sec, 26 inches focal-film distance

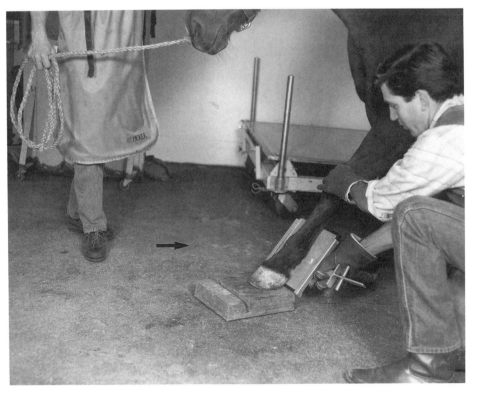

Fig. 3-7
Photograph of the positioning of the foot prior to making the dorsodistal-palmaroproximal view of the fetlock joint. The direction of the central x-ray beam for this view is usually horizontal to the ground but dependent on foot positioning. Use of a cassette holder and strict beam collimation is important in this view. The direction of the 110° angled central x-ray beam (arrow) is marked.

FETLOCK JOINT—LATERAL EXTENDED VIEW
(lateromedial)

Purpose—This view permits determination of the distopalmar (distoplantar) contour of the distal metacarpal bone and especially allows evaluation of the palmar (plantar) aspect of the proximal sesamoid bones.

Preparation—There is no special preparation of the patient other than brushing.

Foot Positioning—The horse is fully weight bearing on the affected limb with the foot placed on the ground or on a positioning block with the cassette against the medial aspect of the joint. The cassette can be in a holder resting on the ground or in a slot in a wooden positioning block. Lift the opposite foot to control motion if necessary (Fig. 3-8).

Tube Positioning—The x-ray tube is positioned directly lateral to the foot with the x-ray beam within a frontal plane through the middle of the limb parallel to the ground. The x-ray beam is directed toward the joint.

Radiographic Technique for Portable Unit (400 speed film-screen system)
- 80 kVp, 10 mA, 0.1 sec, 26 inches focal-film distance
- 80 kVp, 20 mA, 0.06 sec, 26 inches focal-film distance

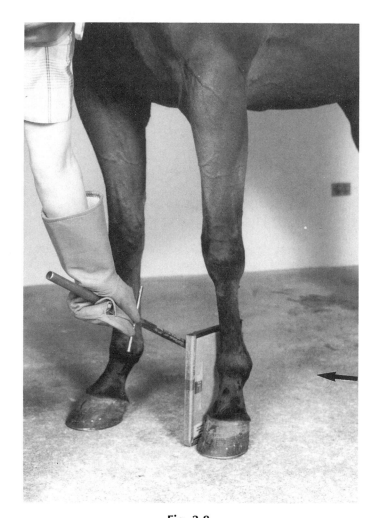

Fig. 3-8
Photograph of the positioning of the foot on the ground preparatory to making the lateromedial view of the fetlock joint. The direction of the central x-ray beam is marked (arrow). It may be helpful with some patients to lift the opposite foot.

FETLOCK JOINT—LATERAL FLEXED VIEW
(lateromedial)

Purpose—The flexed view is especially important since the proximal sesamoid bones are shifted in a proximopalmar (plantar) direction relative to the distal end of the third metacarpal (tarsal) bone and good evaluation of the articular surfaces of these bones is possible. The distal articular surface of the metacarpal (tarsal) bone is more completely evaluated on this view.

Preparation—No special preparation is required

Foot Positioning—The foot is held off the ground at the level of the opposite carpus (tarsus). The fetlock joint is flexed as completely as possible (Fig. 3-9). There is a tendency for the foot to roll medially under the horse. To compensate for this, the foot must be moved laterally or the x-ray beam angled slightly upward. Position the cassette medially using a cassette holder. It is also possible to make this view by resting the dorsum of the foot against a wooden block, however, the degree of flexion is not as great.

Tube Positioning—Position the x-ray machine lateral to the leg and direct the x-ray beam parallel to the ground centering the beam on the fetlock joint or on the proximal sesamoid bones.

> Radiographic Technique for portable unit (400 speed film-screen system)
> • 80 kVp, 10 mA, 0.1 sec, 26 inches focal-film distance
> • 80 kVp, 20 mA, 0.06 sec, 26 inches focal-film distance

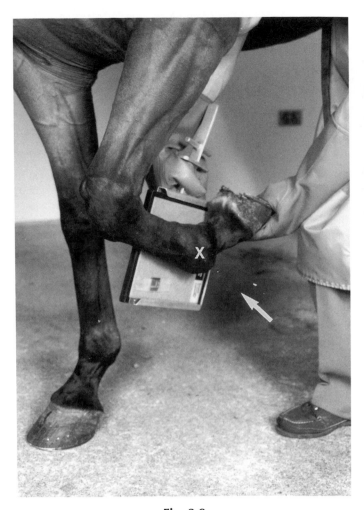

Fig. 3-9
Photograph of the positioning of the foot used to make the flexed lateromedial view of the fetlock joint. The direction of the central x-ray beam (arrow) and point of centering (x) are shown.

FETLOCK JOINT—OBLIQUE VIEWS— (30° dorsolateral-palmaromedial [plantar] or 30° dorsomedial-palmarolateral [plantar])

Purpose—These oblique studies are essential in providing additional views to evaluate the medial and lateral aspects of the dorsal periarticular surfaces of the proximal phalanx, the medial and lateral palmar (plantar) protuberances of the proximal phalanx, and the abaxial surfaces of the proximal sesamoid bones.

Preparation—No special preparation is required except for brushing.

Foot Positioning—The foot is positioned on the ground or on a positioning block with the cassette placed against the lateral aspect of the palmar (plantar) surface for the lateral oblique view (Fig. 3-10) and with the cassette placed against the medial aspect of the palmar (plantar) surface for the medial oblique view (Fig. 3-11). The cassette is held in a cassette holder (Fig. 3-10) or in a slot in the positioning block (Fig. 3-11).

Tube Positioning—The x-ray tube is shifted 45° from the mid-sagittal plane in either medial or lateral direction and is at an angle of 30° to the ground. The central beam is directed at the joint or at the proximal sesamoid bones depending on the area of interest.

> Radiographic Technique for Portable Unit (400 speed film-screen system)
> - 80 kVp, 10 mA, 0.1 sec, 26 inches focal-film distance
> - 80 kVp, 20 mA, 0.06 sec, 26 inches focal-film distance

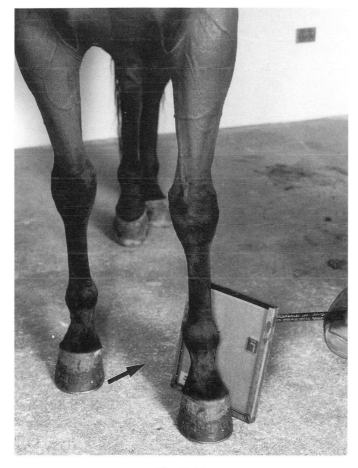

Fig. 3-10
Photograph of the positioning of the foot prior to making the dorsomedial-palmarolateral (lateral) oblique view of the fetlock joint using a positioning block. The direction (arrow) and point of centering of the central x-ray beam are marked.

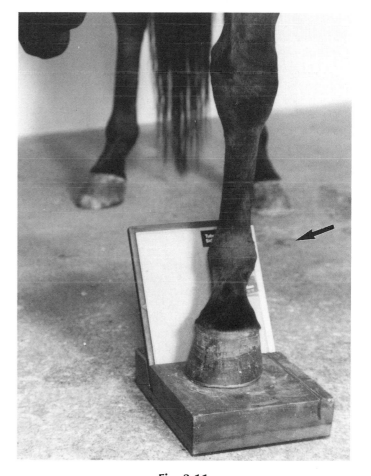

Fig. 3-11
Photograph of the positioning of the foot prior to making the dorsolateral-palmaromedial (medial) oblique view of the fetlock joint using a positioning block. The direction (arrow) and point of centering of the central x-ray beam are shown.

PROXIMAL SESAMOID BONES—
PROXIMOPALMAR-DISTOPALMAR VIEWS
(flexor surface or skyline views)

Purpose—This view has value in examination of both fore- and hindlimbs. It frees the sesamoid bones from overlying bony shadows and has value in the detection of non-displaced sesamoid fractures or in the detection of bony response resulting from tearing of the suspensory ligament attachments from the sesamoid bones.

Preparation—No special preparation is required.

Foot Positioning—The forefoot is placed as far back under the horse as is comfortable while the hindfoot is placed behind the horse. The cassette is placed on the ground in a protecting tunnel and the foot is placed on the tunnel (Fig. 3-12).

Tube Positioning—The x-ray tube is positioned directly behind the palmar (plantar) surface of the metacarpal (metatarsal) bones. The focal-film distance is decreased to 20 inches (50 cm). The beam is directed perpendicular to the ground and centered between the proximal sesamoid bones.

Positioning of the foot and tube is difficult in a study of the forelimb because of being positioned under the horse. While easier to position the foot and tube in a study of the hindlimb, there is danger in being positioned directly behind the horse.

This study can also be made using an oblique view with the tube shifted either medially or laterally and the beam angled so that it passes tangentially along the abaxial surface of the proximal sesamoid bone of interest.

Radiographic Technique for Portable Unit (400 speed film-screen system)
- 80 kVp, 10 mA, 0.1 sec, 20 inches focal-film distance
- 80 kVp, 20 mA, 0.06 sec, 20 inches focal-film distance

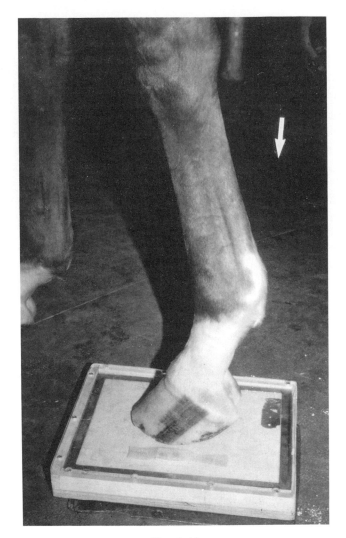

Fig. 3-12

Photograph of the positioning of the foot used to make the skyline view of the proximal sesamoid bones. The direction of the nearly vertical central x-ray beam (arrow) is marked. It is important to have the foot positioned as far caudally as possible to force the sesamoid bones into a position where a tangential view can be obtained. Focal-film distance is decreased for this view.

DISTAL THIRD METACARPAL (Tarsal) BONE—PROXIMODORSAL-DISTODORSAL VIEW (Extensor Surface or Skyline View)

Purpose—This view provides a method for better visualization of lesions just dorsal to the distal end of the third metacarpal bone and the view is essential in providing information for the evaluation of soft tissue mineralization or to detect the character of intra-articular fracture lines that involve the distal metacarpal bone.

Preparation—No special preparation is required.

Foot Positioning—The fetlock joint is fully flexed and the leg positioned slightly forward. The cassette is held against the dorsal surface of the proximal phalanx. Flexion forces the dorsodistal portion of the third metacarpal bone so that it can be studied tangentially (Fig. 3-13). While the study can be performed on the hindlimb, positioning is much more difficult.

Tube Positioning—The x-ray tube is positioned directly above the distal end of the third metacarpal (metatarsal) bone and the focal-film distance is decreased to 20 inches (50 cm). The beam is directed nearly perpendicular to the ground and centered on the dorsodistal end of the third metacarpal (tarsal) bone.

> Radiographic Technique for Portable Unit (400 speed film-screen system)
> • 80 kVp, 10 mA, 0.1 sec, 20 inches focal-film distance
> • 80 kVp, 20 mA, 0.06 sec, 20 inches focal-film distance

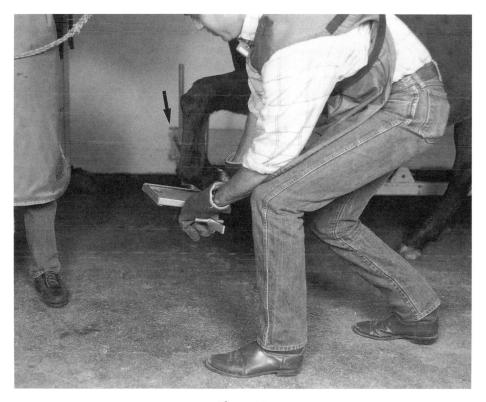

Fig. 3-13
Photograph of positioning of the foot used to make the skyline view of the dorsal surface of the distal end of the third metacarpal (tarsal) bone. The direction of the nearly vertical central x-ray beam (arrow) is marked. It is important to have the fetlock joint fully flexed and positioned cranially as far as is possible to permit projection of the dorsodistal end of the cannon bone. Focal-film distance is decreased for this view.

METACARPAL BONES

This study is often made to evaluate the status of the second and fourth metacarpal bones as well as the larger third metacarpal bone. Usually, the proximal portions of the metacarpal bones are included with the carpal radiographic studies and the distal portions are included with the fetlock studies.

In addition to the dorsopalmar and lateral views, oblique views are of especial value in the examination of the second and fourth metacarpal bones (Fig. 3-14). While the one oblique view projects a splint bone free of superimposed third metacarpal bone, the opposite splint bone is also well evaluated on the same view since it is projected through the uniformly dense medullary cavity of the third metacarpal bone. The second metacarpal bone is larger than the fourth metacarpal bone (Fig. 3-15).

Evaluation of the carpo-metacarpal articulations is important. The second metacarpal bone articulates with the third metacarpal bone and the second and third carpal bones. The fourth metacarpal bone articulates with the third metacarpal bone and the fourth carpal bone.

A different sized cassette is frequently used in radiography of the metacarpal bones. It is best to use a 7 x 17 inch (17 x 43 cm) cassette or to divide a 14 x 17 inch (35 x 43 cm) cassette. The cassette holder may have a leg attached to assist in positioning the heavier cassette without movement during the exposure (Table 3-3). Con-sidering the shortened focal-film distances recommended for use with portable units, it is likely that if the lead aperature if left is position, the radiation field will not cover the length of the cassette.

Cleanliness of the area is not as critical as it was in the examination of more distal portions of the limb. Still it is advisable to brush the leg to remove scurf that creates film artifacts.

Most of these studies are made with the horse weight-bearing without use of any special positioning devices. To ensure there is no motion in the leg being radiographed, it may be necessary to lift the opposite forefoot. If the carpal bones are included in the study, familiarity with the appearance of the carpal bones eliminates the need for a lateral marker or marker identifying the fore- or hindlimbs. It is of value to mark a region of soft tissue swelling, point tenderness, or a small draining tract with a small radiographic marker such as a lead "BB."

The third metacarpal bone forms from two epiphyseal and one diaphyseal ossification centers. The proximal physis closes prior to birth, the distal physeal growth plate closes between 9 and 12 months of age. The second and fourth metacarpal bones have a distal ossification center for the tip or "button" that begins to ossify at 3 months and may remain ununited until during the second year of age. This "button" can be mistaken for a fracture fragment.

Table 3-3
TECHNIQUE FOR RADIOGRAPHIC EVALUATION OF THE METACARPAL BONES

Standard views
  dorsopalmar
  lateromedial
  obliques
Optional views
  cone-down oblique views
Studies of the opposite limb
  until 12-15 months of age
Cassette size
  long enough to include the entire limb
Cassette holders
  specially constructed holders for longer cassettes
Grids
  not necessary
Markers
  lateral
  right or left limb
  fore- or hindlimb

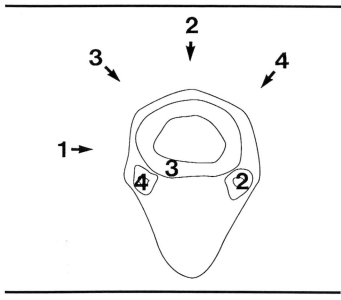

Fig. 3-14
Drawing of a cross-section of the metacarpal region with the second (2), third (3), and fourth (4) metacarpal bones labeled. The arrows show the direction of the x-ray beam for the lateromedial (1), dorsopalmar (2), medial (dorsolateral-palmaromedial) oblique (3), and lateral (dorsomedial-palmarolateral) oblique (4) views of this area.

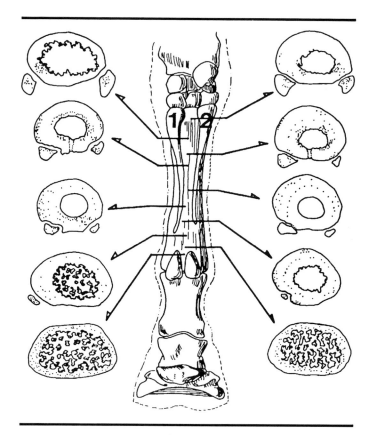

Fig. 3-15
Drawing of the metacarpal region with multiple cross sections that illustrate the relationship of the medial (1) and lateral (2) splint bones with the cannon bone throughout the length of the limb. Note the difficulty in selecting an exact angle for making the oblique views that projects the splint bones without any superimposition by the cannon bone throughout their length.

METACARPAL BONES—
DORSOPALMAR VIEW

Purpose—This standard view should include either the joint proximal or the joint distal to the cannon bone for orientation, or preferably both joints.

Preparation—No special preparation is required other than brushing.

Foot Positioning—The cassette is held against the palmar aspect of the leg in a holder that may include a leg that rests on the ground. The use of a cassette of sufficient length to include the entire bone is helpful.

Tube Positioning—The x-ray tube is positioned in front of the leg, and the central beam is directed parallel to the ground in the mid-sagittal plane and centered on the mid-portion of the metacarpal region or the point of interest (Fig. 3-16).

Radiographic Technique for Portable Unit (400 speed film-screen system)
- 80 kVp, 10 mA, 0.16 sec, 26 inches focal-film distance
- 80 kVp, 20 mA, 0.08 sec, 26 inches focal-film distance

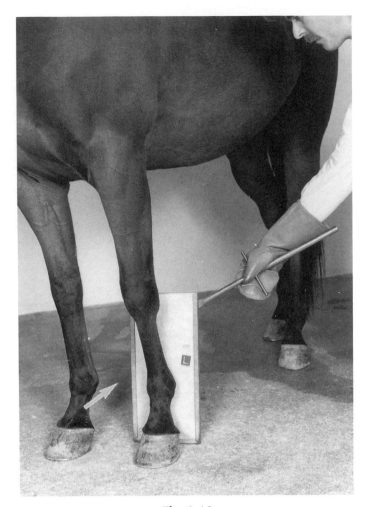

Fig. 3-16
Photograph of the positioning of the forelimb used to make the dorsopalmar view of the metacarpal region. The x-ray beam is centered on the mid-portion of the cannon bone, parallel to the ground, and is within the mid-sagittal plane (arrow). The cassette holder may be rested on the ground or held off the ground depending on the size of the horse, size of the cassette, and the area of greatest interest clinically. A cassette holder is helpful in performing this study.

METACARPAL BONES—
LATERAL VIEW (lateromedial)

Purpose—This is one of the standard orthogonal views for examination of the metacarpal region.

Preparation—No special preparation is required other than brushing.

Foot Positioning—The cassette is held against the medial aspect of the leg in a holder that may use a leg that contacts the ground or the cassette may rest on the ground in examination of a smaller horse.

Tube Positioning—The x-ray tube is positioned lateral to the leg, and the central beam is directed parallel to the ground in the frontal plane and centered on the mid-portion of the metacarpal region (Fig. 3-17).

Radiographic Technique for portable unit (400 speed film-screen system)
- 80 kVp, 10 mA, 0.1 sec, 26 inches focal-film distance
- 80 kVp, 20 mA, 0.06 sec, 26 inches focal-film distance

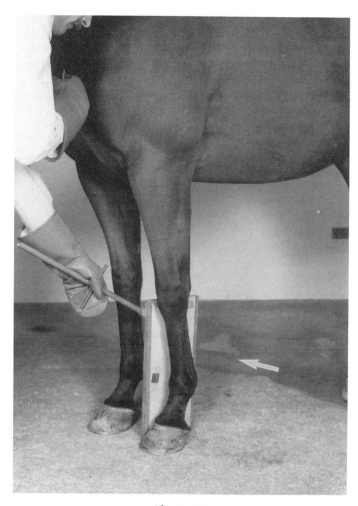

Fig. 3-17
Photograph of the positioning of the forelimb used to make the lateromedial view of the metacarpal region. The x-ray beam is centered on the mid-portion of the cannon bone, is parallel to the ground, and is within the frontal plane (arrow). The cassette holder may rest on the ground or be held off the ground depending on the size of the horse, size of the cassette, and the area of greatest interest. It is safer to stand in front of the horse and hold the cassette for this study.

METACARPAL BONES—
MEDIAL OBLIQUE VIEW
(dorsolateral-palmaromedial)

Purpose—The medial oblique view clearly projects the dorsomedial aspect of the third metacarpal bone, the palmarolateral aspect of the third metacarpal bone, and the lateral splint bone.

Preparation—No special preparation is required other than brushing.

Foot Positioning—The cassette is held against the palmaromedial aspect of the leg in a holder.

Tube Positioning—The x-ray tube is positioned dorsolateral to the leg so that the x-ray beam is directed 45° from the mid-sagittal or lateral plane and is parallel to the ground. The beam is centered on the mid-portion of the metacarpal region or on a point of interest (Fig. 3-18).

Radiographic Technique for Portable Unit (400 speed film-screen system)
- 80 kVp, 10 mA, 0.1 sec, 26 inches focal-film distance
- 80 kVp, 20 mA, 0.06 sec, 26 inches focal-film distance

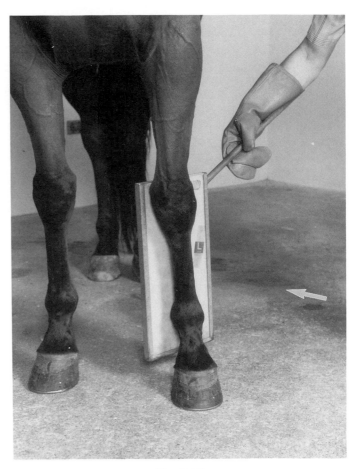

Fig. 3-18

Photograph of the positioning of the forelimb used to make the medial (dorsolateral-palmaromedial) oblique view of the metacarpal region. The x-ray beam is centered on the mid-portion of the cannon bone, is parallel to the ground, and is positioned at a 45° angle from the dorsopalmar or lateral views (arrow). The cassette holder may be rested on the ground or be held off the ground depending on the size of the horse, size of the cassette, and the area of greatest interest.

METACARPAL BONES—
LATERAL OBLIQUE VIEW
(dorsomedial-palmarolateral)

Purpose—The lateral oblique view projects the dorsolateral aspect of the third metacarpal bone, the palmaromedial aspect of the third metacarpal bone, and the medial splint bone.

Preparation—No special preparation is required other than brushing.

Foot Positioning—The cassette is held against the palmarolateral aspect of the leg in a holder.

Tube Positioning—The x-ray tube is positioned dorsomedial to the leg so that the x-ray beam is directed 45° from the mid-sagittal or from the lateral plane and is parallel to the ground. The beam is centered on the mid-portion of the metacarpal region or on the point of interest (Fig. 3-19).

> Radiographic Technique for Portable Unit (400 speed film-screen system)
> • 80 kVp, 10 mA, 0.1 sec, 26 inches focal-film distance
> • 80 kVp, 20 mA, 0.06 sec, 26 inches focal-film distance

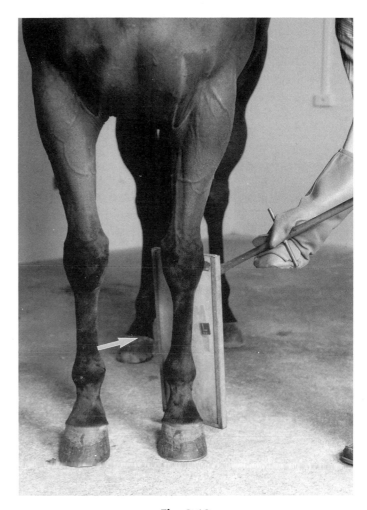

Fig. 3-19
Photograph of the positioning of the forelimb used to make the lateral (dorsomedial-palmarolateral) oblique view of the metacarpal region. The x-ray beam is centered on the mid-portion of the cannon bone, is parallel to the ground, and is at a 45° angle from the dorsopalmar or lateral views (arrow). The cassette holder may be rested on the ground or held off the ground depending on the size of the horse, size of the cassette, and the area of greatest interest.

CARPUS

The carpus of the horse is most commonly composed of seven small, irregularly shaped bones and the interposed hinge-type diarthrodial joints. The antebrachiocarpal and intercarpal joints have a rather large range of motion while motion in the distally located carpometacarpal joint is highly restricted. All joints move essentially as hinge joints and have only limited rotational capability. Because of the conformation of the carpus and the many different ways that traumatic injury can be expressed, it is necessary to make many views to ensure that all bony surfaces and borders and joint surfaces can be studied as completely as possible.

The first and fifth carpal bones may be ossified and seen as normal anatomical variations appearing as small oval dense objects at the level of the carpometacarpal joints on the palmar surface. They should not be mistaken for fracture fragments since their position is predictable and they have a round conformation with smooth borders unlike that seen with fractured fragments. Often, poorly defined concavities in the second and fourth carpal bones adjacent to the first and fifth carpal bones may be misdiagnosed as a site of focal osteomyelitis or as a developmental bone cyst.

The dorsopalmar view can be used to evaluate the degree of closure of the distal radial physis and often this single view of both limbs is made to determine a projected training schedule for young racehorses. In foals with carpal angular deviation, the dorsopalmar view should be made using a longer cassette to enable a complete evaluation of the deviation of the limb from the mid-radial to the mid-metacarpal region. The lateral view permits evaluation of developmental conditions referred to as: "calf kneed," "bucked kneed," and "over at the knees."

The character of the tendons that cross the carpus is clinically important and the grooves defined within the bones are important to evaluate clinically since injury to the distal radius may suggest injury to the tendon or tendon sheath. These are best seen on the skyline views.

The upper portion of the leg is usually clean, but it is still important to determine if leg paints or blisters have been applied, since brushing removes some of this radiopaque debris from the skin. Only right and left markers are required for studies of the carpus, since the medial and lateral aspects of the film can be identified by the unique appearance of the carpal bones. However, until one is familiar with the special projections, a lateral marker may be useful on the oblique views as well as on the skyline views (Table 3-4).

A physeal growth plates separates the small lateral styloid process of the distal ulna which appears as a separate growth center lateral to the distal radial epiphysis. It fuses with the distal epiphysis of the radius by 9 to 12 months. The combined enlarged distal epiphysis of the radius then unites with the metaphysis by 24 to 30 months. The growth center in the proximal metacarpal bone unites prior to birth. A curvilinear physeal plate with variable closure times is present in the accessary carpal bone parallel to the palmar surface.

In an effort to limit tube movement and repositioning of the patient, the following sequence for making the views is suggested: (1) the dorsopalmar view, (2) the medial oblique view made in a dorsolateral-palmomedial direction, (3) the lateral weight-bearing view made in a lateromedial direction, (4) the lateral oblique view made in a palmaro-lateral-dorsomedial direction, and (5) finish with the flexed lateral view made in a lateromedial direction (Fig. 3-20). Skyline views (dorsoproximal-dorsodistal) can be made as indicated. This technique lets you make the first exposure with the tube positioned dorsally and moves the tube consecutively around to the palmarolateral aspect of the leg and then back to the lateral position for the last flexed view. It also keeps you advised of which study is next in the series.

Table 3-4
TECHNIQUE FOR RADIOGRAPHIC EVALUATION OF THE CARPUS

Standard views
  dorsopalmar
  lateromedial extended (weight-bearing)
  lateromedial (flexed)
  medial oblique (dorsolateral-palmaromedial)
  lateral oblique (palmarolateral-dorsomedial)
Optional views
  lateral oblique made in a dorsomedial-palmarolateral
    direction
  dorsoproximal-dorsodistal flexed views (skyline views)
Views of the opposite limb
  dorsopalmar view in a patient less than 24 months
  required if examining a conformational problem in a
    foal
  required if evaluating skeletal maturation, or evaluating
    developmental physitis
  used in evaluation of closure of the distal radial physis
    as an indicator of readiness for training
Cassette size
  small cassette except when evaluating a conformational
    problem in a foal, in which case a longer cassette is
    needed (7 x 17 in, 18 x 43 cm) or divide a larger
    cassette (14 x 17 in, 35 x 43 cm)
Cassette holders
  use even though collimating the primary beam to avoid
    exposure by the primary beam to the leaded glove
    especially in the skyline views
Grid
  not needed except in examination of the heavy draft
    horses or in the exceptional patient with soft tissue
    swelling
Film markers
  right or left limb
  lateral especially on oblique and skyline views

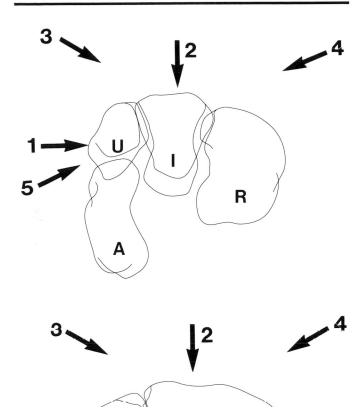

Fig. 3-20
Cross-sectional drawing of the proximal row and distal row of carpal bones with arrows identifying the x-ray beam direction for: (1) lateral (lateromedial), (2) dorsopalmar, (3) medial oblique (dorsolateral-palmaromedial), (4) lateral oblique (dorsomedial-palmarolateral), and (5) lateral oblique (palmarolateral-dorsomedial) views. The radial carpal bone (1), intermediate carpal bone (2), ulnar carpal bone (3), accessary carpal bone (4), second carpal bone (5), third carpal bone (6), and fourth carpal bone (7) are identified.

CARPUS—DORSOPALMAR VIEW

Purpose—This basic view permits good evaluation of the antebrachiocarpal, intercarpal, and carpometacarpal joint spaces and the size, shape, density, and alignment of the carpal bones. The large distally extending radial facet on the distal radius fits into the radial fossa formed by the radial carpal bone on the medial side. The medial and lateral collateral ligaments originate from the large tuberosities located medially and laterally at the distal end of the radius. Sometimes the laterally located scar remaining from the fusion of the distal epiphysis of the ulna to the distal epiphysis of the radius is seen on the dorsopalmar view running in a proximolateral to distomedial direction.

Preparation—No special preparation needed other than brushing.

Foot Positioning—The horse stands with the cassette holder held firmly against the palmar aspect of the leg. The opposite forefoot can be lifted to help control motion.

Tube Positioning—The x-ray tube is positioned dorsal to the carpal region, and the x-ray beam is directed within the mid-sagittal plane, parallel to the ground, and centered on the midcarpal region (Fig. 3-21). A helpful rule of thumb used to determine the exact plane for this view is to draw an imaginary line through the tuberosities on the distal radius that are points of attachment of the medial and lateral collateral ligaments. The beam is centered on a line drawn perpendicular to the midpoint of this line at a distance of one inch (2.5 cm) distal to the "point" of the accessory carpal bone.

Radiographic Technique for Portable Unit (400 speed film-screen system)
- 80 kVp, 10 mA, 0.16 sec, 26 inches focal-film distance
- 80 kVp, 20 mA, 0.08 sec, 26 inches focal-film distance

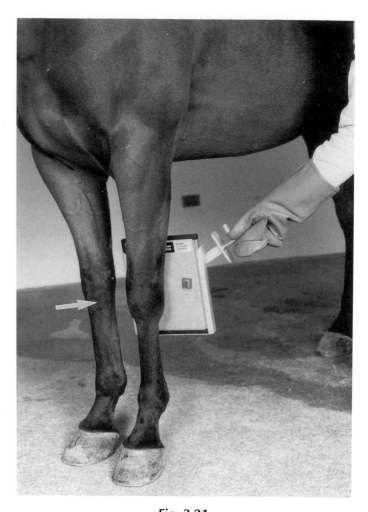

Fig. 3-21
Photograph of the positioning of the forelimb in preparation for making the dorsopalmar view of the carpus. The direction of the horizontal x-ray beam is marked (arrow). It is centered on the carpus within the mid-sagittal plane.

CARPUS—LATERAL EXTENDED VIEW
(lateromedial—weight-bearing)

Purpose—This view permits evaluation of the conformation of this part of the horse's limb as seen laterally. A radiopaque scar often remains at the site of closure of the physeal growth plate in the distal radius. The palmar aspect of the ulnar, third, and fourth carpal bones can be studied. The accessory carpal bone projects in a palmar direction but is usually difficult to evaluate because of overexposure and requires use of a bright light for evaluation. The transverse crest on the caudal surface of the distal radius is a prominent bony shadow. The suspensory ligament originates from the concavity on the palmar surface of the proximal end of the third metacarpal bone and enthesophytes may originate from this area following tearing of the attachment.

Preparation—No special preparation is required other than brushing.

Foot Positioning—The horse is weight bearing with the cassette positioned firmly against the medial aspect of the carpus.

Tube Positioning—The x-ray tube is positioned laterally with the x-ray beam parallel to the ground and directed just distal and dorsal to the prominence created by the easily palpated accessory carpal bone (Fig. 3-22). Determination of the plane of the x-ray beam may be difficult. If there is a conformational problem in the horse, utilizing the foot axis may be unsatisfactory. Palpation of the heads of the splint bones may be helpful in determining the plane of the x-ray beam since they are of similar size and shape.

Radiographic Technique for Portable Unit (400 speed film-screen system)
- 80 kVp, 10 mA, 0.16 sec, 26 inches focal-film distance
- 80 kVp, 20 mA, 0.08 sec, 26 inches focal-film distance

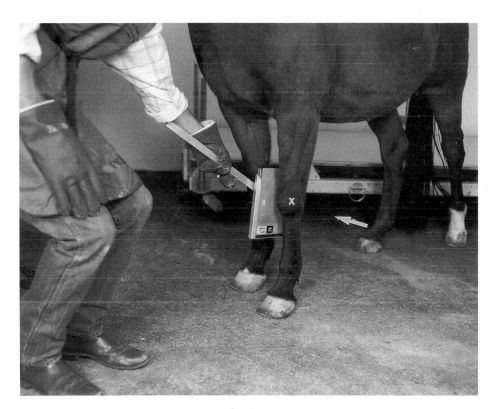

Fig. 3-22
Photograph of the positioning of the forelimb in preparation for making the lateromedial view of the carpus. The direction of the horizontal x-ray beam (arrow) and the point of centering (X) is marked. The bulbs of the heel are marked (open arrow). Laterality of positioning can be insured by having superimposition of the bulbs of the heels.

CARPUS—LATERAL FLEXED VIEW
(lateromedial—flexed)

Purpose—Both articular surfaces of the intermediate and radiocarpal bones as well as the proximal surface of the third and fourth carpal bones and the distal articular surface of the radius can be evaluated. Remember that the intermediate carpal bone appears to be elevated on this view and the radial carpal bone is depressed ("I see you" or "ICU" = intermediate carpal up). Note that the carpometacarpal joint space is a relatively non-movable joint.

Preparation—No special preparation is required other than brushing.

Foot Positioning—The carpus is held flexed to a level of 3/4 full flexion. The foot is held at the level of the carpus of the opposite leg and the carpus is positioned slightly dorsal to the opposite limb (Fig. 3-23). There is a temptation to overflex the carpus in positioning for this view. Also, avoid drawing the carpus medially or laterally. This is especially important as the horse begins to lean on the assistant holding the leg. The positioning of the limb often can be better evaluated by the person holding the horse's head. The cassette is in a holder that is held firmly against the medial aspect of the carpus.

Tube Positioning—The x-ray tube is placed laterally, and the x-ray beam is directed parallel to the ground and centered just dorsal to the accessary carpal bone.

Radiographic Technique for Portable Unit (400 speed film-screen system)
- 80 kVp, 10 mA, 0.16 sec, 26 inches focal-film distance
- 80 kVp, 20 mA, 0.08 sec, 26 inches focal-film distance

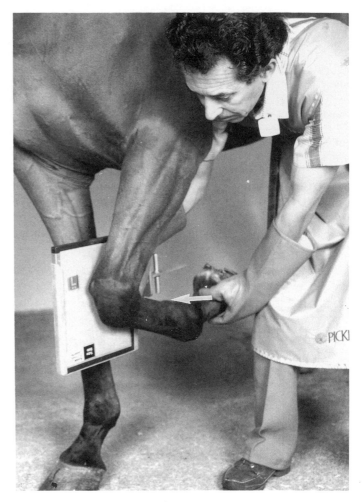

Fig. 3-23
Photograph of the positioning of the forelimb in preparation for making the flexed lateromedial view of the carpus. The direction of the horizontal x-ray beam (arrow) is marked. The person holding the cassette holder can stand either in front or behind the limb.

312

CARPUS—MEDIAL OBLIQUE VIEW
(dorsolateral-palmaromedial)

Purpose—This view permits good visualization of the dorsomedial aspect of the radial and third carpal bones and the palmarolateral aspect of the ulnar and fourth carpal bones and the proximal portion of the fourth metacarpal bone. The accessary carpal bone is projected free from all but a small portion of the distal radius and the ulnar carpal bone.

Preparation—No special preparation is required other than brushing.

Foot Positioning—The horse stands normally with the cassette positioned on the medial aspect of the palmar surface of the leg.

Tube Positioning—The x-ray tube is positioned dorsally and laterally, with the x-ray beam parallel to the ground and centered on the carpal region. The angle of the beam is 60° to 65° from the mid-sagittal plane, 25° to 30° cranial from lateral (Fig. 3-24).

Radiographic Technique for Portable Unit (400 speed film-screen system)
- 80 kVp, 10 mA, 0.16 sec, 26 inches focal-film distance
- 80 kVp, 20 mA, 0.08 sec, 26 inches focal-film distance

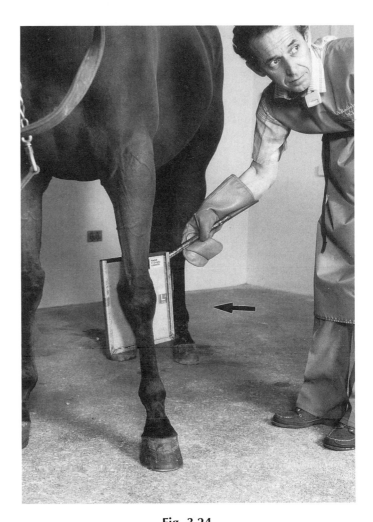

Fig. 3-24
Photograph of the positioning of the forelimb in preparation for making the medial oblique view (dorsolateral-palmaromedial) of the carpus. The direction of the horizontal x-ray beam is marked (arrow). The cassette can be held from in front or beside the horse.

CARPUS—LATERAL OBLIQUE VIEW
(palmarolateral-dorsomedial or dorsomedial-palmarolateral)

Purpose—This view permits good visualization of the dorsolateral aspect of the intermediate and third carpal bones and the palmaromedial aspect of the radial and second carpal bones and the proximal portion of the second metacarpal bone.

Preparation—No special preparation is required.

Foot Positioning—The horse stands normally with the cassette positioned on the lateral aspect of the palmar surface of the leg if the beam is dorsopalmar. The cassette is positioned on the dorsomedial surface of the leg if the beam is directed palmarodorsally.

Tube Positioning—The x-ray tube is positioned dorsally and medially with the x-ray beam parallel to the ground and centered on the carpal region. The angle of the beam is 55° to 60° from the mid-sagittal plane (Fig. 3-25A). It is also possible to make this view by positioning the x-ray tube palmar and lateral (30° to 35° caudal from lateral) and the cassette dorsally and medially (Fig. 3-25B).

Radiographic Technique for Portable Unit (400 speed film-screen system)
- 80 kVp, 10 mA, 0.16 sec, 26 inches focal-film distance
- 80 kVp, 20 mA, 0.08 sec, 26 inches focal-film distance

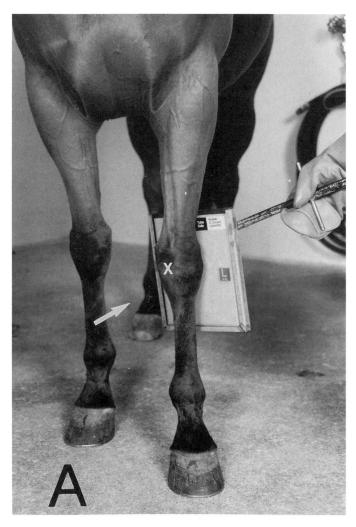 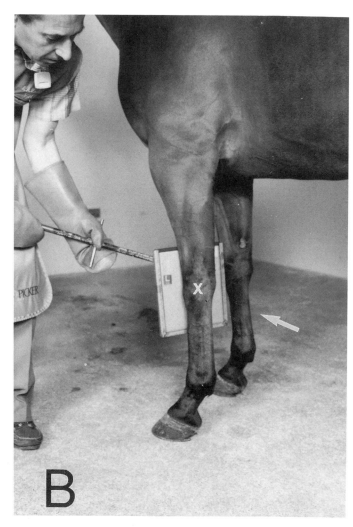

Fig. 3-25

Photographs of the positioning of the forelimb in preparation for making the lateral oblique view of the carpus using a dorsomedial-palmarolateral (A) beam and a palmarolateral-dorsomedial (B) beam. The direction of the horizontal x-ray beams (arrows) and the point of centering (x) are marked.

CARPUS—DORSOPROXIMAL-DORSODISTAL FLEXED VIEWS (skyline views)

Purpose—These three views are made with the carpus held in a flexed position and are primarily used to evaluate the cranial aspect of the distal radius and the dorsal surfaces of the two rows of carpal bones for small or incomplete carpal bone fractures. On the skyline view of the distal radius it is often possible to distinguish the eminences that mark the medially positioned groove that contains the tendon of the extensor carpi radialis muscle and those that mark the laterally positioned groove that contains the tendon of the common digital extensor muscle.

Preparation—No special preparation is required other than brushing.

Limb Positioning—The horse is standing with the carpus held in a flexed position and the metacarpus in a horizontal position.

Tube Positioning—The x-ray tube is positioned proximally and dorsally with the x-ray beam directed in the mid-sagittal plane toward the carpus. The cassette is held against the dorsal surface of the proximal metacarpal bone.

By altering the position of the flexed carpus and x-ray tube, it is possible to ensure that the x-ray beam strikes the anatomical part of interest and projects that bone(s) in a tangential manner on the film. Focal-film distance is shortened for all of these studies, and the radiographic technique is decreased to compensate for the decrease in tissue thickness and the shortened focal-film distance.

Skyline view—distal radius

Hold the leg so that the metacarpus is parallel to the ground, the radius is vertical to the ground, and direct the x-ray beam 65° downward from vertical (Fig. 3-26).

Skyline view—proximal row of carpal bones

Hold the leg so that the radius is angled cranially, the carpus is positioned slightly in front of the carpus on the opposite leg, and the metacarpus is parallel to the ground. Direct the x-ray beam 45° from vertical (Fig. 3-27).

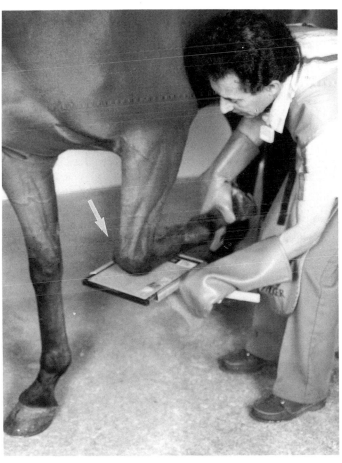

Fig. 3-26
Photograph of the positioning of the forelimb in preparation for making the skyline view (dorsoproximal-dorsodistal) of the distal radius. The direction of the angled vertical x-ray beam is marked (arrow). It is centered on the carpus within the mid-sagittal plane.

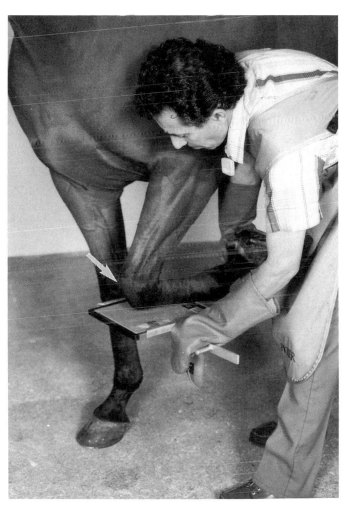

Fig. 3-27
Photograph of the positioning of the forelimb in preparation for making the skyline view (dorsoproximal-dorsodistal) of the proximal row of carpal bones. The direction of the angled vertical x-ray beam is marked (arrow). It is centered on the carpus within the mid-sagittal plane. Note that the carpus is fully flexed and the metacarpus is parallel to the ground.

Skyline view—distal row of carpal bones

Hold the leg so that the radius is angled further cranially than for the skyline view for the proximal row of carpal bones. The carpus is pushed so that it is cranial and proximal to the carpus on the opposite leg, and the metacarpus is parallel to the ground. Direct the x-ray beam so that it is 30° downward from vertical. If you cannot obtain maximum flexion of the joint, you can still obtain a good view of the distal row of carpal bones by directing the x-ray beam at a greater angle (45°) and positioning the flexed knee slightly higher (Fig. 3-28).

Radiographic Technique for Portable Unit (400 speed film-screen system)
- 80 kVp, 10 mA, 0.16 sec, 20 inches focal-film distance
- 80 kVp, 20 mA, 0.08 sec, 20 inches focal-film distance

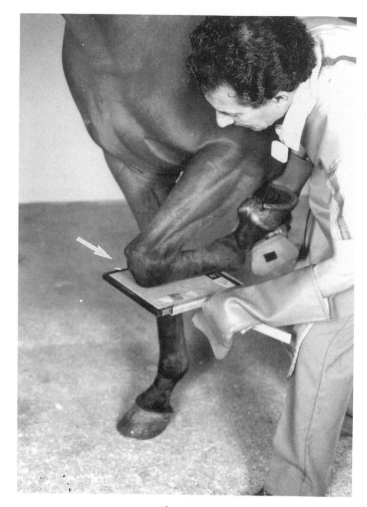

Fig. 3-28

Photograph of the positioning of the forelimb in preparation for making the skyline view (dorsoproximal-dorsodistal) of the distal row of carpal bones. The angulation of the x-ray beam is more nearly vertical in this study than in the study that projects the proximal row of carpal bones (arrow). It is centered on the carpus within the mid-sagittal plane. Note that the carpus is flexed greatly and the metacarpus is parallel to the ground.

RADIUS

A radiographic examination of the radius is much easier to perform in the young horse because of the smaller size or in the recumbent patient because of the greater ease in cassette positioning. Success of the study is dependent on your ability to position the forelimb so that you can position the tube head and cassette satisfactorily. Use of a grid is helpful if it can be used in a correct manner. Film identification is limited to right and left markers. However, lateral markers may be helpful in orientation especially if the entire radius cannot be included on each radiograph. Skin markers are helpful to mark a draining tract or a point of swelling (Table 3-5).

Because of the length of the radius in a mature horse, it is difficult to project the entire bone plus the elbow joint and the antebrachiocarpal joint on the same radiograph. It is always best to make more than a single projection, or include the joint closest to the region of greatest interest.

Table 3-5
TECHNIQUE FOR RADIOGRAPHIC EVALUATION OF THE RADIUS

Standard views
    craniocaudal
    lateral (lateromedial)
Optional views
    caudocranial
    obliques
Views of the opposite limb
    advised in horses with open physes
Cassette size
    use the longest size available (7 x 17 inch, 17 x 43 cm
      size)
Use of a cassette holder
    recommended
Use of a grid
    recommended if x-ray beam direction and cassette
      positioning can be easily controlled
Markers
    lateral
    right and left limb

RADIUS—CRANIOCAUDAL OR CAUDOCRANIAL VIEW

Purpose—This is one of the orthogonal views made of this bone.

Preparation—No special preparation is required except for brushing.

Limb Positioning—The horse stands with the limb extended or in a neutral position. The x-ray tube is positioned in front of the horse with the x-ray beam directed downward in a slightly proximocranial-distocaudal projection. The cassette is held against the caudal aspect of the limb (Fig. 3-29).

If the affected limb is uppermost in a recumbent patient, it is possible to make the study in either a craniocaudal or caudocranial direction. The x-ray tube is positioned appropriately with the cassette against the cranial or caudal aspect of the limb, and the x-ray beam directed parallel to the ground. Correct use of a grid is difficult in either the standing or recumbent patient because of difficulty in obtaining the correct positioning.

With any of the techniques for positioning, attempt to direct the x-ray beam at right angles to the longitudinal axis of the radius.

Tube Positioning—Because of the size of the radius, the x-ray beam is usually centered at a point of soft tissue injury or a point of pain or swelling.

Radiographic Technique for Portable Unit (400 speed film-screen system)
- 80 kVp, 10 mA, 0.16 sec, 26 inches focal-film distance
- 80 kVp, 20 mA, 0.08 sec, 26 inches focal-film distance

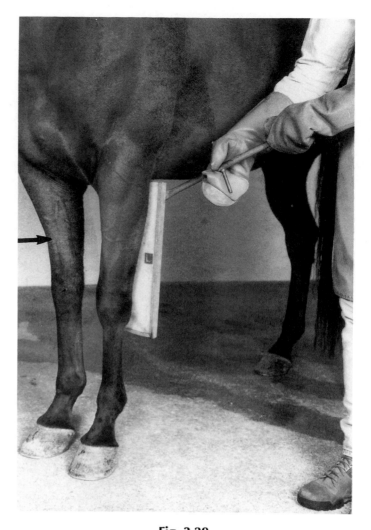

Fig. 3-29

Photograph of the positioning of the forelimb used for making a craniocaudal view of the radius. The x-ray tube is positioned cranially and the x-ray beam is directed slightly downward centering on the radius (arrow). It is advisable to use a cassette holder with a handle.

RADIUS—LATERAL VIEW
(lateromedial or mediolateral)

Purpose—This study is one of the two orthogonal views made.

Preparation—No special preparation is required.

Limb Positioning—If the view is made with the horse standing, the forelimb is in a normal position with the cassette positioned medially. If it is possible to pull the affected limb forward, it may be possible to place the cassette laterally. The study can also be made on the recumbent patient with the affected limb upper-most dictating the need for a lateromedial view with the cassette positioned medially against the upper limb. It is possible that the affected limb may be down and a mediolateral view can be used with the cassette positioned on the ground or table laterally beneath the limb. In any situation, try to position the forelimb as far cranially as is possible to remove it from the thorax.

Beam Center—The x-ray tube is positioned laterally and the beam directed toward the cassette that is held against the medial aspect of the leg (Fig. 3-30). If the lesion is proximal, the beam may be centered proximally and the study be made similar to a lateral view of the elbow joint. The central beam is usually directed at the point of suspected injury, since cassette size is rarely large enough to include the entire radius. There may be unique circumstances in which it is possible to pull the affected limb forward and place the cassette laterally. In that case, the x-ray tube is positioned medially with the beam in a medial to lateral direction and the study made similar to that used for a medial to lateral study of the elbow joint. The x-ray technique should be selected for penetration of the portion of the bone in which interest is the greatest.

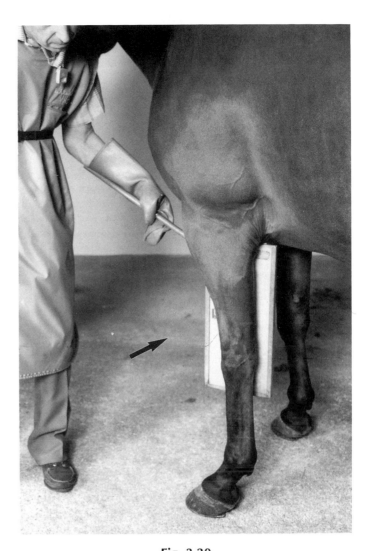

Fig. 3-30
Photograph of the positioning of the forelimb used for making a lateromedial view of the radius in the standing patient. The x-ray tube is positioned laterally and the x-ray beam is directed in a horizontal manner centering on the radius (arrow). Often there is interest only in the proximal radius and the study is centered proximally.

Radiographic Technique for Portable Unit (400 speed film-screen system)
- 80 kVp, 10 mA, 0.16 sec, 26 inches focal-film distance
- 80 kVp, 20 mA, 0.08 sec, 26 inches focal-film distance

ELBOW (Articulatio Cubiti)

The elbow joint (cubital joint) is formed by the humerus, radius, and ulna and is difficult to radiograph in the standing horse because of its size and the difficulty of positioning the cassette in such a manner as to obtain a projection in either a true lateral or true craniocaudal view. If the fracture has marked displacement of the fragments or the joint disease is chronic with marked new bone production, a portable unit may be able to produce a diagnostic study. Certain lesions of the olecranon are clearly identified on the lateral projection because tissue thickness is minimal and the resulting film quality is better. Olecranon injury is difficult to evaluate in the craniocaudal view because tissue thickness is much greater and patient move-ment is a problem. Skyline views (proximodistal) of the olecranon assist greatly in diagnosis of injury to this structure and are a greatly under-utilized radiographic view.

On the craniocaudal view the capitulum (distal humeral lateral condyle) is located laterally where it articulates with the head of the radius (caput radii). The trochlea (distal humeral medial condyle) is located medially where it also articulates with the head of the radius. The lateral tuberosity of the radius is located laterally on the proximal radius and creates a prominent bony mass. The medial and lateral collateral ligaments extend from prominent fossae on the distal humerus to the proximal radius and have no attachment to the ulna. Radio-ulnar ligaments run craniocaudally from the radial head to the ulna distal to the trochlear notch (incisura trochlearis).

On the lateral view, the medial epicondyle of the humerus creates a large shadow distally and caudally. It is superimposed over the smaller lateral humeral epicondyle, a part of the olecranon tuberosity (tuber olecrani), and all of the much smaller anconeal process. Since the medial epicondyle is the origin for the major extensor muscles, it is possible for this to be a site for enthesophyte formation that is an expected aging process. The radial tuberosity is the location of the insertion of the biceps brachii muscle and it is possible to have enthesophyte formation at this point in an older patient that is not related with articular disease. The interosseous space between the radius and ulna creates a radiolucent zone that should not be mis-diagnosed on the radiograph.

There is no special preparation required for this study to prepare the limb for examination. Consideration should be given to the possibility of anesthetizing the patient. However, this creates problems both in dropping the patient and getting it back on its feet during recovery from anesthesia. This is a particular problem in the case of a fracture or injury resulting in non-weight-bearing. While lateral and craniocaudal views are standard, it is sometimes advisable to obtain oblique views because of the nature of a localized lesion or because of unique circumstances determined by the nature of the injury and the limitations on positioning of the limb imposed by the horse (Table 3-6).

Studies of the elbow usually require higher capacity machines than are used for the distal extremities. However, it must be remembered that it is often possible to make lateral views with low capacity machines because the thickness of the limb is often only 10 to 15 cm. This is especially true if the patient is recumbent and the limb can be extended cranially. The limb thickness in the craniocaudal and oblique views is much greater requiring a higher capacity machine to generate an x-ray beam of sufficient energy to penetrate the tissue.

Physeal plates near the elbow generally remain open slightly longer than in the distal part of the limb. The distal humeral physis closes between 12 and 18 months, and the center for the medial epicondyle joins the distal metaphysis of the humerus at 8 to 12 months. The physeal plate in the proximal radius closes about 12 to 18 months, while the apophyseal growth center for the proximal ulna joins the shaft of the ulna between 24 and 30 months.

Table 3-6
TECHNIQUE FOR RADIOGRAPHIC EVALUATION OF THE ELBOW JOINT

Standard views
  craniocaudal (standing)
  mediolateral (standing)
Optional views
  lateromedial
  mediolateral through thoracic cavity
  craniocaudal (recumbent)
  mediolateral (recumbent)
  obliques
  proximodistal (skyline or flexor) view of the olecranon
Views of the opposite limb
  rarely examined except in patients with open physes
Cassette size
  use the largest size that can be easily positioned
Use of a cassette holder
  use for views made with the horse standing
Use of a grid
  not recommended on a standing patient because of problems in positioning
  use on examinations of a recumbent patient
Markers
  right or left limb

ELBOW JOINT—CRANIOCAUDAL VIEW

Purpose—This is a standard view requiring use of a larger x-ray unit. Because of patient size, the study is often limited to visualization of the distal humerus, the joint space, and the proximal radius and ulna.

Preparation—No special preparation is required other than brushing.

Limb Positioning—The horse stands with the affected limb extended and pulled as far cranially as possible. By positioning the foot 8 to 10 inches (20 to 30 cm) off the floor, the elbow is partially separated from the chest wall.

Tube Positioning—The x-ray tube is cranial to the joint and the x-ray beam is directed in a proximocranial-distocaudal direction so that it is perpendicular to the shaft of the radius and the weight bearing portion of the elbow joint can be evaluated. The cassette is held against the radius and ulna (antebrachi) and pushed medially against the rib cage just caudal to the olecranon so that the cassette is perpendicular to the x-ray beam (Fig. 3-31).

A horse with severe injury will not permit having the limb pulled cranially. If the horse holds the limb closely to the chest wall, it is impossible to position the cassette far enough medially to obtain a satisfactory craniocaudal view. If the horse is fully weight-bearing on the limb to be examined, the positioning of the x-ray tube remains cranial but the direction of the x-ray beam is more nearly parallel to the ground. If the horse is recumbent for the examination, the study is easier if the affected limb is uppermost. The elbow can be pulled cranially and the cassette and grid placed just behind the limb. This technique makes centering of the horizontally directed x-ray beam and use of a grid much easier, however, there is still a problem of trying to separate the limb from the chest wall to make positioning of the cassette easier.

A large cassette enables visualization of the greatest area, yet, it may be necessary to use a smaller cassette to obtain the cassette positioning required. Exposure techniques for this view vary because of the great differences in tissue thickness. It is better to obtain an over-exposed radiograph that permits evaluation of the distal humerus and provides penetration so that the olecranon can be studied with a bright light.

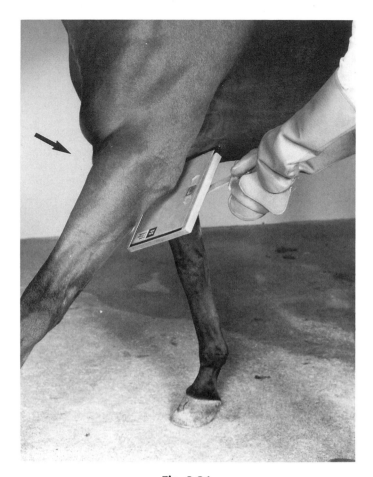

Fig. 3-31

Photograph of the positioning of the forelimb used for making a craniocaudal view of the elbow joint. The foot of the affected limb is elevated and pulled cranially as far as is possible. The x-ray tube is positioned cranially and the x-ray beam is directed downward centering on the elbow joint (arrow). The cassette is within a holder just caudal to the elbow joint and is positioned as far medially as is possible.

Radiographic Technique for Portable Unit (400 speed film-screen system)
 • 80kVp, 10 mA, 0.25-0.35 sec, 26 inches focal-film distance
 • 80kVp, 20 mA, 0.16-0.25 sec, 26 inches focal-film distance

---

ELBOW JOINT—LATERAL VIEW
(mediolateral view)

Purpose—This is the easiest radiographic view to make of the elbow joint and often the only view possible with a portable unit. It produces a radiograph that permits good evaluation of the olecranon and may serve as a survey study.

Preparation—There is no special preparation required other than brushing.

Limb Positioning—With the horse standing, the affected limb should be pulled as far cranially as is possible so that the radius is parallel to the ground.

Tube Positioning—The cassette is positioned laterally and the x-ray tube is just cranial to the opposite forelimb with the x-ray beam parallel to the ground and directed just cranial to the heavy pectoral muscles. The success of this view is determined by the degree of extension of the limb that can be obtained (Fig. 3-32).

In some patients, the limb cannot be adequately extended because of pain or the study must be made with the affected limb in a weight bearing position. In this situation, it may be necessary to position the cassette medial to the elbow joint for a lateromedial view. This technique does not permit placement of the cassette proximally, and

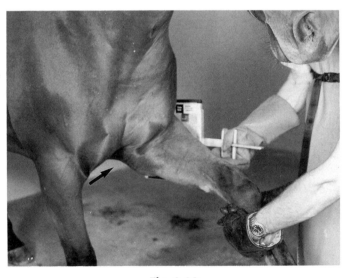

Fig. 3-32

Photograph of the positioning of the forelimb used for making the mediolateral view of the elbow joint. The foot is elevated as much as possible and the limb extended cranially. The tube is positioned medial to the affected limb (lateral to the unaffected limb) and the x-ray beam directed horizontally just cranial to the pectoral muscles (arrow). The central beam is centered on the elbow joint. The cassette is held in a holder lateral to the affected joint.

does not allow complete visualization of the distal humerus or the olecranon. The x-ray tube is positioned laterally to the affected limb for this technique and the x-ray beam is directed parallel to the ground and centered on the elbow joint or olecranon.

Another positioning technique for a lateral view can be made by leaving the affected leg in a normal weightbearing position. This places the elbow adjacent to the cranial lung field and permits the use of this part of the lung field as a "window" for the study. The x-ray technique needs to be increased, but not as much as would be first thought, because of the radiolucency of the lung field. An additional 10 to 15 kVp provides penetration of the overlying muscle. Try to have the patient stand with the affected limb as far caudally as possible so that the musculature of the unaffected limb is cranial and out of the field of exposure. Use of a ceiling suspended cassette holder makes this study much easier.

If the patient is recumbent, the study can be performed with greater ease and effectiveness. The affected leg is positioned in a similar manner whether it is uppermost or on the down side. With the affected leg down, the cassette is more easily positioned on the ground or tabletop next to the affected limb or in a under-table tray. Pull the upper nonaffected limb back and tie it in position. The x-ray tube is positioned over the horse and the x-ray beam is directed vertically and centered on the elbow joint. Use of a grid is easier if the affected limb is down and the cassette and grid are laying on the ground under the horse or are under the tabletop.

With some patients, it is not practical to have the horse laying on the injured limb because of the nature of the injury and the lateral view is made with the affected joint uppermost. However, positioning of the cassette and centering of the x-ray beam are difficult.

Radiography of the recumbent horse is obviously much easier if a table can be used that has an under-table tray that holds the cassette and grid and makes positioning and changing of the cassette much easier.

Flexed and extended lateral views of the elbow may permit a more complete examination of the anconeal process and can be done if the patient is recumbent.

Radiographic Technique for Portable Unit
- 80 kVp, 10 mA, 0.16-0.25 sec, 26 inches focal-film distance
- 80 kVp, 20 mA, 0.1-0.2 sec, 26 inches focal-film distance

ELBOW JOINT—PROXIMODISTAL VIEW
(skyline view)

Purpose—The skyline view of the olecranon is of great value in certain patients, since it provides a third view of the olecranon and one without overlying skeletal structures.

Preparation—There is no special preparation required other than brushing.

Limb Positioning—The leg is held with the elbow joint in complete flexion and the cassette is positioned along the caudal surface of the ulna (Fig. 3-33).

Tube Positioning—The x-ray tube is held over the olecranon adjacent to the thoracic wall using a decreased focal-film distance. The x-ray beam need not be perpendicular to the cassette. This view is made much easier when using a ceiling suspended tubehead.

Radiographic Technique for Portable Unit (400 speed film-screen system)
- 80 kVp, 10 mA, 0.1 sec, 20 inches focal-film distance
- 80 kVp, 20 mA, 0.06 sec, 20 inches focal-film distance

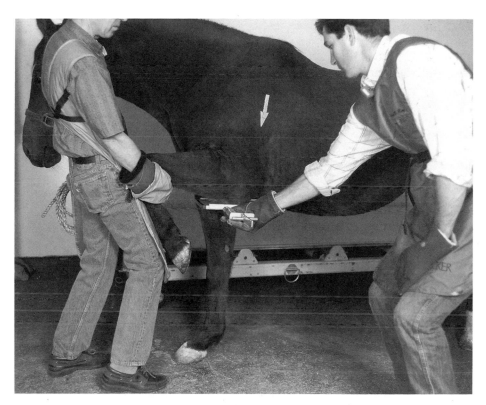

Fig. 3-33

Photograph of the positioning of the forelimb used for making a proximodistal view (skyline view) of the olecranon in a standing horse. The elbow joint is flexed with the radius horizontal to the ground. The x-ray beam is directed vertically (arrow). The cassette is positioned adjacent to the caudal surface of the ulna.

SHOULDER STUDY

Most radiographic examinations of the shoulder joint are made in the young horse when evaluating the humeral head for osteochondrosis. While radiography of the shoulder joint can be made on the standing animal, it is always made easier and the radiographs more diagnostic on the recumbent patient in whom the leg can be more easily positioned through extension. Views are limited to the lateral projections and whatever oblique views can be obtained, since, it is almost impossible to make a cranio-caudal, caudo-cranial, or dorsoventral view. Success of the lateral radiographic view, regardless of patient positioning, is dependent on your ability to position the leg either cranial or caudal to free the shoulder joint from overlying tissues. Use of a grid should be considered, but is difficult (Table 3-7).

The supraglenoid tubercle and coracoid process are apophyseal ossification centers near the cranial aspect of the joint that fuse near 12 months of age along with a center for the cranial part of the glenoid cavity that fuses at a similar time. The age at which ossification center for the greater tubercles of the proximal humerus and the head of the humerus fuse to the body varies widely from 26 to 42 months.

Table 3-7
TECHNIQUE FOR RADIOGRAPHIC EVALUATION OF THE SHOULDER JOINT

Standard view
    mediolateral view
Optional views
    obliques
Views of the opposite limb
    views of the opposite shoulder are suggested when examining for osteochondrosis in the foal
Cassette size
    should be the largest available
Use of a cassette holder
    recommended but may be difficult to use under some circumstances
Use of a grid
    recommended only if correct use is possible
Markers
    right and left limb

SHOULDER JOINT—LATERAL VIEW (mediolateral)

Purpose—This is the most easily obtained view of the shoulder and may be the only view that can be made in many patients.

Preparation—No special preparation is required except to examine the horse carefully and remove dirt and debris attached to the hair coat.

Limb Positioning—The horse stands with the affected limb pulled as far cranially as is possible so that the humeral head is superimposed over the soft tissue of the neck. The cassette is hand-held or held in a cassette holder and is positioned against the lateral aspect of the shoulder joint. The success of the study is dependent entirely on the degree of limb extension that is possible. The unaffected limb is weight-bearing and is positioned as far caudally as is possible to be out of the x-ray field (Fig. 3-34).

Tube Positioning—The x-ray tube is positioned on the opposite side of the horse with the x-ray beam parallel to the ground and centered on the shoulder joint. Direct the beam center more dorsocranially if injury to the supraglenoid process is suspected or more ventrocranial if injury to the tubercles is a possibility.

As with the elbow study, it is also possible to pull the affected limb caudally and use the cranial lung field as a "window" and make a trans-thoracic mediolateral view. In that situation, position the unaffected limb as far cranially as is possible to remove it from the field of view. This is essentially the same positioning as used for the cranioventral position for the thoracic study with the affected limb pulled caudally.

If the patient is recumbent, it is easiest to have the affected limb down with the horse lying on the cassette and grid with the x-ray tube positioned over the patient and the x-ray beam directed vertically.

Radiographic Technique for Portable Unit (400 speed film-screen system)
- 80 kVp, 10 mA, 0.5-0.8 sec, 26 inches focal-film distance
- 80 kVp, 20 mA, 0.4-0.6 sec, 26 inches focal-film distance

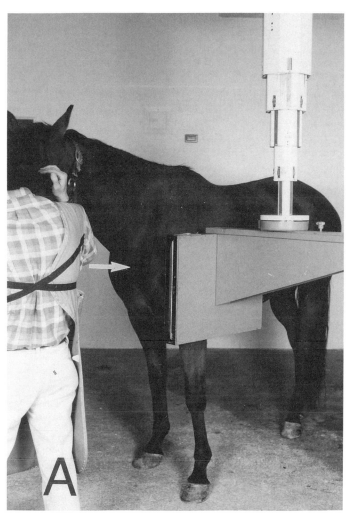

Fig. 3-34
    Photograph of the positioning of the limb used for making the mediolateral view of the shoulder joint. It may be necessary to make the study in a weightbearing manner (A), however, is much better if the foot is elevated and the leg extended cranially (B). The tube is positioned lateral to the normal limb and the x-ray beam directed horizontally (arrow) and centered on the shoulder joint. The cassette is held in a holder lateral to the affected leg.

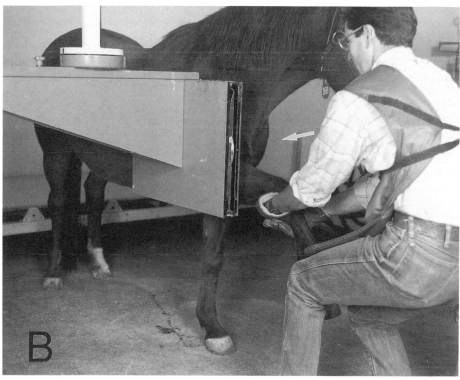

SHOULDER JOINT—OBLIQUE VIEWS

Purpose—Oblique views are usually made to permit evaluation of an area of suspected injury to the point of the shoulder, such as, fracture of one of the three tubercles on the proximal humerus or suspected bicipital bursal injury.

Preparation—No special preparation is required other than brushing.

Limb Positioning—The patient stands with the leg to be examined in a normal standing position.

Tube Positioning—If a caudolateral-craniomedial study is made, the cassette is placed cranial and medial to the affected shoulder joint against the pectoral muscle mass (Fig. 3-35). The x-ray tube is positioned caudally and is lateral to the thorax. The x-ray beam is parallel to the ground or directed downward and centered at the craniolateral aspect of the proximal humerus. A craniomedial-caudo-lateral study may also be made with the cassette placed lateral to the affected shoulder and the x-ray tube cranial and medial to the unaffected leg (Fig. 3-35). The x-ray beam is parallel to the ground or directed slightly upward and is centered at the craniolateral aspect of the proximal humerus. In either positioning technique, the x-ray beam strikes the cassette at a pronounced angle and the resulting radiographic distortion makes evaluation of the underlying bones difficult and use of a grid impossible. This particular positioning can evaluate the distal tip of the spine of the scapula as well.

The x-ray beam is often not directed at the center of the cassette but at the point of interest on the patient. Usually, only the area of the supraglenoid process of the scapula and the greater, intermediate, and lesser tubercles of the humerus are visualized on this oblique view. The character of the shoulder joint space is rarely evaluated clearly. Soft tissues can be evaluated for radiopaque foreign bodies, gas, or calcification/ossification.

Views of this joint made with a portable unit are generally of limited diagnostic quality, but in the event of fractures with marked displacement of the bony fragments, they can be of value.

Radiographic Technique for Portable Unit (400 speed film-screen system)
- 80 kVp, 10 mA, 0.4-0.6 sec, 26 inches focal-film distance
- 80 kVp, 20 mA, 0.2-0.4 sec, 26 inches focal-film distance

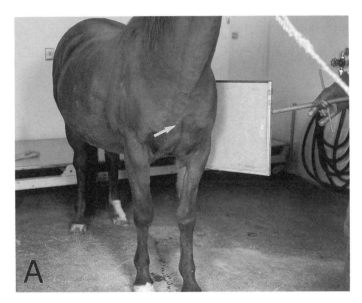 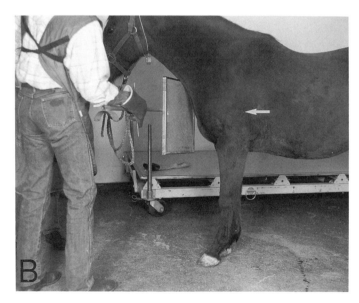

Fig. 3-35
Photograph of the positioning of the limb used for making the oblique view of the shoulder joint. The study is made with the horse weightbearing. The tube is positioned in front of the normal limb and the x-ray beam directed horizontally (arrow) and centered on the shoulder joint (A). The cassette is held in a holder lateral to the affected leg. It is also possible to position the tube lateral to the affected limb with the x-ray beam directed horizontally and centered on the shoulder joint (B). The cassette is held in a holder in a transverse plane cranial to the affected leg.

4. HINDLIMB

Radiographic examinations of the hindlimb distal to the metatarsophalangeal joint are common, although, not used as frequently as examinations of a comparable region of the forelimb. While the radiographic views are usually made in the same manner as in the forelimb, often positioning of the x-ray tube and cassette is more difficult or even dangerous.

Studies proximal to the metatarsophalangeal (fetlock) joint are uncommon except for studies of the tarsus. However, the type of horse seen in your practice greatly influences the examinations made, since, trotters frequently have the tarsal and metatarsal region radiographed. Studies of the stifle are difficult because of the size of the joint, but are often required in the examination of younger horses, where osteochondrosis is common. Most examinations of the pelvis require that the horse be recumbent especially in evaluation of the hip joints.

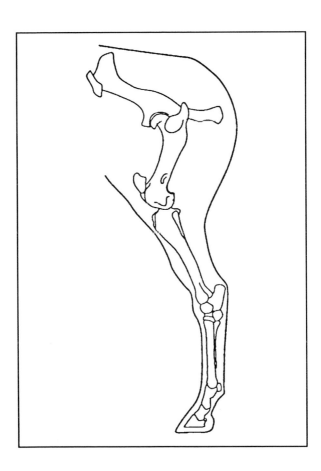

METATARSAL BONES

Studies of the metatarsal bones are performed in essentially the same manner as studies of the metacarpal bones of the forelimb except for differences in angulation of the x-ray beam for the important oblique views. Multiple views are required and the use of long cassettes is recommended (7 x 17 in, 17 x 43 cm) (Fig. 4-1). It is important to include a part of the joints both proximal and distal for purposes of orientation. When using a portable unit at a shortened focal-film distance, the radiation field may not be large enough to cover the entire length of the cassette. If using only 8 by 10 inch (18 x 24 cm) cassettes, it is even more important to include a part of one joint proximal or distal, otherwise, you have no easily recognized anatomical structures for orientation. Cleanliness of the limb is important as it was for radiography of the foot, but is generally limited to careful brushing of the leg. The same radiographic technique can be used for all views except for a slightly increased technique for the dorsoplantar view (Table 4-1).

The third metatarsal bone forms with two epiphyseal centers. The proximal center closes before birth and the distal center closes between 7 and 12 months. The second and fourth metatarsal bones have a distal center that begins to ossify at 3 months and may not close until the horse is a two-year-old.

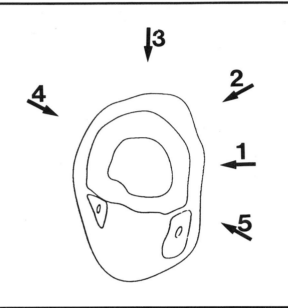

Fig. 4-1
A drawing of a cross-section of the metatarsal region showing the three metatarsal bones. Angles for making the: (1) lateromedial, (2) dorsolateral-plantaromedial (medial) oblique, (3) dorsoplantar, (4) dorsomedial-plantarolateral (lateral) oblique, and (5) plantarolateral-dorsomedial (lateral) oblique views are shown.

Table 4-1
TECHNIQUE FOR RADIOGRAPHIC EVALUATION OF THE METATARSAL BONES

Standard views
dorsoplantar
lateromedal
dorsolateral-plantaromedial (medial) oblique
plantarolateral-dorsomedial (lateral) oblique

Optional views
conedown for cortical stress fractures

Views of the opposite limb
not usually performed

Cassette size
should include the entire metatarsal bones (7 x 17 in, 17 x 43 cm)

Use of a cassette holder
should be used

Use of a grid
not required

Markers
lateral
right or left limb

METATARSAL BONES—DORSOPLANTAR VIEW

Purpose—This is a part of the standard examination for the metatarsus.

Preparation—No special preparation is required other than brushing.

Limb Positioning—The horse stands in a natural position with the cassette placed against the plantar aspect of the metatarsal region (Fig. 4-2). Use of a cassette holder with a "leg" is helpful.

Tube Positioning—The x-ray tube is positioned dorsally and the x-ray beam is angled slightly downward within the midsagittal plane until it is perpendicular to the metatarsal bones. It is centered on the mid-portion of the metatarsal region if a large cassette is used but the beam is centered on the point of interest if a smaller cassette is used.

Radiographic Technique for Portable Unit (400 speed film-screen system)

• 80 kVp, 10 mA, 0.1 sec, 26 inches focal-film distance
• 80 kVp, 20 mA, 0.06 sec, 26 inches focal-film distance

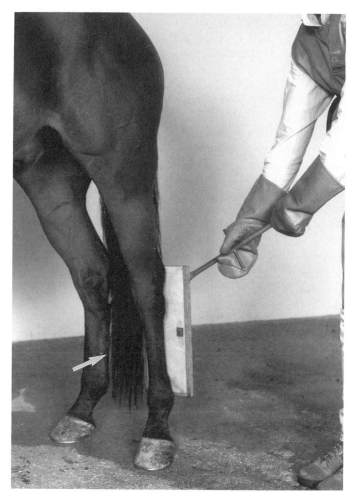

Fig. 4-2

Photograph of the positioning of the hindlimb used for making a dorsoplantar view of the metatarsal bones. The horse is standing normally. The x-ray tube is positioned cranially and the x-ray beam is directed slightly downward (arrow) centering on the midshaft of the cannon bone. The cassette is positioned in a holder.

METATARSAL BONES—LATERAL VIEW
(mediolateral)

Purpose—This view provides an excellent view of the larger lateral splint bone as well as being an orthogonal view for study of the third metatarsal bone.

Preparation—No special preparation is required other than brushing.

Limb Positioning—The horse stands with the hindlimb in a natural position.

Tube Positioning—The x-ray tube is positioned laterally and the cassette is placed against the medial aspect of the leg. Use of a cassette holder is helpful to control motion. The x-ray beam is parallel to the ground and is in the frontal plane and is centered on the midportion of the metatarsal region (Fig. 4-3).

Radiographic Technique for Portable Unit (400 speed film-screen system)

- 80 kVp, 10 mA, 0.1 sec, 26 inches focal-film distance
- 80 kVp, 20 mA, 0.06 sec, 26 inches focal-film distance

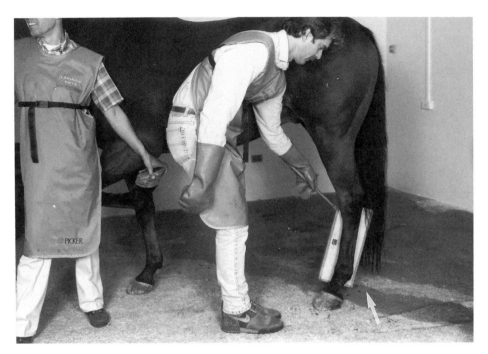

Fig. 4-3
Photograph of the positioning of the hindlimb used for making a lateromedial view of the metatarsal bones. The horse is standing normally. The x-ray tube is positioned laterally and the x-ray beam is horizontal and centered on the midshaft of the cannon bone (arrow). The cassette is positioned in a holder.

METATARSAL BONES—MEDIAL OBLIQUE VIEW (dorsolateral-plantaromedial)

Purpose—This is the special view to demonstrate the fourth, or lateral, metatarsal bone.

Preparation—No special preparation is required other than brushing.

Limb Positioning—The horse stands with the hindlimb in a natural position for this view.

Tube Positioning—The x-ray tube is positioned dorsally and laterally to the limb and the cassette is against the plantar and medial aspect of the metatarsal region. The x-ray beam is angled downward slightly at an angle of 45° to 55° from dorsoplantar (35° to 45° from lateral) so as to be perpendicular to the long axis of the third metatarsal bone and be centered on the midportion of the metatarsal region (Fig. 4-4).

Radiographic Technique for Portable Unit (400 speed film-screen system)

- 80 kVp, 10 mA, 0.1 sec, 26 inches focal-film distance
- 80 kVp, 20 mA, 0.06 sec, 26 inches focal-film distance

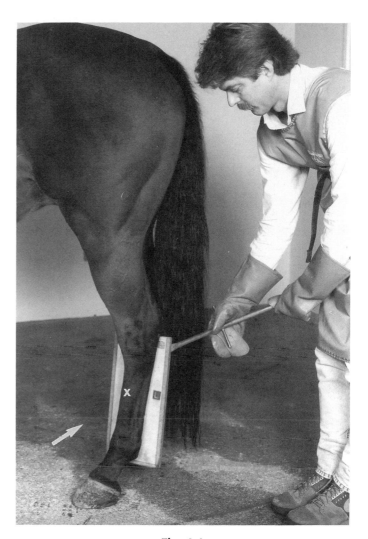

Fig. 4-4
Photograph of the positioning of the hindlimb used for making a dorsolateral-plantaromedial (medial) oblique view of the metatarsal bones. The horse is standing normally. The x-ray tube is positioned dorsally and laterally and the x-ray beam is directed slightly downward (arrow) and centered on the midshaft of the cannon bone. The cassette is positioned in a holder.

METATARSAL BONES—LATERAL OBLIQUE VIEW (plantarolateral-dorsomedial)

Purpose—This is the oblique view that most clearly demonstrates the second, or medial splint bone.

Preparation—No special preparation is required other than brushing.

Limb Positioning—The horse stands with the hindlimb in a natural position for this view.

Tube Positioning—The x-ray tube is positioned caudally and laterally to the limb. The cassette is positioned dorsally and medially and the x-ray beam is directed from behind laterally to in front of the limb medially (plantarolateral-dorsomedial) (Fig. 4-5). The x-ray beam needs to be angled upward slightly to be perpendicular to the long axis of the metatarsal bones. The angle of the x-ray beam is 45° to 55° from dorsoplantar (35° to 45° from lateral) and it is centered on the midportion of the metatarsal region.

To make this projection in a dorsomedial to plantaro-lateral manner requires that the x-ray tube be positioned cranially and medially under the horse making the study more difficult and less safe for the operator. The cassette is positioned against the plantar aspect of the limb laterally (Fig. 4-6).

Other oblique views can be made on a smaller cassette to more clearly outline a lesion suspected from evaluation of the standard views. These oblique views can be made at 5° to 10° increments around the area of interest.

Radiographic Technique for Portable Unit (400 speed film-screen system)

- 80 kVp, 10 mA, 0.1 sec, 26 inches focal-film distance
- 80 kVp, 20 mA, 0.06 sec, 26 inches focal-film distance

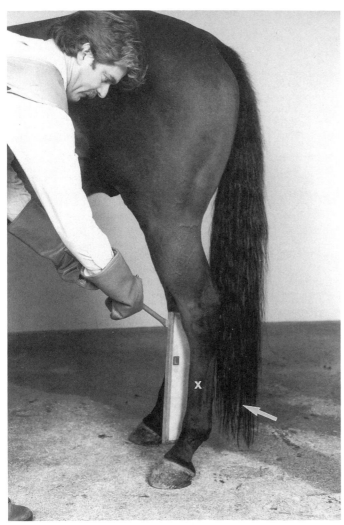

Fig. 4-5
Photographs of the positioning of the hindlimb used for making a plantarolateral-dorsomedial (lateral) oblique view of the metatarsal bones. The horse is standing normally. The x-ray tube is positioned caudally and laterally and the x-ray beam is directed slightly upward (arrow) and centered on the midshaft of the cannon bone.

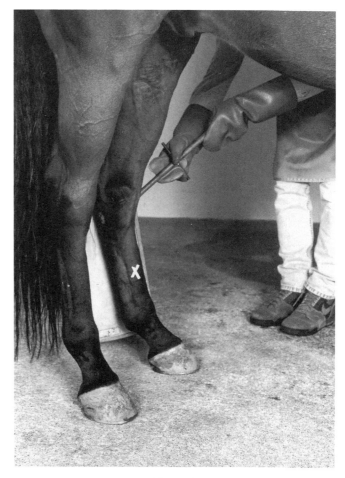

Fig. 4-6
Photographs of the positioning of the hindlimb used for making a dorsomedial-plantarolateral (lateral) oblique view of the metatarsal bones. The horse is standing normally. The x-ray tube is positioned cranial and medially and the x-ray beam is directed slightly downward (arrow) and centered on the midshaft of the cannon bone. The cassette is positioned in a holder.

TARSUS

The tarsus is a hinge type diarthrodial joint composed of 6 or 7 irregularly shaped tarsal bones interposed between the distal tibia and the proximal metatarsus. The shape of the bones results in it being necessary to make many views to ensure that all bony surfaces and joint spaces have been examined as thoroughly as is possible. The tarsus is composed of four major articulations, the: (1) tarsocrural (tibiotarsal), (2) proximal intertarsal, (3) distal intertarsal, and (4) tarsometatarsal joints. The site of major motion within the tarsus is at the tarsocrural (tibiotarsal) joint where the trochlea of the tibiotarsal bone is in contact with the articular surface of the distal end of the tibia where there is a proximomedial to distolateral obliquity of 10° to 15°. This insures lateral movement of the foot during flexion. The distal aspect of the medial trochlea is seen to extend further distally and dorsally than the lateral trochlea while the lateral trochlear ridge is prominently notched distally.

The distal tibia has a physeal plate and there are separate ossification centers for the lateral malleolus, and the calcaneal tuber. The lateral malleolus has a separate center of ossification which unites with the distal epiphyseal center of the tibia at 3 to 8 months and this combined growth center closes at 18 to 24 months of age. The distal growth center in the calcaneus closes at 22 to 36 months. In the mature patient, the lateral malleolus contains a vertical groove for the lateral digital extensor muscle tendon. The medial malleolus is the larger of the two and forms the cranial boundary for the groove for the long digital flexor muscle tendon

The tarsus is relatively high on the leg and the horse is allowed to stand weight-bearing in a normal manner for all but the flexed views, regardless of the type of x-ray machine used. No special technique for preparation is required other than brushing. A cassette holder with a "leg" of some type is valuable in eliminating problems of motion and radiation exposure to the individual holding the cassette. Because the intertarsal joint surfaces are not within a perfectly flat plain, two dorsoplantar views are used for their evaluation. A flexed lateral view can be used as an additional study to the extended, weight bearing, lateral study.

Oblique views are used to study the dorsomedial and dorsolateral aspects of the tarsal region. A special skyline (proximodistal) view of the calcaneus assists in evaluation of the calcaneal tuber. A grid is not necessary in examination of the tarsus in lighter-weight horses, however, in the heavier animals, use of a grid decreases the amount of scatter radiation on the film. Use of lateral markers assists in your orientation of the radiographs until you are familiar with the oblique views (Table 4-2).

Table 4-2
TECHNIQUE FOR RADIOGRAPHIC EVALUATION OF THE TARSAL JOINTS

Standard views
   dorsoplantar (2 views, one horizontal and one at a 10° to 15° angle)
   lateromedial, extended, weight-bearing
   dorsolateral-plantaromedial (medial) oblique
   plantarolateral-dorsomedial (lateral) oblique

Optional views
   lateromedial, flexed
   proximodistal (skyline) of the os calcis (tuber calcaneus)
   dorsomedial-plantarolateral (lateral) oblique

Views of the opposite limb
   not usually needed except if the growth plate in the os calcis in racing horses is used for determination of skeletal maturity to determine training schedules

Cassettes
   small size are usually used

Use of cassette holders
   are of value, especially if they have a supporting "leg" of some type to control motion

Use of a grid
   use is indicated in radiography of heavy breeds
   use is not recommended with a portable unit

Markers
   lateral
   right or left limb

TARSUS—DORSOPLANTAR VIEWS (2)
(10° dorsoproximal-plantarodistal view, horizontal dorsoplantar view)

Purpose—These are standard views used in the examination of the tarsus and two views should be made to provide the most complete evaluation of the intertarsal and tarsometatarsal joints. The 10° downward angled view provides the best projection of the lateral aspect of the joints and the horizontal view provides the best projection of the medial aspect of the joints. The angles used to make the dorsoplantar radiograph can be determined by noting the location of the level of the heads of the metatarsal bones on the radiograph. In the view made with the horizontal beam, the location of the heads of the metatarsal bones is more proximal than when using the 10° view.

The large and clinically important calcaneus is usually not clearly seen on the dorsoplantar views because of failure of the beam to penetrate due to the overlying distal tibia. The talus and the central, third, and fourth tarsal bones are clearly identified on this view.

Preparation—No special preparation is required other than brushing.

Limb Positioning—The horse stands fully weight bearing with the foot pointing outward so that the x-ray tube can be positioned dorsally and slightly laterally and not be under the horse. Elevation of the forefoot on the same side helps to insure that motion is not a problem during the examination. Elevating the opposite forefoot as a means of insuring that you are not kicked during the examination is not a completely satisfactory technique.

Tube Positioning—The x-ray tube is positioned dorsally and slightly laterally and the cassette is held against the plantar aspect of the leg. The x-ray beam is within the midsagittal plane and is either angled downward slightly for view 1, or is horizontal for view 2. The beam is centered on the central tarsal bone for each view and is perpendicular to the long axis of the metatarsal bones (Fig. 4-7).

Radiographic Technique for Portable Unit (400 speed film-screen system)

- 80 kVp, 10 mA, 0.16-0.2 sec, 26 inches focal-film distance
- 80 kVp, 20 mA, 0.08-0.1 sec, 26 inches focal-film distance

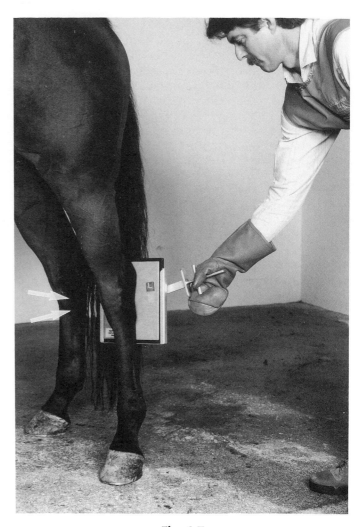

Fig. 4-7

Photograph of the positioning of the hindlimb for the two dorsoplantar radiographs of the tarsal bones. Because the foot is pointed slightly laterally, positioning of the x-ray tube is easier. The x-ray beams (arrows) are directed horizontally or angled downward 10° and centered in the mid-line on the central tarsal bone.

TARSUS—LATERAL VIEW
(lateromedial)

Purpose—Because the head of the fourth metatarsal bone is larger than the second metatarsal bone, it is prominently positioned in a plantar location on this view and the second and fourth metatarsal bones are not seen to be superimposed. Thus, the radiograph made with a true lateral position may appear at first glance to be slightly obliqued. The trochlear ridges of the talus (tibial tarsal bone) are clearly seen to be separated with the medial ridge being larger and projecting further distally and dorsally. The central tarsal bone is seen in the proximal row of tarsal bones and the third tarsal bone occupies most of the distal row of tarsal bones. However, both second and fourth tarsal bones are partially seen on this view. With the help of a bright light, the somewhat overexposed calcaneus can be studied. The articulation between the sustentaculum tali of the calcaneus and the talus is seen on the lateral view. The separate center of ossification for the tuber calcaneus closes at 22 to 36 months of age. Soft tissue shadows may be seen cranially and may be excessively dense due to collection of fluid within the tibiotarsal synovial sac.

Preparation—No special preparation is required other than brushing.

Limb Positioning—The horse stands normally weight-bearing.

Tube Positioning—The x-ray tube is positioned laterally and the cassette is placed against the medial aspect of the tarsus. The top of the cassette includes the most proximal portion of the calcaneus but the x-ray beam should be centered 4 inches (10 cm) distal to the point of the hock (Fig. 4-8). The most common error in positioning is centering the x-ray beam too high on the limb. Since the intertarsal joint spaces are angled, the beam is angled downward 3° to 5°. Determination of the correct positioning of the x-ray tube is difficult and compounded by the tendency for the horse to toe out. Visual examination of the foot can insure that the x-ray beam is correctly positioned for the lateromedial view when you visualize a superimposition of the bulbs of the heel.

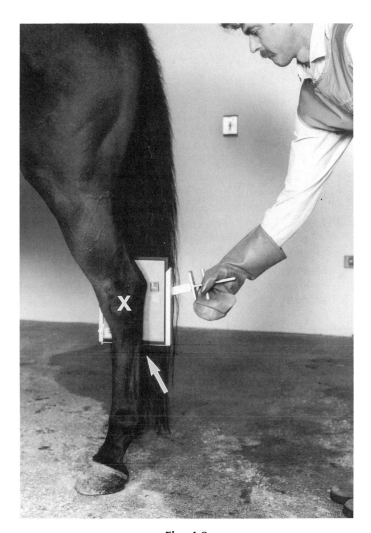

Fig. 4-8
Photograph of the positioning of the hindlimb for an extended lateromedial radiograph of the tarsal bones. The foot is pointed slightly laterally making it easier to position the x-ray tube. The x-ray beam is directed horizontally and centered on the central tarsal bone (arrow). A hand held cassette holder is used.

Radiographic Technique for Portable Unit (400 speed film-screen system)

- 80 kVp, 10 mA, 0.16 sec, 26 inches focal-film distance
- 80 kVp, 20 mA, 0.1 sec, 26 inches focal-film distance

335

TARSUS—LATERAL FLEXED VIEW
(lateromedial)

Purpose—This view permits good evaluation of the tarsocrural joint and the dorsal portion of the calcaneus.

Preparation—No special preparation is required other than brushing.

Limb Positioning—Elevate the foot flexing the fetlock joint as well as the tarsocrural joint. The metatarsal bones are not parallel to the ground but angled downward approximately 30°. The assistant holds the foot in one hand and the cassette holder in the other hand and is somewhat forward for protection in the event that the horse should strike backwards (Fig. 4-9). Using this projection, it is possible to obtain a lateral radiograph in which more of the plantar aspect of the articular surface of the talus can be evaluated.

Tube Positioning—The x-ray tube is placed laterally and the cassette is held against the medial aspect of the tarsal region. The x-ray beam is parallel to the ground and centered cranial to the calcaneus. It is difficult to determine the frontal plane so the position of the location of the x-ray beam may be determined by making it perpendicular to the long axis of the metatarsal bones. In all flexed positions, care must be exercised so that the leg is not abducted since this creates an angle between the x-ray beam and the joints.

Radiographic Technique for Portable Unit (400 speed film-screen system)

- 80 kVp, 10 mA, 0.16 sec, 26 inches focal-film distance
- 80 kVp, 20 mA, 0.1 sec, 26 inches focal-film distance

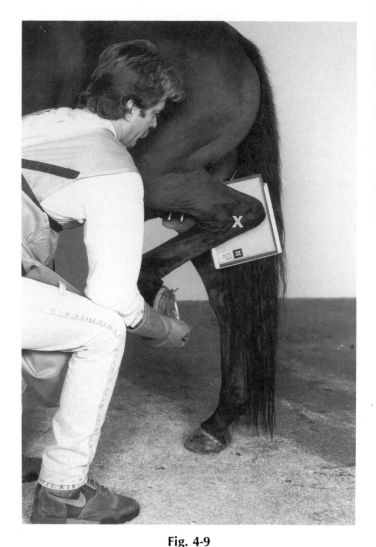

Fig. 4-9
Photograph of the positioning of the hindlimb for a flexed lateromedial radiograph of the tarsal bones. The foot is held with the metatarsal bone angled slightly downward. The x-ray beam is directed horizontally and centered on the central tarsal bone (X). A hand held cassette holder is used.

TARSUS—MEDIAL OBLIQUE VIEW
(dorsolateral-plantaromedial)

Purpose—This view permits good visualization of the dorsomedial aspect of the tarsal region and the proximal portion of the fourth metatarsal bone. This view shows especially: (1) the trochlear ridges of the talus as they fit into the articular surface of the distal tibia (cochlea tibia), (2) the intermediate ridge on the distal tibia that usually contains a shallow synovial fossa, (3) the dorsomedial aspect of the central and third tarsal bones which is the area of attachment of the dorsal tarsal ligament, and (4) a part of the fourth tarsal bone. The proximal portion of the fourth metatarsal bone is seen free of overlying shadows as it articulates with the third metatarsal and fourth tarsal bones. The entire plantar surface of the calcaneus can be studied.

Preparation—No special preparation is required other than brushing.

Limb Positioning—The horse stands normally.

Tube Positioning—The x-ray tube is positioned dorsally and laterally. The cassette is held within a holder firmly placed against the medial and plantar aspect of the tarsus. Try to prevent the horse from leaning laterally. If the horse stands straight, the x-ray beam is directed 3° to 5° downward and is centered on the tarsal region. The beam is angled 45° from midline (45° from lateral). Use of a cassette holder is recommended (Fig. 4-10).

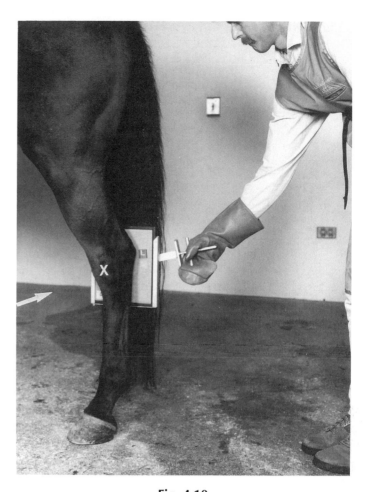

Fig. 4-10
Photograph of the positioning of the hindlimb for a dorsolateral-plantaromedial (medial) oblique radiograph of the tarsal bones. The x-ray beam is directed horizontally (arrow) and centered on the central tarsal bone (X). A hand held cassette holder is used.

Radiographic Technique for Portable Unit (400 speed film-screen system)

- 80 kVp, 10 mA, 0.16 sec, 26 inches focal-film distance
- 80 kVp, 20 mA, 0.1 sec, 26 inches focal-film distance

TARSUS—LATERAL OBLIQUE VIEW
(plantarolateral-dorsomedial)

Purpose—This oblique view permits good visualization of the more dorsal position of the lateral trochlear ridge of the talus with its prominent distal notch, the sustentaculum tali, and the proximal portion of the second metatarsal bone as it articulates with the third metatarsal and first and second tarsal bones. The central and third tarsal bones are well seen along with the second tarsal bone.

Preparation—No special preparation is required other than brushing.

Limb Positioning—The horse stands normally.

Tube Positioning—The x-ray tube is positioned laterally and plantar to the tarsus. The cassette is held firmly against the medial and dorsal aspect of the tarsus. The x-ray beam is directed slightly upward 3° to 5° and is centered on the tarsal region. The beam is angled 55° to 60° from directly behind and 30° to 35° from lateral (Fig. 4-11). Use of a cassette holder is recommended. It is suggested to elevate the forelimb on the same side during the study.

Radiographic Technique for Portable Unit (400 speed film-screen system)

- 80 kVp, 10 mA, 0.16 sec, 26 inches focal-film distance
- 80 kVp, 20 mA, 0.1 sec, 26 inches focal-film distance

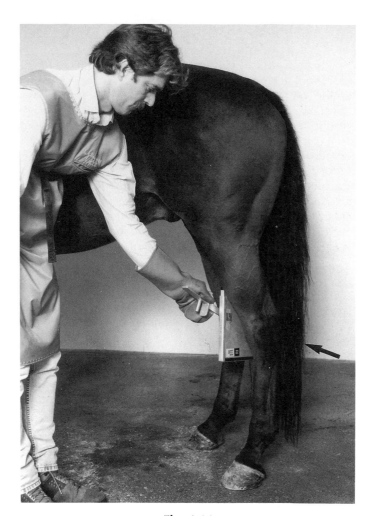

Fig. 4-11
Photograph of the positioning of the hindlimb for a plantarolateral-dorsomedial (lateral) oblique radiograph of the tarsal bones. The x-ray beam is directed horizontally (arrow) and centered on the central tarsal bone. A hand held cassette holder is used.

TARSUS—TUBER CALCANEUS—
PROXIMODISTAL VIEW
(Skyline or Flexor View)

The calcaneus (fibular tarsal bone) is the largest bone of the tarsus, and it functions to extend the tarsocrural (tibiotarsal) joint. At its elongated proximal end is the calcaneal tuber which is attached to the base of the calcaneus by the body or shaft. The tendons of the gastrocnemius and superficial digital flexor muscles insert on the proximal tip of the calcaneus. The calcaneal bursa is located between the superficial flexor tendon and the gastrocnemius tendon. On the plantaromedial aspect of the base of the calcaneus is the important sustentaculum tali. The deep digital flexor tendon and its sheath pass over the sustentaculum tali. A long plantar ligament extends along the plantarolateral aspect of the calcaneus and terminates on the fourth tarsal and the third and fourth metatarsal bones.

Purpose—This view is the only one that enables evaluation of the calcaneus and the sustentaculum tali from a proximal to distal direction without overlying bony shadows.

Preparation—No special preparation is required other than brushing.

Limb Positioning—The foot is elevated off the ground and the tarsal joint is forced into a fully flexed position with the metatarsal bones parallel to the ground.

Tube Positioning—The x-ray tube is positioned above the tarsus and the cassette held in a plane nearly parallel to the ground against the plantar aspect of the calcaneus (Fig. 4-12). The x-ray beam is directed vertically toward the calcaneus with a slightly cranial angulation. The radiographic technique is decreased proportionately because of the shortened focal-film distance as well as the decrease in bony tissue to be penetrated by the primary beam.

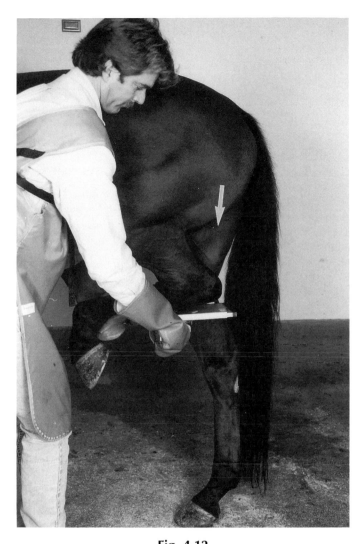

Fig. 4-12
Photograph of the positioning of the hindlimb for a proximodistal (skyline) view of the calcaneus. The x-ray beam is directed nearly vertically (arrow) and is centered on the tuber calcis. The metatarsal bones are positioned in a near horizontal position. A hand held cassette holder is used.

Radiographic Technique for Portable Unit (400 speed film-screen system)

- 80 kVp, 10 mA, 0.1 sec, 20 inches focal-film distance
- 80 kVp, 20 mA, 0.06 sec, 20 inches focal-film distance

TIBIA

Studies of the tibia are generally made using a long cassette so that joints proximal and/or distal can be included in the radiograph for purposes of orientation. A cassette holder is used. Lateromedial and caudocranial (craniocaudal) views are included in the study. Oblique views can be made as required (Table 4-3).

Table 4-3
TECHNIQUE FOR RADIOGRAPHIC EVALUATION OF THE TIBIA

Standard views
    caudocranial
    lateral (lateromedial)

Optional views
    craniocaudal
    oblique

Views of the opposite limb
    rarely radiographed

Cassette size
    7 x 17 inch (17 x 43 cm) cassette or 14 x 17 inch (34 x 43 cm) cassette divided

Use of cassette holders
    are helpful to reduce both the physical danger in performing the study and the radiation exposure

Use of a grid
    not required

Markers
    lateral
    right and left limb

TIBIA—CAUDOCRANIAL OR CRANIOCAUDAL VIEW

Purpose—This is one of the two standard orthogonal views of the tibia.

Preparation—No special preparation of the horse is required other than brushing.

Limb Positioning—The horse is permitted to stand normally.

Tube Positioning—The cassette is held against the cranial aspect of the leg and the x-ray tube positioned caudally. The caudocranially directed x-ray beam is directed slightly downward (Fig. 4-13). The x-ray beam is within the midsagittal plane of the limb and is centered on a point of soft tissue injury, pain, or swelling. It is difficult to include the entire bone on a single radiograph.

It is also possible to make this study with the cassette held against the caudal aspect of the limb and the x-ray tube positioned cranially. The object-film distance is greater when using this technique and it is not as safe to position the x-ray tube cranial to the limb and to hold the cassette caudal to the limb.

Radiographic Technique for Portable Unit (400 speed film-screen system)

- 80 kVp, 10 mA, 0.2-0.25 sec, 26 inches focal-film distance
- 80 kVp, 20 mA, 0.1-0.16 sec, 26 inches focal-film distance

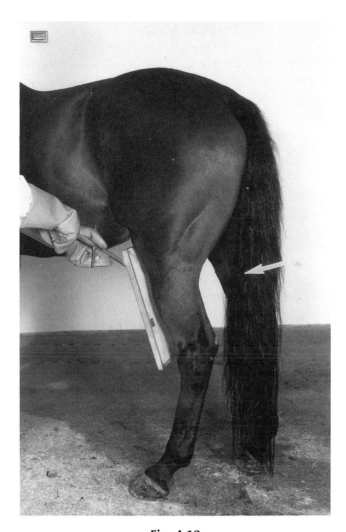

Fig. 4-13
Photograph of the positioning of the horse prior to a caudocranial view of the tibia. The x-ray beam is directed slightly downward (arrow) and is centered on the midshaft of the tibia.

TIBIA—LATERAL VIEW
(lateromedial)

Purpose—This is one of the two standard orthogonal views of the tibia.

Preparation—No special preparation of the horse is required other than brushing.

Limb Positioning—The horse is permitted to stand normally with the limb examined pointing in external rotation slightly.

Beam Center—The x-ray beam is directed horizontally, within the frontal plane of the limb, and is centered on the middle of the tibia or on a point of interest. The cassette is held against the medial aspect of the limb and the x-ray tube positioned laterally (Fig. 4-14).

Radiographic Technique for Portable Unit (400 speed film-screen system)

- 80 kVp, 10 mA, 0.16 sec, 26 inches focal-film distance
- 80 kVp, 20 mA, 0.08 sec, 26 inches focal-film distance

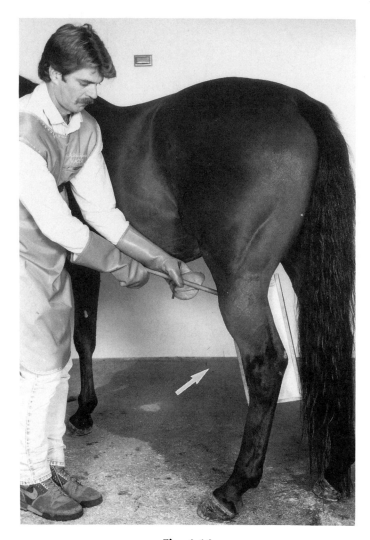

Fig. 4-14
Photograph of the positioning of the horse prior to a lateromedial view of the tibia. The x-ray beam is directed horizontally (arrow) and centered on the midshaft of the tibia or area of interest.

STIFLE JOINT

The medial and lateral femorotibial and femoropatellar joints combine to form the stifle joint. Radiographic studies of the stifle joints are made commonly and can be highly informative if the views are technically adequate. The caudolateral-craniomedial oblique view demonstrates the medial condyle and is of value in the diagnosis of osteochondrosis of the medial condyle. The lateral projection of the stifle joint is most informative in diagnosing osteochondrosis of the medial or lateral ridges of the trochlea. The lateral view can be made with the stifle joint in a semiflexed position with the distal limb extended caudally and has been suggested as a method of improving the view. All views are of value in the detection of periarticular lipping which is diagnostic of secondary joint disease. The special views of the patella and femoropatellar joint surfaces require different positioning of cassette and central beam and a change in radiographic technique and are valuable to demonstrate both traumatic and degenerative changes (Table 4-4).

The distal growth center of the femur closes at 20 to 30 months. The apophyseal center of the tibial tuberosity joins the proximal tibial growth center at 9 to 12 months and the combined growth centers join the tibial shaft at 20 to 30 months.

Table 4-4
TECHNIQUE FOR RADIOGRAPHIC EVALUATION OF THE STIFLE JOINT

Standard views
  caudocranial
  lateral (lateromedial) stifle joint (semi-flexed)
  caudolateral-craniomedial (lateral) oblique
  lateral (lateromedial) patella

Optional views
  craniocaudal
  caudomedial-craniolateral (medial) oblique
  proximodistal (skyline or flexor) patella
  caudocranial distal femur
  lateral (lateromedial) distal femur

Views of the opposite limb
  views should be made in a study for osteochondrosis

Cassette size
  large size should be used for views of the stifle joint
  small cassettes should be used for views of the patella

Use of cassette holders
  difficult to use

Use of the grid
  is indicated because of tissue thickness but it is impractical to use because of problems in beam direction and because of the required increase in exposure time

Markers
  lateral
  right and left limb

STIFLE JOINT—CAUDOCRANIAL VIEW

Purpose—It is difficult to position the cassette for this view because of increased tissue thickness but the resulting radiograph offers a good opportunity for detection of new bone formation indicative of secondary joint disease as well as an opportunity to evaluate joint width. It is difficult to control the amount of flexion of the stifle joint during this exposure.

Preparation—No special preparation is required other than brushing.

Patient Positioning—The horse stands normally, however, it is usually a requirement to lift the forefoot on the same side to enable positioning of the cassette in the flank region.

Tube Positioning—Because of a desire to limit the object-film distance, this projection is made with the x-ray tube behind the horse and the cassette held cranially against the patella (Fig. 4-15). Center the beam on the "cleft" seen in the soft tissues on the cranial aspect of the joint. The degree of flexion of the joint makes it difficult to know in what plane to direct the x-ray beam. The average patient is not completely weight-bearing, making it desirable to have the beam parallel to the ground or directed downward (proximodistally) at a 5° angle. It is possible to direct the beam downward to a greater degree and project the intercondylar region to better advantage and obtain a "tunnel" view. It may be desirable to make several caudocranial views using different beam angles. It is extremely difficult to use a grid properly because the grid and cassette pivot against the point of the patella and are usually angled with the distal part of the cassette pushed further medially and caudally. It is possible to made this view in a similar manner on the recumbent patient with the affected limb uppermost.

A major problem in obtaining a diagnostic radiograph using the caudocranial view is the result of the marked increase in tissue thickness proximally. This means that if the joint space and proximal tibia are correctly exposed, the distal femur is markedly underexposed. Since it may be important to evaluate the distal femur, joint surfaces, as well as the proximal tibia, it may be necessary to make two radiographs using two different exposure settings.

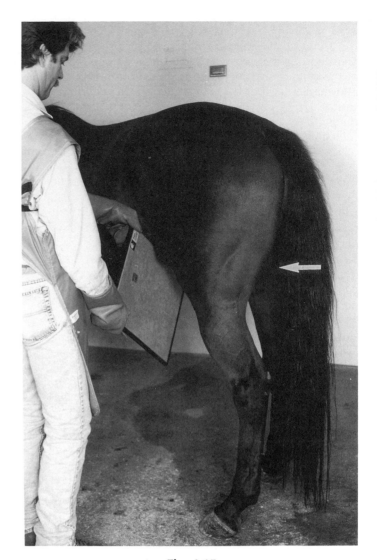

Fig. 4-15

Photographs of the positioning of the horse prior to a caudocranial radiograph of the stifle joint. The horse stands naturally with the cassette positioned in the flank region and the x-ray tube positioned caudally. The x-ray beam (arrow) is directed horizontally or slightly downward and centered on the joint space. Lifting the forefoot on the same side assists in positioning the horse for this examination.

Radiographic Technique for Portable Unit (400 speed film-screen system)

- 80 kVp, 10 mA, 0.6-0.8 sec, 26 inches focal-film distance
- 80 kVp, 20 mA, 0.3-0.4 sec, 26 inches focal-film distance

STIFLE JOINT—LATERAL VIEW
(lateromedial)

Purpose—This view provides good evaluation of the articular surfaces of the femorotibial joints. Both ridges of the distal femoral trochlea are seen at least partially on this view and developmental anomalies in this region can be evaluated. The femoral condyles usually are superimposed but a large cystic lesion due to osteochondrosis in one of the condyles may still be identified.

Preparation—No special preparation is required other than brushing.

Patient Positioning—The horse stands weight-bearing and the cassette is cautiously placed medial to the stifle joint by forcing it as far into the flank as is possible (Fig. 4-16). This usually induces the horse to pick up the foot, sometimes rather quickly, so it is best to lift the forefoot on the same side prior to positioning the cassette. It is also possible to make this view with the foot elevated and carried a short distance caudally. This creates a semiflexed position permitting good evaluation of the femoral condyles and proximal tibia.

Tube Positioning—The x-ray tube is positioned laterally with the x-ray beam directed parallel to the ground and centered distal and caudal to the patella. Center the beam on the joint space regardless of how far proximally you have been able to position the cassette.

It is also possible to make this study on a recumbent patient. If the affected leg is uppermost on the recumbent horse, the cassette can be relatively easily pushed into the flank region medial to the joint. The x-ray tube is placed over the horse with the beam directed vertically. With the affected limb down, the cassette is placed beneath the horse and the upper, nonaffected limb can be flexed and pulled cranially to remove it from the field of exposure. If the horse is positioned on a table, the cassette can be placed in an undercarriage tray with a grid making it relatively easy to position the cassette.

A major problem in centering for the lateromedial view of the stifle joint, regardless of patient positioning, is the temptation to center the beam on the patella which is proximal and cranial to the femorotibial joint surfaces resulting in a badly obliqued view of the joint surfaces. Another problem comes from centering the beam on the cassette instead of the patient when the positioning of the cassette is compromised.

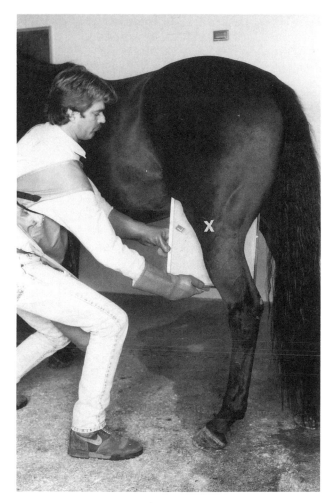

Fig. 4-16
Photograph of the positioning of the horse for a lateromedial radiograph of the stifle joint. The horse stands naturally with the cassette positioned in the flank and the x-ray tube positioned laterally. The x-ray beam is directed horizontally and centered (x) distal to patella.

Radiographic Technique for Portable Unit (400 speed film-screen system)

- 80 kVp, 10 mA, 0.3-0.4 sec, 26 inches focal-film distance
- 80 kVp, 20 mA, 0.16-0.2 sec, 26 inches focal-film distance

STIFLE JOINT—LATERAL OBLIQUE VIEW
(caudolateral-craniomedial)

Purpose—This view is the best for evaluation of osteochondrosis-like lesions in the medial condyle and in the lateral ridge of the trochlea in the distal femur.

Preparation—No special preparation is required other than brushing.

Patient Positioning—The horse stands naturally with the forefoot on the same side lifted to control the horse during this examination.

Tube Positioning—The x-ray tube is positioned caudally and laterally and the cassette pushed as far medially as possible so that it rests against the medial ridge of the trochlea (Fig. 4-17). The beam is centered on the caudal aspect of the intercondylar region and is parallel to the ground, directed 35° lateral to medial from the midsagittal plane. This view is made without a grid.

Radiographic Technique for Portable Unit (400 speed film-screen system)

- 80 kVp, 10 mA, 0.3-0.4 sec, 26 inches focal-film distance
- 80 kVp, 20 mA, 0.16-0.2 sec, 26 inches focal-film distance

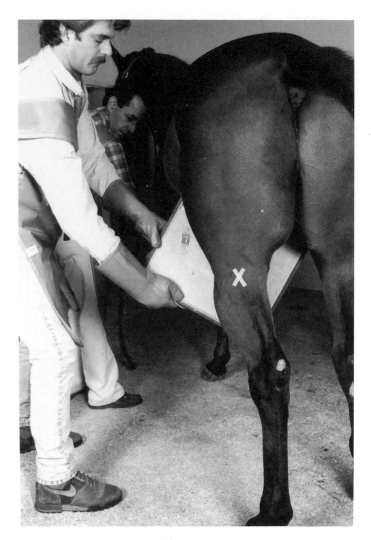

Fig. 4-17

Photograph of the positioning of the horse for a caudolateral-craniomedial (lateral) oblique radiograph of the stifle joint. The horse stands naturally with the cassette positioned as far into the flank as is possible and the x-ray tube positioned caudally and laterally. The x-ray beam is directed horizontally and centered (x) on the lateral aspect of the intercondylar region.

STIFLE JOINT—MEDIAL OBLIQUE VIEW
(caudomedial-craniolateral)

Purpose—This view is of importance in evaluation of the lateral femoral condyle, but is not made commonly and is dangerous because of the positioning required for the x-ray tube.

Preparation—No special preparation is required other than brushing.

Patient Positioning—The horse stands comfortably weight bearing on the affected limb.

Tube Positioning—The x-ray tube is positioned medially behind the horse and the cassette is held cranially and laterally (Fig. 4-18). Positioning the cassette for this view is easier than for the opposite oblique view because it does not have to be pushed into the flank region. The x-ray beam is directed parallel to the ground or slightly downward, angled at a 45° angle from the caudocranial view, and centered on the intercondylar region.

Radiographic Technique for Portable Unit (400 speed film-screen system)

- 80 kVp, 10 mA, 0.3-0.4 sec, 26 inches focal-film distance
- 80 kVp, 20 mA, 0.16-0.2 sec, 26 inches focal-film distance

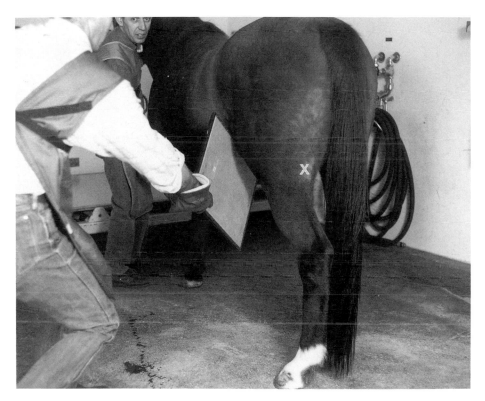

Fig. 4-18

Photograph of the positioning of the horse for a caudomedial-craniolateral (medial) oblique radiograph of the stifle joint. The horse stands naturally with the cassette positioned cranially and laterally and the x-ray tube positioned caudally and medially. The x-ray beam is directed horizontally and centered (x) on the medial aspect of the intercondylar region.

STIFLE JOINT—LATERAL PATELLAR VIEW
(lateromedial)

Purpose—This view of the patella and the femoropatella articulation is important in the detection of developmental, traumatic or degenerative disease.

Preparation—No special preparation is required other than brushing.

Patient Positioning—The horse stands naturally.

Tube Positioning—The x-ray tube is positioned laterally and a small cassette is held medially but further proximally and cranially than for the regular lateromedial view (Fig. 4-19). The x-ray beam is parallel to the ground and centered on the patella approximately 3 1/2 to 5 inches (9 to 13 cm) proximal to the tibiofemoral cleft. The radiographic technique is decreased for this view because of the decrease in thickness of the bony structures.

Radiographic Technique for Portable Unit (400 speed film-screen system)

- 80 kVp, 10 mA, 0.16 sec, 26 inches focal-film distance
- 80 kVp, 20 mA, 0.08 sec, 26 inches focal-film distance

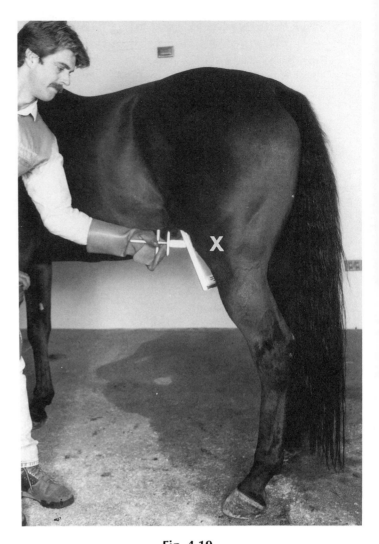

Fig. 4-19
Photograph of the positioning of the horse for a lateromedial radiograph of the patella. The horse stands naturally with the cassette positioned in the flank and the x-ray tube positioned laterally. The x-ray beam is directed horizontally and centered (x) on the patella proximal to the soft tissue cleft. By decreasing the radiographic technique, the patella and its articulation with the femur are clearly seen.

STIFLE JOINT—PROXIMODISTAL PATELLAR VIEW (Flexor or Skyline View)

Purpose—This view permits evaluation of the femoro-patellar joint space as well as being the only view of value in the detection of nondisplaced fractures of the patella.

Preparation—No special preparation is required other than brushing.

Patient Positioning—This view of the patella is accomplished with the horse standing naturally and one assistant flexing the stifle joint. Success of the view is dependent on being able to hold the stifle joint completely flexed with the limb pulled caudally so the tibia is as near horizontal as is possible. The hock joint may either be flexed or fully extended.

Tube Positioning—The x-ray tube is positioned above the patella lateral to the lumbar spine with the x-ray beam directed vertically toward the patella with the beam angled proximocranial-distocaudal from the vertical at approximately 35° to 45°. The cassette is held against the proximal tibia but positioned far enough proximally (cranially) to permit projection of the patella on the film. This positioning makes the cassette at an angle relative to the central beam (Fig. 4-20). The object-film distance is decreased to 20 to 25 inches (40 to 60 cm). The decreased tissue thickness permits the study to be made without use of a grid. It is also possible to make this view with the horse recumbent.

Radiographic Technique for Portable unit (400 speed film-screen system)

- 80 kVp, 10 mA, 0.16 sec, 26 inches focal-film distance
- 80 kVp, 20 mA, 0.08 sec, 26 inches focal-film distance

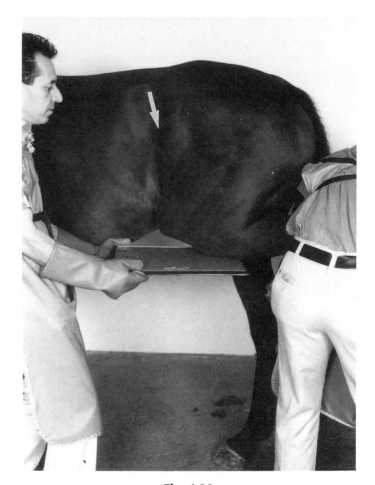

Fig. 4-20
Photograph of the positioning of the horse for the proximodistal (flexor or skyline) radiograph of the patella. Notice the placement of the cassette under the stifle joint against the proximal tibia. The x-ray tube is overhead with the closely collimated beam directed downward at a slight angle (arrow).

PELVIS AND HIP JOINTS

Studies of the bony pelvis and hip joints for bone or joint disease are required rather often in the foal following trauma. The radiographic studies may also be directed to include the sacro-iliac joints as well as the lumbosacral region in an effort to explain the etiology of back pain in horses. These anatomic regions are more difficult to visualize on radiographs of larger horses.

In the smaller patients, ventrodorsal views of the pelvis with oblique views of the hip joints are not difficult to achieve using only sedation since it is possible to position a small patient onto the cassette. Similar studies of the pelvis and hip joints in the adult horse can usually be made only if the horse is positioned in dorsal recumbency under general anesthesia with the hindlimbs in a "frogleg" position with the cassette positioned under the horse. Because of the increased size, a single view is made for the bony pelvis and an oblique view for each hip joint. Use of a "tunnel" device or cassette tray under the tabletop makes movement and replacement of cassettes much easier. It is relatively easy to use a grid and accurately center the central beam (Table 4-5).

The x-ray unit must have a capacity for high kVp exposures. The length of the exposure is not important because patient motion is relatively well controlled and breathing during the exposure usually does not cause movement of the bony pelvis. The major problems of radiography of the hip joints and pelvis include the: (1) difficulty in making studies on the standing horse that are diagnostic, (2) difficulty in positioning the cassette and grid without a table and undertable tray when the horse is recumbent, and (3) problems in anesthesia and recovery from the anesthesia in the event of fracture or luxation.

Physeal closure of the pelvic bones at the acetabulum occurs between 18 and 24 months but the pelvic symphysis remains open until 2 to 7 years of age. The proximal femoral physis closes between 24 and 30 months. The apophyseal center for the greater trochanter joins the femoral shaft at 18 to 30 months while the time for union of the apophyseal center for the lesser trochanter is inconsistent.

Table 4-5
TECHNIQUE FOR RADIOGRAPHIC EVALUATION OF THE PELVIS AND HIP JOINTS

Standard views
    ventrodorsal
    ventrodorsal oblique for each hip

Optional views
    ventrodorsal for lumbosacral region
    ventrodorsal oblique for each sacroiliac joint
    standing lateral views

Views of the opposite limb
    both hip joints should be included for comparison in all studies

Cassettes
    use the largest size cassette available

Use of cassette holder
    use of an undertable tray is helpful in positioning the cassette

Use of a grid
    use of a grid is necessary to control the level of radiation fog in all patients

Marker
    right and left

PELVIS AND HIP JOINTS—
VENTRODORSAL VIEW

Purpose—This is the best view for evaluation of the hip joints and bones of the pelvis as well as the lumbosacral region and sacro-iliac joints.

Preparation—If possible, feces should be removed from the rectum. This may result in an air-filled ballooned rectum that helps in further decreasing tissue density. It may be necessary to anesthetize all but the youngest patients.

Patient Positioning—The horse is placed in dorsal recumbency with the hindlimbs positioned in a flexed manner. The legs do not come in contact with the tabletop or ground but are angled between 20° and 30° from the surface. It is important that both limbs are positioned as nearly in the same position as is possible to provide the same projection of each hip joint (Fig. 4-21).

Tube Positioning—The tube is positioned over the patient with the beam directed vertically. The positioning is dependent on the size of the patient and the area of clinical interest. If the horse is small enough, the tube may be centered and the entire pelvis including both hip joints can be included on one radiograph. In the larger horses, the tube is shifted laterally and the tube is centered on each hip joint. Interest may center on the lumbosacral or sacroiliac joints, the tuber coxae, or the ischial tuberosities, in which case the tube is shifted either cranially or caudally. The radiographic technique needs to be increased if the areas of interest have greater tissue density.

Radiographic Technique for Portable Unit for Foal—
150-200 lbs (70-90 kg) (400 speed film-screen system)

- 80 kVp, 10 mA, 0.5 sec, 26 inches focal-film distance
- 80 kVp, 20 mA, 0.25 sec, 26 inches focal-film distance

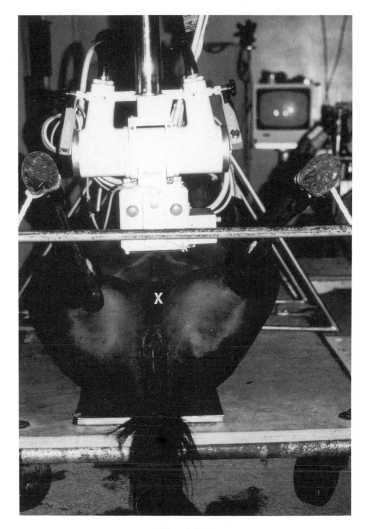

Fig. 4-21

Photograph of the positioning of the horse for a ventrodorsal radiographic study of the pelvis. It is not possible to extend the limbs of a mature horse and a "frog-leg" position is used. The x-ray beam is directed vertically and centered on the mid-line between the hip joints (x). Note the cassette and grid positioned directly under the horse if a cassette tray is not available for use.

PELVIS AND HIP JOINTS—VENTRODORSAL OBLIQUE VIEW

Purpose—The purpose of this view is to provide a second projection of the individual hip joint. While not orthoganol, the two views are supportive.

Preparation—No special preparation is required. Because of positioning the patient at an oblique angle, the rectal contents are not of as great concern since they are displaced and are not superimposed over the hip joints.

Patient Positioning—The horse is placed in dorsal recumbency with the hindlimbs positioned in a flexed manner. The pelvis is then obliqued by 10° to 20° with the unaffected side elevated off the tabletop (Fig. 4-22). The degree of obliquity is not as important as is your ability to reproduce a similar positioning when radiographing the opposite limb.

Tube Positioning—The tube is positioned over the hip joint lateral to the midline and the central beam directed vertically. It is possible to center the x-ray beam further laterally and radiograph the proximal femur using this position.

Radiographic Technique for Portable Unit for Foal—150-200 lbs (70-90 kg) (400 speed film-screen system)

- 80 kVp, 10 mA, 0.5 sec, 26 inches focal-film distance
- 80 kVp, 20 mA, 0.25 sec, 26 inches focal-film distance

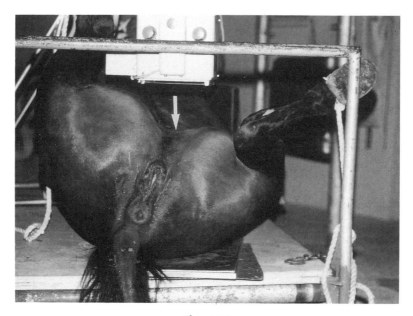

Fig. 4-22
Photograph of the positioning of the horse for oblique ventrodorsal radiographs of the pelvis for evaluation of the hip joint. It is not possible to extend the limbs of a mature horse and a "frog-leg" position is used. The horse is rolled toward the side being examined with the unaffected side elevated. Different methods can be used to immobilize the hindlimbs. The x-ray beam is directed vertically (arrow) and centered laterally from the mid-line over the hip joint of interest.

5. SINUS TRACK

Horses often have puncture wounds in which knowledge of the depth and extent of the soft tissue injury is helpful in determining treatment and prognosis. Other injuries progress with the development of chronic draining tracts of unknown cause and information about the location of the tract and the presence of possible foreign bodies is important to assist in the surgical planning. Some of these patients are easily examined radiographically by use of tract injections using either air or a positive contrast agent or a combination of the two.

The principles of the study are similar even though the tissue injury examined may vary widely. Non-contrast studies are made prior to injection to determine the presence of radiopaque foreign bodies or associated bony injury. The wound or tract is examined clinically and probed to determine the nature of the wound. For a sinus tract injection, the device used for injecting the contrast medium may be rigid, such as a teat cannula, or may be flexible as a soft catheter. Select a catheter that allows you to probe the depth of the tract and determine the number of channels

that can be injected with contrast material. If it is possible, remove as much of the debris blocking the openings to the tracts as is possible so that the contrast agent can flow freely. It may be helpful to use a catheter with an inflatable bulb to provide a seal at the skin surface that prevents drainage of the contrast agent. Usually that is not as helpful as it might appear and it is often better to elevate the foot or limb so that the contrast agent drains dependently into the depth of the wound or tract ensuring good filling (Fig. 5-1). However, if the wound is high on the limb, this type of positioning is not possible. If there is drainage from the tract following injection and you are concerned about the amount of positive contrast that remains, it may help to follow the injection of the positive contrast material by an injection of air. This double contrast technique insures that at least some of the positive contrast agent remains coating the wall of the tract while the air fills the uppermost part of the tract. The addition of air in a tract injection often converts a study with a poorly visualized tract of little value into a diagnostic study with identification of the complete tract or identification of a foreign body. Regardless of the location or contrast technique to be used, try to probe as

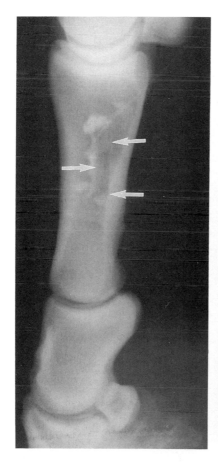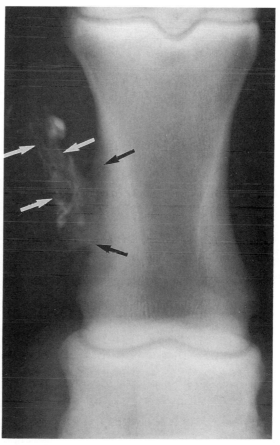

Fig. 5-1
Lateromedial and dorsopalmar views of the digit in a 10-year-old Saddlebred stallion with a history of injury to the front foot 5 months ago. Drainage had been noted for the last 3 months. Following injection of a positive-contrast agent, the foreign body is visualized (white arrows). Surgical removal of the wooden splinter followed the radiographic study. Note the bony response to the chronic inflammatory process (black arrows).

many tracts as is possible and try to fill each one with positive contrast agent or consider use of a double contrast technique.

The volume of positive contrast agent to use varies with the size of the wound or tract and the amount of agent that is lost at the time of injection. There is no maximum amount of contrast agent to use and repeated radiographs may require injection of additional amounts of contrast agent. Between 5 ml and 25 ml of contrast are often used for the first injection. If the positive contrast agent drains from the opening, wipe it away carefully since it is radiopaque and compromises the study by casting heavy white shadows on the radiograph.

Any of the positive contrast agents that are recommended for parenteral injection can be used to fill a draining tract. Most of these are water-soluble and tend to flow rather quickly from the tract opening. Some other agents not used for parenteral injection are oily and may coat the wall of the tract better, but they are more difficult to inject. Air is best used in conjunction with water soluble products. Barium sulfate should not be used since it does not flow easily, is difficult to inject, blocks the tracts, and remains after the injection. Try to use as clean a technique as possible for the injection, recognizing that in most patients the site is obviously infected. In the event of a recent puncture wound, the importance of a clean or even sterile technique is more easily understood, since it is possible that you might extend contamination from the skin by your probing and injections.

It may be valuable to use a metallic rigid probe in the examination of some injuries such as a puncture wound through the sole of the foot. Radiography following placement of a probe shows the depth and direction of the injury (Fig. 5-2). However, remember that a rigid probe may only demonstrate one aspect of the sinus tract. Later, if the foot presents with drainage, it may be more informative to use the protocol described above in an attempt to outline all of the branches of the tract and their depth.

The nature of the radiographic views to be used is dependent on the anatomical site injected. Obviously, a second orthogonal view always provides more information since it is possible to generate the third dimension in your mind of the location of the tract. However, in many patients it is impossible to obtain a second view. A study of a draining sinus tract in the withers, shoulder, or chest wall is probably limited to a single lateral or oblique radiographic view. The withers or shoulder region are examples of a lesion with marked differences in tissue thickness and two exposures using different machine settings may be needed.

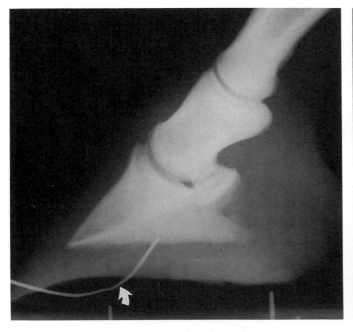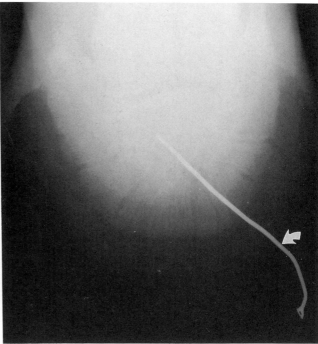

Fig. 5-2
Lateromedial and dorsopalmar views of the third phalanx following placement of a metallic probe (arrows) that demonstrated the depth and direction of a draining tract following a "street nail" injury in a 5-year-old Quarter Horse mare. In this patient, the injury is limited to the soft tissues of the foot and there are no bony changes noted radiographically.

6. HEAD

Radiography of the horse's head requires skill and imagination to achieve diagnostic radiographs of the area of interest. Radiography is an important diagnostic procedure for diagnosing: (1) dental disease, (2) diseases of the nasal cavity, and (3) diseases of the paranasal sinuses in the horse. Because the head is large, many oblique radiographic views are made with the x-ray beam in a tangential plain to the area of interest in an effort to decrease tissue thickness and remove superimposed tissues that compromise radiographic interpretation. Use of an oblique of the opposite unaffected dental arcade as a "normal control" is highly recommended because of the variation in the radiographic appearance of teeth as they age. The best "normal" radiograph for comparison is the one you make of the opposite dental arcade of the same horse.

Due to the thickness of the skull and density of the teeth, true lateral radiographs are often not of great diagnostic value, however, they can be used as a reference view. Dorsoventral (ventrodorsal) studies can be of value but are difficult to obtain in the standing horse because of the great tissue thickness and because of the problem of having to position an x-ray tube either over or under the horse's head. Occlusal views are difficult to obtain, but are of great value especially in studies of the incisor teeth. Collimation of the x-ray beam is more difficult when examining the head because of the oblique angles of the x-ray beam to the head and the fact that the beam often does not strike the cassette at a right angle. Because of beam angulation, object distortion is often seen on the resulting radiograph.

The nature of x-ray tube suspension determines whether it is convenient or even possible to use some of the positions described. Use of a ceiling-suspended tube makes movement of the tube easier but prevents you from positioning the tube under the horse's head. A portable unit on wheels can be moved easily to the horse and it is possible to position the tube under the head, but is difficult to use in a stall. Holding a box-type portable while radiographing the head is difficult because of the weight of the tube-head.

There is little preparation required in radiography of the head. Markers for right or left are required in addition to metallic markers that indicate drainage tracts or other clinically evident lesions. Markers that indicate the positioning of the cassette are helpful when studying fluid levels within the paranasal sinuses.

In the standing patient, the head is free to move in any direction. Thus, while it is possible to describe the position of the x-ray tube and cassette rather specifically, remember that the object you are radiographing is continually moving until the time of the exposure. Therefore, it may be difficult to reproduce exact positioning and a great deal of ingenuity and freedom in choice of technique must be exercised in making these examinations.

Restraint is difficult because of placement of the tube and cassette around the horse's head. It is often of some value to cover the horse's eye so that a cassette can be placed more easily against the head. Remember to remove any hands within the primary x-ray beam after the cassette is in position and just prior to the exposure. It is possible to place the patient in stocks, but it is still necessary to control the head. Use of a halter may be helpful, but in some views it is necessary to at least partially remove the halter or modify its position so that it does not create artifactual shadows on the film. Use of a rope halter is strongly recommended so that if it is within the primary beam, a part of the anatomy beneath the halter can still be visualized. Grasping the tongue and pulling it to the side often opens the mouth for special views, however, this places the hands near the primary x-ray field and thus, is not as acceptable a procedure. Tranquilization or sedation is always beneficial in performing a radiographic examination of the skull. Using the ears to control the horse is possible, but permission should be obtained from the owner.

Size of cassette is not critical and, in fact, it is probably better to use several smaller cassettes than one large one because of object distortion due to the varying object-film distances. It is important to use cassette holders around the head because of the radiation hazard from scattered radiation. Because of the difficulty of coordinating the positioning of the x-ray tube, direction of the x-ray beam, and positioning of the cassette and because most views include air-filled nasal passages and sinuses that have a low tissue density, a grid is not recommended for these studies. This means that it is possible, and often desirable, to have the x-ray beam oblique to the face of the cassette. Focal-film distance is difficult to ascertain because of the continued movement of the horse's head and it may be helpful to have a previously measured small wooden dowel or string attached to the tube head or collimator that allows you to quickly determine the correct distance to the tube head.

The radiographic examinations of the head are divided depending on the area of greatest interest as suggested by clinical signs. Some of these anatomical regions include: (1) maxillary sinuses and nasal passages (Table 6-1, Fig. 6-1), (2) frontal studies (Table 6-2, Fig. 6-2), (3) incisors (Table 6-3, Fig. 6-3), (4) maxillary check teeth (Table 6-4, Fig. 6-4), (5) mandibular check teeth (Table 6-5, Fig. 6-5), and (6) oro- and nasopharynx, larynx, and guttural pouch (Table 6-6). Some of the views used in evaluation of a certain anatomical structure are also used to study other anatomical structures with only slight changes in radiographic technique or angulation of the x-ray beam.

The maxillary sinus is identified dorsal to the upper molar teeth and the caudal root of the fourth upper check tooth. The bony septum between the cranial and caudal compartments of the maxillary sinus originates near the second molar (fifth upper check tooth). It can usually be visualized by vertically directed bony sheets, but changes in appearance from study to study occur because lack of repeatable positioning causes the x-ray beam to interact differently with the bones. The bony infraorbital canal is superimposed over the central portion of the maxillary sinus and the nasolacrimal canal is positioned at the dorsal rostral border of the maxillary sinus. The size of the maxillary sinus

Table 6-1
TECHNIQUE FOR RADIOGRAPHIC EVALUATION OF THE MAXILLARY SINUSES AND NASAL CAVITY

Standard views
   lateral
   dorsoventral
   oblique

Optional views
   coned-down

Views of the opposite side
   oblique of the opposite side should be made so that a comparison can be made

Cassette size
   varies depending on size of horse and purpose of examination

Use of cassette holders
   used when possible

Use of a grid
   not required

Markers
   right or left
   lead locational markers

Table 6-2
TECHNIQUE FOR RADIOGRAPHIC EVALUATION OF THE FRONTAL REGION

Standard views
   lateral
   oblique

Optional views
   dorsoventral or ventrodorsal views can be made in an anesthetized patient

Views of the opposite side
   oblique view of the opposite side should be made so that a comparison can be made

Cassette size
   varies depending on size of horse and purpose of examination

Use of cassette holders
   used when possible

Use of a grid
   not required

Markers
   right or left
   lead locational markers

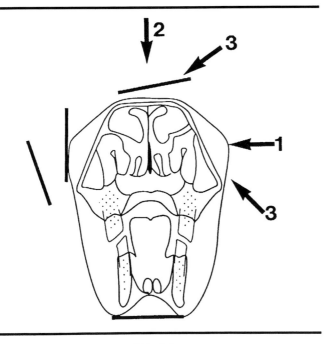

Fig. 6-1
Drawing of the cross-section of the head showing the direction of the x-ray beam for: (1) lateral views, (2) ventrodorsal views, and (3) oblique views of the nasal cavity and maxillary sinuses. The position of the cassettes is indicated (black lines).

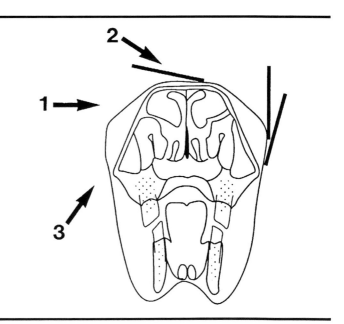

Fig. 6-2
Drawing of the cross-section of the head showing the direction of the x-ray beam for: (1) lateral views, (2) dorsoventral oblique views, and (3) ventrodorsal oblique views of the frontal sinuses. The position of the cassettes is indicated (black lines).

Table 6-3
TECHNIQUE FOR RADIOGRAPHIC EVALUATION OF THE INCISOR REGION

Standard views
  lateral
  oblique

Optional views
  dorsoventral (ventrodorsal)
  occlusal

Cassette size
  small size is adequate

Use of cassette holders
  used when possible

Use of a grid
  not required

Markers
  right or left
  upper or lower arcade

Table 6-4
TECHNIQUE FOR RADIOGRAPHIC EVALUATION OF THE UPPER DENTAL ARCADE (Maxillary Teeth)

Standard views
  lateral
  oblique

Optional views
  dorsoventral

Opposite dental arcade
  oblique of the opposite side should be made so that a comparison can be made

Cassette size
  should be large size
  size determines the region evaluated

Use of cassette holders
  used when possible

Use of grid
  not required

Markers
  right or left
  lead markers to identify site of injury or drainage

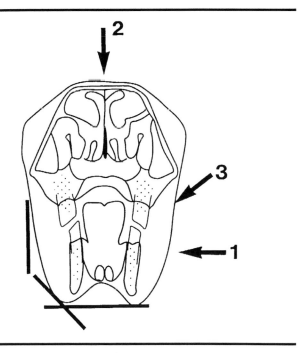

Fig. 6-3
Drawing of the cross-section of the head showing the direction of the x-ray beam for: (1) lateral views, (2) dorsoventral views, and (3) dorsoventral oblique views of the incisor teeth. The position of the cassettes is indicated (black lines).

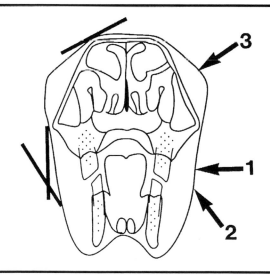

Fig. 6-4
Drawing of the cross-section of the head showing the direction of the x-ray beam for: (1) lateral views, (2) ventrodorsal oblique views, and (3) dorsoventral oblique views of the upper cheek teeth. The position of the cassettes is indicated (black lines).

Table 6-5
TECHNIQUE FOR RADIOGRAPHIC EVALUATION OF THE LOWER DENTAL ARCADE (Mandibular Teeth)

Standard views
    lateral
    oblique

Optional views
    dorsoventral
    lateral for the vertical ramus of the mandible

Views of the opposite arcade
    oblique of the opposite side should be made so that a comparison can be made

Cassette size
    use largest available

Use of cassette holders
    use is helpful

Use of grid
    may be required on the dorsoventral view

Markers
    right or left
    lead location markers

Table 6-6
TECHNIQUE FOR RADIOGRAPHIC EVALUATION OF THE ORO- AND NASOPHARYNX AND GUTTURAL POUCH

Standard view
    lateral

Optional views
    opposite lateral
    oblique with the beam directed rostrocaudally or caudorostrally

Cassette
    as large as possible

Use of grid
    not necessary but should be used if a suspended cassette holder is available

Use of cassette holder
    should be used

Markers
    right or left side
    Mitchell markers assist in determining cassette positioning

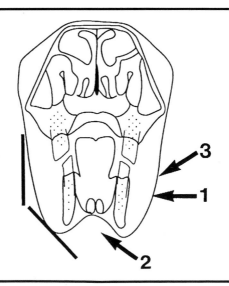

Fig. 6-5
Drawing of the cross-section of the head showing the direction of the x-ray beam for: (1) lateral views, (2) ventrodorsal oblique views, and (3) dorsoventral oblique views of the lower cheek teeth. The position of the cassettes is indicated (black lines).

appears to increase as the horse ages because of the decrease in size of the roots of the molars. The x-ray beam is usually directed toward the fourth premolar or first molar (third or fourth upper cheek teeth) in these views. If the site of the lesion is known, the x-ray beam is directed toward this particular point of interest. The view of the opposite upper arcade for comparison should be made attempting to use the same beam centering and beam angulation.

Abnormalities due to fluid accumulation within the paranasal sinuses are often recognized by horizontal air-fluid interfaces, irregular bordered fluid opacities due to trapped fluid, or smooth bordered fluid opacities due to abscessation. Horizontal air-fluid levels are seen most commonly in the maxillary sinuses, but may also be identified in the frontal sinuses. The position of the head is critical when evaluating free fluid since it shifts in location dependent on the position of the head. In the maxillary sinus, a minimal amount of fluid may be obscured by superimposed cheek teeth. Thus, the amount of fluid within the sinus and the size of the roots have a great affect on your ability to visualize free fluid within the maxillary sinus.

The frontal sinus is outlined dorsally and caudally by the frontal bone and rostrally by the maxillary sinus. The orbit is difficult to identify but is a round bony structure superimposed over the ethmoturbinates which are recognized as a spherical structure with a laminated appearance somewhat like a sliced onion. The spheno-palatine sinus is ventral and caudal to the ethmoturbinates, but is difficult to see because of superimposition from the vertical ramus of the mandible.

The horse has "hypsodont" teeth with enamel that covers both the crown and root and are different from the "brachydont" teeth of the dog and cat. The incisor teeth have deep indentations or infundibula on the occlusal surfaces with cementum and enamel covering the inner surface of the infundibula. The deciduous dental formula is 3/3 incisors, 1/1 canine teeth, and 3/3 check teeth. The most common permanent dental formula is 3/3 incisors, 1/1 canine teeth, 3/3 premolar teeth, and 3/3 molar teeth. The first premolar teeth are present uncommonly and are referred to as "wolf" teeth. If present, they are much smaller than the other three premolars.

Eruption of the permanent teeth causes resorption of the roots of the three deciduous cheek teeth and the creation of "caps" that represent the residual of the deciduous teeth that are located "capping" the occlusal surface of the erupting permanent teeth. These are normally broken off or may remain in position causing problems in eruption of the permanent teeth. The permanent teeth continue to grow with lengthening of the roots until six years of age, at which age, the teeth appear to shorten due to attrition with the creation of long, tapered roots.

The periodontal space is identified by the radiolucent zone between the cementum/enamel on the root and the trabecular bone forming the alveolus around the root. Identification of the periodontal space is relatively easy in the younger patient but becomes a less easily visualized structure as the horse ages. The radiolucent space around the tooth continues around the apex of the root creating a rounded radiolucent pocket in the younger horse. With age, this radiolucent pocket disappears and is replaced by sparse bony trabeculae surrounding the thin, tapering roots of the older horse. However, the periodontal space in the older horse remains as a thinner radiolucent zone around the proximal portion of the roots.

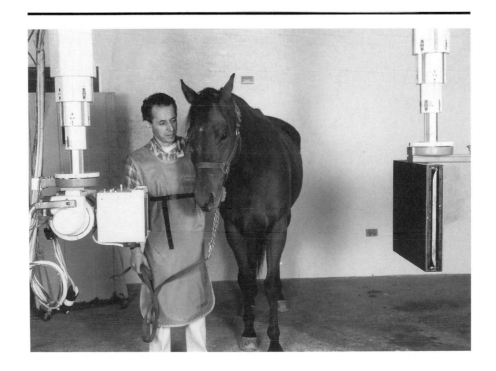

HEAD—LATERAL VIEW

Purpose—This view permits evaluation of the air-filled paranasal sinuses and nasal passages. The sinuses are superimposed and laterality of a lesion may not be determined from the radiographic study, but injury to the surrounding bone may be identified. Both bone lesions and fluid-filled sinuses are contrasted nicely with the aerated portions of the head. Rostral or caudal malalignment of the incisor teeth following developmental anomaly or traumatic injury can seen. The two large dental arcades are superimposed on this view and dental disease is difficult to identify.

Preparation—No special preparation is required other than brushing the haircoat.

Patient Positioning—The horse stands naturally with removal of the halter if possible or use of a less radiopaque round or flat rope halter.

Tube Positioning—The x-ray tube is positioned laterally on one side of the head and the cassette against the affected side. The x-ray beam is parallel to the ground and is directed toward the area of interest or near the site of the first molar if the study is to be of a survey nature. It is best to use a ceiling-suspended or hand held cassette holder (Figs. 6-6, 6-7). In the absence of a cassette holder, avoid standing directly behind the cassette in this view and even consider using two people to hold the cassette so that neither is within the primary beam. Large movable plate-holding devices are available that can be rolled into position.

Radiographic Technique for Portable Unit for the Lateral view of the Nasal Cavity and Maxillary Sinuses (400 speed film-screen system)

- 80 kVp, 10 mA, 0.1 sec, 26 inches focal-film distance
- 80 kVp, 20 mA, 0.06 sec, 26 inches focal-film distance

Radiographic Technique for Portable Unit for Lateral View of the Frontal Region (400 speed film-screen system)

- 80 kVp, 10 mA, 0.1 sec, 26 inches focal-film distance
- 80 kVp, 20 mA, 0.06 sec, 26 inches focal-film distance

Radiographic Technique for Portable Unit for the Lateral View of the Incisor Region (400 speed film-screen system)

- 80 kVp, 10 mA, 0.16 sec, 26 inches focal-film distance
- 80 kVp, 20 mA, 0.08 sec, 26 inches focal-film distance

Radiographic Technique for Portable Unit for the Lateral View of the Upper Dental Arcade (Maxillary Teeth) (400 speed film-screen system)

- 80 kVp, 10 mA, 0.25-0.3 sec, 26 inches focal-film distance
- 80 kVp, 20 mA, 0.12-0.16 sec, 26 inches focal-film distance

---

Radiographic Technique for Portable Unit for the Lateral View of the Lower Dental Arcade (Mandibular Teeth) (400 speed film-screen system)

- 80 kVp, 10 mA, 0.25-0.3 sec, 26 inches focal-film distance
- 80 kVp, 20 mA, 0.12-0.16 sec, 26 inches focal-film distance

---

Radiographic Technique for Portable Unit for Lateral View of the Mandible (400 speed film-screen system)

- 80 kVp, 10 mA, 0.2 sec, 26 inches focal-film distance
- 80 kVp, 20 mA, 0.1 sec, 26 inches focal-film distance

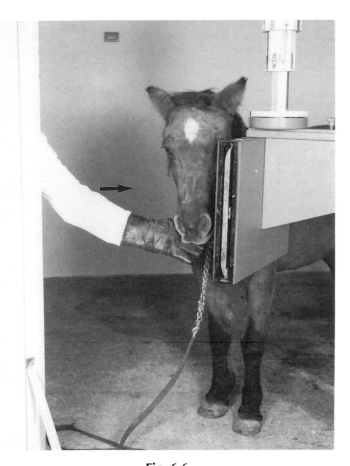

Fig. 6-6

Photograph of the positioning of the head used for making a lateral view especially for the paranasal sinuses. The horse is standing normally. The x-ray tube is positioned laterally and the x-ray beam is directed horizontally (arrow). The central beam is directed at the first upper molar or at an area of interest. The cassette is positioned either by a ceiling-suspended holder or in a hand-held holder.

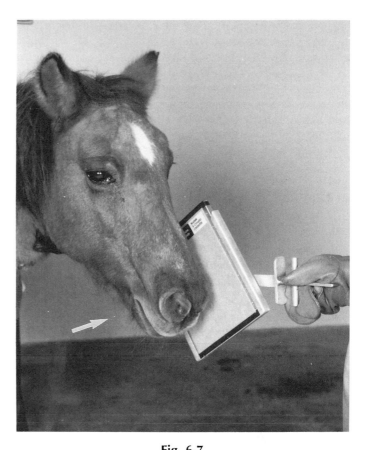

Fig. 6-7

Photograph of the positioning of the head used for making a lateral view of the incisor region. The horse is standing normally. The x-ray tube is positioned laterally and the x-ray beam is directed horizontally (arrow). The central beam is directed at the incisors. The cassette is positioned in a hand-held holder.

HEAD—DORSOVENTRAL (ventrodorsal) VIEW

Purpose—This view permits comparison of one side of the head with the other and permits detection of differences in size, shape, and density of individual anatomical structures. Identification of density differences are important because of the common finding of fluid-filled sinuses or soft tissue masses within the nasal cavity. Bony differences are more difficult to appreciate because of the presence of superimposed dense dental structures. Because of the density of the teeth, they are not usually studied using this view. However, since they are seen "en face", the surrounding alveoli can often be studied.

Preparation—No special preparation is required other than brushing the haircoat.

Patient Positioning—The horse stands naturally but with the head depressed as far as is possible so that the x-ray tube can be placed in front of the head.

Tube Positioning—The x-ray tube is positioned in front and dorsally over the head and the cassette is placed against the ventral aspect of the mandible. Use a cassette holder if possible. The x-ray beam is directed toward the ground being centered on the midline of the head on the area of interest (Figs. 6-8, 6-9). There may be rare situations in which it is desirable to position the x-ray tube under the head and place the cassette dorsally against the maxilla and nasal bones but this is more difficult.

Radiographic Technique for Portable Unit for Dorsoventral View of the Nasal Cavity and Maxillary Sinuses (400 speed film-screen system)

- 80 kVp, 10 mA, 0.3-0.4 sec, 26 inches focal-film distance
- 80 kVp, 20 mA, 0.16-0.2 sec, 26 inches focal-film distance

Radiographic Technique for Portable Unit for the Dorsoventral View of the Incisor Region (400 speed film-screen system)

- 80 kVp, 10 mA, 0.16 sec, 26 inches focal-film distance
- 80 kVp, 20 mA, 0.08 sec, 26 inches focal-film distance

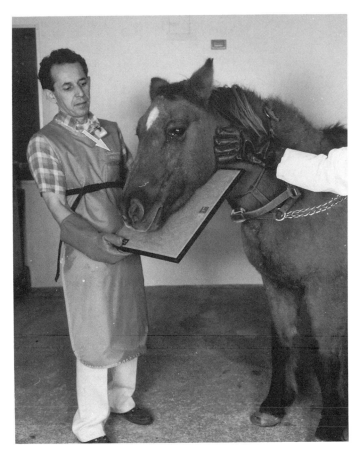

Fig. 6-8
Photograph of the positioning of the head used for making a dorsoventral view. The horse is standing normally. The x-ray tube is positioned cranially and dorsally and the x-ray beam is directed vertically so it is nearly perpendicular to the face of the cassette (arrow). Positioning of the tube is somewhat dependent on how high or low the horse holds its head. The central beam is directed between the first upper molars (fourth upper cheek teeth) or at an area of interest. It may be difficult to position the cassette in a holder, and, therefore, it is often hand-held. Good collimation of the primary beam is required in either situation.

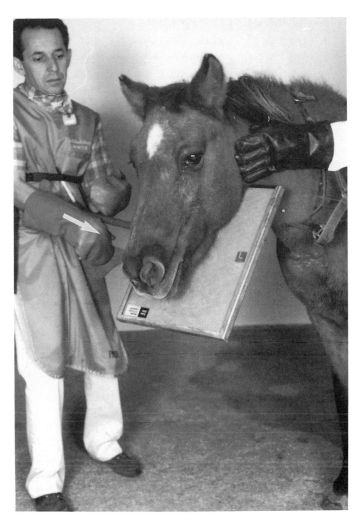

Fig. 6-9
Photograph of the positioning of the head used to make the dorsoventral radiograph of the incisor teeth. The cassette is held against the body (horizontal ramus) of the mandible and the x-ray beam (arrows) is directed so that it is perpendicular to the face of the cassette and centered on the incisor region. Try to let the head remain in a neutral position. Remove the halter if it is possible to control the head in another way. The size of the cassette used for this study may vary.

HEAD—OBLIQUE VIEW
(dorso 45° lateral-ventrolateral D45L-VLO or dorso 60° lateral-ventrolateral D60L-VLO)

Purpose—These views produce the best radiographs for evaluation of the maxillary sinuses, frontal sinuses, and both dental arcades. Bilateral studies should be made because there is great variation in the appearance of the teeth with age, and having the unaffected side to compare with the affected one is most helpful. Oblique views are important in evaluation of the roots of the cheek teeth since they are projected free of other bony or dental structures. This provides good visualization of the ventral portion of the maxillary sinus and the middle of the frontal sinus without superimposition of the orbit or ethmoturbinates.

Preparation—No special preparation is required other than brushing the haircoat.

Patient Positioning—The horse can stand naturally.

Tube Positioning—To visualize the maxillary sinuses and the nasal passages, the cassette is placed ventrally against the affected side of the head and the x-ray tube is positioned dorsolaterally above the head on the opposite unaffected side. The x-ray beam is directed downward toward the head centering on the third and fourth cheek teeth on the affected side. The cassette is angled against the head at approximately 45° (Fig. 6-10).

To visualize the incisor region, the cassette is positioned below the affected jaw and laterally with the x-ray tube positioned above and laterally. It is also possible to position the cassette above the affected jaw and laterally with the x-ray tube positioned below and laterally. The x-ray beam is directed at a 45° angle.

To visualize the upper dental arcade, the cassette is placed against the affected side of the head and the x-ray tube is placed laterally against the unaffected side of the head dorsally. The x-ray beam is directed downward at a 45° angle and is centered on the region of interest. The oblique of the normal side is made in a similar manner. It is also possible to make this oblique view with the x-ray tube positioned laterally and ventrally below the head on the affected side with the cassette against the unaffected side dorsally. In this technique, the x-ray beam is divided upwardly.

To visualize the lower dental arcade, the cassette is placed against the unaffected side of the head ventrally. The x-ray tube is placed laterally to the affected side of the head dorsally and the x-ray beam is directed downward at a 45° angle. It is also possible to make this oblique view by directing the x-ray beam in an upward direction aiming at the intermandibular area. The cassette is positioned dorsally and laterally to the affected side.

To visualize the frontal region, the cassette is placed against the horse's head on the affected side slightly ventrally and the x-ray tube is placed on the opposite unaffected side slightly above the head. The x-ray beam is obliqued downward approximately at a 30° angle and centered on the midline just behind the eye on the affected side.

Radiographic Technique for Portable Unit for the Oblique View of the Maxillary Sinuses and Nasal Passages (400 speed film-screen system)

- 80 kVp, 10 mA, 0.1 sec, 26 inches focal-film distance
- 80 kVp, 20 mA, 0.06 sec, 26 inches focal-film distance

Radiographic Technique for Portable Unit for the Oblique View of the Frontal Region (400 speed film-screen system)

- 80 kVp, 10 mA, 0.1 sec, 26 inches focal-film distance
- 80 kVp, 20 mA, 0.06 sec, 26 inches focal-film distance

Radiographic Technique for Portable Unit for the Oblique View of the Incisor Region (400 speed film-screen system)

- 80 kVp, 10 mA, 0.16 sec, 26 inches focal-film distance
- 80 kVp, 20 mA, 0.08 sec, 26 inches focal-film distance

Radiographic Technique for Portable Unit for the Oblique View of the Upper Dental Arcade (400 speed film-screen system)

- 80 kVp, 10 mA, 0.16-0.2 sec, 26 inches focal-film distance
- 80 kVp, 20 mA, 0.08-0.12 sec, 26 inches focal-film distance

---

Radiographic Technique for Portable Unit for the Oblique View of the Lower Dental Arcade (400 speed film-screen system)

- 80 kVp, 10 mA, 0.16-0.2 sec, 26 inches focal-film distance
- 80 kVp, 20 mA, 0.08-0.12 sec, 26 inches focal-film distance

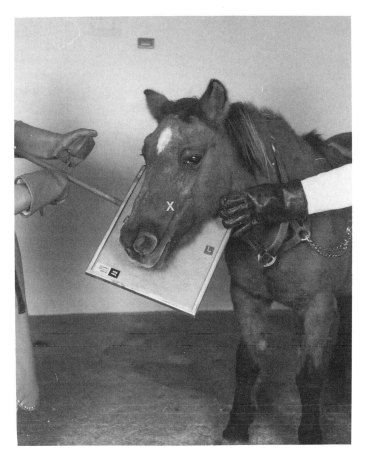

Fig. 6-10

Photograph of the positioning of the head used for making an oblique view of the nasal cavity and maxillary sinuses (dorsolateral-ventrolateral). The horse is standing normally. The x-ray tube is positioned above the head and adjacent to the unaffected side. The x-ray beam is directed obliquely downward so that it is nearly perpendicular to the face of the cassette. The central beam is directed at the first upper molar or at an area of interest (x). It is imperative that the beam be closely collimated so that hands are outside of the primary beam.

INCISOR TEETH—OCCLUSAL VIEW

Purpose—This view is difficult because it requires that the cassette be placed within the horses mouth. Still, it is worth attempting because it demonstrates a lesion involving the incisors with the greatest clarity because there are no overlying bone or dental structures.

Preparation—The horse usually requires chemical restraint to be able to position the cassette within the mouth, otherwise, it is possible to attempt to use a specially constructed cassette holder that includes some type of a speculum device to protect the cassette.

Patient Positioning—The horse can be standing or recumbent.

Tube Positioning—For the upper incisors, the x-ray tube is positioned over the head with the beam directed downward. For the lower incisors, the x-ray tube is positioned below the head with the beam directed upward. The x-ray beam is directed toward the intra-oral cassette and is perpendicular to its surface. This can be accomplished by following the angle of the head as the horse as it is raised or lowered. Focal-film distance may be decreased for this view.

Radiographic Technique for Portable Unit (400 speed film-screen system)

- 80 kVp, 10 mA, 0.06 sec, 20 inches focal-film distance
- 80 kVp, 20 mA, 0.04 sec, 20 inches focal-film distance

ORO- AND NASOPHARYNX AND GUTTURAL POUCH

These structures can be evaluated with a lateral view using x-ray machines with minimal capabilities because they are soft tissue structures, contain air, and the tissue thickness is not great. Findings of greatest interest are the character of the epiglottis and the arytenoid folds, presence of fluid or thickening of the lining of the guttural pouches, laryngeal masses, and the character of the soft palate (Fig. 6-11). The head should be held slightly extended so as to move the vertical ramus of the mandible so it isn't superimposed over areas of interest. A lateral view centering on the area of interest is the only view that can be made. The structures to be evaluated are on the midline, but it may still be helpful to compare the opposite lateral view in localizing a lesion based on its magnification due to differing object-film distances. Use of a suspended cassette holder makes this study relatively easy (Table 6-6).

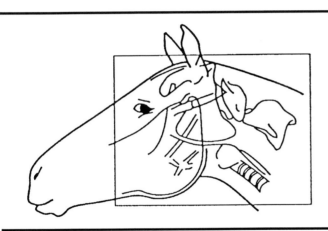

Fig. 6-11
Drawing of the head of a horse showing location of the guttural pouch relative to the nasopharynx, oropharynx, and larynx. The x-ray beam is centered on the caudal aspect of the mid-portion of the mandibular ramus.

ORO- AND NASOPHARYNX AND GUTTURAL POUCH—LATERAL VIEW

Purpose—This is the only view that is regularly made of the soft tissues in the neck.

Preparation—No special preparation is required other than brushing the haircoat.

Patient Positioning—The horse stands naturally. Rarely the study can be made in lateral recumbency. Remember that positioning of the head determines how fluid within the guttural pouch will be visualized radiographically.

Tube Positioning—The cassette is positioned against one side of the neck. Since the structures are near or are on the midline, use of either lateral view usually produces a diagnostic radiograph. If the lesion appears to be located to one side, the cassette should be against the affected side if this is possible. The x-ray tube is placed on the opposite side of the neck. In the standing patient, the x-ray beam is parallel to the ground and centered just caudally to the mid-portion of the ramus of the mandible.

Radiographic Technique for Portable Unit (400 speed film-screen system)

- 80 kVp, 10 mA, 0.3 sec, 26 inches focal-film distance
- 80 kVp, 20 mA, 0.16 sec, 26 inches focal-film distance

Table 6-6
TECHNIQUE FOR RADIOGRAPHIC EVALUATION OF THE ORO- AND NASOPHARYNX AND GUTTURAL POUCH

Standard view
    lateral

Optional views
    opposite lateral
    oblique with the beam directed rostrocaudally or caudorostrally

Cassette
    as large as possible

Use of grid
    not necessary but should be used if a suspended cassette holder is available

Use of cassette holder
    should be used

Markers
    right or left side
    Mitchell markers assist in determining cassette positioning

7. TRACHEA AND ESOPHAGUS

Studies of the soft tissues of the horse's neck provide information concerning the air-filled trachea and esophagus. Only lateral views can be made on the standing horse. Oblique views made on a recumbent patient are more diagnostic than ventrodorsal views because of the positioning of the endotracheal tube. Flexion and extension studies add information to that seen on the neutrally positioned lateral views since they may be helpful in repositioning the trachea relative to a soft tissue mass (Table 7-1).

If the x-ray tube is ceiling mounted and a cassette holder is attached, lateral views of the cervical region in a standing patient are relatively easy to make. Markers are placed ventrally on the neck to be away from a suspected lesion. If a portable unit is used, it is more difficult to elevate both tube and cassette so that the central beam is centered on the cassette.

Because the trachea is filled with air, it is easily seen radiographically without use of any contrast agent. Radiographic techniques are determined by the tissue density to be penetrated, with less exposure required for the trachea and esophageal studies than for the spinal studies. Usually large cassettes are used so there can be some continuity in evaluation of the various regions of the neck. Overlapping films produce a series of radiographs that permit evaluation of the entire cervical trachea. Soft tissues localization markers make this orientation easier. Studies of the esophagus are suggested in patients with dysphagia. The esophagus is normally collapsed and does not contain air or radiodense material and is, therefore, not normally identified on a non-contrast film. It can be visualized in the pathological state if intra- or extraluminal air is present or if a radiopaque foreign body in lodged in the esophagus. The best visualization of the esophagus follows administration of a positive contrast agent alone or combined with air.

Ventrodorsal or oblique views are usually made only in a recumbent horse and right or left markers are needed. Use of a grid is not required on the lateral views, but may be important if ventrodorsal or oblique views are made on a large patient in a recumbent position. Usually three overlapping exposures permits evaluation of the entire cervical esophagus. Visualization of the esophagus at the thoracic inlet is always difficult because of the presence of the skeletal structures and muscles in this region.

Table 7-1
TECHNIQUE FOR RADIOGRAPHIC EVALUATION OF THE TRACHEA AND ESOPHAGUS

Standard views
  lateral

Optional views
  opposite lateral may be helpful
  oblique may be made if the patient is recumbent
  flexion and extension may be made

Cassette size
  largest cassettes available should be used

Use of cassette holders
  the study is much easier performed with ceiling-suspended holders on a standing patient

Use of grids
  not necessary

Markers
  right or left

TRACHEA—LATERAL VIEWS

Purpose—The size, shape, and location of the air-filled trachea and the integrity of the tracheal wall can be determined, in addition to the presence of intraluminal, mural, or extra-mural lesions.

Preparation—No preparation is required other than brushing the haircoat.

Patient Positioning—The horse can stand normally so that the x-ray beam can be centered on the cervical region. Try to elevate the head so that the mandible isn't superimposed over the larynx.

Tube Positioning—The x-ray tube is placed laterally. In the standing patient, the x-ray beam is parallel to the ground and centered just caudal to the mid-portion of the ramus of the mandible. The cassette is held against the opposite side of the neck. The most cranial studies are centered on the larynx, while the other studies are centered on the mid-cervical trachea and at the thoracic inlet.

Radiographic Technique for Portable Unit (400 speed film-screen system)

- 80 kVp, 10 mA, 0.1 sec, 26 inches focal-film distance

- 80 kVp, 20 mA, 0.06 sec, 26 inches focal-film distance

ESOPHAGUS—LATERAL VIEWS

Purpose—Evaluation of a patient may be helpful to determine the cause of dysphagia. Use of a positive contrast agent alone or with air greatly improves the quality of the study.

Preparation—No preparation is required for the non-contrast study. In the event of a dilated proximal esophagus, it is helpful to empty it of food and fluid prior to administration of a positive contrast agent. Otherwise, you are simply adding the contrast agent to a fluid filled esophagus and the contrast agent cannot outline the point of obstruction, stricture, or ulceration.

Patient Positioning—The study is usually limited to lateral views made with the horse standing. If the horse is tranquilized, the head is often held down. If alert, the head is more often held high making the study more difficult especially when trying to administer a liquid contrast agent.

Tube Positioning—The cassette is held against the side of the neck. The x-ray tube is placed on the opposite side of the neck and the x-ray beam directed parallel to the ground and centered on the cassette.

The non-contrast radiograph is made as a control study prior to administration of the contrast agent. The contrast media is then given by use of a dose syringe or through a tube. Barium sulfate liquid is rather easily administered through a dose syringe and the exposure is made just after swallowing. Hold the horse's head high in the air after putting the contrast solution in the mouth to avoid receiving a "white" shower. For the first films, it is recommended to administer between 100 and 150 cc of barium sulfate solution for a suspected high cervical lesion. After evaluation of the first view, additional contrast agent may be added. It is also possible to pass a stomach tube to a point of stricture and infuse a smaller amount of the barium sulfate suspension through the tube at this point of interest. This technique requires use of much less barium sulfate mixture and avoids having the potential mess that results after trying to administer a large amount of contrast agent through a dose syringe. Additional radiographs can be made after several swallowing attempts. Radiographs that show the contrast solution both proximal and distal to the stricture are of greatest value since they can be of value in determining the length and character of the stenotic lesion. If a tube is used to administer the contrast agent, it should be withdrawn prior to the last exposure.

Esophatrast is a thicker barium sulfate preparation that tends to coat the mucosal surface of the esophagus and is of value in the determination of mural or mucosal lesions. It can be used to better advantage in the event of a suspected esophageal lesion that is not characterized by stricture or intraluminal obstructive mass. Dependent on size, it requires about 1/2 to 3/4 tube of esophatrast or 200 to 400 gm (300 to 600 cc) of a thick liquid barium sulfate suspension to study the esophagus of a single patient. (Esophatrast is available in a 16 ounce, 800 gm, tube.)

If the radiographs suggest a normal passage of the liquid barium solution, it may then be valuable to mix the contrast agent with grain or concentrate and feed it with the intent of evaluating swallowing function and to evaluate if there is sufficient esophageal distention to permit passage of a solid bolus.

Air can also be used as the contrast agent. It does not coat the mucosal surface, but distends the esophagus and is of value in determination of esophageal stricture. The air contrasts nicely with the esophageal wall following administration of barium sulfate solution and creates a double-contrast study when performed in this manner. It may not be possible to penetrate a solid column of barium sulfate solution with the x-ray beam and identify an intraluminal lesion. The double-contrast contrast column permits identification of intraluminal lesions as well as mucosal pattern because of its decreased density.

Radiographic Technique for Portable Unit (400 speed film-screen system)

- 80 kVp, 10 mA, 0.1 sec, 26 inches focal-film distance
- 80 kVp, 20 mA, 0.06 sec, 26 inches focal-film distance

---

8. SPINE

CERVICAL SPINE

Studies of the cervical vertebra may be required because of cervical pain with or without neurological deficits and are most commonly made in the foal that has suffered an acute traumatic event and sustained a fracture/dislocation. In the yearling or 2-year-old, suspected developmental cervical spondylopathy is often a reason for radiographic examination. The overlapping series of films provides good evaluation of the bony segments and the interposed radiolucent intervertebral discs.

Most studies of the cervical spine are made in the standing patient and are done without special preparation. If the patient is recumbent it is important to place pads under the head to position the spine parallel to the ground or parallel to the tabletop. Difficulty may be encountered in positioning the cassettes under the neck unless a table with a cassette tray is available. In positioning the suspected trauma patient, care should be taken to avoid potential injury to the spinal cord. It may be possible to position the horse in dorsal recumbency and make ventrodorsal views of the cervical spine. If this is done, it must be recognized that the neck arches greatly with the horse in this position and padding must be used to reduce this arching. In addition, the x-ray beam should be angled caudal to cranial to obtain the best projection of the disc spaces. Regardless of positioning, several radiographs are needed to evaluate the entire cervical spine (Table 8-1).

Table 8-1
TECHNIQUE FOR RADIOGRAPHIC EVALUATION OF THE CERVICAL SPINE

Standard views
   multiple lateral views made in the standing or recumbent patient

Optional views
   multiple flexed and extended lateral
   ventrodorsal
   oblique

Cassettes
   large size should be used

Use of grid
   difficult to use in lateral views of standing patients
   helpful in lateral views of recumbent patients
   necessary for ventrodorsal studies

Use of cassette holders
   difficult to use in standing patients unless ceiling suspended

Markers
   locational markers and numbers are needed to identify cervical segments

CERVICAL SPINE—LATERAL VIEWS

Purpose—This is often used as a survey study and is helpful in determination of the diagnosis or prognosis of a severely affected horse.

Preparation—If the horse is ambulatory, there is probably no need for special preparation. If the horse is recumbent, take special care to clean the neck especially on the down side and use positioning devices such as foam wedges to make the cervical spine parallel to the ground or tabletop.

Patient Positioning—Positioning is dependent on whether the patient is standing or is recumbent.

Tube Positioning—In the standing patient, the cassette is held against the side of the neck with the x-ray tube on the opposite side. The x-ray beam is parallel to the ground and the most cranial view is centered on C-2 (Fig. 8-1A), the second view is centered on C-4 (Fig. 8-1B), and the caudal view is centered on C-6 (Fig. 8-1C). Place lead markers on the neck so that the similarly appearing cervical segments can be identified without question. Increases in the radiographic technique are necessary for the caudal view because of the increased thickness of the neck at the thoracic inlet. Additional flexed and extended studies can be made with the head depressed or elevated, although, this may be difficult in the standing animal.

If the patient is recumbent, it is much easier to position the x-ray tube over the horse with the beam directed vertically. It may be difficult to place the cassette under the horse unless you have a cassette tray under the table. Because of the thickness of the shoulders, the head and neck in the recumbent animal are much lower and are in an oblique position relative to the tabletop or ground. Large wedge pads need to be used to elevate the head so the cervical spine is parallel to the tabletop or the ground. Flexed and extended lateral views are more easily made in the anesthetized horse. Drawings assist in understanding these views (Fig. 8-2).

CERVICAL SPINE—CRANIAL PORTION
Radiographic Technique for Portable Unit (400 speed film-screen system)

- 80 kVp, 10 mA, 0.2 sec, 26 inches focal-film distance
- 80 kVp, 20 mA, 0.1 sec, 26 inches focal-film distance

CERVICAL SPINE—MIDDLE PORTION
Radiographic Technique for Portable Unit (400 speed film-screen system)

- 80 kVp, 10 mA, 0.3-0.4 sec, 26 inches focal-film distance
- 80 kVp, 20 mA, 0.2-0.25 sec, 26 inches focal-film distance

CERVICAL SPINE—CAUDAL PORTION
Radiographic Technique for Portable Unit (400 speed film-screen system)

- 80 kVp, 10 mA, 0.5 - 0.8 sec, 26 inches focal-film distance
- 80 kVp, 20 mA, 0.35 - 0.5 sec, 26 inches focal-film distance

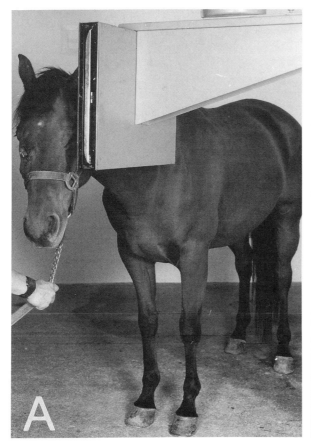

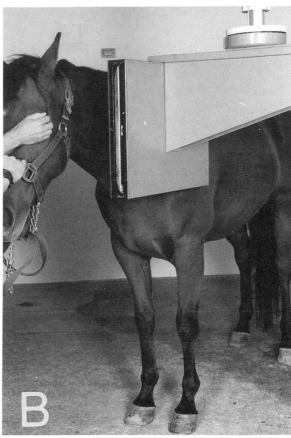

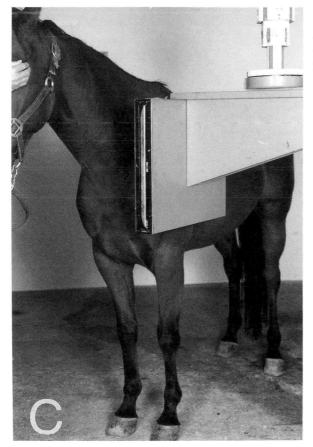

Fig. 8-1
Photographs showing positioning of the standing horse for lateral cervical studies centered on C-2 (A), C-4 (B), and C-6 (C). Use of a suspended cassette holder makes this study on a standing horse much easier. The x-ray beam is directed in a horizontal plane centered appropriately for each view.

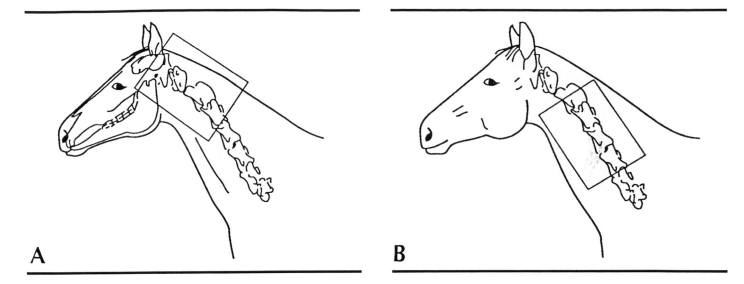

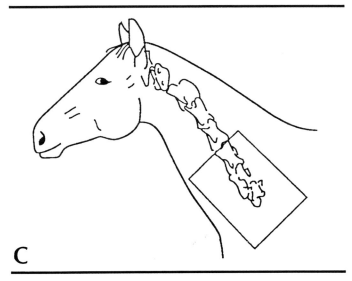

Fig. 8-2
Drawings showing positioning of the recumbent horse for lateral cervical studies centered on C-2 (A), C-4 (B), and C-6 (C).

CERVICAL MYELOGRAPHY

This special procedure requires: (1) the patient be anesthetized, (2) a method be established for easily and quickly changing cassettes, (3) a grid holder or tray be available, (4) positioning of the head that insures that the cervical spine is parallel to the tabletop or cassette holder, and (5) availability of assistants that are available to move the horse as is required. It is a valuable technique for ascertaining the degree, nature, and location of spinal cord lesions of the cervical spine causing transverse myelopathy. These lesions are often associated with developmental cervical spondylopathy or an acute or healed fracture. Metrizamide (Amipaque, Winthrop-Breon Laboratories, New York, NY), Iohexol (Omnipaque, Winthrop-Breon Laboratories, New York, NY), and Iopamidol (Isovue, E.R.Squibb & Sons Co, Princeton, NJ) are all water-soluble, nonionic, triiodinated benzoic acid-derivatives that can be safely used in horses as well as in dogs and cats. Iohexol is used at concentrations of 180 or 240 mgs of I/ml while iopamidol has been safe and effective at concentrations of 200 mg of I/ml. Iopamidol is used at a concentration of 300 mg of I/ml without adverse effects. Both iohexol and iopamidol are available in multidose sterile vials.

Prior to the myelogram, physical and neurological examinations and a non-contrast cervical radiographic study are performed. The non-contrast radiographic study is most easily made following anesthesia, just prior to the myelogram. A basic rule in diagnostic radiology is to never inject a contrast agent unless a diagnostic non-contrast study has been performed first.

Following anesthesia, cerebrospinal fluid (CSF) is collected from the cisterna magna at the time of spinal needle positioning and may be evaluated for cell count, differential determination, and protein content prior to injection of the contrast agent. Permit as much CSF to flow from the needle as is possible, since removal of CSF lessens the increase in pressure that results from the injection. Inject the contrast medium at a rate of 10 to 12 ml/minute over a 4 to 5 minute period to achieve the injection of the required 40 to 60 ml. A 3/4 inch plywood board or similar positioning device is placed under the head and neck to elevate the head for 5 minutes following the injection to insure that the contrast agent flows into the spinal subarachnoid space rather than around the brain.

The series of radiographic views is the same as that used for examination of the cervical spine (Fig. 8-2). Flexed and extended views are carefully used to temporarily exaggerate spinal cord compression and maximally demonstrate the site of maximum injury. Ventrodorsal and oblique views are difficult to make in the anesthetized horse, but may serve to support the findings noted on the lateral views and may demonstrate laterally located compressive lesions that are not visible on the lateral views.

CRANIAL PORTION
Radiographic Technique for Portable Unit (400 speed film-screen system)

- 80 kVp, 10 mA, 0.2 sec, 26 inches focal-film distance
- 80 kVp, 20 mA, 0.1 sec, 26 inches focal-film distance

MIDDLE PORTION
Radiographic Technique for Portable Unit (400 speed film-screen system)

- 80 kVp, 10 mA, 0.3-0.4 sec, 26 inches focal-film distance
- 80 kVp, 20 mA, 0.2-0.25 sec, 26 inches focal-film distance

CAUDAL PORTION
Radiographic Technique for Portable Unit (400 speed film-screen system)

- 80 kVp, 10 mA, 0.5-0.8 sec, 26 inches focal-film distance
- 80 kVp, 20 mA, 0.35-0.5 sec, 26 inches focal-film distance

THORACIC SPINE

The study is most easily performed in younger horses searching for hematogenous spondylitis characterized by collapse of vertebral bodies with marked shortening noted radiographically, or vertebral fractures that may appear with a similar pattern of vertebral collapse. The study is limited to lateral views in most patients.

With portable equipment, this study can be performed on smaller patients who are standing, while higher powered equipment and a ceiling suspended x-ray tube and cassette holder are required to examine larger horses in a standing position. On patients who are anesthetized, and motion can be controlled, lower powered equipment may be adequate for any size patient. In the adult horse, only a few vertebral segments can be included on each lateral view.

In the standing patient, the x-ray beam is horizontal and centered on the segment(s) of interest. In the recumbent patient, the x-ray beam is directed vertically being centered on the region of interest. Use of a grid improves the quality of the resulting radiograph and should be used where possible in all patients.

Studies of the spinous processes are a helpful study in the older patient with a history of trauma to the region of the withers or a history of a draining tract over the back. The patient is usually radiographed standing with the cassette positioned further dorsally and is more easily perform if some type of cassette holder can be used. A grid is usually not used for these studies. It is possible to prepare a cassette with intensifying screens of different speeds to compensate for the difference in tissue thickness. By having a slower speed screen dorsally and a faster speed screen ventrally, it is possible to use one exposure and obtain a satisfactory radiograph of the entire spinous process. Otherwise, it is necessary to use different exposure settings for two views to permit visualization of both the base of the spinous processes as well as the tips (Table 8-2).

Table 8-2
TECHNIQUE FOR RADIOGRAPHIC EVALUATION OF THE THORACIC SPINE

Standard views
  multiple lateral views made in the standing or recumbent patient

Optional views
  centering on tips of the spinous processes with decreased technique

Cassettes
  large size should be used

Use of grid
  difficult to use in lateral views of standing patients
  helpful in lateral views of recumbent patients

Use of cassette holders
  difficult to use in standing patients unless ceiling suspended

Markers
  locational markers may be used

DORSAL PORTION OF THE WITHERS
Radiographic Technique for Portable Unit (400 speed film-screen system)

- 80 kVp, 10 mA, 0.2 sec, 26 inches focal-film distance
- 80 kVp, 20 mA, 0.1 sec, 26 inches focal-film distance

VENTRAL PORTION OF THE WITHERS
Radiographic Technique for Portable Unit (400 speed film-screen system)

- 80 kVp, 10 mA, 0.4 - 0.5 sec, 26 inches focal-film distance
- 80 kVp, 20 mA, 0.2 - 0.3 sec, 26 inches focal-film distance

9. THORAX

Studies of the thorax have become more common with the development of equipment with tubes of greater heat-capacity capabilities and more satisfactory methods of providing chemical restraint for the horse. Exposure times can be decreased by the use of faster rare-earth film-screen systems. A major problem in thoracic radiography is the need for a linkage system between the x-ray tube and the cassette holder so that the x-ray beam can be quickly changed in position and remain directed toward the center of the cassette. This type of synchronous movement is relatively easy to obtain with ceiling supported systems (Fig. 8-1) that place the horse between the x-ray tube and the cassette. One danger inherent in the use of these systems is that the patient may move laterally and strike either the x-ray tube or the suspended cassette holder.

A combination of views are made in the adult patient. Radiography in the foal is easier to perform and the study can be accomplished with one film. The side suspected of being diseased is placed next to the cassette to obtain the smallest object-film distance between the lesion and the film. By comparing two opposite lateral radiographs made with the right and left sides against the cassette, it is possible to locate a lesion within the chest cavity. Good grid systems are necessary to clean up the scattered radiation that would otherwise fog the film. Use a lead marker at the 11th interspace so that the distance between the ribs can serve as an indicator of the stage of respiration. This marker also serves as a reference point for thoracocentesis or for directing an ultrasound study.

Focal film distances used for thoracic radiography are usually 40 inches (100 cm) to 60 inches (150 cm). This distance can be increased to 80 inches (200 cm) and an airgap of 6-8 inch (9 to 20 cm) distance between the patient and the cassette be used to decrease the amount of scatter radiation rather than use a grid. This savings in radiographic technique obtained by not using the grid can be used to compensate for the increase in technique that is needed due to the increased focal-film distance (Table 9-1).

Ventrodorsal radiographs cannot be made in the adult patient, but they can be made in the small foal. While not technically excellent, they are still of great assistance in especially for evaluation of the caudal lung lobes.

Table 9-1
TECHNIQUE FOR RADIOGRAPHIC EVALUATION OF THE THORAX

Standard views
    multiple lateral

Optional views
    ventrodorsal in small patients

Opposite lateral views
    may be helpful in localizing pulmonary or pleural lesions

Cassette size
    must be large

Use of cassette holder
    almost mandatory

Use of grid
    grid system must be good or airgap utilized to control scatter radiation

Markers
    needed to mark ribs for orientation

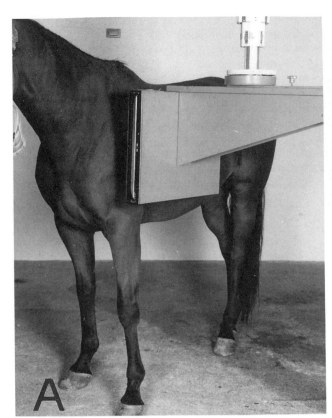

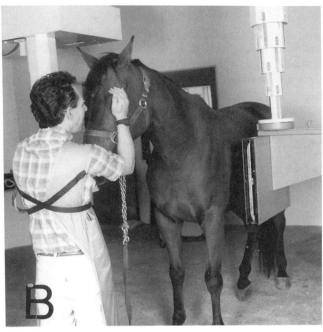

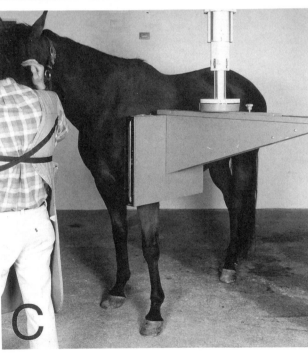

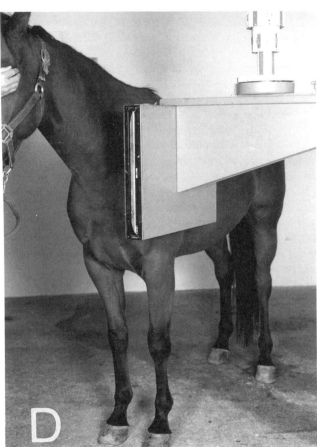

Fig. 9-1

Photographs of patient and cassette positioning for the four views commonly used in lateral radiography of the mature horse's thorax. Suspended and cross-connected x-ray tube and cassette holder are illustrated. The four regions of the thorax are caudodorsal (A), caudoventral (B), cranioventral (C), and craniodorsal (D).

THORAX—LATERAL VIEW

Purpose—This is usually the only view(s) made of the thorax.

Preparation—No special preparation is required other than brushing the haircoat.

Patient Positioning—The average horse tends to stand with the elbows well under the chest. Therefore an effort must be made to extend the forelimbs cranially as far as is comfortable, to move the heavy triceps musculature from the field of interest. Otherwise, the horse stands naturally.

Tube Positioning—The x-ray tube is placed laterally and the beam is directed parallel to the ground in all views. The cassette is positioned on the opposite side and three or four exposures are made (Figs. 9-1, 9-2). If the patient is small, the study may be made with a single exposure (Fig. 9-2). Greater radiographic exposure is needed for both cranial views.

DORSOCAUDAL REGION—FOAL
Radiographic Technique for Portable Unit without grid—150-200 lbs (70-90 kg) (400 speed film-screen system)
- 80 kVp, 10 mA, 0.1 sec, 26 inches focal-film distance
- 80 kVp, 20 mA, 0.06 sec, 26 inches focal-film distance

VENTRAL REGION—FOAL
Radiographic Technique for Portable Unit without grid—150-200 lbs (70-90 kg) (400 speed film-screen system)
- 80 kVp, 10 mA, 0.3 sec, 26 inches focal-film distance
- 80 kVp, 20 mA, 0.16 sec, 26 inches focal-film distance

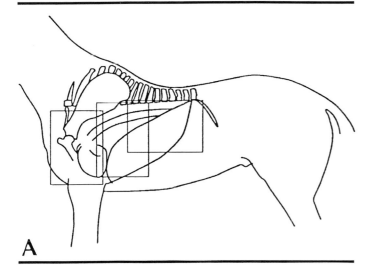 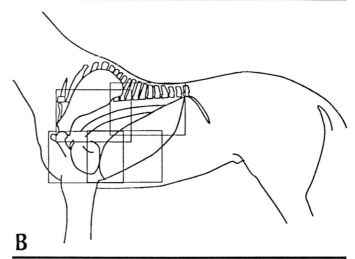

Fig. 9-2

Drawings of the location of the exposure fields commonly used in lateral radiography of the horse's thorax. Three views may be adequate in a smaller horse (A) while four views are required in a larger horse (B).

10. ABDOMEN STUDY

To perform lateral studies of the abdomen in the standing horse with any consistency of quality of the resulting radiographs, a ceiling-suspended x-ray tube and cassette-holder with grid are necessary (Table 10-1). Other systems of centering the x-ray beam can be improvised but they require a much longer time to perform the study. A large x-ray generator is required to produce an x-ray beam sufficiently strong enough to penetrate the abdomen of a horse. Use of high-speed rare-earth type film-screen systems is important. High-quality grid systems are important because of the massive amount of scatter radiation that is produced. The x-ray beam is centered at the last rib in the small patient. In the larger horse, more than one exposure should be made with the x-ray beam centered cranioventral, mid-abdominal, and caudodorsal (Fig. 10-1).

Abdominal studies in a foal are much easier and the lateral view can be made standing or recumbent. A ventrodorsal view can be made with the foal in dorsal recumbency. Because of the decrease in tissue thickness these studies can be made with medium powered equipment. It is still helpful to use a grid.

Radiographic Technique in a Foal for Portable Unit Without Grid-100 lbs (40 kg) (400 speed film-screen system)

- 80 kVp, 10 mA, 0.2 - 0.25 sec, 26 inches focal-film distance
- 80 kVp, 20 mA, 0.16 sec, 26 inches focal-film distance

Table 10-1
TECHNIQUE FOR RADIOGRAPHIC EVALUATION OF THE ABDOMEN

Standard views
    multiple lateral

Optional views
    dorsoventral in small patients

Opposite lateral views
    not helpful since most lesions lie on the midline and cannot be localized

Cassette size
    must be large

Use of cassette holder
    use of holder connected to tube is almost imperative

Use of grid
    use of a grid system is almost imperative

Markers
    may be used to indicate the site of a palpable soft-tissue lesion

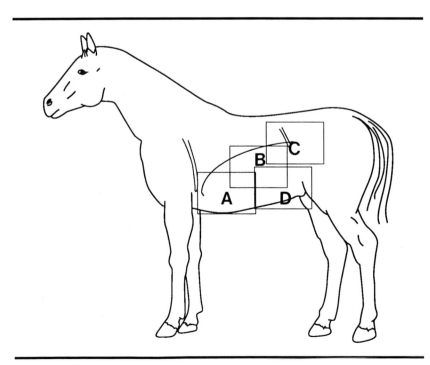

Fig. 10-1
A drawing demonstrates cassette positioning (A, B, C, and D) and x-ray beam centering for lateral abdominal studies on a large horse.

SELECTED EQUINE REFERENCES

Adams WM and Thilsted JP. Radiographic apearance of the equine stifle from birth to 6 months. Vet Radiol 26: 126, 1985.

Ammann Von K and Fackelman G. Zur Röntgendiagnose geschwulstartiger Prozesse der Nasengänge und Nasennebenhöhlen beim Pferd. Wien Tierärztl, Mschr 58:151-3, 1971.

Arnbjerg J. Contrast radiographs of joints and tendon sheaths in the horse. Nord Veterinaermed 21:318, 1969.

Bargai U. The radiological examination of the digestive system of the horse. Acta radiol Suppl 319:59, 1972.

Brown MP and MacCullum FJ. Anconeal process of ulna: Separate centre of ossification in the horse. Br Vet J 130:434, 1974.

Brown MP and MacCallum FJ. A system of grading ossification in limbs of foals to assist in radiologic interpretation. Am J Vet Res 36:655, 1975.

Calislar T and St Clair LE. Observations on the navicular bursa and the distal interphalangeal joint cavity in the horse. J Am Vet Med Assoc 154:410, 1969.

Campbell JR and Lee R. Radiographic techniques in the diagnosis of navicular disease. Eq Vet J 4:138, 1972.

Cook WR. Skeletal radiology of the equine head. Vet Radiol 11:35, 1970.

Denoix JM. Radiographic examination of the equine stifle. Point vet 18:17, 1986.

DeHaan CE O'Brien TR and Koblik PD. A radiographic investigation of third carpal bone injury in 42 racing thoroughbreds. Vet Radiol 28:88, 1988.

Dik FJ and Gunsser I. Atlas of Diagnostic Radiology of the Horse. Part 1. Diseases of the Front Limb. WB Saunders Co. Schlütersche Verlagsanstalt und Druckerei, Hannover, 1987.

Dik FJ and Gunsser I. Atlas of Diagnostic Radiology of the Horse. Part 2. Disease of the Hind Limb. WB Saunders Co. Schlütersche Verlagsanstalt und Druckerei, Hannover, 1989.

Dik FJ and Gunsser I. Atlas of Diagnostic Radiology of the Horse. Part 3. Diseases of the Head, Neck and Thorax. W.B. Saunders Co. Schlütersche Verlarsanstalt und Druckerei, Hannover, 1990.

Dixon RT. Radiography of the equine carpus. Aust Vet J 45:171, 1969.

Farrow CS. Radiography of the equine thorax: Anatomy and technic. Vet Rad 22:62, 1981.

Farrow CS. Equine thoracic radiology. J Am Vet Med Assoc 179:776, 1981.

Farrow CS McNeel SV and Morgan JP. Visualization of the tuber calcaneus and sustentaculum in the horse. Calif Vet 30:14, 1976.

Gabel AA Spencer CP and Pipers FS. A study of correlation of closure of the distal radial physis with performance and injury in the standardbred. J Am Vet Med Assoc 170:188, 1977.

Gibbs C. The equine skull: Its radiological investigation. J Am Vet Radiol Soc 15:70, 1974.

Gibson KT McIlwraith CW and Park RD. A radiographic study of the distal interphalangeal joint and navicular bursa of the horse. Vet Radiol 31:22, 1990.

Habel RE Barrett RB Deisem CD and Roenigk WJ. Nomenclature for radiologic anatomy. J Am Vet Med Assoc 142:38, 1963.

Hago BED and Vaughan LC. Use of contrast radiography in the investigation of tenosynovitis and bursitis in horses. Eq Vet J 18:375, 1986.

Heinze CD and Lewis RE. Radiographic diagnosis of the equine pelvis. Case reports: J Am Vet Med Assoc 159:1328, 1971.

Hannas CM O'Brien TR and Linford RL. Distal phalanx fractures in horses—A survey of 274 horses with radiographic assessment of healing in 36 horses. Vet Rad 29:98, 1988.

Hornof WJ and O'Brien TR. Radiographic evaluation of the palmar aspect of the equine metacarpal condyles: a new projection. Vet Rad 21:161, 1980.

Hornof WJ O'Brien TR and Pool RR. Osteochondritis dissecans of the distal metacarpus in the adult racing thoroughbred horse. Vet Rad 22:98, 1981.

Jeffcott LB and Kold SE. Radiographic examination of the equine stifle. Eq Vet J 14:25, 1982.

Kealy, JK. Principles of radiographic interpretation. Eq Vet. J 2:78, 1970.

Kneller SK and Losonsky JM. Misdiagnosis in normal radiographic anatomy: Nine structural configurations simulating disease entities in horses. J Am Vet Med Assoc 195:1272, 1989.

Koblik PD O'Brien TR and Coyne CP. Effect of dorsopalmar projection obliquity on radiographic measurement of distal phalangeal rotation angle in horses with laminitis. J Am Vet Med Assoc 192:346, 1988.

Koblik PD and Toal R. Portable veterinary x-ray support systems for field use. J Am Vet Med Assoc 199:186, 1991.

Lewis RE and Heinze CD. Radiographic examination of the equine pelvis: Technique. J Am Vet Med Assoc 159:1387, 1971.

Losonsky JM and Kneller SK. Variable locations of nutrient foramina of the proximal phalanx in forelimbs of Standardbreds. J Am Vet Med Assoc 193:671, 1988.

MacCallum FJ Brown MP and Goyal HO. An assessment of ossification and radiological interpretation in limbs of growing horses. Brit Vet J 134:366, 1978.

MacCallum FJ Latshaw WK and Kelly RE. Identification of postnatal ossification sites: A contribution to radiographic interpretation. Br Vet J 127:83, 1970.

Mason TA and Bourke JM. Closure of the distal radial epiphysis and its relationship to unsoundness in two year old thoroughbreds. Aust Vet J 49:21, 1973.

Mattoon JS and O'Brien TR. Radiographic evaluation of the calcaneus in the horse: a retrospective study. Proc Am Assoc Equine Pract p369, 1988.

Mendenhall A and Cantwell HD. Equine Radiographic Procedures. Lea and Febiger. Philadelphia 1988.

Monfort TN. A radiographic survey of epiphyseal maturity in Thoroughbred foals from birth to three years of age. Proc Am Assoc Equine Pract pp33, 1967.

Morgan JP. Radiographic study of the distal ulna of the horse. J Am Vet Rad Soc 6:78, 1965.

Morgan JP Neves J and Baker T. Equine Radiography, Iowa State University Press, Ames Iowa, 1991.

Morgan JP and Silverman S. Techniques of Veterinary Radiography. 4th ed Iowa State University Press, Ames Iowa, 1984.

Münzer B. Röntgendiagnostik der Thoraxorgane beim Pferd. Tierärztliche Praxis 7:475, 1979.

Myers VS. Confusing radiologic variations at the distal end of the radius of the horse. J Am Vet Med Assoc 147:1310, 1965.

Myers VS and Emmerson MS. The age and manner of epiphyseal closure in the forelegs of two Arabian foals. J Am Vet Rad Soc 7:39, 1966-67.

Nilsson, G and Olsson S-E. Radiologic and patho-anatomic changes in the distal joints and the phalanges of the standardbred horse. Acta Vet Scand Suppl 44:1, 1973.

O'Brien TR. Radiographic interpretation of the equine tarsus. Proc Am Assoc Equine Pract p289, 1987.

O'Brien TR. Disease of the thoroughbred fetlock joint—A comparison of radiographic signs with gross pathologic lesions. Proc Am Assoc Equine Pract p367, 1977.

O'Brien TR. Radiology of the equine stifle. Proc Am Assoc Equine Pract, 1973.

O'Brien TR. Radiographic diagnosis of the 'hidden' lesions of the third carpal bone. Proc Am Assoc Equine Pract p343, 1977.

O'Brien TR and Baker TW. Distal extremity examination: How to perform the radiographic examination and interpret the radiographs. Proc Am Assoc Equine Pract p553, 1982.

O'Brien TR DeHaan CE and Arther RM. Third carpal bone lesions of the racing thoroughbred. Proc Am Assoc Equine Pract p515, 1985.

O'Brien TR Millman TM Pool RR and Suter PF. Navicular disease in the thoroughbred horse: a morphologic investigation relative to a new radiographic projection. J Am Vet Rad Soc 16:39, 1975.

O'Brien TR Hornof WJ and Meagher DM. Radiographic detection and characterization of palmar lesions in the equine fetlock joint. J Am Vet Med Assoc 178:231, 1981.

O'Brien TR Baker TW and Koblik P. Stifle Radiology: How to perform an examination and interpret the radiographs. Proc Am Assoc Equine Pract p531, 1986.

O'Brien TR Morgan JP Wheat JD and Suter PF. Sesamoiditis in the thoroughbred: a radiographic study. J Am Vet Rad Soc 12:75, 1971.

O'Brien TR Morgan JP Park RD and Lebel JL. Radiology in equine carpal lameness. Cornell Vet 61:666, 1971.

Olsson S-E and Giers E. A multipurpose x-ray unit for veterinary use. J Am Vet Rad Soc 6:82, 1965.

Orsini PG Rendano VT and Sack WO. Ectopic nutrient foramina in the third metatarsal bone of the horse. Eq Vet J 13:132, 1981.

Oxspring GE. The radiology of navicular disease with observations on its pathology. Vet Rec 15:1433, 1936.

Palmer SE. Radiography of the abaxial surface of the proximal sesamoid bones. J Am Vet Med Assoc 181:264, 1982.

Park RD Morgan JP and O'Brien TR. Chip fractures in the carpus of the horse: a radiographic study of their incidence and location. J Am Vet Med Assoc 157:1305, 1970.

Pezzoli G and Del Bue M. Valutazione radiografica del grado di sviluppo scheletrico nel cavallo trottatore in rapporto all'attivita' atletica. Folia vet 5:399, 1975.

Phillips DF. Radiology in your practice: choosing the right equipment. Vet Med 587, 1987.

Pool RR Meagher DM and Stover SM. Pathophysiology of navicular syndrome. Equine Pract 5:109, 1989.

Poulos PW and Smith MF. The nature of enlarged "vascular channels" in the navicular bone of the horse. Vet Radiol 29:60, 1988.

Reid CF. Radiography of the alimentary canal of the horse. Jl S Afr Vet Ass 46:69, 1975.

Rendano VT and Grant B. The equine third phalanx: its radiographic appearance. J Am Vet Rad Soc 19,125, 1978.

Rendano VT and Ryan G. Technical assistance in radiology. Part II. Basic considerations and radiation safety. Cont Ed 9:547, 1988.

Rick MC O'Brien TR Pool RR and Meagher D. Condylar fractures of the third metacarpal bone and third metatarsal bone in 75 horses: Radiographic features, treatments, and outcome. J Am Vet Med Assoc 183:287, 1983.

Rose J Taylor BJ and Steel JD. Navicular disease in the horse: An analysis of seventy cases and assessment of a special radiographic view. J Equine Med Surg 2:492, 1978.

Schebitz H and Wilkens H. Atlas of Radiographic Anatomy of the Horse. 3rd ed WB Saunders Co. Philadelphia 1978.

Shively MJ. A comparison of unofficial and proper anatomic terms: Bones of the thoracic limb. J Am Vet Med Assoc 180:849, 1982.

Shively MJ and Smallwood JE. Radiographic and xero-radiographic anatomy of the equine tarsus. Eq Pract 2:19, 1980.

Shively MJ. Normal radiographic anatomy of the equine digit. Southwestern Vet 36:227, 1985.

Shively MJ. Normal radiographic anatomy of the equine digit. J Eq Med Surg 2:77, 1978.

Smallwood JE Shively MJ Rendano VT and Habel RE. A standardized nomenclature for radiographic projections used in veterinary medicine. Vet Radiol 26:2, 1985.

Smallwood JE and Shively MJ. Nomenclature for radiographic views of limbs. Eq Pract 1:41, 1979.

Smallwood JE and Shively MJ. Radiographic and xero-radiographic anatomy of the equine carpus. Eq Pract 1:22, 1979.

Smallwood JE Albright SM Metcalf MR Thrall DE and Harrington BD. A xerographic study of the developing quarterhorse foredigit and metacarpophalangeal region from six to twelve months of age. Vet Rad 31:254, 1990.

Smallwood JE Albright SM Metcalf MR Thrall DE and Harrington BD. A xerographic study of the developing equine foredigit and metacarpophalangeal region from birth to six months of age. Vet Rad 30:98, 1989.

Smallwood JE and Holladay SD. Xeroradiographic anatomy of the equine digit and metacarpophalangeal region. Vet Rad 28:166, 1987.

Stick JA Jann HW Scott EA and Robinson NE. Pedal bone rotation as a prognostic sign in laminitis of horses. J Am Vet Med Assoc 180:251, 1982.

Stilson AE Herring DS and Robertson JT. Contribution of the nasal septum to the radiographic anatomy of the equine nasal cavity. J Am Vet Med Assoc 186: 590, 1985.

Svalastoga E. Navicular disease in the horse: A micro-radiographic investigation. Nord Vet Med 35:131, 1983.

Swanstrom OG and Lewis RE. Arthrography of the equine fetlock. Proc Am Assoc Equine Pract p221, 1969.

Thrall DE. Textbook of Veterinary Diagnostic Radiology. WB Saunders Co. Philadelphia, 1986.

Thrall DE Lebel JL and O'Brien TR. A five-year survey of the incidence and location of equine carpal chip fractures. J Am Vet Med Assoc 158:1366, 1971.

Tohara S. Radiological studies on the ossification of legbones of horses. Jap J Vet Sci 12:1, 1950.

Travenor WD and Vaughan LC. Radiography of horses and cattle. Brit Vet J 118:359, 1962.

Turner TA Kneller SK Badertscher RR et al. Radiographic changes in the navicular bones of normal horses. Proc Am Assoc Equine Pract p309, 1986.

Van de Watering CC and Morgan JP. Chip fractures as a radiologic finding in navicular disease of the horse. J Am Vet Radiol Soc 16:206, 1975.

Verschooten F and DeMoor A. Tendinitis in the horse: Its radiographic diagnosis with air-tendograms. J Am Vet Rad Soc 19:23, 1978.

Walker M and Goble D. Barium sulfate bronchography in horses. Vet Rad 21:85, 1980.

Webbon PM. Problems associated with the use of radiography in the examination of a horse for a purchaser. Eq Vet J 13:15, 1981.

Widmer WR. Iohexol and iopamidol: New contrast media for veterinary myelography: J Am Vet Med Assoc 194, 1714, 1989.

Williams FL and Campbell DY. Tendon radiography in the horse. J Am Vet Med Ass 139:224, 1961.

Young A O'Brien TR and Pool RR. Exercise-related sclerosis in the third carpal bone of the racing thoroughbred. Proc Am Assoc Equine Pract p339, 1988.

Zeskov B. A study of discontinuity of the fibula in the horse. Am J Vet Res 20:852, 1959.

SECTION F

RADIOGRAPHY OF THE BOVINE

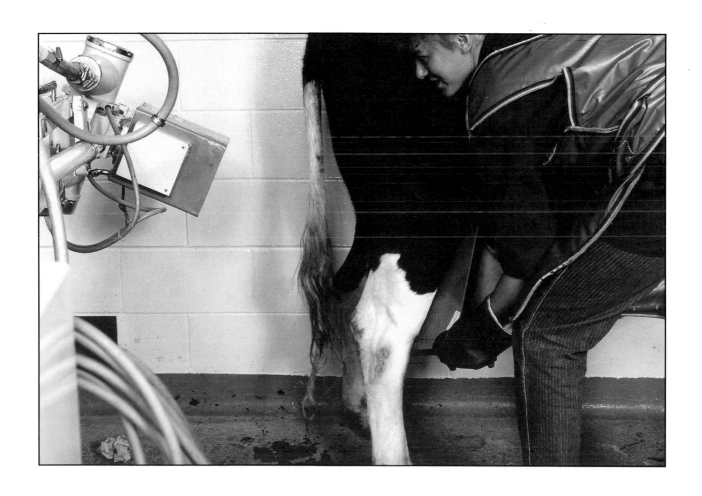

1. INTRODUCTION

Bovine radiology has been a neglected and little explored area of veterinary radiology. Many food animal practices do not have radiographic equipment, and it is not always economically realistic to use diagnostic radiology in cattle. However, recent technical advances in radiography (rare earth screens, more powerful portable and mobile x-ray machines) have made their use in bovine medicine today more practical and feasible. Also, there can now be a significant difference between the value of a pure-bred calf or a high-producing dairy or beef cow and the value of its carcass after emergency slaughter. It can therefore be advantageous to make use of every means to obtain an accurate diagnosis and prognosis, and hence to ensure correct and effective surgical or medical care of a bovine patient.

The logistics involved in radiography of the bovine patient may be time-consuming and complicated because the animals are often difficult to work with compared to a dog or a horse. The introduction of excellent, fast-acting sedatives for cattle has considerably reduced handling problems during radiographic examination. These sedatives are useful even in cows in early pregnancy, but are contraindicated in late pregnancy or in patients with known liver disease. General anesthesia is a possibility in veterinary hospitals, but is probably not indicated in a practice environment.

USES OF BOVINE RADIOGRAPHY

Radiography in the trauma patient is often necessary for making an accurate diagnosis and prognosis. Radiography is essential to detect developmental diseases of the skeleton in young animals, such as nutritional deficiencies and osteochondrosis. The application of radiological examination in cattle has proved itself particularly rewarding under the following specific clinical situations:

Feet: Lameness in adult cattle usually arises from foot problems such as foreign body penetration into the sole, sole abscesses, interdigital dermatitis, septic arthritis and distal phalangeal (P-III) fractures. All of these conditions may assume a chronic nature, be accompanied by complications, and may eventually require surgery. Radiographic examination permits assessment of the extent of the lesion, its nature, and the most likely prognosis. Surgical procedures such as amputation or arthrodesis should always be preceded by radiographic examination.

Legs: Radiographic examination is valuable in establishing the nature of the joint swellings which are so common in bulls, especially those housed in insemination centers. The distinction between serous arthrosis (hydroarthrosis) and degenerative joint disease (DJD) in the tarsus of heavy-breed bulls may determine the possibility of continued use of these animals, and often indicates the course of treatment required. Young cattle frequently suffer from septic arthritis, the severity of which can be more accurately evaluated by radiography than by clinical examination. Older animals may have a chronic inflammatory, non-infectious gonitis with DJD due to rupture of cruciate or patellar ligaments; these lesions need to be differentiated from infectious arthritis if treatment is to be appropriate. Calves which are non-ambulatory following forced extraction at parturition may have any of a number of lesions which can best be differentiated by radiography; these lesions include femoral nerve paresis, pelvic fractures, femoral head luxation, fractures of the femoral capital epiphysis, and femoral diaphyseal fractures.

Head: Radiographic examinations of mandibular and sub-mandibular hard swellings may identify lesions due to actinobacillosis or actinomycosis, or those that are the result of a tooth root infection or abscess. The paranasal and frontal sinuses are other common sites of infection, often not producing clear clinical signs, and radiography helps to determine whether surgery is required for drainage or whether the lesion may be treated medically

Chest: Thoracic structures are easily defined by radiography, both in young and adult cattle. Pulmonary infections, diseases of the esophagus, pleuritis, and pericarditis may be diagnosed radiographically.

Abdomen: Penetrating foreign bodies involving the reticulum are a well known clinical syndrome in cattle. Without radiography, only clinical impressions are possible, with blood counts that may substantiate diagnosis and suggest the need for surgery. Radiography is a means of exact diagnosis, making it possible to determine not only the presence of metal objects in the reticulum, but also the extent of wall penetration and whether secondary abcessation is present. Abomasal sand, or omasal-abomasal impaction by plastic twine and sand, is a common finding in certain types of feeding regimens.

Reproductive organs: Radiography has proved to be valuable in breeding soundness examinations in bulls. Radiography of the testes demonstrates calcified lesions, such as old hematomas or cysts, which block the seminiferous tubules or vas deferens. Contrast radiography is valuable as a means for visual demonstration of the level of teat obstruction and its nature.

2. EQUIPMENT

X-RAY MACHINES

As in equine radiography, portable, heavier mobile, and stationary x-ray machines are available for bovine radiography and each have their own advantages and limitations.

The portable x-ray machine is a unit which may be packed, moved, and reassembled at the side of the animal to be examined. These machines may therefore be considered "cow-side" x-ray units (Fig. 2-1). These units produce up to 90 kVp at 10 mA, or alternatively, higher mA (up to 30 mA) at lower kVp. These machine settings limit the usefulness of the machine to radiography of the extremities, although improvisations also permit its use for radiography of parts of the neck and skull.

The heavier mobile x-ray machine is built in a permanent casing on wheels, and may be self-propelled by an electric motor or moved manually. These units are much heavier than the portable machines, generally weighing several hundred kilograms (Fig. 2-2). The x-ray tube has a rotating anode, enabling production of higher milliamperage. These machines can produce up to 125 kVp at up to 45 mAs, and are able to provide these values at an exposure time of several hundredths of a second. Such machines are designed with a versatile tube suspension arm, which may be rotated and directed in any direction, thus making the radiographic examination of both standing and recumbent cows relatively easy. Excellent diagnostic radiographs may be obtained of the skull, neck, chest, and heavier parts of the upper extremities. Radiographs of good quality may

also be made of the lumbar vertebrae and the abomasum and reticulum of cows. With the use of rare-earth screens, special techniques such as use of an air-gap to reduce the effect of scatter radiation, and a 24-hour starvation of the patient, it is possible to obtain diagnostic radiographs of lumbar vertebrae of 1000-1200 kg bulls.

The major disadvantage of the mobile unit is that it can only be moved on hard, smooth flooring such as concrete or tile, and a bovine patient housed in a cow-shed or barn with straw or soft bedding must be brought to the machine. Therefore, it is advisable for large dairy or beef operators and insemination centers to construct a special area for radiography, including a stanchion in a cow-shed with smooth concrete flooring near a convenient power supply.

Stationary units in a veterinary hospital offer the most versatile method of radiographing bovine patients, but

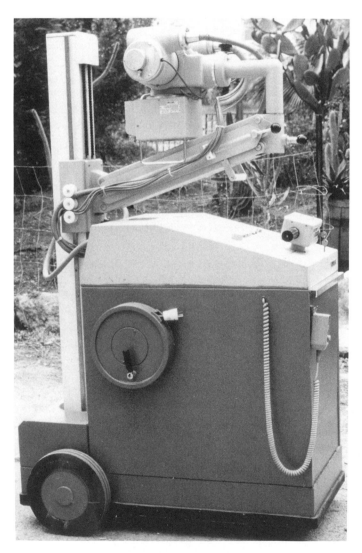

Fig. 2-1
An old "box-portable" type x-ray machine with controls limited to an on-off switch with a mechanical timer that is spring-loaded. The tube may be supported by a small portable stand (arrow) or may be hand-held. A unit of this type can be useful for radiography of the feet of the cow.

Fig. 2-2
A mobile condenser-discharge x-ray machine seen in a folded position ready to be moved on the site or to be loaded into a mobile laboratory for long distance moving. A unit of this type requires a firm smooth surface on which to roll.

require that the patients be transported to a clinic for radiography. A ceiling suspended tube and a separately suspended, but interconnected, cassette holder make radiography of the thorax and abdomen of the standing patient much easier. The capabilities of these units are usually 125 kVp, 300 to 500 mA, and exposure times of less than 1/30 second, and higher powered units are available.

PROCESSING EQUIPMENT

Processing may be performed using the wet-tank or the automatic processor methods. The wet-tank system is a reliable and reasonable processing method for farm use when processing a small number of radiographs. However, tabletop automatic processors are light-weight (no more than 50 kg), and may be easily set up on a table or installed on a countertop. Their advantages seem to justify the additional expense in large cattle operations, insemination centers, and bovine veterinary practices.

RADIOGRAPHIC ACCESSORIES

Conventional screen cassettes with relatively slow film-screen speed, are recommended for radiography of the foot of cattle to provide the higher film detail useful to diagnose bone and joint disease.

Rare-earth screen cassettes with much faster film-screen speeds, are essential for radiographic examination of the thick parts of bovine patients, such as the thorax, abdomen, lumbar vertebrae, and pelvis. These cassettes can effectively decrease the mAs required to radiograph larger animal parts from 100 to 120 mAs down to 25 to 30 mAs.

Film must be selected to match the speed and type of intensifying screen to be used. A slow film provides higher detail and can be used in radiography of the feet. A much faster film is used in radiography of thicker anatomical parts to permit a decrease in the amount of radiation necessary for the exposure.

Portable grids control scatter radiation and permit radiography of thicker abdominal parts of the cow. These are placed in front of the cassette during an exposure, and absorb the scatter radiation which would fog the radiograph and decrease film contrast. Grids are indispensable for chest radiographs since anatomic detail is small and sharp definition is essential.

Radiation protection practices include: (1) use of lead gloves, aprons, and thyroid collars; (2) collimation of the primary beam; (3) never standing or placing any part of your body in the primary beam; (4) positioning yourself behind the machine during the exposure; (5) rotating personnel holding the animal or cassette; and (6) using cassette holders whenever possible to keep helpers hands and body outside the primary x-ray beam (Fig. 2-3).

Patient positioning is easier achieved in radiography of cattle in the hospital, either by a stanchion, headgate, or other mechanical devices, whereas, radiography on the farm requires more improvisation and use of accessories. The use of sedative drugs is strongly advised. Special positioning devices include foot stands, cassette holders, and grid cassette stands that are valuable in radiography of the foot.

Proper film marking is best achieved at the time of radiography by placing lead numbers and letters, lead tape, or other devices on the cassette before exposure.

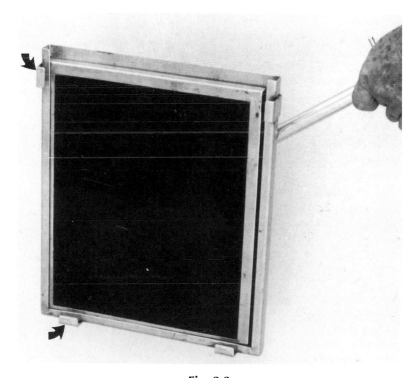

Fig. 2-3
Metal cassette holder with handle that has guides (black arrows) that can be used to hold a portable grid.

3. VIEWS AND POSITIONING

FOOT

Clinically, the foot of the bovine consists of all parts below the metacarpo (tarsal) phalangeal or fetlock joint. Since these parts of the leg constantly come in contact with the ground, they are the most frequently traumatized and consequently the most frequently radiographed. The common clinical conditions which affect the foot include osteomyelitis, sequestrum formation, septic arthritis, paronychia, fractures of mature bone, physeal fractures, traumatic joint disease, degenerative joint disease, penetration by foreign objects, and soft tissue calcification. Other conditions include lameness of an obscure nature, soft tissue swelling, joint effusion, chronic deformation of the feet, chronic ulceration, fistulas, and surgical complications. Radiography is also indicated when no definite clinical diagnosis can be made or when there is no response to treatment.

Unlike in equine radiography, where clinical examination and diagnostic nerve blocks usually direct attention at a very specific anatomical region, in bovine radiography the entire foot is most often included in a single examination, especially in calves. This point should be kept in mind, even though the following sub-sections describe the radiography of specific regions.

Another difference in comparison with equine radiography is that the lateromedial view in the bovine is frequently of little diagnostic value because superimposition of the digits tends to obscure lesions: conversely, this lateromedial superimposition makes comparative oblique views essential for lesion identification or confirmation in most examinations of the bovine foot.

RADIOGRAPHY OF THE DISTAL PHALANX (Ungular Bone, Pedal Bone, Os Pedis, Third Phalanx, Coffin Bone, P-III) AND DISTAL INTERPHALANGEAL JOINT (Coffin Joint)

It is relatively easy to position the x-ray tube for examinations of the distal phalanx when they are performed on the forelimb. It can be difficult to position the tube and cassette when examining the pelvic limb unless the animal adopts a "toed-out" stance; it is often possible to induce this stance by means of a rope tied around the distal metatarsus. Usually the study can be made in a weight-bearing manner. Positioning blocks and cassette holders are needed only for the lateral view. Close collimation of the primary x-ray beam is the best method to reduce radiation exposure to assistants. Preparation of the patient is important in achieving a diagnostic study and includes brushing and cleaning the foot, as well as trimming the hoof wall and cleaning the sole of the foot.

A basic study of the distal phalanx consists of dorsopalmar (plantar), and lateral views. Oblique views may be considered optional until a definite lesion is identified, either on physical examination or radiographically, that might be better evaluated by these special views (Table 3-1).

The markers for studies of the digit are not unique, but it is important that some method be used to identify medial and lateral aspects of the radiograph. Remember to select the identification of one side or the other and follow that convention regularly. In this manual, all markers are placed laterally, if possible.

Table 3-1
TECHNIQUE FOR RADIOGRAPHIC EVALUATION OF THE DISTAL PHALANX

Standard views
  dorsopalmar (plantar) 45°
  lateromedial

Optional views
  oblique
  lateral view of a single claw with film positioned between the claws
  dorsopalmar (plantar) 65°

Views of the opposite limb
  dorsopalmar (plantar) view of opposite limb if radiographing calves

Cassette size
  8 x 10 inches (18 x 24 cm)

Cassette holder
  consider use on the lateral view
  use a tunnel on the dorsopalmar view to protect the cassette

Grid
  use of a grid not indicated

Markers
  fore or hind foot
  right or left foot
  medial or lateral aspect

DISTAL PHALANX—DORSOPALMAR (plantar) VIEW (45° dorsoproximal-palmarodistal)

Purpose of study: This view is most valuable for detection of fractures or bone or joint infection involving the distal phalanx and/or distal interphangeal joint.

Preparation: Clean the hoof wall and sole since the presence of dirt or rocks or roughening of the sole create artifacts on the radiograph.

Positioning: The foot is placed on the cassette which is on the ground slightly in front of the normally standing patient possibly using a cassette tunnel (Fig. 3-1).

Beam location: The tube is positioned in front of the foot approximately 24 in (60 cm) off the ground and angled at approximately 45° so that the central x-ray beam in centered on the coronary band on the midline (mid-sagittal plane). The closely collimated beam is at a right angle to the hoof wall in a foot that is correctly trimmed. In the patient with feet that are uncared for, the angle of intercept with the hoof wall changes as the toe lengthens.

It is possible to use non-screen technique on the dorso-palmar (plantar) view of the distal phalanx since the patient is weightbearing and there is little chance of motion during the longer exposure. In this event, it is essential to use a tunnel to protect the non-screen film. This technique is especially valuable in studies where high-detail is of valuable in the detection of an undisplaced fracture. Using a portable unit, exposure times for the adult are 2 to 3 seconds and are 1 to 2 seconds for the calf.

In the event of an unexplained shadow on the standard dorsopalmar (plantar) radiograph, it is possible to alter the angle of the x-ray beam to 65° dorsoproximal-palmarodistal. This creates a different projection of the solar margin and body of the distal phalanx and slightly changes the appearance of the body of the distal phalanx. A shadow on the radiograph that shifts in position on the second view is due to irregularities in density or shape of the sole or bulbs of the heel or is on the hoof wall. If the finding is in fact a lesion in the bone, it remains in the same position relative to the distal phalanx on both projections.

Normal radiograph and drawing are shown (Fig. 3-2).

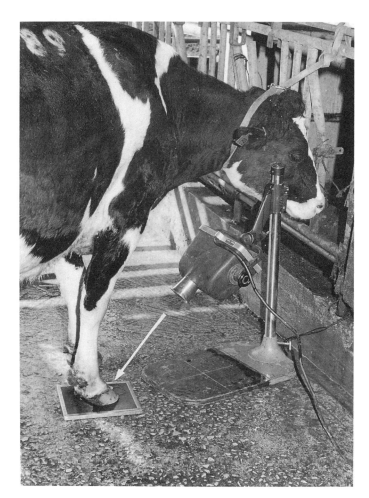

Fig. 3-1

Positioning used for dorsopalmar (plantar) radiography of distal phalanx (PIII). The foot is placed on the cassette which is on the ground slightly in front of the standing patient. The central beam (arrow) is at a 45° angle to the ground and centered on the coronary band.

Radiographic Technique for Portable Unit (400 speed film-screen system)
- 80 kVp, 10 mA, 0.06 sec, 24 inches focal-film distance
- 100 kVp, 10 mA, 0.04 sec, 24 inches focal-film distance

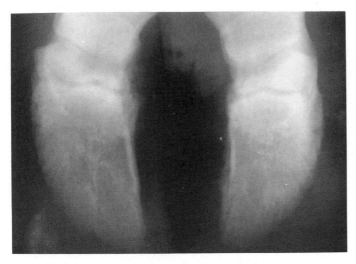

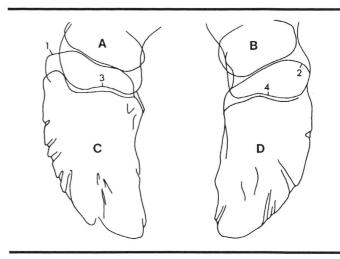

Fig. 3-2
Radiograph and drawing of the distal phalanx (PIII) as seen on the dorsopalmar (plantar) view. Anatomical structures are labelled (A,B—distal sesamoid bones, C,D—distal phalanges, 1,2—proximal border of the distal phalanges, 3,4—distal border of the second phalanx).

DISTAL PHALANX—LATERAL VIEW
(lateromedial)

Purpose: Major reasons for using the lateral view are to localize foreign bodies in the foot and to identify fractures of the distal phalanx. The distal interphalangeal joint space can be identified if the projection is a true lateral. Superimposition of the digits often creates major problems in analyzing and interpreting the radiographs.

Preparation: The routine preparation for cleaning the foot is required.

Positioning: The foot is positioned on some form of block so that the foot is elevated sufficiently so that the x-ray beam is directed in a horizontal plane and centered on the distal phalanx. It is convenient for the block to have a slot that holds the cassette in addition to elevating the foot. Using a cassette holder eliminates the need for an assistant to hold the cassette.

Beam location: The tube head is positioned laterally with the x-ray beam parallel to the ground surface. The beam is centered on the coronary band (Fig. 3-3).

Radiographic Technique for Portable Unit (400 speed film-screen system)
- 80 kVp, 10 mA, 0.06 sec, 24 inches focal-film distance
- 100 kVp, 10 mA, 0.04 sec, 24 inches focal-film distance

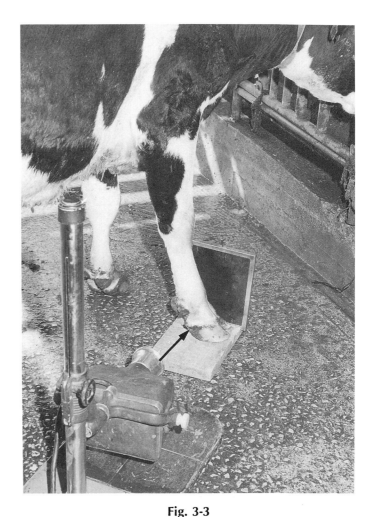

Fig. 3-3
Positioning used for lateral radiography of distal phalanx (PIII). The foot is placed on a block so that the foot is elevated sufficiently so the x-ray beam can be directed in a horizontal plane and centered on the hoof wall. The direction of the central beam is marked (arrow).

DISTAL PHALANX—LATEROMEDIAL VIEW (mediolateral) WITH AN INTERDIGITAL FILM

Purpose: The interdigital view permits evaluation of the distal phalanx of a single claw without superimposition of the other claw. The use of oblique views often eliminates the need for this view.

Preparation: No special preparation is required except to insure that the interdigital region is cleaned.

Positioning: This view is most easily accomplished with the patient in a lateral recumbent position, however, it can be made with the bovine standing with the foot supported off the ground.

Beam location: Use of a non-screen film is recommended. It is placed in the interdigital space (Fig. 3-4) and the tube is positioned laterally to radiograph the lateral claw and medially to radiograph the medial claw. The film is enclosed in an additional plastic envelope to prevent it from becoming wet or dirty. Exposure values must be increased approximately ten-fold because of the slow speed of the non-screen system.

Normal radiograph and drawing are shown (Fig. 3-5).

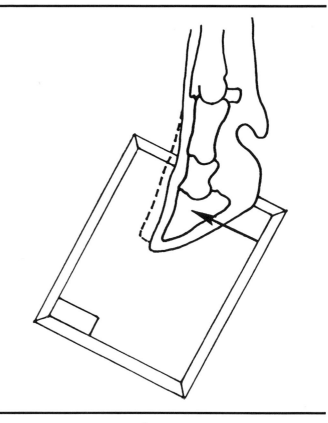

Fig. 3-4
Drawing illustrating the positioning used for lateral radiography when using an interdigital film. The direction of the central beam is marked (arrow)

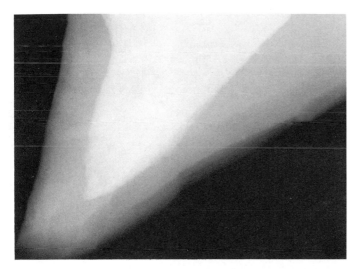 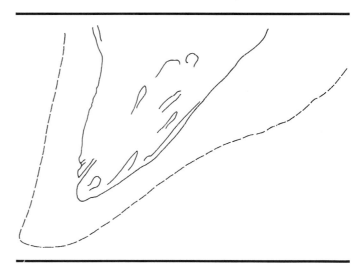

Fig. 3-5
Radiograph and drawing of a distal phalanx (P-III) of one digit as made using an interdigital technique illustrating the value of the technique. Because of low exposure values, soft tissues are well seen. Higher exposure value provide more details of the bone, but overexpose the soft tissues.

DISTAL PHALANX— MEDIAL OBLIQUE VIEW (dorsolateral-palmaro [plantaro])

Purpose: The oblique views enable visualization of the distal phalanges of the two claws without superimposition of the other claw. It is especially useful for identifying relatively transverse P-111 fractures and for assessing joint or navicular bone involvement in septic conditions.

Preparation: The routine preparation used for cleaning the foot is required.

Positioning: The patient stands normally with the foot on the positioning block used for the lateral view. The cassette is placed in a slot in the positioning block or is held vertically in a holder.

Beam location: The tube head is positioned 45° lateral to that location used for the dorsopalmar view and the beam is angled 45° to the ground and centered on the digit of interest. Both oblique views of the digits are usually made for the purpose of comparison.

Radiographic Technique for Portable Unit (400 speed film-screen system)
- 80 kVp, 10 mA, 0.06 sec, 24 inches focal-film distance
- 100 kVp, 10 mA, 0.04 sec, 24 inches focal-film distance

Table 3-2
TECHNIQUE FOR RADIOGRAPHIC EVALUATION OF THE PROXIMAL AND MIDDLE PHALANGES (P-I and P-II) AND PASTERN JOINT (Proximal Interphalangeal Joint)

Routine views
  dorsopalmar (plantar)
  lateral

Optional views
  oblique

Views of the opposite limb
  required under 9 months of age

Cassette size
  small cassette satisfactory (8 x 10 in, 18 x 24 cm)

Cassette holder
  useful to decrease exposure to scattered radiation exposure

Grids
  not needed in radiography of the phalanges

Film markers
  right or left
  medial or lateral
  fore- or hindlimb

PROXIMAL AND MIDDLE PHALANGES (P-I and P-II) AND PASTERN JOINT (Proximal Interphalangeal Joint)

Studies of the phalangeal area include the proximal (os compedale) and middle (os coronale) phalanges and center on the proximal interphalangeal joint (pastern joint) but may include the metacarpophalangeal joint (fetlock joint) and distal interphalangeal joint (coffin joint) as well. The study usually evaluates acute or chronic trauma, inflammation of bone or joint, or secondary joint disease. Following acute injury, the study is of value in identification of a fracture and often only dorsopalmar and lateral views are needed to fully appreciate the nature of the fracture line(s). Periosteal new bone that has formed secondarily to acute or chronic injury can be noted on all views. Infectious joint disease produces localized destructive changes that may be evident on all views, but are often best appreciated by comparing mediolateral oblique and lateromedial oblique views.

Tendons and ligaments attach to these bones and enthesophyte production at the site of these attachments is often secondary to chronic injury In older animal, enthesophytes are often seen as incidental findings where the cruciate ligaments attach distally on the axial cortices of the proximal phalanges.

This is a relatively easy study to perform, and errors in positioning are minimal and usually related to conformational problems in the patient. The foot is placed on the ground and the patient stands normally with the x-ray tube positioned dorsally.

Identification of the film requires marking right or left and fore- or hindfoot. The medial or lateral aspect should be identified consistently by the use of one of these markers. In this manual, the lateral marker is always used where possible (Table 3-2).

Proximal growth plates of the proximal and middle phalanges close between 6 to 9 months of age. Comparison studies of the opposite foot in calves permit evaluation of the stage of physeal closure and avoid the erroneous diagnosis of developmental or traumatic disease in normal patients.

PROXIMAL AND MIDDLE PHALANGES (P-I and P-II) AND PASTERN JOINT (Proximal Interphalangeal Joint)— DORSOPALMAR VIEW (45° dorsoproximal-palmarodistal)

Purpose: The 45° dorsopalmar (plantar) view is a standard part of the study.

Preparation: No specific preparation of the digit is required except for brushing the hair coat.

Positioning: The foot is positioned on the ground with the patient standing normally with the cassette positioned close behind the digit and held in a cassette holder that is resting on the floor. A positioning block is used if the entire foot is being included in the study.

Beam location: The x-ray tube is placed in front of the digit with the central beam directed within the mid-sagittal plane. The angle of the beam is dependent on the positioning of the foot, but is usually 45° to the ground. Attempt to place the foot so the x-ray beam is perpendicular to the foot axis. The beam is centered on the proximal interphalangeal joint or a point of interest.

Radiographic Technique for portable unit (400 speed film-screen system)
- 80 kVp, 10 mA, 0.1 sec, 24 inches focal-film distance
- 100 kVp, 10 mA, 0.08 sec, 24 inches focal-film distance

PROXIMAL AND MIDDLE PHALANGES (P-I and P-II) AND PASTERN JOINT (Proximal Interphalangeal Joint)— LATERAL VIEW (lateromedial)

Purpose: In addition to learning of the character of the bone and joints in the digit, the lateral view provides valuable information on the character of the foot axis.

Preparation: No special preparation is required.

Positioning: The foot is placed on the ground with the patient standing normally. Cassette is held vertically, medial to the fetlock and rests on the floor. The combination of tube head type and foot position must ensure that the x-ray beam is parallel to the ground. If this is a problem, the foot can be elevated by placing it on a block.

Beam location: The x-ray tube is positioned laterally and the cassette is held vertically medial to the fetlock and resting on the floor with the beam centered on the middle phalanx or point of interest.

Radiographic Technique for Portable Unit (400 speed film-screen system)
- 80 kVp, 10 mA, 0.1 sec, 24 inches focal-film distance
- 100 kVp, 10 mA, 0.08 sec, 24 inches focal-film distance

PROXIMAL AND MIDDLE PHALANGES (P-I and P-II) AND PASTERN JOINT (Proximal Interphalangeal Joint)— MEDIAL OBLIQUE VIEW (dorsolateroproximal-palmaromediodistal)

Purpose: The oblique view is used to evaluate the middle phalanges and to detect areas of new bone production.

Preparation: No special preparation is required.

Positioning: The foot is positioned in a similar manner as used for the dorsopalmar (plantar) view. A positioning block is used if the entire foot is being included.

Beam location: The cassette is held vertically and rests on the floor behind the medial dew claw. The x-ray tube should be in a location so that the central beam is perpendicular to the foot axis. The x-ray beam is angled downward at an angle of 45° to the ground, and the tube is rotated 45° lateral from the position used for the dorsopalmar view. The beam is centered on the middle phalanx or point of interest.

It is also possible to make a lateral oblique view with the tube held medially and the cassette positioned next to the lateral dew claw, however, the positioning is more difficult, as the x-ray tube must be on the opposite side of the animal, which may be prevented by the restraint system employed.

Radiographic Technique for Portable Unit (400 speed film-screen system)
- 80 kVp, 10 mA, 0.1 sec, 24 inches focal-film distance
- 100 kVp, 10 mA, 0.08 sec, 24 inches focal-film distance

FETLOCK JOINT
(Metacarpo- or Metatarsophalangeal Joint) AND PROXIMAL SESAMOID BONES

The metacarpo (tarso)-phalangeal joint (fetlock area) of the leg, although not coming in direct contact with the ground, is still vulnerable and often involved traumatically. It is a complicated area anatomically because of the articulations between the metacarpal (tarsal) bone, the first phalanges, and the proximal sesamoid bones. In addition, it contains the flexor tendons, the suspensory ligament, and several sesamoidian ligaments. These ligamentous structures are often over-flexed or over-extended, especially in young heifers, resulting in clinical lameness and distension of the joint. In addition, the fetlock joint capsule is a much larger capsule and thus more clinically vulnerable than those of the interphalangeal joints.

Infections of the soft tissues of the foot may extend along the phalanges into the fetlock joint, causing swelling of the joint. Many cases of septic arthritis of the fetlock joint which cannot be traced directly to a local origin are hematogenous. In the young animal, the growth plates are prone to both traumatic and infectious diseases, the latter often hematogenous. Growth-plate separations or fractures are quite common and may result in marked deformity of the bone. Because of the frequency of these conditions, radiography is indicated in any clinical involvement of the fetlock area which is not resolved after a few days of treatment. Clinically, most fetlock trauma involves soft tissue swelling, non-supporting lameness, and pain manifested on palpation. The radiographic signs vary markedly with the pathologic process involved.

Routine radiographic views include dorsopalmar (plantar), lateromedial, and dorsopalmar (plantar) oblique views. It is possible to make the oblique views either with the tube held medially and the cassette positioned next to the lateral dew claw or with the tube held laterally and the cassette positioned next to the medial dew claw (Table 3-3).

Preparation of the patient is relatively easy requiring only brushing of the ankle. Film identification requires indicating whether the leg is right or left and fore or hind.

The distal physis of the third metacarpal (metatarsal) bone closes between 6 and 12 months while the proximal physis of the first phalanges closes between 4 and 9 months. The proximal sesamoid bones each form from a single ossification center. Growth plates in the hindlimbs close at a slightly older age than in the forelimbs.

Table 3-3
TECHNIQUE FOR RADIOGRAPHIC EVALUATION OF THE FETLOCK JOINT (Metacarpo- or Metatarsophalangeal Joint) AND PROXIMAL SESAMOID BONES

Standard views
    dorsopalmar
    lateromedial
    oblique

Studies of opposite limb
    necessary only under the age of 12 months

Cassette size
    small cassette can be used (8 x 10 in, 18 x 24 cm); larger if entire foot is included
    rare earth screens should be used

Cassette holders
    valuable to use to decrease exposure from scatter radiation

Grid
    not needed in radiography of the fetlock joint.

Film markers
    right or left
    fore- or hindlimb
    medial or lateral

FETLOCK JOINT
(Metacarpo- or Metatarsophalangeal Joint)
AND PROXIMAL SESAMOID BONES—
DORSOPALMAR (plantar) VIEW

Purpose: the dorsopalmar view is a standard view for examination of both the fetlock joint and the proximal sesamoid bones. The radiographic technique may be altered slightly if greater penetration is required to visualize the proximal sesamoid bones.

Preparation: Only brushing of the ankle is required.

Positioning: The foot is placed on the ground with the bovine fully weight-bearing and the cassette positioned against the palmar (plantar) surface (Fig. 3-6).

Beam location: The x-ray tube is placed in front of the foot, and the x-ray beam is directed in the mid-sagittal plane parallel to the ground. The cassette is held in contact with the digit. The beam is centered at the fetlock joint.

Normal radiograph and drawing are shown (Fig. 3-7).

Radiographic Technique for Portable Unit (400 speed film-screen system)
- 80 kVp, 10 mA, 0.1 sec, 24 inches focal-film distance
- 100 kVp, 10 mA, 0.08 sec, 24 inches focal-film distance

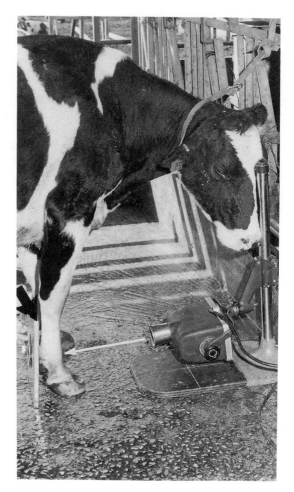

Fig. 3-6
Positioning used for dorsopalmar (plantar) radiography of the metacarpophalangeal (metatarsophalangeal) joint. The cassette is placed erect on the ground just behind the standing patient. The central beam is horizontal (arrow).

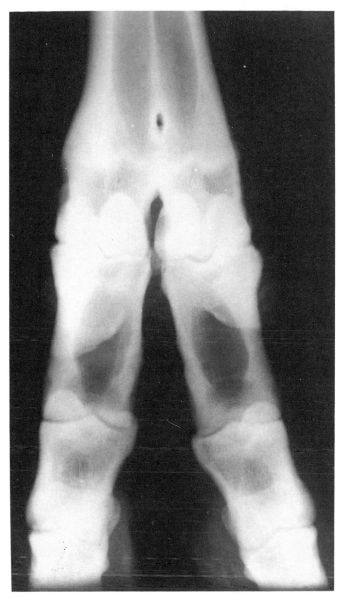
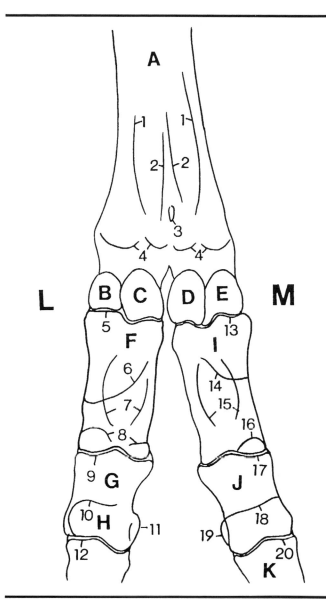

Fig. 3-7

Radiograph and drawing of the foot as seen on the dorsopalmar (plantar) view with the anatomical structures labeled on the drawing.

A. Metacarpus
B. Proximal lateral sesamoid bone of the lateral digit.
C. Proximal medial sesamoid bone of the lateral digit.
D. Proximal medial sesamoid bone of the medial digit.
E. Proximal lateral sesamoid bone of the medial digit.
F. 1st phalanx of the lateral digit.
G. 2nd phalanx of the lateral digit.
H. Distal sesamoid bone (navicular bone) of the lateral digit.
I. 1st phalanx of the medial digit.
J. 2nd phalanx of the medial digit.
K. 3rd phalanx of the medial digit.

1. Cortex metacarpus.
2. Fusion line of 3rd and 4th metacarpal bones
3. Nutrient foramen.
4. Calcified distal metacarpal growth plate.
5. Metacarpophalangeal joint space of lateral digit.
6. Dew claw of lateral digit.
7. Cortex of 1st phalanx of the lateral digit.
8. Proximal caudal border of 2nd phalanx of the lateral digit.
9. Proximal interphalangeal joint space of the lateral digit.
10. Proximal border of the distal sesamoid bone of the lateral digit.
11. Border of the distal sesamoid bone of the lateral digit.
12. Distal interphalangeal joint space of the lateral digit
13. Metacarpophalangeal joint space of the medial digit.
14. Dew claw of medial digit.
15. Cortex of 1st phalanx of the medial digit.
16. Proximal border of the 2nd phalanx of the medial digit.
17. Proximal interphalangeal joint space of medial digit.
18. Proximal border of the distal sesamoid bone of the medial digit.
19. Border of the distal sesamoid bone of the medial digit.
20. Distal interphalangeal joint space of the medial digit.

FETLOCK JOINT
(Metacarpo- or Metatarsophalangeal Joint)
AND PROXIMAL SESAMOID BONES—
LATERAL VIEW

Purpose: The lateral view permits good evaluation of the fetlock joint axis. The proximal sesamoid bones are not superimposed on the third metacarpal (tarsal) bone, but are superimposed on each other.

Preparation: Only brushing of the ankle is required.

Positioning: The patient is fully weight bearing on the affected limb with the foot on the ground and the cassette held against the medial aspect of the joint. The cassette can be in a holder resting on the ground (Fig. 3-8).

Beam location: The x-ray tube is positioned directly lateral to the foot with the x-ray beam parallel to the ground and directed toward the fetlock joint.

Normal radiograph and drawing are shown (Fig. 3-9).

Radiographic Technique for Portable Unit (400 speed film-screen system)
- 80 kVp, 10 mA, 0.1 sec, 24 inches focal-film distance
- 100 kVp, 10 mA, 0.08 sec, 24 inches focal-film distance

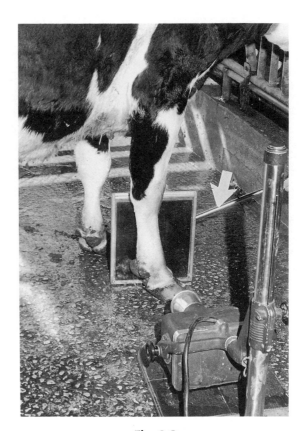

Fig. 3-8
Positioning used for lateral radiography of the fetlock joint and proximal sesamoid bones. The central beam is parallel to the ground and centered on the area of interest. Notice the use of a cassette holder (white arrow).

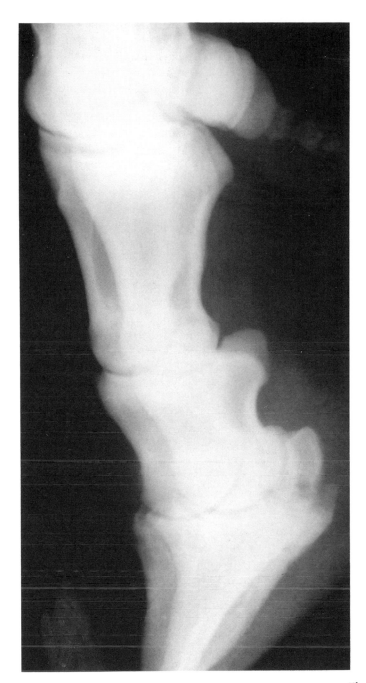
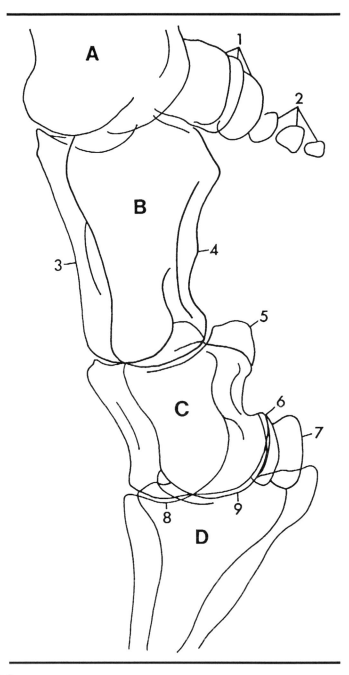

Fig. 3-9

Radiograph and drawing of the foot as seen on a lateral radiograph with the anatomical structures labelled on the drawing.

A. Distal metacarpus (metatarsus)
B. Proximal phalanges (PI) (superimposed)
C. Middle phalanges (PII) (superimposed)
D. Distal phalanges (PIII) (superimposed)

1. Proximal sesamoid bones (superimposed)
2. Rudimentary bones of the dewclaws
3. Dorsal cortex of medial proximal phalanx
4. Palmar cortex of lateral proximal phalanx
5. Proximopalmar eninence of lateral middle phalanx
6. Palmar border of medial distal sesamoid bone
7. Palmar border of lateral distal sesamoid bone
8. Distal interphalangeal joint, medial digit
9. Distal interphalangeal joint, lateral digit

FETLOCK JOINT
(Metacarpo- or Metatarsophalangeal Joint)
AND PROXIMAL SESAMOID BONES—
MEDIAL OBLIQUE VIEW
(30° dorsolateral—palmaromedial [plantar])

Purpose: This oblique view is essential as the first phalanges and the sesamoid bones form a part of the fetlock joint and are superimposed over each other in a true lateral view and therefore cannot be completely evaluated. Oblique studies are essential in providing additional methods to evaluate both productive and destructive bony changes as well as changes of arthrosis.

Preparation: Only brushing of the ankle is required.

Positioning: The foot is positioned on the ground with the cassette placed against the medial aspect of the palmar (plantar) surface of the joint. The cassette rests on the ground and is held in a cassette holder.

Beam location: Oblique views require that the tube be positioned dorsolaterally and the cassette be shifted to a palmar (plantar) location by approximately 45° from the position used for the lateromedial view. The x-ray tube is shifted 45° laterally from the mid-sagittal plane and is directed parallel to the ground. The central beam is directed at the fetlock joint or at the proximal sesamoid bones depending on the area of interest.

The opposite oblique view made with the tube positioned dorsomedially and the cassette palmarolaterally is normally also made.

Radiographic Technique for Portable Unit (400 speed film-screen system)
- 80 kVp, 10 mA, 0.1 sec, 24 inches focal-film distance
- 100 kVp, 10 mA, 0.08 sec, 24 inches focal-film distance

CARPUS

The carpus of the bovine is most commonly composed of six small, irregularly shaped bones and the interposed hinge-type diarthrodial joints. The two proximal joints have a rather large range of motion while motion in the distally located carpometacarpal joint is highly restricted. All joints move essentially as hinge joints and have only limited rotational capability. Because of the conformation of the carpus and the many different ways that traumatic injury can be expressed, it is difficult to evaluate all bony surfaces and borders completely.

The two standard views of the carpus are the dorsoplamar and lateromedial extended made using 10 x 12 in (24 x 30 cm) cassettes. With a portable machine, the focal-film distance is recommended to be 24 in (60 cm). With a rotating anode tube, the focal-film distance is increased to 40 in (100 cm). Use of a grid is recommended and is a requirement in radiography of the carpus of heavier bulls. Use of rare-earth intensifying screens is recommended to enable use of shorter exposure times (Table 3-4).

While other views of the carpus may be made, oblique or flexed views are not routinely made in the bovine since "slab" fractures or interarticular corner fractures are rarely, if ever, identified.

The upper portion of the leg is usually cleaner, but brushing often removes some of the objectionable dirt and debris from the skin. Only right and left markers are required for studies of the carpus. The medial and lateral aspects of the film can be identified by the unique appearance of the carpal bones.

The physeal growth plates are easily identified on the radiographs. The distal epiphysis of the radius unites with the metaphysis by 24 to 30 months. The large lateral styloid process of the distal ulna appears as a separate growth center lateral to the distal radial epiphysis and unites at about 36 months.

Table 3-4
TECHNIQUE FOR RADIOGRAPHIC EVALUATION OF THE CARPUS

Standard views
  dorsopalmar
  lateromedial extended

Optional views
  oblique views
  lateromedial flexed

Views of the opposite limb
  dorsopalmar view helpful in a calf or heifer less than 24 months

Cassette size
  medium cassette (10 x 12 in, 24 x 30 cm) except when evaluating a conformational problem, in which case a longer cassette is needed (7 x 17 in, 18 x 43 cm) or may divide a larger cassette (14 x 17 in, 35 x 43 cm)

Cassette holders
  use where possible

Grid
  highly recommended

Film markers
  right or left

CARPUS—DORSOPALMAR VIEW

Purpose: The dorsopalmar view is a basic view of the carpal region, and other films are compared with it. It permits good evaluation of the character of the antebrachiocarpal, intercarpal, and carpometacarpal joint spaces and the size, shape, and density of the carpal bones. This view is most valuable in determining alignment of the carpal bones and forelimb deviation. The prominent distal ulna is noted radiographically.

Preparation: No special preparation needed.

Positioning: The bovine stands normally with the legs even and the cassette holder is held firmly against the palmar aspect of the leg (Fig. 3-10).

Beam location: The x-ray tube is positioned in front of the carpal region, and the x-ray beam is directed within the mid-sagittal plane, parallel to the ground, and centered on the readily palpable intercarpal joint space. Because the bovine stands with the legs slightly rotated externally, the dorsoplamar view is made with the tube positioned slightly lateral to the longitudinal axis of the cow so the tube appears to be positioned as for a slightly obliqued view.

Normal radiograph and drawing are shown (Fig. 3-11).

Radiographic Technique for Portable Unit (400 speed film-screen system)
- 80 kVp, 10 mA, 0.1 sec, 24 inches focal-film distance
- 100 kVp, 10 mA, 0.08 sec, 24 inches focal-film distance

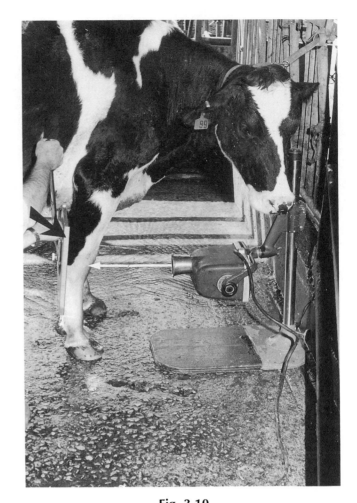

Fig. 3-10
Positioning used for dorsopalmar radiography of the carpus. The central beam (arrow) is parallel to the ground and centered on the carpus. Notice the use of a cassette holder (arrow).

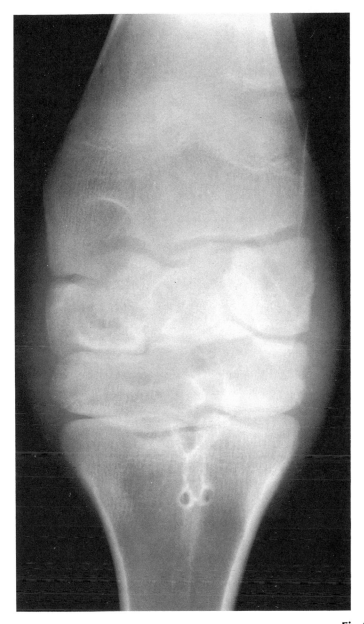

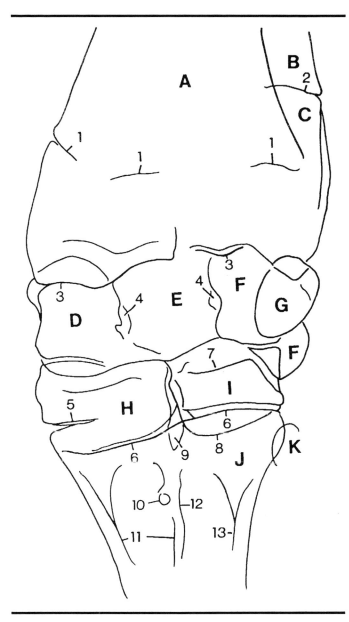

Fig 3-11

Radiograph and drawing of the carpus as seen on the dorsopalmar view with anatomical structures labeled on the drawing.

A. Radius
B. Ulna—metaphysis
C. Ulna—epiphysis
D. Radial carpal bone
E. Intermediate carpal bone
F. Ulnar carpal bone
G. Accessory carpal bone
H. Third carpal bone
I. Fourth carpal bone
J. Fused third and fourth metacarpal bones
K. Fifth metacarpal bone

1. Distal growth plate of the radius
2. Distal growth plate of the ulna
3. Radiocarpal joint space.
4. Intercarpal joint spaces between the radial carpal, intermediate, and ulnar carpal bones
5. Mediodorsal edge of the third metacarpal bone
6. Carpometacarpal joint space
7. Proximopalmar border of the fourth carpal bone
8. Distal edge of the fourth carpal bones
9. Third and fourth carpal joint space
10. Nutrient foramen
11. Cortex of third metacarpal bone
12. Junction of the third and fourth metacarpal bones
13. Cortex of the fourth metacarpal bone

CARPUS—LATERAL VIEW (weight-bearing) EXTENDED (lateromedial)

Purpose: This is the second basic view and it is essential for demonstrating the accessory carpal bone, which is occasionally involved in carpal lesions.

Preparation: No special preparation is required.

Positioning: The patient is weight bearing with the cassette positioned firmly against the medial aspect of the carpus (Fig. 3-12).

Beam location: The x-ray tube is positioned laterally with the x-ray beam parallel to the ground and directed just distal and dorsal to the prominence created by the easily palpated accessory carpal bone

Normal radiographs and line-drawings are shown (Fig. 3-13).

Radiographic Technique for Portable Unit (400 speed film-screen system)
- 80 kVp, 10 mA, 0.1 sec, 24 inches focal-film distance
- 100 kVp, 10 mA, 0.08 sec, 24 inches focal-film distance

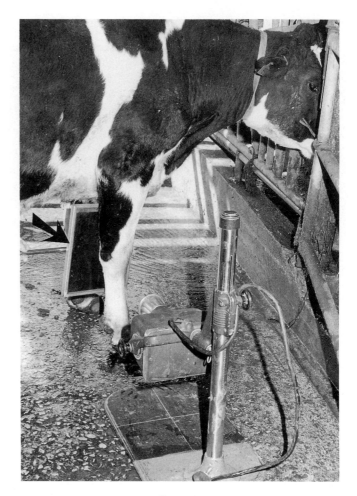

Fig. 3-12

Positioning used for lateral radiography of the carpus. The central beam is parallel to the ground and centered on the carpus. Notice the use of a cassette holder (arrow).

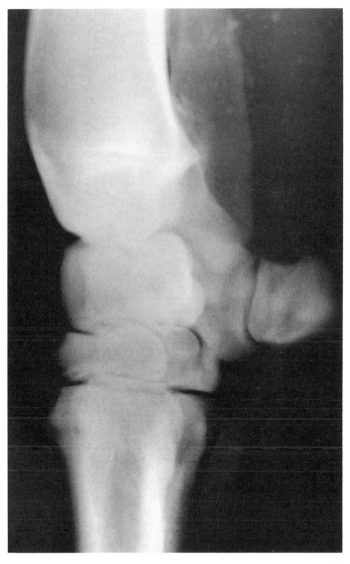
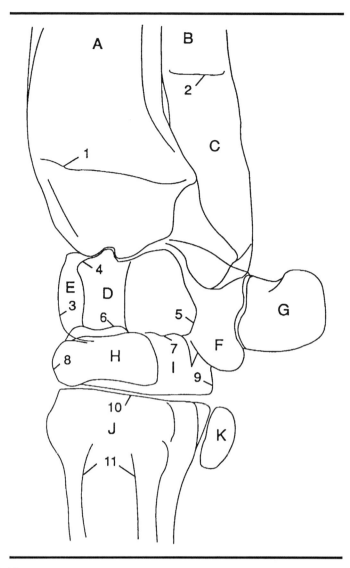

Fig. 3-13
Radiograph and drawing of the carpus as seen on the lateral radiograph with anatomical structures labeled on the drawing.

A. Radius
B. Ulna—metaphysis
C. Ulna—epiphysis
D. Radial carpal bone
E. Intermediate carpal bone
F. Ulnar carpal bone
G. Accessory carpal bone
H. Fused second and third carpal bone
I. Fourth carpal bone
J. Fused third and fourth metacarpal bones
K. Fifth metacarpal bone

1. Distal growth plate of the radius
2. Distal growth plate of the ulna
3. Radiocarpal joint space.
4. Dorsal border of third carpal bone
5. Palmar border of third carpal bone
6. Intercarpal joint space—proximal aspect
7. Intercarpal joint space—distal aspect
8. Dorsal border of second and third carpal bones
9. Palmar border of fourth carpal bone
10. Carpometacarpal joint space
11. Cortex of metacarpal bone

ELBOW JOINT (Humeroradial Joint) (Articulatio Cubiti)

The elbow joint (cubital joint) is formed by the humerus, radius, and ulna. The elbow joint is difficult to radiograph in the standing bovine because of its size and the difficulty of positioning the cassette in such a manner as to obtain a projection in either a true lateral or true craniocaudal view. Still, it is a study that needs to be made occasionally because of need to evaluate for possible bone or joint injury secondary to a puncture wound or because of suspected sprain or fracture.

Fractures of the olecranon are more easily evaluated on the lateral view because tissue thickness is much less and a film of good diagnostic quality is thus more easily made; a portable unit may be able to produce a satisfactory lateral study of the olecranon. Olecranon injury is difficult to evaluate in the craniocaudal view because tissue thickness is much greater and patient movement is a problem.

The nutrient foramen in the humerus is at the junction of the middle and distal thirds medially and is seen on a craniocaudal view of the elbow joint in which the cassette is positioned proximally. On the craniocaudal view the capitulum (distal humeral lateral condyle) is located laterally where it articulates with the head of the radius (caput radii). The trochlea (distal humeral medial condyle) is located medially where it also articulates with the head of the radius.

On the lateral view, the medial epicondyle of the humerus creates a large shadow distally and caudally. It is superimposed over the smaller lateral humeral epicondyle, the olecranon process, and part of the olecranon tuberosity (tuber olecrani).

There is no special preparation required for this study. While lateral and craniocaudal views are standard, oblique views are sometimes necessary to define suspect lesions. Use of a grid improves the quality of the radiograph, however, it is usually difficult to position the grid correctly. Identification of the film is limited to right or left markers. Using a special lead marker to identify a soft tissue injury or soft tissue tract is helpful (Table 3-5).

Studies of the elbow usually require higher capacity machines than the portable units that are used for the distal extremities. This is especially true in the patient with a swollen elbow. However, it may be possible to make lateral views with low capacity machines because the thickness of the limb is often only 4 to 6" (10 to 15 cm). The limb thickness in the craniocaudal and oblique views is much greater, usually requiring a higher capacity machine to generate an x-ray beam of sufficient energy to penetrate the tissue.

Rare-earth screens are highly recommended for use in studies of the elbow to decrease exposure time. Use 10 by 12 in (24 x 30 cm) cassettes. Use of 40 in (100 cm) focal-film distance is suggested with a rotating anode tube.

Physeal plates near the elbow generally remain open longer than in the distal part of the limb. The center for the medial epicondyle joins the distal metaphysis of the humerus at 8 to 12 months and the distal humeral physis closes between 12 and 18 months. The proximal growth center for the radius closes about 12 to 18 months. The single growth center for the proximal ulna closes between 24 and 30 months.

Table 3-5
TECHNIQUE FOR RADIOGRAPHIC EVALUATION OF THE ELBOW JOINT

Standard views
    caudocranial
    lateromedial

Optional views
    craniocaudal
    obliques

Views of the opposite limb
    rarely examined except in patients with open physes

Cassette size
    use a 10 x 12 in (24 x 30 cm) cassette

Use of a cassette holder
    use for views made with the patient standing

Use of a grid
    not recommended on a standing patient

Markers
    right or left

ELBOW JOINT—CAUDOCRANIAL VIEW

Purpose: The caudocranial view is a standard view and often requires use of a larger x-ray unit. Because of patient size, the study is often limited to visualization of the distal humerus, the joint space and the proximal radius and ulna. This compromised study is still sufficient from which to make many diagnoses.

Preparation: No special preparation is required.

Positioning: The bovine stands normally.

Beam location: The x-ray tube is caudal to the joint and the caudocranial x-ray beam is directed parallel to the ground so that it is perpendicular to the shaft of the radius. The cassette is held just cranial to the joint and the cassette is at an angle to the x-ray beam (Fig. 3-14).

Cassette size: The cassette size needs to be determined by the particular case. A large cassette enables visualization of the greatest area. However, if the site of the injury is known, a smaller cassette may be positioned more easily. The difference in tissue thickness makes it impossible to optimally visualize all of the tissues. It is better to obtain an over-exposed radiograph that permits evaluation of the distal humerus and provides penetration so that the olecranon can be visualized. Use of a bright-light always assists in the evaluation of the over-exposed portions of these radiographs.

It is possible to make this view in a craniocaudal manner. The cassette is placed in a holder at the caudal aspect of the olecranon, parallel to it, and at a right angle to the lateral chest wall. The tube is placed cranially and the central beam is directed toward the cassette from the cranial aspect of the elbow joint. The central beam is directed upward at a 20° to 30° angle from craniodistal to caudoproximal. This position reduces the tissue width between the tube and cassette and thus the angled beam demonstrates the joint space more clearly.

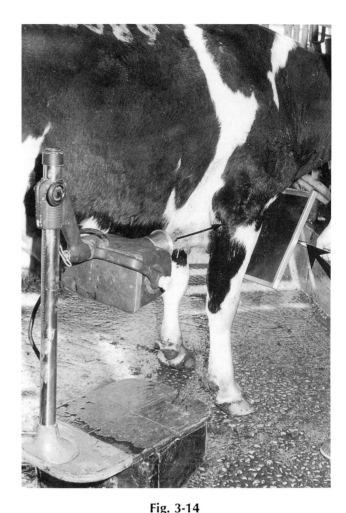

Fig. 3-14
Positioning for caudocranial radiography of the humeroradial (elbow) joint. The central beam (long black arrow) is parallel to the ground and perpendicular to the shaft of the radius. Notice the use of a cassette holder (black arrow).

Radiographic Technique for Portable Unit (400 speed film-screen system)
- 80 kVp, 10 mA, 0.25-0.35 sec, 24 inches focal-film distance
- 100 kVp, 10 mA, 0.1-0.15 sec, 24 inches focal-film distance

800 speed film-screen system)
- 90 kVp, 20 mA, 0.2-0.3 sec, 30 inches focal-film distance

ELBOW JOINT—LATERAL VIEW
(lateromedial)

Purpose: The lateral view is the easiest radiographic view to make of the elbow joint and often the only view possible with a portable unit. It produces a radiograph that permits good evaluation of the olecranon and serves as a survey study for the elbow joint.

Preparation: There is no special preparation required.

Positioning: The bovine stands normally.

Beam location: The cassette is within a holder and is positioned medially and the x-ray tube is lateral with the x-ray beam parallel to the ground (Fig. 3-15).

OLECRANON—LATEROMEDIAL VIEW

Purpose: Often an injury involves only the olecranon and the radiographic study can be limited to a lateral view of that more easily examined portion of the elbow.

Preparation: There is no special preparation required.

Positioning: The bovine stands normally.

Beam location: The cassette within the holder is in the same position as for the lateral view of the elbow joint except that the upper edge of the cassette is placed slightly above the olecranon. The tube is positioned laterally and the central beam is parallel to the ground and centered on the olecranon. A grid is not used because of the decreased tissue thickness. Either 24 in (60 cm) or 40 in (100 cm) focal-film distance can be used.

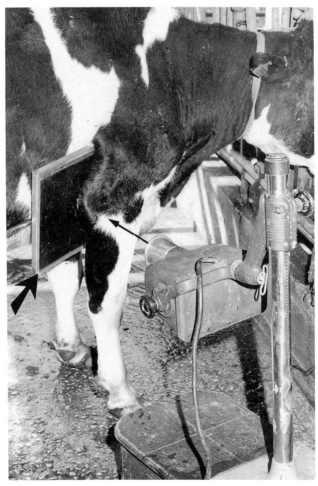

Fig. 3-15
Positioning for lateral radiography of the humeroradial (elbow) joint. The central beam (long black arrow) is parallel to the ground and directed at the elbow joint. Notice the use of a cassette holder (black arrow).

SHOULDER JOINT
(Scapulohumeral Joint)

Radiographic examination of the shoulder joint is a rarely used study. Avulsion fractures of the supraglenoid tuberosity of the scapula due to pulling of the biceps brachii muscle or traumatic fractures involving the proximal humeral tubercles are a possible cause of lameness that can be identified radiographically. Post-traumatic calcification or ossification of the tendon of the biceps brachii muscle can be identified on the lateral radiograph.

Radiography of the shoulder joint is limited to mediolateral projections on a recumbent patient and whatever oblique views can be obtained on the standing patient, since, it is almost impossible to make a craniocaudal, caudocranial, or dorsoventral view. Use of a grid is almost impossible. No special preparation of the patient is needed. Film identification is limited to right and left markers (Table 3-6).

Any study of the shoulder joint requires use of a rotating anode tube. The focal-film distance should be 40 in (100 cm). Use of rare-earth screens is recommended. Use a 10 by 12 in (24 x 30 cm) cassette.

The scapula has a group of ossification centers near the cranial aspect of the joint. These are the supraglenoid tubercle and coracoid process that fuse near 12 months of age and the cranial part of the glenoid cavity that fuses at a similar time. The ossification center for the greater tubercles of the proximal humerus and the head of the humerus fuse to the body at 26 to 42 months. Because of the difficulty in obtaining high quality radiographs of these bones, they are not easily visualized radiographically and the ages of physeal closure have not been well studied.

Table 3-6
TECHNIQUE FOR RADIOGRAPHIC EVALUATION OF THE SHOULDER JOINT

Standard view
  obliques (on standing patient)

Optional views
  mediolateral view (on recumbent patient)

Views of the opposite limb
  views of the opposite shoulder are suggested when examining a calf

Cassette size
  should be the largest available

Use of a cassette holder
  recommended for a standing patient, but may be difficult to use; if the cassette is handheld, the largest cassette available should be used and the x-ray beam collimated so that the gloved hands are well away from the field of exposure
  for the recumbent lateral view, a tunnel should be used to protect the cassette

Use of a grid
  not recommended for a standing patient; may be used for recumbent mediolateral view

Markers
  right and left limb

SHOULDER JOINT—
TANGENTIAL OBLIQUE VIEWS

Purpose: Oblique views are usually made to permit evaluation of an area of suspected injury to the point of the shoulder. The views are often used to determine fracture of one of the tubercles on the proximal humerus or suspected bicipital bursal injury. Tissues deep to the surface are not well visualized on the radiograph.

Preparation: No special preparation is required.

Positioning: The patient stands with the limb to be examined in a normal standing position.

Beam location: If a caudolateral-craniomedial study is made, the cassette is placed in a vertical position cranial to the shoulder in the standing animal and pushed medially so that half of its width is medial to the protruding lateral tuberosity of the humerus. The x-ray tube is positioned caudally and is lateral and slightly dorsal to the middle of the thorax. The x-ray beam is angled downward and centered at the craniolateral aspect of the proximal humerus (Fig. 3-16).

In this positioning technique, the primary beam strikes the cassette at an angle making use of a grid impossible because of severe grid cutoff that would result. Scatter radiation is extensive because of the amount of soft tissue. The x-ray beam is often not directed at the center of the cassette but at the point of interest on the patient. Usually, only the area of the acromion process of the scapula and the lateral tubercles of the humerus are visualized on this oblique view. The character of the shoulder joint space is rarely evaluated clearly. Soft tissues can be evaluated for radiopaque foreign bodies, gas, or calcification/ossification. Film identification is limited to right or left markers.

This is often a nonproductive study, but is may be worth the effort if it provides even limited evaluation concerning a lesion on the point of the shoulder because this is such a difficult region to evaluate clinically. Evaluation of the oblique view, however, is best combined with an evaluation of a lateral view made in the recumbent patient.

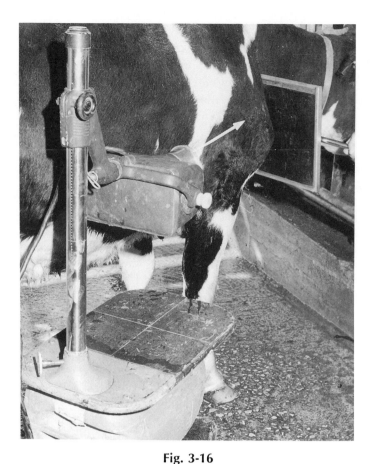

Fig. 3-16
Positioning for oblique radiography of the humeroscapula (shoulder) joint using a caudolateral-craniomedial beam. The central beam is marked (arrow).

Radiographic Technique for Portable Unit (400 speed film-screen system)
- 80 kVp, 10 mA, 1.0-1.5 sec, 24 inches focal-film distance
- 100 kVp, 10 mA, 0.4-0.5 sec, 24 inches focal-film distance

SHOULDER JOINT—LATERAL VIEW
(mediolateral)

Purpose: The mediolateral view can only be made if the bovine is in a lateral recumbent position.

Preparation: No special preparation is required except to examine the patient carefully for dirt and debris attached to the hair coat.

Positioning: The patient lies with the affected or down limb pulled as far cranially as is possible so that the humeral head is superimposed over the soft tissue of the neck. The neck and head should be extended and pulled dorsally to avoid having the caudal cervical spine superimposed over the shoulder joint. The upper, unaffected limb is positioned as far caudally as is possible to be out of the x-ray field. The cassette is positioned on the ground under the affected limb. The success of the study is dependent entirely on the degree of limb extension that is possible.

Beam location: The x-ray tube is positioned above the patient with the x-ray beam perpendicular to the ground and centered on the shoulder joint. Direct the central beam more dorsocranially if injury to the supraglenoid process is suspected or more ventrocranially if injury to the tubercles is a possibility.

The resulting radiographs are dependent on the age and size of the patient and the positioning technique utilized. In a smaller patient, it is possible to obtain high quality radiographs while in the larger patient the study is more compromised.

Radiographic Technique for Portable Unit (400 speed film-screen system)
- 80 kVp, 10 mA, 0.4-0.6 sec, 24 inches focal-film distance (non-grid standing)
- 100 kVp, 10 mA, 0.4-0.5 sec, 24 inches focal-film distance (non-grid standing)
- 100 kVp, 10 mA, 0.3-0.4 sec, 24 inches focal-film distance (non-grid recumbent)
- 100 kVp, 100 mA, 0.03-0.04 sec, 40 inch focal-film distance (non-grid standing)
- 100 kVp, 100 mA, 0.02 sec, 40 inch focal-film distance (non-grid recumbent)

(800 speed film-screen system)
- 90 kVp, 20 mA, 0.2-0.3 sec, 30 inches focal-film distance (non-grid standing)

TARSUS

The tarsus of the bovine is the site of numerous clinical conditions which appear at varying ages. The nature of the lesions range from congenital deformities and inherited musculoskeletal disease, such as spastic paresis seen in young calves, to various traumatic conditions which may appear at all ages. Degenerative lesions occur with higher prevalence in bulls.

Within the tarsus are a tarso-crural (tibiotarsal) hinge type diarthrodial joint, 5 irregularly shaped tarsal bones interposed between the distal tibia and the proximal metatarsus, and intertarsal and tarsometatarsal joints. The site of major motion within the tarsus is at the tarsocrural (tibiotarsal) joint where the proximal trochlea of the tibiotarsal bone (talus) is in contract with the articular surface of the distal end of the tibia. Unlike the horse, the bovine talus also has a distal trochlea, so the proximal intertarsal joint of the bovine also permits considerable motion.

On the dorsoplantar views the proximal portion of the large and clinically important calcaneus is not usually seen due to the overlying distal tibia. The talus, the fused central and fourth tarsal bones, and the fused second and third tarsal bones are identified on this view. On the lateral view, the small first tarsal bone located plantar to the fused second and third tarsal bone and the metatarsal sesamoid bone (rudimentary second metatarsal) are also visible.

The bovine is allowed to stand weight-bearing in a normal manner for all views, regardless of the type of x-ray machine used. No special technique for preparation is required other than brushing. A cassette holder with a "leg" of some type is valuable in eliminating problems of cassette motion and radiation exposure to the individual holding the cassette. Because the intertarsal joint surfaces are not within a perfectly flat plain, two dorsoplantar views are used for their evaluation in cases where this is critical.

Oblique views of the tarsus with the tube positioned lateral or medial to that position used for the dorsplantar view are not commonly used unless it is thought that they will more clearly demonstrate a lesion suspected on physical examination or on another radiograph.

All views of the tarsus can be made using 10 by 12 in (24 by 30 cm) cassette. With a portable machine, the focal-film distance is recommended to be 24 in (60 cm). With a rotating anode tube, the focal-film distance can be increased to 40 in (100 cm). Use of a grid is highly recommended and is a requirement in radiography of large cows. Use of rare-earth intensifying screens is recommended to permit shortening of exposure times. Film identification is limited to right or left markers. Use of medial or lateral markers may assist in your orientation of the radiographs until you are familiar with the oblique views (Table 3-7).

The growth plate for the distal tibia closes at 18 to 24 months of age. The lateral malleolus remains as a separate center of ossification in the adult bovine, articulating with the distal tibia, talus , and calcaneus. On lateromedial views, the calcaneus is clearly visible with the proximal growth plate closing at 22 to 36 months.

Table 3-7
TECHNIQUE FOR RADIOGRAPHIC EVALUATION OF THE TARSAL JOINTS

Standard views
> dorsoplantar (2 views using different dorsoplantar angles)
> lateromedial

Optional views
> dorsolateral-plantaromedial (medial) oblique
> plantarolateral-dorsomedial (lateral) oblique

Views of the opposite limb
> not usually needed except in radiography of calves

Cassettes
> medium size are usually used—10 by 12 in (24 by 30 cm)

Use of cassette holders
> are of value, especially if they have a supporting "leg" of some type to control motion

Use of a grid
> use is indicated in radiography of heavy breeds
> use is not recommended with a portable unit

Markers
> right or left
> medial or lateral

TARSUS—DORSOPLANTAR VIEWS (2)
(10° dorsoproximal-plantarodistal, horizontal dorsoplantar)

Purpose: The two dorsoplantar views are standard views used in the examination of the tarsus and both views should be made to provide the most complete evaluation of the intertarsal and tarsometatarsal joints.

Preparation: No special preparation is required.

Positioning: The patient stands fully weight bearing with the foot pointing outward slightly. With the foot in this position, the x-ray tube can be positioned dorsally and slightly laterally and not be under the patient (Figs. 3-17, 3-18).

Beam location: The cassette is placed within a holder and held against the plantar aspect of the tarsus parallel to the calcaneus. The x-ray tube is positioned dorsally and slightly laterally, is within the midsagittal plane, and is directed toward the cassette and centered on the palpable trochlea. For the first view that demonstrates the tarsometatarsal joint space the beam is parallel to the ground. For the second view that demonstrates the

intertarsal joint spece, the beam is directed at a right angle to the cassette, is perpendicular to the shaft of the metatarsal bone, and is angled downward in a dorsoproximal to plantarodistal angle. The two different beam angles are used so that the nature of both the intertarsal and tarsometatarsal joint spaces is visualized. The beam is centered on the palpable trochlea for each view.

Normal radiograph and line-drawings are shown (Fig. 3-19).

Radiographic Technique for Portable Unit (400 speed film-screen system)
- 80 kVp, 10 mA, 0.2 sec, 24 inches focal-film distance
- 100 kVp, 10 mA, 0.1-0.12 sec, 24 inches focal-film distance

---

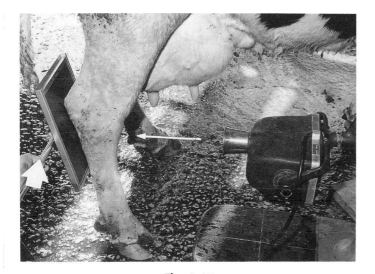

Fig. 3-17
Positioning for dorsoplantar radiography of the tarsus. The central beam (arrow) is parallel to the ground for view #1. Notice the use of a cassette holder (arrow).

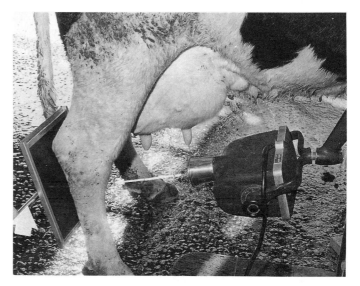

Fig. 3-18
Positioning for dorsoplantar radiography of the tarsus. The central beam (arrow) is angled toward the ground and is perpendicular to the long axis of the metatarsal bone for view #2. Notice the use of a cassette holder (arrow).

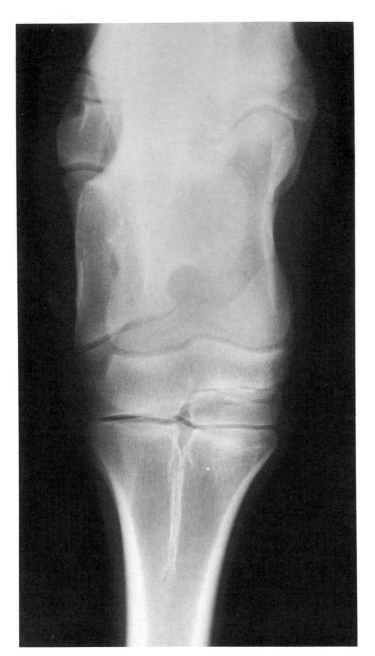
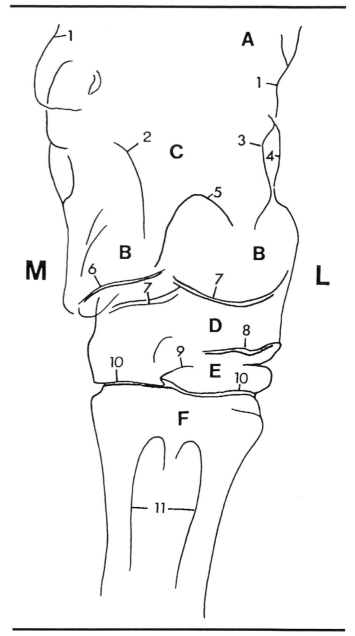

Fig. 3-19

Radiograph and drawing of the tarsus as seen on the dorsoplantar view with anatomical structures labelled on the drawing.

A. Tibia
B. Trochlea (tibiotarsal bone)
C. Calcaneus (fibulotarsal bone)
D. Fused central and fourth tarsal bone
E. Fused second and third tarsal bones
F. Fused third and fourth metatarsal bones

1. Lateral and medial aspects of tibia
2. Medial aspect of distal calcaneus
3. Lateral aspect of distal trochlea
4. Lateral aspect of distal trochlea
5. Dorsal articulating facets of trochlea
6. Plantar aspect of distal trochlea
7. Proximal intertarsal joint space
8. Joint space between fused second and third tarsal bones and fused central and fourth tarsal bones
9. Medial aspect of fused second and third tarsal bones
10. Tarsometatarsal joint space
11. Cortex of fused second land third metatarsal bones

TARSUS—LATERAL VIEW (lateromedial)

Purpose: The first tarsal bone is visualized on the lateral view and with the help of a bright light, the somewhat overexposed calcaneus can be studied. The articulation between the sustentaculum tali of the calcaneus and the talus is seen. In the younger patient the separate center of ossification for the tuber calcaneus can be identified. This closes at 22 to 36 months of age. Soft tissue shadows may be seen cranially.

Preparation: No special preparation is required.

Positioning: The patient stands normally weight-bearing with the x-ray tube positioned laterally and the cassette is placed against the medial aspect of the tarsal region (Fig. 3-20).

Beam location: The top of the cassette should include the most proximal portion of the calcaneus, but the x-ray beam should be centered 4 inches (10 cm) distal to the point of the hock. The most common error in positioning is centering the x-ray beam too high on the limb.

Normal radiograph and line-drawings are shown (Fig. 3-21).

Radiographic Technique for Portable Unit (400 speed film-screen system)
- 80 kVp, 10 mA, 0.15 sec, 24 inches focal-film distance
- 100 kVp, 10 mA, 0.08-0.1 sec, 24 inches focal-film distance

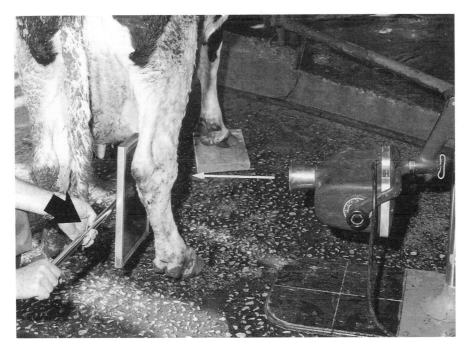

Fig. 3-20
Positioning for lateral radiography of the tarsus. The central beam (arrow) is parallel to the ground and is centered on the tarsal bones. Notice the use of a cassette holder (arrow).

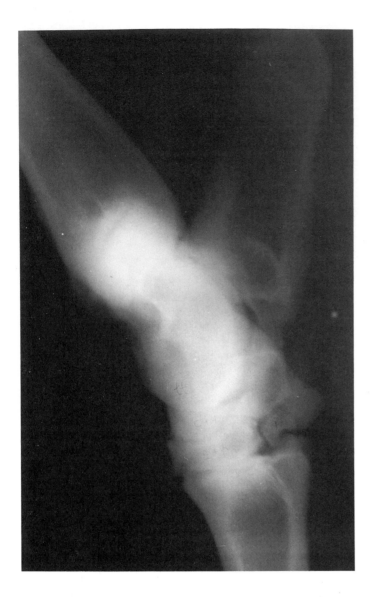
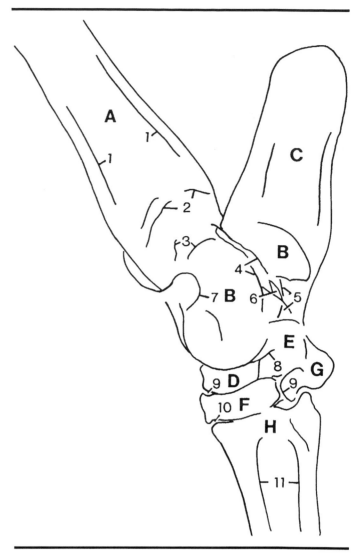

Fig. 3-21

Radiograph and drawing of the tarsus as seen on the lateral view with anatomical structures labelled on the drawing.

A. Tibia
B. Trochlea (tibiotarsal bone)
C. Calcaneus (fibulotarsal bone)
D. Fourth tarsal bone
E. Central tarsal bone
F. Fused second and third tarsal bones
G. First tarsal bone
H. Fused third and fourth metatarsal bones

1. Cortex of tibia
2. Distal growth plate of tibia
3. Articulating facet of trochlea
4. Articulating facet of calcaneus
5. Plantar aspect of calcaneus
6. Articulating facet of trochlea
7. Cranial aspect of trochlea
8. Joint space between central and fourth tarsal bones
9. Intertarsal joint space
10. Tarsometatarsal joint space
11. Cortex of fused third and fourth metatarsal bones

STIFLE JOINT (Femorotibial Joint) AND PATELLA

The femoro-tibial joint is the largest joint of the body and is divided into 3 separate compartments, the lateral femorotibial, the medial femorotibial, and the femoropatellar. In the bovine, this joint is the site of numerous traumatic, degenerative and septic conditions. Though quite remote from the ground, it is one of the most traumatized joints in cattle. The additional structure of support, the patella, makes the joint more vulnerable to trauma.

Radiography is an essential part of a complete examination for diagnosis, treatment, and prognosis of lesions involving this joint. The anatomy of this joint is such that there are several soft tissue structures not recognized on a normal stifle radiograph, but which are often the sites of lesions. These are; 1) lateral and medial menisci, 2) cranial and caudal cruciate ligaments, and 3) cranial (straight), medial and lateral patellar ligaments. Since these are radiolucent structures, trauma may only be deduced indirectly through a good working knowledge of their points of origin and insertion and resulting new bone production at these sites.

Clinical stifle problems in the suckling calf or during the first six months of life are rarely encountered. However, growing calves entering the estrous cycle are most susceptible to stifle problems. The conditions observed in these calves, as well as in heifers, are; 1) patellar luxation, 2) rupture of the cranial cruciate ligament, 3) tibial tuberosity avulsion, 4) joint effusion, and 5) collateral ligament trauma. Most of these lesions occur during the heat cycle, when the calf in heat slips when mounted, or the mounting calf slips when dismounting. The fact that these cases occur more often on concrete floors supports the hypothesis of heat cycle-related etiology of these lesions. Rare cases of septic arthritis of the stifle, probably of hematogenic etiology, do occur.

Radiographic studies of the stifle joints are made commonly and can be highly informative if the views are technically adequate. The caudocranial view is of value in the detection of periarticular new bone which is diagnostic of secondary joint disease. The special views of the patella and femoropatellar joint surfaces require different positioning of cassette and central beam and a different radiographic technique. They are valuable to demonstrate both traumatic and degenerative changes in this joint (Table 3-8).

All views of the stifle joint can be made on a 10 by 12 in (24 by 30 cm) cassette. A grid is used on the caudocranial and lateromedial views. Tissue thickness warrants the use of a grid, but it is very difficult to make the central beam perpendicular to the plane of the cassette, and malposition of the tube results in severe grid cut-off. Rare-earth intensifying screens are recommended. These views are best made with a rotating anode tube at 40 in (100 cm) focal-film distance.

The distal growth center of the femur unites at 20 to 30 months while the apophyseal center of the tibial tuberosity joins the proximal tibial growth center at 9 to 12 months and the combined growth centers join the tibial shaft at 20 to 30 months. Because of the thickness of the joint, the resulting radiographs often lack in film quality. It is for this reason in part that there is a lack of information on the specific ages of physeal closure.

Table 3-8
TECHNIQUE FOR RADIOGRAPHIC EVALUATION OF THE STIFLE JOINT

Standard views
    caudocranial
    lateromedial stifle joint

Optional views
    lateromedial patella
    craniolateral-caudomedial (medial) oblique

Views of the opposite limb
    probably not indicated

Cassette size
    large size should be used for the views of the stifle joint 10 by 12 in (24 by 30 cm) and smaller cassettes for the views of the patella

Use of cassette holders
    difficult to use

Use of the grid
    indicated because of tissue thickness but difficult to use correctly

Markers
    right and left

STIFLE JOINT—CAUDOCRANIAL VIEW

Purpose: The caudocranial view is essential for diagnosis of patellar displacement and allows diagnosis of degenerative joint disease, particularly, the identification of new bony production on the inner aspect of the intercondylar region that is not seen on other views. Reducing the tube-cassette distance (focal-film distance) may be necessary to penetrate the tissue thickness on this view. Use of a cone or other collimating device is important to decrease the effect of scatter radiation on the film This is especially important since it is difficult to use a cassette holder to make this view and the helper must not be within the primary beam. The caudocranial view cannot be achieved by conventional portable radiographic equipment, but requires a rotating anode unit.

Preparation: No special preparation is required.

Positioning: Because of a desire to limit the object-film distance, this projection is made with the x-ray tube behind the patient and the cassette held cranially against the patella. The cassette is held vertically in front of the joint at a right angle to the body wall. It must be placed as far proximal and pushed as far medially as the size of the cow's abdomen allows. The tube is positioned caudal to the joint and the central beam is directed caudoproximal to craniodistal from a point above the level of the joint. The joint space is thus projected in an oblique manner. The cassette without a grid is usually angled with the distal part of the cassette pushed further medially and caudally.

Beam location: The x-ray tube is positioned caudal to the joint with the beam directed downward thus projecting the intercondylar region to better advantage and obtain a "tunnel" view of the distal femur.

A major problem in obtaining a diagnostic radiograph using the caudocranial view is the result of the marked increase in tissue thickness proximally. This means that if the joint space and proximal tibia are correctly exposed, the distal femur is badly underexposed. Since it may be important to evaluate the distal femur, joint surfaces, as well as the proximal tibia, it may be necessary to make two radiographs using two different exposure settings.

Radiographic Technique for Portable Unit (400 speed film-screen system)
- 80 kVp, 10 mA, 0.6-0.8 sec, 24 inches focal-film distance
- 100 kVp, 10 mA, 0.3-0.4 sec, 24 inches focal-film distance
- 100 kVp, 100 mA, 0.1 sec, 40 inches focal-film distance

(800 speed film-screen system)
- 90 kVp, 20 mA, 0.15-0.2 sec, 30 inches focal-film distance

STIFLE JOINT—LATERAL VIEW (lateromedial)

Purpose: The lateral view is the easiest view of the stifle joint to make and provides good evaluation of the articular surfaces of the femorotibial joints. Both ridges of the distal femoral trochlea are seen at least partially on this view. The position of the patella is demonstrated as well as the relationship of the intercondylar eminence of the tibia to the condyles of the femur. In dairy cattle with a large udder, this view is complicated by an inability to position the cassette far enough proximally. Thus, the femoral condyles and patella are often only partially visualized. However, the distal portion of the femoral condyles and the intercondylar eminence of the tibia are always seen. These structures are important when rupture of the cranial cruciate ligament is suspected.

Preparation: No special preparation is required other than brushing the hair coat.

Positioning: The patient stands weight-bearing and the cassette is placed medial to the joint, between the leg and udder, and pushed proximally as much as possible (Fig. 3-22).

Beam location: The x-ray tube is positioned laterally with the x-ray beam directly parallel to the ground and centered distal and caudal to the patella. Use of a collimator is important since the beam must be smaller than the size of the cassette because of the difficulty in using a cassette holder for this view.

On a recumbent patient, the affected limb can be placed down and the cassette placed beneath the patient and the upper, nonaffected limb can be flexed and pulled cranially and proximally to remove it from the field of exposure. If the patient is positioned on a table, the cassette can be placed in an undercarriage tray making it relatively easy to change cassettes. The use of a table also makes it easy to use a grid with the resulting improvement of radiographic technique.

A major problem in centering for the lateromedial view of the stifle joint, regardless of patient positioning, is the temptation to center the beam on the patella which is proximal and cranial to the femorotibial joint surfaces. This results in a badly obliqued view of the joint surfaces. Another problem comes from centering the beam on the cassette instead of the patient when the positioning of the cassette is compromised.

The appearance of the anatomical structures on the lateromedial radiographs of the stifle joint varies widely because of the differences in positioning the cassette. In some studies the distal femoral condyles and patella are clearly projected, while in other studies the distal femur and patella are only seen in part.

Radiographic Technique for Portable Unit (400 speed film-screen system)
- 80 kVp, 10 mA, 0.3-0.4 sec, 24 inches focal-film distance
- 100 kVp, 10 mA, 0.15-0.2 sec, 24 inches focal-film distance
- 100 kVp, 100 mA, 0.05 sec, 40 inches focal-film distance

(800 speed film-screen system)
- 90 kVp, 20 mA, 0.2-0.3 sec, 30 inches focal-film distance

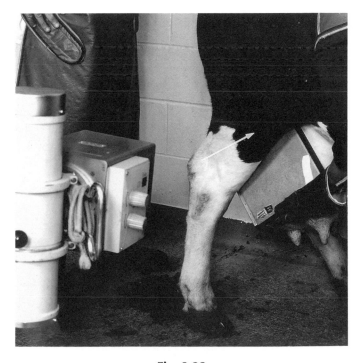

Fig. 3-22
Positioning used for lateral radiography of the stifle joint. The central beam is parallel to the floor (arrow).

STIFLE—LATEROMEDIAL PATELLAR VIEW

Purpose: The lateral view of the patella should be used as a standard view in evaluation of this part of the stifle joint. Being able to evaluate the patella and the femoropatella articulation is important in the detection of degenerative, traumatic, or degenerative disease.

Preparation: No special preparation is required.

Positioning: The bovine stands normally.

Beam location: The x-ray tube is positioned laterally and the cassette held medially but further proximally and cranially than for the regular lateromedial view. The x-ray beam is parallel to the ground and centered on the patella.

A smaller cassette is used for this view permitting it to be positioned more cranially. The radiographic technique is decreased for this view because of the decrease in thickness of the bony structures.

Radiographic Technique for Portable Unit (400 speed film-screen system)
- 80 kVp, 10 mA, 0.06-0.15 sec, 24 inches focal-film distance
- 100 kVp, 10 mA, 0.06 sec, 24 inches focal-film distance
- 100 kVp, 100 mA, 0.03 sec, 40 inches focal film distance

(800 speed film-screen system)
- 90 kVp, 20 mA, 0.1-0.2 sec, 30 inch focal-film distance

PELVIS

In the adult, pelvic radiography can only be done on a deeply sedated or anesthetized animal, whereas radiography of the calf is much easier. Suspect pelvic or hip joint injury is the most common indication for pelvic radiography in bovines of any age. Conditions which may occur include femoral nerve paresis, pelvic fractures, femoral head luxation, and, in calves, fractures of the femoral capital epiphysis ("slipped" capital femoral epiphysis), or greater trochanter

The animal must be in dorsal recumbency, with both hindlegs extended laterally as much as possible. Note that the legs are not extended caudally nor are they flexed as might be done in radiography of a dog or cat (Fig. 3-23). In a calf, however, it is frequently useful to make two ventrodorsal views for comparison, one with the limbs abducted laterally and one with the limbs flexed craniad. This often permits detection of femoral epiphyseal fractures, which may not be displaced on one of these views. In a dairy cow, the udder should be pushed cranially as much as possible to decrease the soft tissue thickness to be penetrated. The cassette is placed beneath the patient and the central beam is aimed at the center of the cassette. This permits the making of ventrodorsal or, if desired, slightly obliqued views. It is possible to oblique the patient slightly to one side to shift the position of the udder to decrease tissue thickness. This obliquity also permits good visualization of a single hip joint. An oblique view of the opposite hip should then be made for comparison.

A grid is used because of the tissue thickness to be penetrated. Rare-earth screens permit decrease in exposure time. Only a rotating anode tube produces sufficient radiation to make this examination. A focal-film distance of 40 in (100 cm) is recommended.

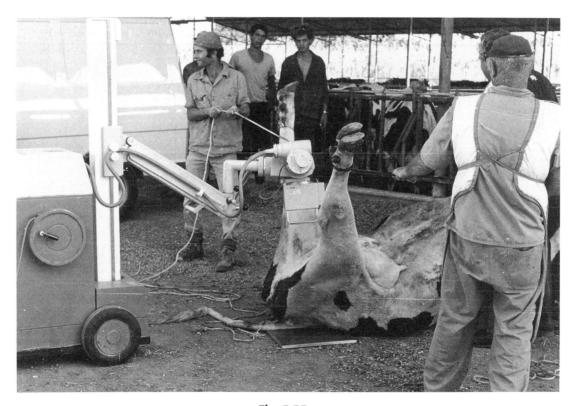

Fig. 3-23
Positioning used for ventrodorsal radiography of the pelvis in a recumbent patient using a mobile condenser-discharge x-ray machine.

HEAD

The head region is so anatomically complex that it is quite difficult to avoid having some structures of interest superimposed upon other structures on any given radiographic view. The many different views which are described indicate the effort which can be made to evaluate certain structures without confusing superimposed shadows.

Radiography of the head is used to evaluate the bones that make up the skull and the mandible, but in the bovine it is most often used to evaluate the teeth and sinuses. The studies are important in the evaluation of a patient that refuses to eat because of pain on chewing. Nasal discharge that is nonresponsive to treatment can be further evaluated by radiography of the head. In such cases, paired or comparative oblique lateral views are frequently the most useful studies, as these views best project the teeth and maxillary sinuses.

ROSTROCAUDAL OR FRONTAL VIEW

Purpose: This study is made primarily to evaluate the character of the frontal sinuses, either for infection or to evaluate radiographic evidence for polled versus non-polled status.

Preparation: No special preparation is required.

Positioning: The bovine stands normally with the head restrained.

Beam location: The cassette is placed flat against the dorsal aspect of the neck with the upper edge of the cassette slightly above the poll. The tube is positioned above the patient's nose and the beam is directed towards the cassette at a slight angle. The beam is centered on midline about halfway between the orbits and the pool (Fig. 3-24).

It is not necessary to use a grid because of the decreased tissue density in the air-filled sinuses. In addition, the thickness of the tissue to be examined is not great. Therefore, it is possible to make this study with a portable unit using slow-speed screens at 24 in (60 cm). Use of a rotating anode and rare-earth screens makes shorter exposure time and use of 40 in (100 cm) focal-film distance possible. Use a 10 by 12 in (24 by 30 cm) cassette.

This study has also been described using a rostrally directed beam directed toward a cassette held against the frontal region of the head. Some restraint device (head-gates) would prevent using this technique easily.

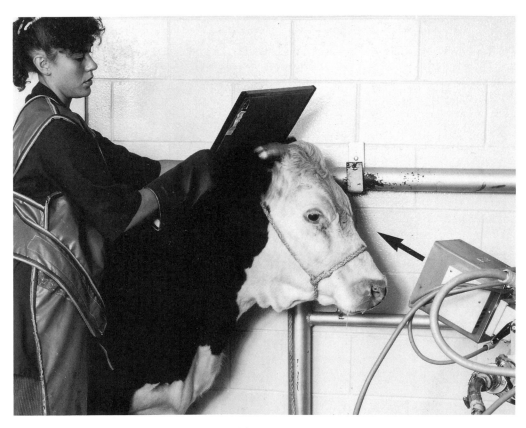

Fig. 3-24
Positioning used for rostrocaudal radiography of the head (frontal sinuses). The tube is positioned above the patient's nose and the beam (arrow) is directed towards the cassette at a slight ventrodorsal direction.

MAXILLARY SINUS AND UPPER TEETH—LATERAL VIEW

Purpose: This study is made primarily to evaluate the character of the upper cheek teeth, the maxillary sinuses, and the maxilla. This view is especially important in the visualization of gas/fluid levels within the sinuses.

Preparation: No special preparation is required.

Positioning: The patient stands normally.

Beam location: This is made in the same fashion as the lateral view of the caudal mandible except the cassette is positioned more cranial and dorsal. The cassette is placed next to the head on the side of the suspected lesion with the cassette parallel to the sagittal plane of the head. The tube is positioned on the opposite side of the head and the central beam is directed at right angles to the center of the cassette. Use a 14 by 17 in (34 by 42 cm) cassette with a grid. Use of rare-earth screens and a 40 in (100 cm) focal-film distance is recommended.

MAXILLARY SINUS AND UPPER TEETH—DORSOVENTRAL (DV) VIEW

Purpose: This study is made primarily to evaluate suspected fractures and the character of the maxillary sinuses. It is of little value for examining the teeth because of superimposition of the upper and lower arcades.

Preparation: No special preparation is required.

Positioning: The bovine stands normally with the head restrained.

Beam centering: Cassette is placed beneath the mandible so that the cassette is in contact with the ventral aspect of both rami. The tube is placed above the rostral part of the head with the beam directed at a right angle to the cassette. The central beam is directed on the dorsal midline of the head. If the beam remains within the midsagittal plane of the head, the angle of the beam with the cassette can vary widely without compromising the study. This view best demonstrates the paranasal sinuses, the rostral portion of the mandibular bodies, and the roots of the incisors. The study is made without a grid. Regular-speed screens in a 14 by 17 in (34 by 42 cm) cassette are adequate. The focal-film distance is 24 in (60 cm) with a portable unit or 40 in (100 cm) with a rotating anode tube.

MAXILLARY SINUS AND UPPER TEETH: DORSOVENTRAL OBLIQUE VIEW

Purpose: This study is made primarily to evaluate the character of the upper cheek teeth, the maxillary sinuses, and the maxilla.

Preparation: No special preparation is required.

Positioning: The patient stands normally.

Beam location: The cassette is placed next to the suspected affected maxillary sinus, so its plane is parallel to that of the head. The tube is positioned on the opposite side of the head and above. The central beam is directed in a dorsal-to-ventral direction so it strikes the cassette at an angle (Fig. 3-25). The beam is centered on the site of the suspected lesion.

This view demonstrates the maxillary sinus and the roots of the premolar and molar teeth on the affected side. Slow-speed screens are adequate. A grid cannot be used because of centering problems due to angulation of the beam. A 14 by 17 in (34 by 42 cm) cassette is recommended, and either 24 in (60 cm) or 40 in (100 cm) focal-film distance can be used.

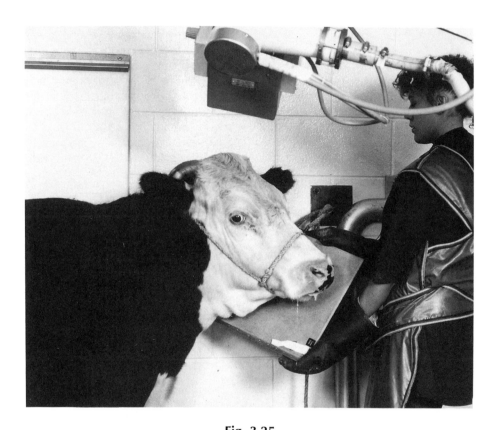

Fig. 3-25
Positioning used for dorsoventral oblique radiography of the maxillary sinus and upper teeth. The central beam is directed in a dorso-to-ventral direction so it strikes the cassette at an angle.

CAUDAL MANDIBLE (pars mandibuli)— LATERAL VIEW

Purpose: This study is made primarily to evaluate the character of the lower cheek teeth and the body of the mandible.

Preparation: No special preparation is required.

Positioning: The patient stands normally.

Beam location: The cassette is placed against the head next to the side affected, with the cassette parallel to the sagittal plane of the head. The tube is positioned on the opposite side of the head and the central beam is directed at right angles to the cassette. Use a 14 by 17 in (34 by 42 cm) cassette with a grid. Use of rare-earth screens and a 40 in (100 cm) focal-film distance is recommended.

ROSTRAL PORTION OF THE MANDIBLE (pars incisiva)—LATERAL VIEW

Purpose: This study is made primarily to evaluate the character of the incisor teeth and the rostal portion of the mandible.

Preparation: No special preparation is required.

Positioning: The patient stands normally.

Beam location: The cassette is placed adjacent to the mandible on the side of the suspected lesion. The tube is directed from the opposite side, centering the beam on the suspected lesion site. The true lateral view is usually limited in demonstration of the lesion because of superimposition of the opposite mandibular ramus. Thus, a slightly obliqued view is often more diagnostic because the rami of the mandible are separated. Use a 10 by 12 in (24 by 30 cm) cassette. Regular-speed screens can be used. The focal-film distance with a portable unit should be 24 in (60 cm) or 40 in (100 cm) with a rotating anode tube. A grid is not necessary because of the minimal tissue thickness and density.

CAUDAL MANDIBLE (pars mandibuli)— VENTRODORSAL OBLIQUE VIEW

Purpose: This study is made primarily to evaluate the character of the lower cheek teeth and the body of the mandible.

Preparation: No special preparation is required.

Positioning: The patient stands normally.

Beam location: The cassette is placed on the lateral aspect of the head and the tube is positioned ventral to the mandible with the central beam angled toward the cassette. The central beam is directed in a ventral to dorsal direction with the beam centered on the intermandibular space. Do not use a grid. Usually the beam is centered on the site of injury, so a 10 by 12 in (24 by 30 cm) cassette is adequate. Rare-earth screens are not needed. Either 24 in (60 cm) or 40 in (100 cm) focal-film distance can be used.

A similar oblique view of the mandible can be made with the cassette placed against the lateral aspect of the head with the x-ray tube positioned above and the beam angled dorsoventrally. Some magnification and blurring results from increased subject-film distance, but this loss of detail is often acceptable and the positioning is often easier.

A comparative oblique view of the opposite mandible is frequently useful, especially to evaluate the teeth.

ROSTRAL PORTION OF THE MANDIBLE (pars incisiva)—VENTRODORSAL VIEW

Purpose: This study is made primarily to evaluate injury to the lower incisors, mandibular symphyseal fractures, or fractures of the rostral portions of the mandible.

Preparation: The study is easier performed on an anesthestized or heavily sedated animal.

Positioning: The cow may be standing or recumbent.

Beam location: This study is made with the cassette positioned in the cow's mouth and must be made with the cow in a recumbent position or sedated. Open the mouth with a nose-lead and push the cassette into the cow's mouth with the cassette front facing downward. An equine mouth speculum can also be used in a sedated cow to create space for the cassette. The tube is directed toward the cassette from the ventral aspect of the head with the beam at a right angle to the cassette. Use a 8 by 10 in (20 by 24 cm) cassette. Slow-speed screens can be used. The focal-film distance can be 24 in (60 cm) or less. A grid is not needed.

SPINE

Radiographic diagnosis of spinal disease in the bovine most often depends on lateral views. Traumatic and infectious lesions are the most common presumptive diagnoses. The studies are always easier made of a recumbent cow. However, in a larger cow, the studies must usually be made with the animal standing using a stanchion and a cassette holder Multiple films are required to study the areas of interest. Even on lateral views, the abdominal viscera may be superimposed over the spine in all but young or thin calves. This is especially true if the animal is radiographed in lateral recumbency. This superimposition of gas- and ingesta-filled bowel may make diagnosis of some lesions difficult or impossible.

Ventrodorsal views can be made of small-to-medium calves; however, they are of limited value except in the cervical region. This is because of the large amount of overlying tissues (mediastinum and sternum in thoracic region, gas and ingesta in lumbar region), and because of the low tissue density of the vertebrae. Only marked changes in alignment or shape are likely to be detectable on ventrodorsal views. Thus, clinically significant changes in bone density and architecture may go undetected.

In small calves up to 3 months of age, spinal radiographs can include the entire spine and be made with portable equipment (Fig. 3-26). In older calves and adults, a rotating anode tube is necessary and the cervical and lumbar regions are most usually radiographed (Fig. 3-27). Rare-earth screens are recommended. When radiographing the cervical region, use of a grid is not required regardless of age of the patient. In the thoracolumbar region, it is necessary to use a grid at all times. The choice of a focal-film distance and use of a stationary or rotating anode depends on the size of the patient. It is recommended that a 14 by 17 in (34 by 42 cm) cassette be used in all patients. In both projections, the beam is centered on the area of interest.

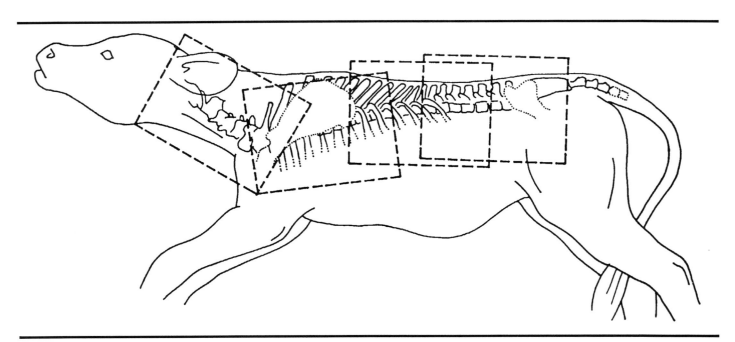

Fig. 3-26
Drawing showing positioning used for lateral radiography of a calf spine. Cassette positions are indicated by broken lines. Notice that the caudal cervical spine and the cranial thoracic spine are considerably ventral to the dorsal body surface.

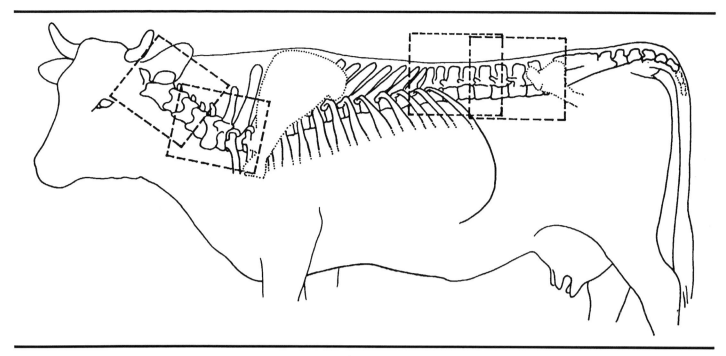

Fig. 3-27
Drawing showing positioning used for lateral radiography of an adult bovine spine. Cassette positions are indicated by broken lines. The cervical spine angles sharply caudoventrally from the poll towards the shoulder. Two large films are necessary to study the entire cervical or the entire lumbar region.

THORAX

The most common radiographic study of the bovine thorax consists of a single lateral view made on a large 14 by 17 in (34 by 42 cm) film with the animal standing. In the calf, this single view usually includes the entire thorax (Fig. 3-28). If a calf is radiographed in lateral recumbency, making both left and right lateral radiographs is sometimes useful to counteract the effect which postural atelectasis has in reducing the visibility of lesions in the dependent or "down" lung. Dorsoventral or ventrodorsal views may also be made with small calves.

In large calves and adult cattle, thoracic studies require use of a rotating anode tube and rare-earth screens to decrease exposure times so that motion can be controlled. A focal-film distance of 100 cm (40 in) should be used along with a grid to decrease scatter radiation. A single radiograph may be used and include only the caudodorsal portion of the thorax. In patients with extensive lung disease, this limited caudodorsal study is often sufficient for diagnosis and prognosis. However, in patients with focal lung disease it is possible to create a "mosaic" of 2 to 3 films with overlapping fields can be very helpful (Fig. 3-29). The areas usually seen with the different views are described:

View #1—dorsocaudal lung field: The field is bounded dorsally by a line parallel to the back of the cow, 10 cm below the dorsal midline. Caudally, the field is bounded by the 12th rib. The central beam is directed to the 10th rib, which is most easily detected by counting from the last rib cranially. This view demonstrates the diaphragmatic lung lobes, the ventral aspect of the thoracic vertebrae, and the dorsal aspect of the diaphragmatic line.

View #2—central lung field: The field is bounded cranially by a point 3 to 5 cm caudal to the shoulder joint. Ventrally, it is bounded by a line about 10 cm proximal to the point of the elbow. The central beam is directed to the 5th rib. This view demonstrates the major vessels in the thorax and the cranial lung lobes.

View #3—ventrocaudal lung field: The field is bounded ventrally by the ventral body wall and cranially by the point of the elbow, which should be included in the field. The central beam is directed to the 6th rib. This view demonstrates the caudal border of the heart, the intermediate lung field caudal to the heart, and the ventral aspect of the line of the diaphragm.

In large patients, image geometry has an effect on the study. Only lesions in the lung nearest the cassette are clearly seen. Lesions in the lung furthest from the cassette are magnified and may be blurred beyond recognition by unfavorable image geometry. One may let clinical findings (auscultation and percussion) determine the site to be radiographed, and place that portion of the lung next to the cassette. Alternatively, one may make both left and right lateral radiographs of similar anatomic regions. The protocol followed most commonly is to make the first lateral thoracic radiograph by placing the cassette on the right side of the cow and the tube on the left side. This serves as a survey study. If a lesion is detected, the second radiograph is made by placing the cassette on the left side of the cow and the tube on the right side. A comparison of the size and appearance of a lesion will permit an estimation of the location of the lesion. This is because of the change in the size of the lesion that occurs as the object-film distance is altered. Since adult cattle are usually radiographed while standing, postural atelectasis is avoided.

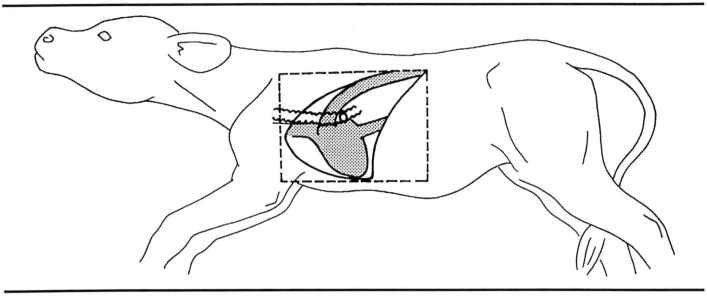

Fig. 3-28
Drawing showing positioning used for lateral radiography of the calf thorax. Cassette position is indicated by broken lines. In small calves radiographed in lateral recumbency with the forelimbs pulled cranially, all thoracic structures can be seen.

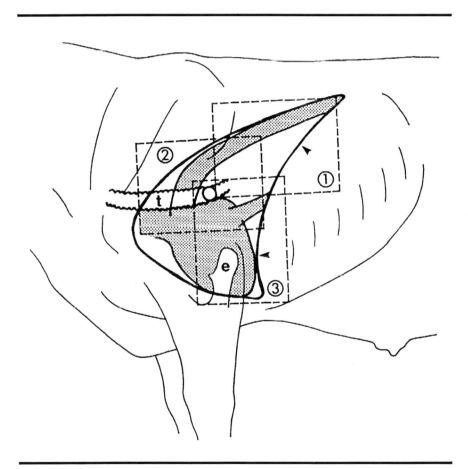

Fig. 3-29
Drawing showing positioning used for lateral radiography of adult bovine thorax. Cassette positions are indicated by broken lines. (t=trachea; e=elbow/olecranon; arrowheads indicate line of diaphragm). View 1 is the most used single view of the dorsocaudal lung field. View 2 is used to evaluate the base of the heart and dorsocranial lung field. View 3 is oriented vertically and demonstrates the caudal border of the heart, the intermediate lung field caudal to the heart, and the ventral aspect of the diaphragm.

429

ABDOMEN

The most common radiographic study of the bovine abdomen consists of a single lateral view on a large 14 by 17 in (34 by 42 cm) film. In an adult cow, the largest standard film includes only a portion of the abdomen. Because disorders in the region of the reticulum are the major adult bovine conditions for which radiography is indicated, the cranioventral portion of the abdomen is radiographed (Fig. 3-30).

Radiography may be done with the animal either standing or in lateral recumbency. With the cow standing, the cassette is placed on the right side of the cow. The field is bounded ventrally by the ventral body wall, and cranially by a line just caudal to the point of the elbow. The central beam is directed towards the 7th rib. This view demonstrates the reticulum and the ventral aspect of the diaphragmatic line.

In a young calf, the entire abdomen can be visualized on one or two large radiographs (Fig. 3-31). Ventrodorsal views may also be made in calves.

Only rotating anode units can be used for abdominal radiography. Use of rare-earth screens is recommended along with the use of a grid. The largest film size available should be selected. Difficulty may be experienced in the centering of the beam on the center of the cassette.

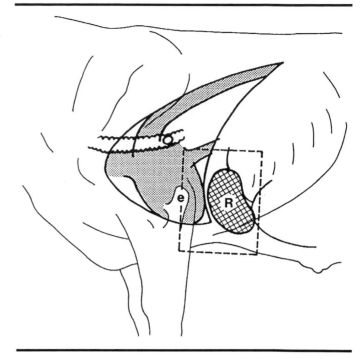

Fig. 3-30
Drawing showing positioning used for lateral radiography of an adult bovine abdomen (reticulum). Cassette position is indicated by broken lines. The reticulum (R) lies caudad to the heart (shaded) and extends ventral to the heart apex. (e=elbow/olecranon)

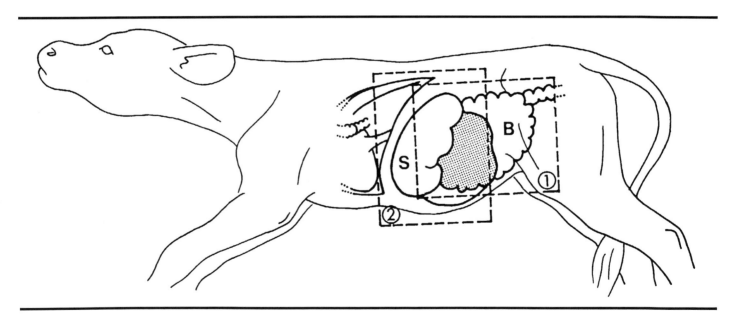

Fig. 3-31
Drawing showing positioning used for lateral radiography of a calf's abdomen. Cassette positions are indicated by broken lines. (S=stomach; B=bowel; shaded region indicates stomach-bowel superimposition). A longitudinally oriented cassette (1) may include all abdominal organs in a small calf. A vertically oriented cassette (2) is more appropriate in a larger calf to include all cranial abdominal organs.

REFERENCES

Bargai U Pharr J and Morgan J P. Bovine Radiology. Iowa State University Press, Ames, Iowa. 1989.

Bargai U. A complete mobile radiology laboratory for large animal field work. Vet Rad 28: 66-71, 1987.

Bargai U. Radiographic diagnosis of 152 cases of chronic, non-responsive lameness in cattle. Refuah Vet 32:137-139, 1975.

Bargai U. The radiological findings of diseased legs in intensive dairy cattle in Israel. Proc 6th World Congress of Buiatrics (Cattle Dise), pp. 214-217, 1974.

Burt J Myers VS Hillman D J and Getty R. The radiographic locations of epiphyseal lines in bovine limbs. J Am Vet Med Ass 152:168, 1968.

Chandra IS Deshpande K Nigram J M and Singh A P. Cerebral contrast ventriculography in bovines. Indian J Vet Surg 2:86-89, 1981.

Chandra IS Nigam J M and Sharma D N. Radiographic visualization of lower bowel by retrograde barium study in buffalo calves. Indian J Vet Surg 3:18-21, 1982.

Chandra IS Singh A P and Nigram J M. Retrograde orbital angiography in Bovines. Indian Vet J 59: 895-897, 1982.

Diesem CD Hockman M and Burt JK. Age determination and structural changes in calves. J Am Vet Med Ass 158:1542, 1971.

Dougherty RW and Meredith C D. Cinefluorographic studies of the ruminant stomach and of eructation. Am J Vet Res 16:96, 1955.

Ducharme NG Dill S G and Rendano V T. Reticulography of a cow in dorsal recumbency; an aid in the diagnosis and treatment of traumatic reticuloperitonitis. J Am Vet Med Assoc 182:585-588, 1983.

Emara M. Some observations on epiphyseal union of long bones in young Egyptian cattle and its importance as an aid in estimation of age. Vet Rec 49:1534-1537, 1937.

Fuentes O and Pedroso M. Pulmonary radiography in healthy and pneumonic calves. Revista de la solud animal 6:5-11, 1984.

Gajraj Singh M M and Kumar R. Contrast radiography in the diagnosis of teat affections. J Am Vet Rad Soc 16:11-12, 1975.

Glossop C A and Ashdown R R. Cavernosography and differential diagnosis of impotence in the bull. Vet Rec 118:357-360, 1986.

Gogoi S N Nigam J M and Singh A P. Angiographic evaluation of bovine foot abnormalities. Vet Radiol 23:171-174, 1982.

Jonson G Jacobson S O Strömberg B and Olsson S-E. Radiological changes in epiphyseal lines and metaphysis of young bulls on intensive feeding. Acta Radiologica Supp. Proc. 2nd Int. Cong. Vet Rad, 1970.

Koper S and Mucha M. Radiographic diagnosis of thoracic organ diseases in cows. Medycyna Weterynaryjna 35:472-477, 1979.

Lee R. Bovine respiratory disease: Its radiological features. J Am Vet Rad Soc 15:41-48, 1974.

Lindsay FEF Boyd J S and Hogg D A. A preliminary radiographic study of the time of appearance of the loci of ossification of the distal sesamoids of the young calf. Res Vet Sci 10:586, 1969.

Lindsay FEF. Observation on the loci of ossification in the prenatal and neonatal bovine 1. The appendicular skeleton. Br Vet J 125:101, 1969.

Lindsay FEF. Observation on the loci of ossification in the prenatal and neonatal bovine skeleton. III The vertebral column. Br Vet J 128:121, 1972.

MacCallum FJ Latshaw W K and Kelly RE. Identification of post-natal ossification sites: A contribution to radiographic interpretation. Br Vet J 127:83, 1970.

Nagel E. Transrectal and vaginal routes for radiography of the hip joint of horses and cattle. Proc. International meeting of orthopedics of hoofed and small cloven animals. Oct 1983. Wien. Hanover 12-16, 1985.

Pasquin C. Atlas of Bovine Anatomy. Sudz Publishing, Eureka, California, 1982.

Shively J J and Smallwood J F. Normal radiographic and xerographic anatomy of the bovine manus. Bov. Prac. 14:74-82, 1979.

Singh A P Singh J T Williamson H D Peshin P K and Nigam J M. Radiographic visualization of the ruminant upper urinary tract by a double contrast technique. Vet Radiol 24:106-111, 1983.

Singh AP Peshin P K Chawla S K Chanda I S and Singh J. Contrast radiography of alimentary tract in calves. Indian J Anim. Sci 55:854-859, 1985.

Smallwood J E and Shively M J. Radiographic and xerographic anatomy of the bovine tarsus. Bov Prac 2:28-45, 1981.

Stowater J L Francis J J and Pickard J R. Dental radiography in cattle. Technique and application for age determination. J Am Vet Rad Soc 19:213-217, 1978.

van Weeren P R Klein W R and Voorhout G. Urolithiasis in small ruminants. II.Cystourothrography as a new aid in diagnosis. Vet Q 9:76-83, 1987.

Verschooten F and Oyaert W. Radiographic diagnosis of esophageal disorders in the bovine. J Am Vet Rad Soc 23:85-89, 1977.

Verschooten F Oyaert W and Drubbel R. Radiographic diagnosis of lung disease in cattle. J Am Vet Rad Soc 15:49-59, 1974.

Weaver A S Anderson L De Laistre Banting A Demerzis P N Knezevic P E Petersen D J and Sankovic R. Review of disorders of the ruminal digit with proposals for anatomical and pathological terminology and recording. Vet Rec 108:117-120, 1981.

Webbon P M and Ramsey L J. Survey of x-ray machines in veterinary practice. Vet Rec 112, 224-227, 1983.

Witzig P and Hugelshofer J. Diagnosis of teat stenosis in the cow by means of double-contrast radiography. Schwezer archiv für tierhenkunde 109:507-515, 1984.

SECTION G

AVIAN RADIOGRAPHY

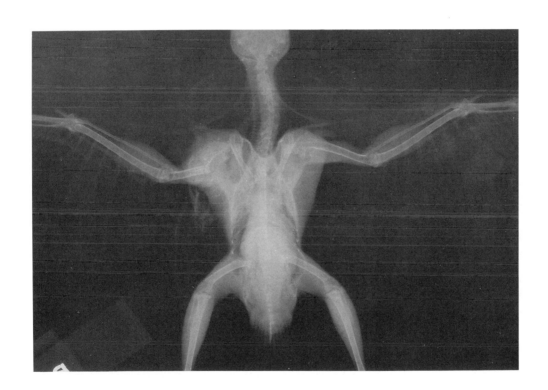

1. INTRODUCTION

Radiography is a frequently used routine diagnostic procedure performed on avian patients and plays an important role in diagnosis of avian disease, partially because the large air sacs provide such good contrast between the body organs. The size and character of the birds make radiography different than it is performed on mammals and certainly makes it a challenging study. It is the purpose of this section to provide basic information to encourage many to consider greater use of this diagnostic technique.

Many anatomical features of the bird are different from those of mammals and many clinicians have not had extensive training in the anatomy of the avian species. Many features not present in mammals are of great importance in radiology of birds. The multiple paired and unpaired air sacs are perhaps the best example of this difference. They are easily visualized by their absence of tissue density and consequently provide negative contrast for the abdominal and thoracic organs. The smaller, dorsally located lungs are much more difficult to evaluate in the bird. They appear as a honeycombed structure and have much less importance in radiographic diagnosis when compared with mammalian lungs.

Even the skeletal system in birds has a different appearance. The prominent thoracic girdle is composed of the scapula, caracoid and clavicular bones (furcula). The presence of the notarium, synsacrum, and pygostyle make examination of the vertebral column a challenge while the sacrum is a disproportionately large structure with minimal tissue density. Pneumatized bones along with the estrogenic and androgenic driven deposition of medullary bony tissue prior to egg-laying are other examples of obvious differences in the bird.

The kidneys, adrenal glands, and gonads are crowded into the dorsal portion of the mid and caudal abdomen and are often difficult to separate on the radiograph. The kidneys are tightly embedded in depressions on the ventral surface of the synsacrum and in the renal fossa of each ilium and are practically invisible radiographically without the use of special procedures. Avian urography can be performed following intravenous injection of iodinated contrast agents and subsequent radiography. The digestive system is rather well seen radiographically with the long esophagus leading to the ingluvies (crop) at the thoracic inlet. The proventriculus is a tubular shaped organ while the ventriculus (gizzard) is round or oblong and usually identified by the radiodense grit it contains. The intestines are composed of the tubular duodenum, jejunum, ileum, ceca, and rectum that are difficult to separate on the survey radiograph. This system is rather easily examined by positive-contrast radiography.

The heart and liver fill the cranioventral portion of the body cavity and often blend into one single shadow on the radiograph. Just caudal and slightly dorsal to the liver shadow is the rounded splenic shadow that is clearly identified on most studies.

Variations between the species are marked and just when you learn that the ovary and oviduct are usually unpaired and on the left side, you read that paired ovaries and oviducts may be found in some birds of prey. Large paired ceca are well-developed in the duck, goose, turkey, and chicken and occupy space caudally, but are vestigial in the canary and pigeon, and absent in the budgerigar. Typically there are three toes pointing forward and one toe pointing backwards as an adaptation for perching in many species, however, the parrot and budgerigar have two toes pointing forward and two toes pointing backward as an adaption for climbing and grasping.

2. RADIOGRAPHIC EQUIPMENT

A machine with a maximum capacity of 100 mA and 80 kVp is adequate for avian radiography. Exposure times must be brief in avian radiography to avoid motion. A small focal spot provides better detail when radiographing smaller birds, and if you have a focal spot of 0.3 mm, it is possible to increase the object-film distance in an effort to obtain a magnification study. This is discussed in greater detail later. While a higher kVp may be needed for the larger birds such as the raptors, many of the smaller birds are examined using rather low range kVp settings. For this reason removal of the filter from the tubehead decreases exposure time markedly since removal prevents the absorption of the lower-energy photons that are needed to produce the radiograph. In many units it is not possible to remove the added filtration. Regulations may require that no person be in the examination room if the filter is not in place during use of the machine. Use of a high-detail film-screen system is helpful in avian radiography and the best radiographic detail can be achieved if a non-screen film system is used. It is possible to use a closely collimated beam for all studies of birds.

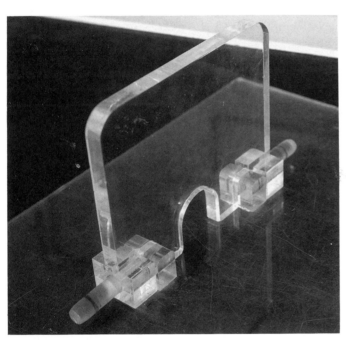

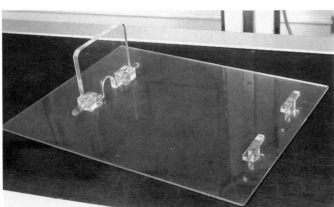

Figs. 3-1

3. RESTRAINT

Restraint of the birds is important and the readers are referred to the many articles written on this subject. The selection of the anesthetic agent is based on the age and general condition of the bird and the restraint required for the study. The use of atropine can be considered. Ketamine hydrochloride (Vetalar, Parke Davis) is often used intramuscularly. Many clinics may make the decision that sedation is not sufficient for avian radiography and that an inhalation anesthesia is necessary. Anesthesia prevents further stressing of the patient, struggling that results is fractures, and having assistants bitten during positioning. Many of the avian patients have a high monetary value that makes the use of inhalation anesthesia desirable. Isofluorane can be used for this purpose.

The patient can be restrained on a plastic sheet or positioning board using masking tape since it is more radiolucent than other types of tape, is less traumatic to skin and feathers, and can be removed rather easily. The use of velcro strips is generally unsatisfactory because the bird can pull the wings free. Use care in the use of a single strip of tape on wings of large birds since it is possible for them to rotate the body in an effort to become free and fracture the mid-shaft of the humerus. To avoid this, place a second tape over the mid-part of the wing. Often the restraint board uses a block device to hold the head and neck making this part of the body difficult to evaluate (Fig. 3-1 and Fig. 3-2).

Many of the wild birds are found in a depressed state because of not eating. These patients can be positioned rather easily without sedation and seem to not become stressed by this. It is rare that these birds struggle during the radiographic procedure and it can be performed safely. Other birds, especially the raptors, can be positioned with the use of a hood as the only form of restraint along with the positioning board.

The technique chart developed for use with birds should be made with the plastic sheet or positioning plate in position. A portion of the chart can be made with removal of the filter from the tubehead, if this is possible. Recognize the loss of body heat with any form of sedation or anesthesia and use heating pads and/or heated recovery cages following the radiographic study.

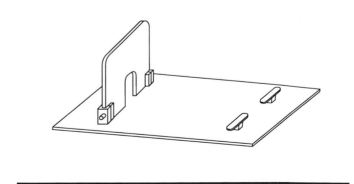

Fig. 3-2

4. RADIOGRAPHIC VIEWS

LATERAL VIEW WHOLE BODY

This view provides a lateral projection of the body as well as lateral projection of the wings, legs, cervical region, and head. It is obtained by placing the patient in lateral recumbency and extending the wings dorsally and the legs ventrally. The neck is fastened to the plastic plate with masking tape or the block device. Both wings and legs are separated slightly so they are not superimposed. The dependent wing and leg is positioned cranially for identification. Avoid excessive traction on the upper leg since this produces rotation of the patient's body. Tape is placed over both wing tips, both wings, the neck, and both feet (Fig. 4-1).

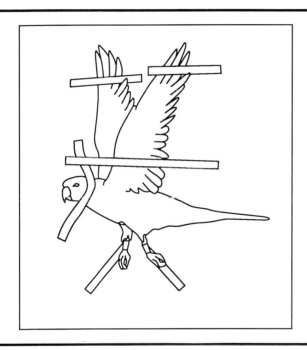

Fig. 4-1

VENTRODORSAL VIEW OF THE WHOLE BODY

This view provides a ventrodorsal projection of the body as well as a craniocaudal view of the legs. The wings are seen in a lateral view and the cervical region and head are usually obliqued. The view is obtained by placing the patient in dorsal recumbency with both wings fully and equally extended. Position the body so that the sternum and spine are superimposed. The legs are pulled caudally, however, it may not be possible to fully extend the legs because of the strength of the bird. The positioning board may have tie-down cleats to assist in positioning the legs. Two strips of masking tape are placed over each wing using the outermost primary feathers. One strip of tape is placed over the neck, and a strip is placed over each foot. Additional tape can be placed over the tip of the tail in a large bird (Fig. 4-2).

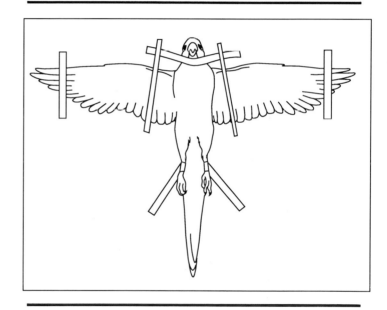

Fig. 4-2

CAUDOCRANIAL VIEW OF THE WING

This view provides the only method of obtaining the opposite projection of the wing since both views of the whole body show the wings in lateral projection. Unfortunately, this view requires that the bird be held by hand to obtain correct positioning.

The bird is positioned upside down with the long axis of the body parallel to the vertically directed x-ray beam. The wing to be studied is extended fully with the cranial or leading edge in contact with the cassette (Fig. 4-3).

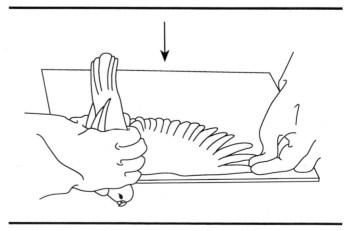

Fig. 4-3

5. RADIOGRAPHIC TECHNIQUE

Since most members of a given species are of similar size, it is convenient to separate the technique chart by species rather than requiring measurement of the bird. The species are conveniently placed into three groups: (1) small, (2) medium-sized, and (3) large birds. Since the studies are whole body studies, the entire bird can be evaluated on each film. It is possible to decrease the radiographic technique by 5 kVp when noting extreme emaciation of the patient.

All of the exposures are estimated using a focal-film distance of 40 inches (100 cm), a filter in place, and a 50 speed screen-film system (such as the Quanta extremity system) (Table 5-1).

6. MAGNIFICATION RADIOGRAPHY

Magnification techniques can be used if you have an x-ray tube with a small focal-spot of 0.3mm in size or smaller. Lower the x-ray tube so that the distance to the tabletop is 30 inches (75cm). Place the patient on the table using a plastic sheet or positioning board. Using some form of wooden or cardboard box, position the film 10 inches (25cm) below the tabletop. This provides a magnification of 130%. It is possible to use a focal-object distance and object-film distance of 20 inches (50cm) to obtain greater magnification. Use the same radiographic technique as with the conventional tabletop technique. Magnification can be used with either high-detail screen film system or non-screen film.

Magnification radiography is of greatest value in radiography of the head and in some skeletal studies.

Table 5-1
EXPOSURE CHART

Species	kVp	mA	Exposure time
Small sized species			
Parakeet	50 - 54	100	1/20 - 1/15 sec
Finches			
Medium sized species			
Canary			
Cockatiel			
Quail	54 - 58	100	1/20 - 1/15 sec
Kestrals			
Yellow-napped parrot			
African gray parrot			
Large sized species			
Raptors			
Macaws	58-64	100	1/20-1/15 sec
Larger parrots			
Chickens			
Caudocranial view of wing			
All species	50-54	100	1/20-1/15 sec

7. AVIAN GASTROINTESTINAL RADIOGRAPHY

Definition

A positive contrast medium can be used to assist in the evaluation of the gastrointestinal tract of birds. Gastrointestinal signs in birds may be due to infectious diseases, parasites, toxins, and metabolic disturbances associated with kidney and liver diseases. Therefore, a complete medical history, thorough physical examination, non-contrast radiographs, and laboratory data are indicated prior to considering contrast radiography of the gastrointestinal tract.

Indications

1. acute, chronic, or nonresponsive regurgitation
2. vomition
3. diarrhea
4. palpation of an abnormal crop or abdomen
5. hemorrhagic diarrhea
6. distention of the gastrointestinal tract with gas and fluid as seen on non-contrast radiographs (usually due to infection or toxicity)
7. organ displacement seen on non-contrast radiographs

Contraindications

1. regurgitation that is only associated with sexual display or affection toward an owner
2. polyurea that is the cause of loose droppings
3. tranquilizers and anesthetics since the effects on gastrointestinal motility in birds is not well known
4. study should not be performed if bird will be severely stressed

Equipment

1. a type of plexiglas immobilization board
2. mouth speculum
3. barium sulfate suspension diluted to 10-20% w/w
4. catheter—infant feeding tubes or soft rubber urethral catheters are superior to rigid metal catheters—size selected so that it passes easily into the cervical esophagus
5. syringe of appropriate size

Technique

1. make non-contrast radiographic studies
2. withhold food and water for about 4 hours if the crop is to be evaluated
3. proceed if only small amount of seeds remain in the crop or proventriculus
4. warm barium sulfate suspension to 80° F.
5. use of a speculum is determined by the size of the bird—a padded hemostat can be used with cockatiels, conures, or lovebirds while a nasal speculum is used on parrots
6. pass catheter to crop or mid-esophageal region
7. palpate to verify catheter location to avoid introducing catheter into trachea
8. slowly inject the warmed barium sulfate suspension using a volume that fills the crop (the volume varies with size of the bird and is generally based on a dosage of 25ml/kgbw)

canary, finch—	0.25-0.5 ml
parakeet—	1.0-3.0 ml
cockatiel, conure, lovebird—	3.0-5.0 ml
smaller parrots—	10 ml
larger parrots—	15 ml

9. administer the barium sulfate suspension into the crop unless bird is without a crop, in which patients the suspension is injected into the esophagus or proventriculus
10. place gentle digital pressure on the midcervical region over the esophagus and remove the catheter to prevent regurgitation
11. make ventrodorsal and lateral radiographs at 0 time, 30 minutes, 60 minutes, 2 hours (usually the contrast meal is within the cloaca within 2 hours)
12. make additional studies at 4 hours, and 24 hours following administration of contrast medium if the passage of the contrast meal is delayed

Comments

1. estimate movement of the contrast meal—the proventriculus, ventriculus, and proximal portion of the small intestine should be filled with the barium meal within 15 to 30 minutes in the normal patient
2. estimate transit time to cloaca—the barium meal should be in the cloaca in 60 to 120 minutes in the normal patient
3. estimate emptying time of the crop—the barium meal should have emptied from the crop within 4 hours in the normal patient

8. AVIAN UROGRAPHY

Definition
Usage of an intravenous contrast medium for the evaluation of the urinary tract of birds is particularly of value in patients in which there is a homogeneous soft tissue mass obscuring the normally discernible outlines of the liver and intestines. A complete medical history, thorough physical examination, non-contrast radiographs, and laboratory data are indicated prior to contrast radiography of the urinary tract.

Indications
1. abdominal distention
2. unilateral or bilateral paresis of the toes and legs
3. droppings that are less frequent but voluminous or extremely watery
4. palpation of an abnormal mass

Contraindications
1. if use of anesthesia or sedation is not appropriate
2. study should not be performed if the bird will be severely stressed by the procedure

Equipment
1. a type of plexiglas immobilization board
2. needle and syringe
3. water-soluble iodinated contrast agent used for urography

Technique
1. use chemical restraint (IM ketamine hydrochloride)
2. make a non-contrast radiographic study
3. inject contrast agent into the brachial vein undiluted at a dosage of 1.5 mg of I/gram of body weight
4. make ventrodorsal views at 10 seconds, 60 seconds, and 2 minutes following completion of the injection
5. additional views at 5 to 7 minutes show the contrast medium either expelled from the cloaca or filling the rectum

Comments
1. findings on the non-contrast studies may suggest that lateral views are more valuable

REFERENCES

Altman RB. Avian anesthesia. Comp Cont Ed 2:38-43, 1980.

Evans SM. Avian radiographic diagnosis. Comp Cont Ed 3:660-6, 1981.

Kollias GV. Avian anesthesia—Principles, practice and problems. AAHA 49th Annual Meeting Proceedings. 1982, pp13-14.

Lafebre TJ. Radiography in the caged bird clinic. Am An Hosp Assoc 4:41-8, 1968.

McMillan MC. Avian gastrointestinal radiography. Comp Cont Ed 5:273-8, 1983.

McMillian MC. Avian gastrointestinal radiography. Comp Cont Ed 4:173-8, 1982.

McMillian MC. Avian radiology, in Petrak ML (ed): Diseases of Cage and Aviary Birds, 2nd ed. Lea & Febiger, Philadelphia. 1982, pp 329-360.

McNeel SV and Zenoble RD. Avian urography. J Am Vet Med Assoc 178:366-8, 1981.

Paul-Murphy JR Koblik PD Stein G and Penninck DG. Psittacine skull radiography. Vet Rad 31:218-224, 1990.

Rübel GA Isenbügel E and Wolvekamp P. Atlas of Diagnostic Radiology of Exotic Pets. WB Saunders Co., Philadelphia. 1991.

Silverman S. Avian radiographic technique and interpretation, in Kirk RW (ed): Current Veterinary Therapy VII. WB Saunders Co., Philadelphia. 1980, pp 649-52.

Smith SA and Smith BJ. Atlas of avian radiographic anatomy. WB Saunders Co., Philadelphia. 1992.

SECTION H

EXOTIC SPECIES RADIOGRAPHY

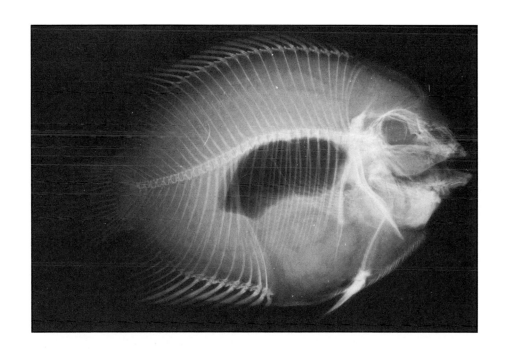

1. SMALL MAMMALS

Many owners with pets acquire an attachment to these animals that leads to their being radiographed in connection with diagnosis and treatment of disease. A great amount of information can be gained from whole body studies even though you may not be familiar with normal radiographic anatomy.

Several methods of mechanical restraint are used to immobilize small mammals for radiographic studies. Mechanical methods are often used without sedation or anesthesia, and are highly successful in patients who are accustomed to be handled. Tape, gauze, or padded forceps may be used to hold limbs in position for the lateral view or used to extend the limbs on the dorsoventral or ventrodorsal views. However, some form of chemical restraint is recommended in conjunction with mechanical restraint to achieve radiography most easily. Ketamine hydrochloride given intramuscularly is the most commonly used method of restraint. Dosages range from 10 mg/kgbw to 80 mg/kgbw dependent on the species. The ketamine may be combined with xylazine in some species.

Tabletop technique is used most commonly because of the small size of the patients. While non-screen film technique can be used, it is also possible to use high-detail film-screen systems. If the kVp to be used is below 60 kVp, the filter may be removed from the tubehead if this is possible. The same technique can usually be used for both views in the whole body study. Because of the small size of the patients, whole body studies are usually made that include the extremities as well. Descriptions of positioning in the sections on radiography of the dog and cat can be directly used in radiography of some small mammals.

Respiratory rates are rapid in this group of animals, especially when stressed, therefore, use the shortest exposure time possible. Hopefully, this is 1/60 second or shorter.

WHOLE BODY—LATERAL VIEW

Patient positioning: Place the patient in right lateral recumbency with the limbs extended and held by gloved hands, sandbags, rope, tape, or gauze. Tape is used most often. Avoid over-extension of the limbs cranially and caudally since this frequently causes obliquity of the body. Extend the forelimbs so the elbows are cranial to the thoracic cavity. Tape over the neck helps in positioning the head (Fig. 1-1).

Beam center: Using a vertically directed beam, center on the midportion of the body.

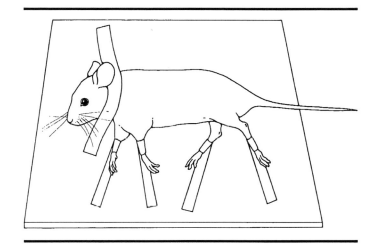

Fig. 1-1

WHOLE BODY—VENTRODORSAL VIEW

Patient positioning: Place the patient in dorsal recumbency with the limbs held by a gloved hand, sandbags, rope, tape, or gauze. Extend the limbs as far as is possible. Position the forelimbs so the elbows are cranial to the thoracic cavity. Strips of tape can be placed across the body. The head and neck are extended so they are not superimposed over the cranial portion of the thorax. Tape can be used to hold the head in position (Fig. 1-2).

Beam center: Using a vertically directed beam, center on the midportion of the body.

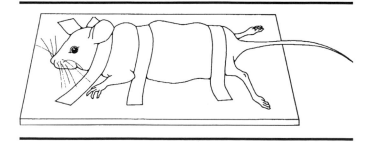

Fig. 1-2

WHOLE BODY—DORSOVENTRAL VIEW

A dorsoventral view can be made only if the patient is large enough to hold with gloved hands.

Patient positioning: Place the patient in ventral recumbency with the limbs held by a gloved hand or by rope. Extend the limbs as far as is possible. Position the forelimbs so the elbows are cranial to the thoracic cavity. The head may need to be flexed to avoid positioning it over the cranial portion of the thorax. It is possible to use a strip of tape to hold the head against the cassette.

Beam center: Using a vertically directed beam, center on the midportion of the body.

EXTREMITIES

Views of the extremities are made using the same positioning as for the whole body studies. With the animal in lateral position, the affected limb is pulled as far as possible using tape fastened around the foot, and lateral views are made. Separate the arms or legs so they are not superimposed on the lateral views. With the patient in ventrodorsal position, the affected limb is extended as far as possible using tape fastened around the foot, and craniocaudal or caudocranial views are made.

Table 1-1
RADIOGRAPHIC TECHNIQUE
(40 inches FFD tabletop technique using a 50 speed film-screen system without a grid)

species	kVp	mA	exposure time	mAs
mouse	48	200	1/60	3.3
rat	48	200	1/60	3.3
hamster	48	200	1/60	3.3
ferret	50	400	1/60	6.6
guinea pig	50	400	1/60	6.6
chinchilla	50	400	1/60	6.6
rabbit	56	400	1/60	6.6

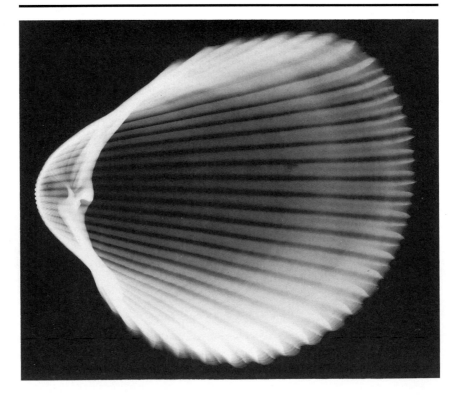

2. NONHUMAN PRIMATES

Almost all nonhuman primates are sedated or anesthetized for radiographic examinations. This reduces the probability of injury to the assistant and facilitates the use of mechanical restraint devices. The use of an especially constructed restraint board eliminates the possibility of accidental x-ray exposure to the assistants. The restraint device also serves as a positioning device and standardizes positioning techniques. The restraint boards are most easily used in patients who have been preconditioned to their use.

Two views are used to complete the radiographic study of either the thorax or the abdomen. Thoracic studies of the sedated or anesthetized patient can be made without the use of a restraint board, however, positioning is more difficult. While the thoracic studies are best made with the patient erect, the abdominal and pelvic studies are usually made with the patient recumbent. Studies of the head require the use of a special head restraint device. Studies of the arms and legs can be made with the patient recumbent on the table using the restraint techniques used for the abdomen. Separate the arms or legs so they are not superimposed on the lateral views. Ropes can be used to extend the limbs for craniocaudal views.

The thoracic conformation varies greatly between species and must be considered when calculating exposure factors. Even two species with identical external thoracic measurements may require different exposures due to the different ratios of the thoracic wall thickness to the thoracic cavity volume. The upper abdomen (substernal) region is much thicker than is the lower abdominal (prepelvic) region in both lateral and ventrodorsal measurements. The exposure factors should be adjusted to allow visualization of the region of greatest interest. A technique chart is necessary for radiography of nonhuman primates to accommodate the variety of ages, sizes, and shapes of the patients to be examined.

Use of focused grids is recommended for patients over 15 cm thick. It may be possible to use a greater focal-film distance for erect thoracic studies such as 80 inches (200 cm) in association with use of an air-gap technique to control the effect of scatter radiation.

Because of patient stress, respiratory rates are rapid and the exposure times should be 1/60 second or faster and the exposure should coincide with maximum inspiration.

There is no preparation required for the thoracic studies, however, it is helpful to fast the patient, if possible, for 12 hours prior to the abdominal studies. The relatively large cecum is difficult to empty and fills the right side of the abdominal cavity on the radiograph in many species.

THORAX STUDY—ERECT LATERAL VIEW

Positioning: The sedated patient is placed next to the plastic restraint and positioning device in the erect position with the left side next to the film holder. The patient's hands are tied above its head and secured to the restraint device. The elbows are pulled behind the head and tied close together with cotton gauze. Gentle traction is placed on the cords tied around the patient's ankles to minimize spinal curvature. These cords are then secured to the lower end of the restraint device. It is sometimes necessary to place radiolucent sponges between the restraint board and the sternum and midlumbar areas to prevent patient rotation. A radiolucent wedge can be placed under the chin to extend the head and neck to prevent them from being superimposed on the upper thorax (Fig. 2-1).

Beam center: Center the horizontally directed x-ray beam between the spine and sternum at the level of the 5th rib.

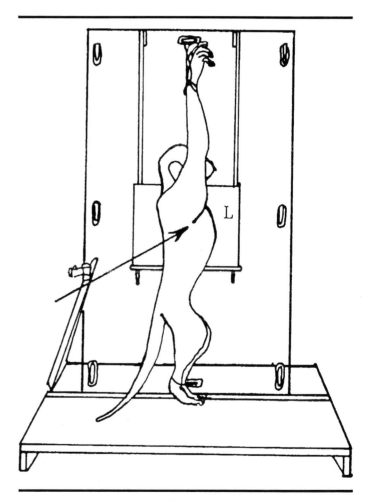

Fig. 2-1

THORAX STUDY—
ERECT VENTRODORSAL VIEW

Positioning: The sedated patient is placed next to the plastic restraint and positioning device in the erect position facing the horizontally directed x-ray beam. The patient's hands are secured above its head and secured to the restraint device. Gentle traction is placed on the cords tied around the patient's ankles and the legs are fastened to the bottom of the restraint device in a comfortably extended position. It is necessary to place radiolucent sponges or a roll of radiolucent material under the chin to prevent the head from falling forward and being superimposed on the upper thorax (Fig. 2-2).

Beam center: Center the horizontally directed x-ray beam between the spine and sternum at the level of the 5th rib.

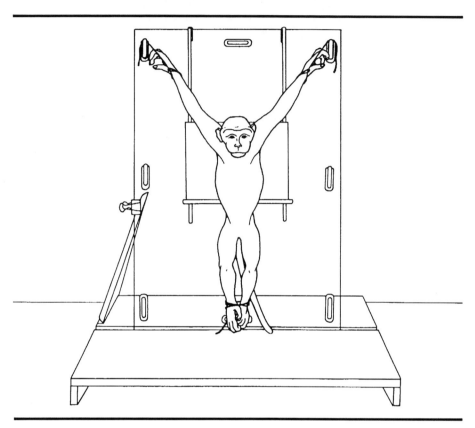

Fig. 2-2

ABDOMINAL STUDY—
RECUMBENT LATERAL VIEW

Positioning: The sedated patient is placed in left lateral recumbency. The patient's hands are tied above its head and secured by ropes or sandbags. Position the elbows behind the head. Gentle traction is placed on the patient's ankles to minimize spinal curvature. The legs are then secured to the table by ropes or immobilized using sandbags. It is sometimes necessary to place radiolucent sponges between the table and the sternum and midlumbar areas to prevent patient rotation (Fig. 2-3).

Beam center: Center the x-ray beam on the mid-abominal region.

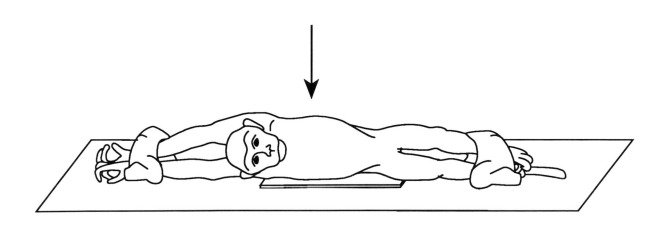

Fig. 2-3

ABDOMINAL STUDY—
RECUMBENT VENTRODORSAL VIEW

Positioning: The sedated patient is placed on the table in dorsal recumbency. The patient's hands are secured above its head and secured to the tabletop or held with sandbags. Gentle traction is placed on the cords tied around the patient's ankles and the legs are fastened to the table or held by sandbags (Fig. 2-4).

Beam center: Center the x-ray beam on the mid-abdominal region.

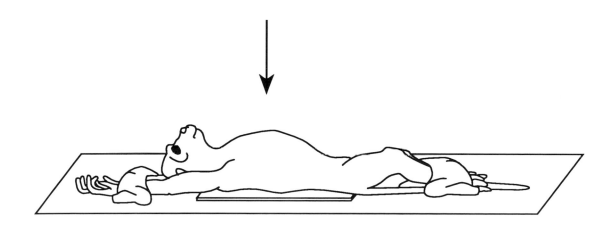

Fig. 2-4

3. REPTILES AND AMPHIBIANS

TURTLES AND TORTOISES

In the United States the following distinction is made between the terms turtle and tortoise. A tortoise is a land dwelling turtle with a high domed shell and columnar elephant-shaped hindlimbs. They go to water only to drink or to bathe. There are three species of tortoises in the United States; the desert tortoise, the Texas tortoise, and the gopher or Florida tortoise. In contrast, the word "turtle" is used for other turtles who spend much time in water, such as: pond turtles, river turtles, box turtles, musk turtles, and sea turtles.

Since most turtles and tortoises are rather lethargic, they are rather easily positioned for radiographic studies. Smaller patients can be placed within paper or cardboard boxes. These restraint boxes can be fastened to the face of the cassette. Larger patients can be taped to the cassette face or tabletop. This group of animals presents some unique problems to the radiographer because of the presence of the shell which surrounds the thoracic and abdominal regions. The presence of the shell makes it difficult to radiograph the appendicular skeleton because the limbs are retracted into the shell so easily. However, the patient often extends its head and limbs from its shell if taped to the cassette and otherwise left undisturbed. It is usually beneficial to gradually lower the environmental temperature in the patient's enclosure to decrease the patient's activity without severely altering its metabolic rate.

Many of the problems caused by the presence of the shell can be circumvented by the judicious use of horizontal beam techniques. The patient can be taped to a sponge block and held for a lateral and craniocaudal view. If it is not possible to position the tube to perform a cross-table study, the sponge block with the animal taped to the top can be positioned on its side to make a lateral view of the animal with a vertically directed x-ray beam. The block is then placed on end so the craniocaudal view can be made with a vertically directed x-ray beam. Appreciate that the views made with the vertical beam require that the animal be positioned "on edge" or "on end" which permits free fluid to shift in position or permits body organs to move. It is important to understand that views made with the vertical beam are not as valuable as those made with the horizontal beam.

You should attempt to make a minimum of three views of each patient: (1) a dorsoventral view made with a vertical beam, (2) a lateral view made with a vertical or horizontal beam, and (3) a craniocaudal view made with a vertical or horizontal beam.

Use non-screen technique for the smaller patients and a high-detail screen system for the larger ones. A grid is not needed except for the much larger species.

It is possible to do positive-contrast studies of the gastrointestinal tract of turtles or tortoises using barium sulfate suspension, however, the transit time is long and makes evaluation of the study difficult. It can be best used to locate the parts of the gastrointestinal system.

WHOLE BODY STUDY— LATERAL VIEW USING HORIZONTAL BEAM

Positioning: Place the patient on the cassette and immobilize it using masking tape or confine it in a paper box to restrict movement. Position the patient so the lateral edge of the shell is placed in contact with the cassette. Make the exposure when the extremities are extended from the shell (Fig. 3-1).

Beam center: Using a horizontally directed beam, center on the midportion of the body.

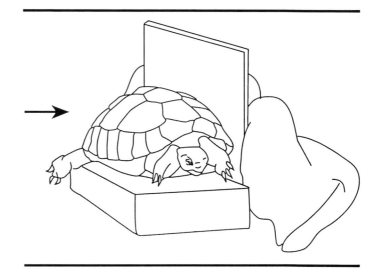

Fig. 3-1

WHOLE BODY STUDY—
LATERAL VIEW USING VERTICAL BEAM

Positioning: Immobilize the patient by taping it to the top of a sponge block and placing the sponge on edge. The lateral edge of the shell rests on the face of the cassette. Make the exposure when the extremities are extended from the shell (Fig. 3-2).

Beam center: Using a vertically directed beam, center on the midportion of the body.

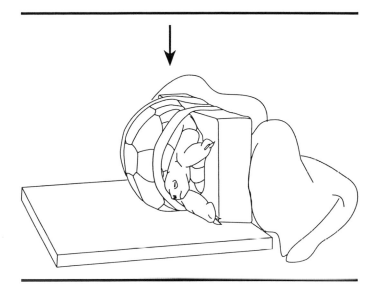

Fig. 3-2

WHOLE BODY STUDY—
CRANIOCAUDAL VIEW USING
HORIZONTAL BEAM

Positioning: Immobilize the patient using masking tape or confine it in a paper box to restrict movement. The cassette is directly behind the patient and the tube is re-positioned to be in front of the animal with the x-ray beam directed through the long axis in a craniocaudal direction. Make the exposure when the extremities are extended from the shell (Fig. 3-3).

Beam center: Using a horizontally directed beam, center on the head.

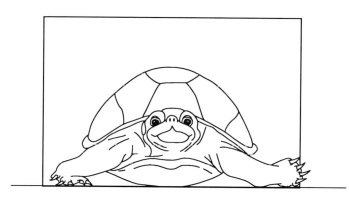

Fig. 3-3

Table 3-1
TECHNIQUE CHART FOR TURTLES
(40 inches FFD tabletop technique using a 50 speed film-screen system without a grid)

size	beam direction	kVp	mA	exposure time	mAs
5 cm thick	lateral view	58	400	1/60	6.6
	dorsoventral view	62	400	1/60	6.6
	craniocaudal view	60	400	1/60	6.6
10 cm thick	lateral view	58	400	1/40	10
	dorsoventral view	62	400	1/40	10
	craniocaudal view	60	400	1/40	10
15 cm thick	lateral view	64	400	1/20	20
	dorsoventral view	62	400	1/20	20
	craniocaudal view	66	400	1/20	20

(the techniques are the same for both vertically directed or horizontally directed beam)

WHOLE BODY STUDY—CRANIOCAUDAL VIEW USING VERTICAL BEAM

Positioning: Immobilize the patient by taping it to the top of a sponge block and placing the sponge on end. The patient is "standing" on the cassette and the tube is above with the x-ray beam directed vertically through the long axis of the patient in a craniocaudal direction. Make the exposure when the extremities are extended from the shell (Fig. 3-4).

Beam center: Using a vertically directed beam, center on the head.

WHOLE BODY STUDY—DORSOVENTRAL VIEW USING VERTICAL BEAM

Positioning: Immobilize the patient on the cassette using masking tape or confine it in a paper box to restrict movement. Make the exposure when the extremities are extended from the shell (Fig. 3-5, 3-6).

Beam center: Using a vertically directed beam, center on the midportion of the body

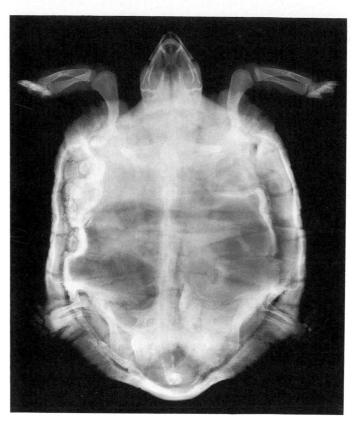

Fig. 3-5

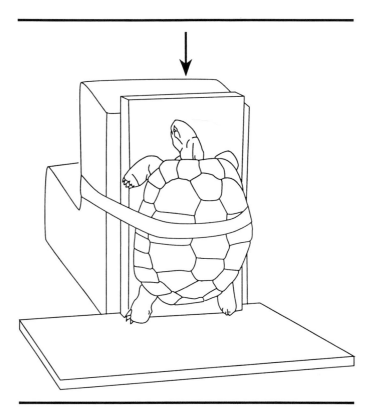

Fig. 3-4

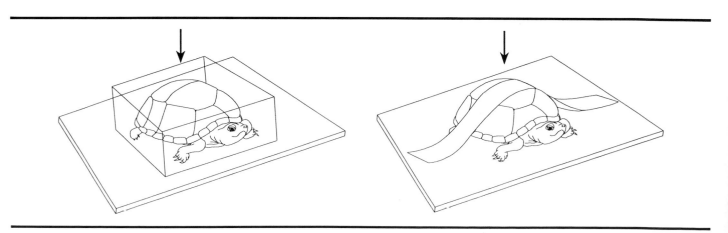

Fig. 3-6

LIZARDS

The patients are usually rather easy to position especially if they are lethargic because of a carefully lowered environmental temperature. Masking tape can be used to position the more active patient. It can be placed over the neck, caudal to the forelimbs, and over the pelvis. Contrast studies of the gastrointestinal tract can be performed (Fig. 3-7).

WHOLE BODY STUDY— DORSOVENTRAL VIEW—VERTICAL BEAM

Positioning: Place the patient directly on the cassette in sternal recumbency. Minimal scoliosis of the spine does not cause a problem in diagnosis. If the patient is active, masking tape can be used for restraint with tape over the neck, thorax, and pelvis. The tail of the larger lizards can be taped in position (Fig. 3-8).

Beam center: Center the vertical beam on the center of the body.

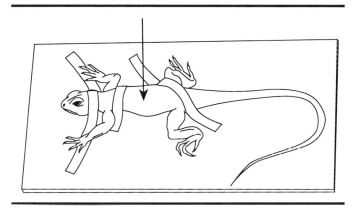

Fig. 3-8

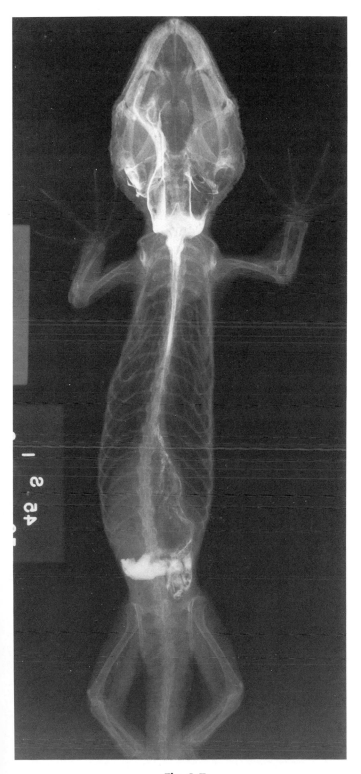

Fig. 3-7

WHOLE BODY STUDY—LATERAL VIEW—HORIZONTAL BEAM

Positioning: Place the patient in sternal recumbency directly on a sponge block or plastic sheet that can be elevated from the tabletop. Position the cassette on edge using sandbags to hold it against the patient's body. Try to keep the spine as straight as possible since scoliosis alters object film distance. If the patient is active, masking tape can be used for restraint with tape over the neck, thorax, and pelvis. The tail of the larger lizards can be taped in position (Fig. 3-9).

Beam center: Center the horizontal beam on the center of the body.

It is very difficult to position the patient in lateral recumbency on the cassette for examination with a vertical beam. If your tubehead does not rotate, it may be necessary to attempt this positioning to obtain the second view.

EXTREMITIES—VERTICAL BEAM

Positioning: Place the patient in sternal recumbency directly on the cassette. If the patient is active, masking tape can be used for restraint with tape over the neck, thorax, and pelvis. The tail of the larger lizards can be taped in position. Extend the limb of interest and position it in an extended position using masking tape or rope of appropriate size.

Beam center: Center the vertical beam on the limb of interest

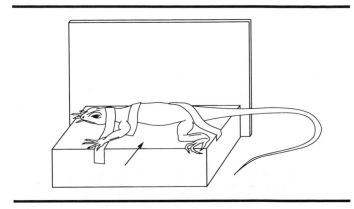

Fig. 3-9

Table 3-2
TECHNIQUE CHART FOR SKINKS, IQUANAS, AND MONITOR LIZARDS
(40 inches FFD tabletop technique using a 50 speed film-screen system without a grid)

beam direction	kVp	mA	exposure time	mAs
lateral view	54-56	400	1/60	6.6
dorsoventral view	54-56	400	1/60	6.6

Table 3-3
TECHNIQUE CHART FOR SNAKES
(40 inches FFD tabletop technique using a 50 speed film-screen system without a grid)

size	beam direction	kVp	mA	exposure time	mAs
Small (5 cm body diameter)	both views	50	400	1/60	6.6
Medium (10 cm body diameter)	both views	54	400	1/60	6.6
Large (15 cm body diameter)	both views	58	400	1/60	6.6

SNAKES

Restraint is similar for snakes as for the other exotic species. If the snake is small it can be coiled on the cassette where it remains because of a lethargic nature or because of a box serving as a mechanical restraint. The other possibility is to stretch the snake and tape it to a long plastic sheet. This permits repositioning the plastic to make dorso-ventral and lateral views. It is helpful to mark body segments by taping differing numbers of metallic pellets on the body. This enables you to compare anatomical locations on consecutive films.

To evaluate the respiratory system, the cranial two-thirds of the body need to be included. To study the gastro-intestinal system, the entire body needs to be included.

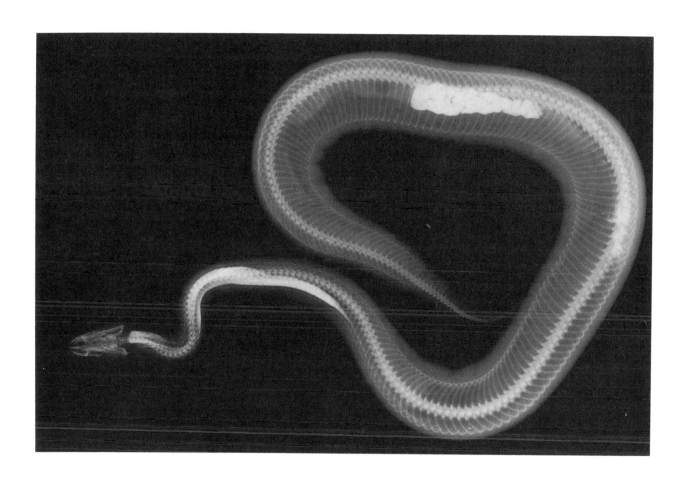

REFERENCES

Gibbs C and Hinton MH. Radiological examination of the rabbit. 1. The head, thorax and vertebral column. J sm Anim Pract 22:687-703, 1981.

Holt PE. Radiological studies of the alimentary tract of two Greek Tortoises (Testudo graeca). Vet Rec 103:198-200, 1978.

Jackson OF and Fasal MD. Radiology in tortoises, terrapins and turtles as an aid to diagnosis. J sm Anim Pract 22:705-16, 1981.

SECTION I

ULTRASOUND

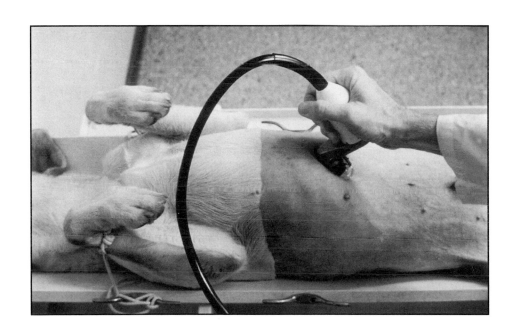

1. INTRODUCTION

Diagnostic ultrasound was first used clinically in the early 1960's and this imaging modality is still growing and evolving each year. This chapter is intended to give a basic introduction into the world of diagnostic ultrasound including scanning procedures, techniques (do's and don't's) of scanning, a brief discussion of normal and abnormal anatomy as seen on ultrasound, as well as a variety of other considerations. The intent is not to be the all encompassing text, but rather to give you, the student or practitioner, a comprehensive starting point. Ultrasound, like no other imaging modality, requires an unparalleled interaction between operator and equipment. One must dedicate a large amount of time in order to be adequate in scanning and interpretations. Ultrasound requires that you use all the information available, history, physical exam, serology, chemistry, and radiographs, along with what can be seen on the ultrasound screen, to make an accurate diagnosis.

2. BASIC PHYSICS AND NOMENCLATURE

The piezoelectric (pressure electricity) material has unique properties which make ultrasound possible. The piezoelectric effect was first described by Pierre and Jacques Curie in 1880. The principle of the physics is exhibited in certain materials, in diagnostic ultrasound the piezoelectric material is usually a man-made ferro-ceramic wafer made out of lead zirconate titanate (PZT). When an electric field is applied to a piezoelectric crystal it changes shape (only a few microns), and when the electric field is applied in a series of pulses, the material vibrates like a cymbal producing waves of sound. The wavelength and frequency of these sound waves generated are a function of the material's thickness. Conversely, when pressure from a sound wave returning to the transducer strikes the crystal, an electrical charge is generated, is interpreted by a computer and produces an image. The modern ultrasound machine is based upon this principle (Fig. 2-1).

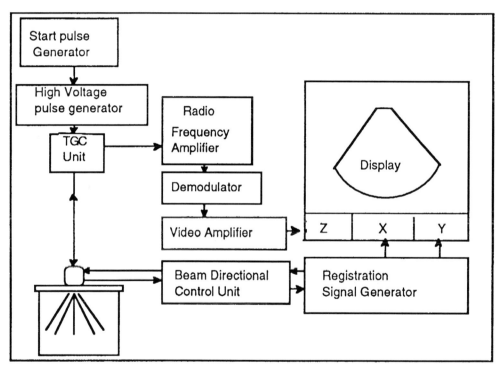

Fig. 2-1
Diagram showing the basic components found within ultrasound equipment.

3. DEFINITIONS OF TERMS OF INTEREST IN ULTRASOUND

ATTENUATION (dB—non-used attenuation)—Attenuation is the reduction in the intensity of an ultrasound beam as it travels through a medium.

ATTENUATION COEFFICIENT (a)—Attenuation coefficients are numerical values that express how different materials attenuate an ultrasound beam per unit path length (dB cm^{-1} MHz^{-1}).

ACOUSTIC IMPEDANCE (Z)—A measure of how easily acoustic waves can be formed as they pass through a particular medium which impedes the waves passage depending on its density. Acoustic impedance is the product of the velocity (C) of the acoustic energy and the density (p) of the medium through which it is traveling. At acoustic interfaces, the greater the variation in acoustic impedance between two media, the greater the acoustic reflection. Ultrasound machines are calibrated for an average velocity of 1540 meters/second.

ACOUSTIC INTERFACE—The plane of contact between media of different acoustic impedance's (related to the density of the tissue and the velocity of sound). At this interface, a portion of the ultrasonic pulse is transmitted, reflected, and refracted.

ARTIFACT—A signal in the normal signal mix that seems to be originating from tissues being scanned but <u>does not</u> have an anatomical correlation in the tissues. Artifacts can come from external noise, reverberations, multipath reflections, and <u>maladjusted equipment</u>. They can also come from the ultrasonic beam geometry and unusual changes in beam intensity.

EXAMPLES OF ARTIFACTS:
Resolution artifacts:
<u>Acoustic noise</u>—Specular echoes thought the image—Gain set to high
<u>Section thickness</u>—Beam thickness is 1-2mm, this can lead to mis-representing the edge of an object.
<u>Axial resolution</u>—Most accurate representation of an objects true size along the axis of the beam. A principle of imaging—not a true artifact.
<u>Lateral resolution</u>—Objects measured from side-to-side is less accurate than a top-to-bottom measurement. A principle of imaging which can result in mis-representation of objects. In current ultrasound equipment Axial and Lateral resolution artifacts are a very minor problem.

Propagation path artifacts:
<u>Reverberation</u>—Echoes bounce off the face of the transducer and return to the tissues or bounce off the under surface of reflecting structures on the return to the transducer. Commonly seen in the urinary bladder and other anechoic structures.

<u>Mirror image</u>—An air interface reflects all sound back to the transducer, where a substantial portion is reflected off the transducer face back to the air interface then back to the transducer. The computer interprets the echoes returning from the second, reflected sound wave as being beyond the air interface due to the time lag. This produced a mirror image of the tissue that is between the transducer and the air interface. Commonly when scanning the liver, there appears to be liver on the thoracic side of the diaphragm.

Attenuation artifacts:
<u>Shadowing</u>—The beam encounters a structure which absorbs a large portion of the sound, thus producing a hypoechoic area (tail) behind the object.
<u>Enhancement</u>—As the beam travels thru a hyper or anechoic region, the sound reaching the far side of the structure is stronger, producing a bright or enhanced surface on the far side of the structure. This can be of great advantage when trying to determine whether a structure is solid or cystic. Also known as Posterior Acoustic Enhancement.
<u>Edge shadowing</u>—Sound which encounters the tangential portion of a curved wall has significant refraction of the sound waves traveling thru the margin, thus the beam distal to the edge is weaker (darker).

Miscellaneous artifacts:
<u>Comet-tail</u>—Forms from reverberation when a strong reflector is encountered (air bubble or metal). Appears as a trail of increased echogenicity behind the structure. Also called 'ring-down artifact'.
<u>Apparent Enhancement</u>—Tissue in the focal zone displays greater intensity than tissue not in the focal zone.

DAMPING—A technique using mechanical or electronic methods to reduce the duration, or ring-down time, of the transducer crystal after excitation. The damping process decreases the transmitted pulse width and thus improves the axial resolution and beam intensity.

ECHO DROP-OUT—The disappearance of signals, typically resulting from lack of penetration of the ultrasound beam.

ECHOGENICITY—This term refers to the "brightness" of tissues being displayed.
<u>Anechoic</u>—a structure with no echoes (black).
<u>Hypoechoic</u>—fewer echoes than expected.
<u>Isoechoic</u>—"normal" amount of echoes (shades of gray).
<u>Hyperechoic</u>—more echoes than expected (white).

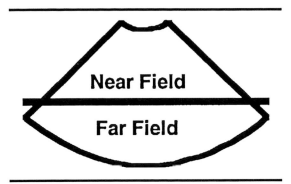

FAR FIELD—The portion of an ultrasound beam that diverges as a function of distance along the beam axis. In the far field, the beam diverges in a regular pattern. It is also known as the Fraunhofer zone because the diffraction processes are described by Fraunhofer light diffraction physics.

FOCAL LENGTH—The distance along the ultrasound beam axis from the center of the transducer to the focal point.

FOCAL POINT—That point in a focused ultrasound beam that has the highest intensity when measured in a non-attenuating medium. In diagnostic imaging, the closer the structures of interest are to the focal point, the greater is the resolution.

FOCAL ZONE—That portion of a focused ultrasound beam extending axially on either side of the focal point in which the amplitude of an echo from a standard echo source is not reduced more than 6dB. The focal zone is the region of optimal resolution.

FREQUENCY—Refers to the number of vibrations cycles per second, measured in hertz (Hz). Diagnostic ultrasound is in the range of 1 million cycles per second (megahertz = MHz) to 20MHz. (Note: <u>Frequency and resolution have a direct relationship, while frequency and penetration have an inverse relationship</u>), most ultrasound transducers are in the range of 2.5MHz to 10MHz.

VARIOUS CATEGORIES OF SOUND:

Name	Frequency range
Infrasound	Below 20 Hz
Audible sound	20-20,000 Hz
Ultrasound	Above 20,000 Hz
Diagnostic Ultrasound	1,000,000-20,000,000 Hz

GAIN—The amount of amplification applied to signal output. Gain may be expressed in decibels or as a ratio of the output signal to the input signal. The amount of acoustic energy transmitted by the transducer into the tissues provides energy for the returning echoes. Increasing this setting produces a beam which penetrates deeper into tissues, but also results in increased scattering of the beam and increased acoustic noise, resulting in lower resolution. Therefore, use the minimum power setting which adequately penetrates to the desired depth and avoid excessive levels!

NEAR FIELD—The portion of a beam of ultrasound within which that beam can remain in parallel, from the face of the transducer to the beginning of field divergence. Also known as the Fresnel zone.

REJECTION—A technique whereby returning echoes below a certain threshold are not displayed. Rejection is often used to remove small, non-structural signals from an image without removing the larger anatomical signals.

RESOLUTION—A system's ability to distinguish two objects that are positioned closely side by side. It is primarily a function of the narrowness of the ultrasonic beam. Acoustic lenses, which narrow the ultrasonic beam can improve lateral resolution.

TGC (Time Gain Compensation)—The change of signal amplification to compensate for ultrasound beam attenuation, transducer focusing, and pulse frequency. The purpose of TGC is to permit display images of equal echogenicity so that they appear with equal brightness regardless of depth. Hence, echoes from greater depth require more gain than echoes from shallower depths.

TGC controls typically include: <u>Gain (power)</u> which controls the overall signal strength or output of the ultrasound beam; <u>Near Gain</u> which controls the degree of amplification applied to signals returning from the near field; <u>Slope Delay</u> which determines the depth where TGC should begin (the TGC ramp); and <u>Slope Rate</u> which determines the rate of change of signal gain with respect to depth.

4. EQUIPMENT

There are many types of diagnostic ultrasound equipment including types of transducers. The principle types of equipment in use today are:

A-MODE—A method of presenting echo information from a single beam of ultrasound in which the amplitude of the signals usually appears on the "Y" axis, and depth is shown on the "X" axis. The "A" stands for amplitude. This type of ultrasound is still used widely today in Opthalmic Ultrasound.

M-MODE—The "M" stands for motion. A display mode in which a B-mode trace is formed and moved as a function of time to present motion of the echo sources. This form of display is used primarily for studying cardiac dynamics, but is not limited to that use.

B-MODE—A display mode in which the signal is displayed as a dot with its intensity proportional to the signal strength (amplitude) and its position corresponding to the target's distance from the transducer. The brightness of the dot varies with signal strength unless adjusted by the TGC controls. The two types of B-MODE are Static and Dynamic or (Real-Time) imaging.

STATIC B-MODE—An ultrasound device that makes single frame, stationary, two-dimensional images of the body interior by movement of a singe transducer attached to a position-sensing arm. The image is built by storing each B-mode trace as the transducer is moved. The accumulated B-mode traces make the resulting two-dimensional image. Static B-Mode is now almost extinct, due to the difficulty in obtaining quality images (mostly due to artifacts).

REAL-TIME IMAGING—Typically referred to as 2D. An imaging technique in which the image is created by a rapid succession of B-mode traces. The image is remade so rapidly that, as acoustic interfaces move in the ultrasound field, the image changes, depicting motion in real time.

DOPPLER—A signal processing technique that detects or separates the Doppler shift frequency from the received radio frequency (rf) signal. Most often used for detection of direction and rate of flow within an artery or vein.

DUPLEX—This imaging method includes both 2D and one of three signals displayed simultaneously. These are M-Mode, Doppler (these two methods are displayed in conjunction with the 2D image), or Color Doppler (this image is displayed on top of the 2D image and gives information about both direction and velocity using a color overlay).

TRANSDUCERS—The transducer is a hand-held probe composed of the piezoelectric crystal, etc. The crystal serves as both the sender of the ultrasound beam (<1% of the time) and the receiver of the reflected sound (>99% of the time). Several types of transducers are in use today.

MECHANICAL SECTOR—A 2D sector display of real-time images generated by motor-driven ultrasonic transducers oscillating or rotating over the image field There are one to four crystals in this transducer.

ANNULAR ARRAY—Transducer configuration in which the transducer elements are arranged in concentric rings around a central disc. Because the elements are time-phase stimulated, the ultrasound beam can be variably focused over a range of depths during transmission and reception.

LINEAR ARRAY—An assemblage of transducers arranged in a line parallel to each other. Parallel image elements can be generated by pulsing them sequentially either singly or in groups, generating a line of B-mode echoes. Together, these B-mode echoes form a 2D Linear image.

PHASED ARRAY—As generally used, a multi-element transducer in which the elements are electronically time-phase coordinated to generate a steered and focused wavefront. The steering and focusing are achieved by timing the transmission and reception of pulses to and from each of the arrayed elements. This is the most popular type of transducer at present, the image quality is very good, and there are no moving parts to wear out.

BASIC EQUIPMENT NEEDED

As you can see there is quite a variety of equipment available. An ultrasound machine can have one, some, or all of the above equipment, of course the more options you have, the higher the price. The price of new ultrasound equipment varies from around $20,000 to more than $300,000. The old adage that "you get what you pay for" is usually true here. Typically the image quality goes up with the more expensive equipment.

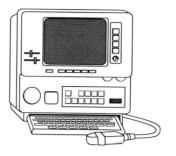

A good basic unit for a general small animal practice should include an ultrasound machine with a 7.5MHz, 5.0MHz, and 3.0MHz transducers (these usually are sector phased array types of scanners). With this range of transducers, you can image animals that range in size from a small cat to a large dog. A recording device is also needed and a standard VCR does nicely for most examinations. Still copies are nice for client relations or to send to a referring veterinarian. There are a variety of printers (gray scale to color) that are available.

It is also important to consider the "footprint" of a transducer. This is the term used to describe the area of contact needed to create an image. Some transducers have such a large footprint that they are essentially useless for veterinary ultrasonography.

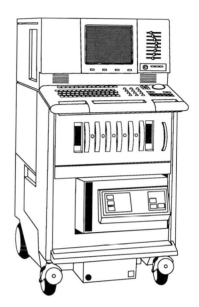

The equipment previously listed may be supplemented in the following ways:

1) Cardiac: M-Mode is very useful and more accurate for measurement of the heart than 2D (normal values can be found in the references).
2) Doppler: This mode of imaging is useful for both cardiac and abdominal studies.
3) Large animal practice: A linear array transducer will be helpful for pregnancy and tendon exams.

5. SUMMARY OF PROCEDURE

Learning the practice of ultrasound is a long and intensive process and adding M-Mode and/or Doppler adds a great deal of time to the learning curve. This is said not to discourage you, but to advise you that ultrasound is not something that can be learned within a week, or a month. The average practitioner requires several months to a year of using ultrasound on a daily basis to become a "good" ultrasonographer.

Ultrasound is not intended to replace any other tools that the practitioner uses, but rather to add additional information to assist in making a diagnosis. Remember that you are training your brain to recognize a new set of signals, be consistent and be patient.

Ultrasound examinations should be considered a part of the diagnostic process, it is in no way intended to be the sole test used to make a diagnosis. Ultrasound reveals the appearance of the anatomy of the organs scanned. It is important to convert the visualization of any organ scanned using 2D and convert this into a 3D image within your brain.

Ultrasound requires that you know the anatomical features including the size and texture of individual organs being scanned. Ultrasound has been described as "like trying to explore Carlsbad Caverns by using only a pen-light". This is true if you do not know the anatomical features (or if you have never been in Carlsbad Caverns). However, if you have a very good map and are familiar with Carlsbad Caverns in your mind (know the appearance of the organs), it is easy to find your way around using only a pen-light.

6. HOW TO PERFORM THE EXAMINATION

TECHNICAL CONSIDERATIONS

Lesions can easily be missed or misinterpreted by using the incorrect transducer, improper TGC settings, poor screen contrast, and scanning in a brightly lit room. On the other hand a poor image can also result in over diagnosis. Poor images and an overactive imagination can result in misdiagnosis. The most common error in learning ultrasound is to over diagnose!

When starting the exam, always use the highest frequency transducer appropriate for the exam being performed. After an initial pass (exam) is made, then a lower frequency transducer can be used to view what was missed while scanning with the higher frequency transducer. Always use only the amount of "pressure" needed to visualize the structure, it is the tendency of new ultrasonographers to press very hard on the patient causing a great deal of discomfort.

The power setting should be set so that the most distal structure can be seen, then use the TGC to dampen the near field so that the image is of uniform brightness. Use the lowest power setting possible, this helps to keep the image quality high.

Always scan in a darkened room. This is because there is a glare off the screen in a brightly lighted room. This glare, along with the tendency to use to much power to produce a "brighter" image, often renders the image useless.

PATIENT PREPARATION

The best way to determine if an ultrasound exam is indicated is to follow a problem oriented approach in working-up each patient. The timing of the ultrasound examination in the course of the diagnostic work-up varies according to the clinician and the individual patient's signs. If, for example, the physical exam reveals an abdominal mass, ultrasound may be indicated immediately. At other times, clinical laboratory results and survey radiographs may offer more diagnostic information than the ultrasound examination. The need for ultrasound should be determined on an individual case basis.

Relatively little patient preparation is needed. It can be helpful to fast the patient overnight but is not absolutely mandatory. If the gastrointestinal tract contains large amounts of gas and food, complete examination is difficult. Fasting is highly recommended if the ultrasound exam is being performed specifically for the gastrointestinal tract, and/or pancreas. Enemas are not recommended because they usually introduce large amounts of air into the gastrointestinal tract. Remember that image quality is of poorer quality in emaciated and obese patients and those with gas-filled bowel.

All patients need to have the haircoat clipped in order to get quality images. Remember that ultrasound can not pass thru air and without shaving there is a great deal of air trapped within the hair. A number 40 clipper blade is sufficient in preparing the patient. If clipping is not possible alcohol can be liberally applied then ultrasound gel.

Tranquilization is rarely needed except for biopsies. Agents that promote panting (oxymorphone for example), or acepromazine that can lead to significant splenic enlargement should be avoided. A commonly used and very effective combination is ketamine and valium. However the patients condition and illness should dictate what if anything is used for sedation.

PATIENT POSITIONING
Abdominal Scanning

Place the patient in dorsal recumbency in a padded V shaped trough (a surgery table for example), with the head located at the far end of the table (towards the ultrasound machine). Place the machine so that your dominant hand does the scanning and your non-dominant hand has easy access to the control panel. Be consistent in positioning the patients, since this makes learning ultrasound easier.

Cardiac Scanning

The patient is scanned from both sides (right and left). A table allows the heart to fall against the chest wall, giving a better window for the exam. The table can be made from almost any material with wood and plexiglas being the most commonly used (Fig. 6-1).

SCREEN IMAGE ORIENTATION

Always use the correct orientation of images when scanning since this aids in learning ultrasound, as well as aiding when referring your exams to a radiologist (Fig. 6-2).

It is often difficult to know the orientation of an image when it is presented on hardcopy or videotape and therefore, it is extremely important that you keep the appropriate orientation in mind when scanning. When recording your images, always label the orientation.

USE OF TWO PLANES

Since the ultrasound beam gives only a limited view of anatomy, an organized systematic scanning pattern is essential. The exact order of organ scanning is not as crucial as is proper bi-planar imaging of each structure. Each structure should be examined in at least two planes, usually longitudinal and transverse planes. Many times oblique views may be useful in producing diagnostic images. Use as many views from as many angles as necessary to gain the diagnostic information needed. All exams should be complete, it only requires a few extra minutes to look at the total abdomen.

Basic rules for ultrasound scanning are reviewed below (Table 6-1).

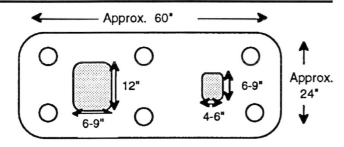

The larger hole is for dogs and the small hole is for cats.

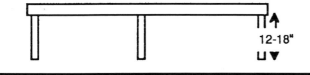

Fig. 6-1
Drawing of a model of a table that can be used for cardiac scanning. These dimensions are only suggestions.

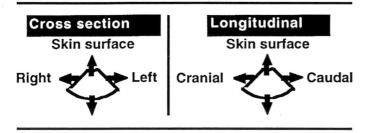

Fig. 6-2
The diagrams represent the standard orientation used for ultrasound scans.

Table 6-1
BASIC RULES FOR ULTRASOUND SCANNING

Always scan in a dimly lighted room.

Always remove hair and maintain good transducer-skin contact with liberal amounts of coupling gel to help avoid artifacts.

Always position the animal on the exam table in a consistent orientation.

Always position the image on the screen with the proper orientation. Know where cranial, caudal, left, and right are; if you are confused—stop—and reorientate yourself.

Slowly perform the scan.

All structures visualized in each image must be identified.

Always scan each organ in at least two planes (Longitudinal and Sagittal).

Perform an ultrasound examination consistently using the same technique for each examination.

Consistency in performing the examination helps train your brain to recognize a new set of visual signals.

7. GENERAL CONSIDERATIONS AND GUIDELINES

Use the highest frequency transducer which penetrates to the area which needs to be imaged. Maintain proper adjustment (control) of power, TGC, screen brightness and contrast.

A "good" ultrasound image is of uniform brightness, the TGC is adjusted properly giving a high quality uniformly diagnostic image.

Problems and Solutions:

1) Too many echoes generally
   A) Turn down the gain (power)
   B) Use the TGC controls to suppress the image, but remember that this also increases contrast because the smaller echoes are attenuated disproportionately to the stronger echoes.
   C) Change to a higher frequency transducer.

2) Too many echoes proximally
   A) Add or increase slope delay.
   B) Decrease slope.
   C) Due to the focal zone of a transducer, a stand-off may be needed to visualize structures near the transducer. There are several commercially available stand-off pads, one that is not quite as good but is easily available is a plastic bag of IV fluids. Remember to use gel on both sides of the bag. If information from deeper structures is not needed, switching to a higher frequency transducer also helps.

3) Too many echoes distally
   A) Decrease slope.
   B) Use a higher frequency transducer.

4) Too few echoes generally
   A) Check to ensure there is adequate coupling, use enough gel.
   B) Check the slope and slope delay, set them to have minimal effect.
   C) Increase the gain or power.
   D) Use a lower frequency transducer.

5) Too few small amplitude echoes
   A) Check to ensure there is adequate coupling, use enough gel.
   B) Check the slope and slope delay, set them to have minimal effect.
   C) Increase the gain or power.
   D) Use a lower frequency transducer.

6) Too few echoes proximally
   A) Reduce slope delay.
   B) Increase slope.

7) Too few echoes distally
   A) Check slope and slope delay.
   B) Use a lower frequency transducer.

8) Too many echoes in suspected cyst
   A) Decrease gain or power.
   B) Check slope and slope delay.
   C) Use a higher frequency transducer.
   D) The suspected cyst may not be a cyst.

8. ABDOMINAL ULTRASOUND

A complete ultrasound examination consists of imaging all major organ systems and abdominal regions. The following list of organs and structures should be readily identifiable:

Liver
    Parenchyma
    Gall bladder
    Portal veins
    Hepatic veins
    Diaphragm

Spleen
    Parenchyma
    Splenic vein

Kidneys
    Cortex
    Medulla
    Renal artery and vein
    Fat within the renal pelvis

Adrenal glands
    Left adrenal (usually seen)
    "Region" of the right adrenal (may or may not be seen)

Genital system
    Uterine body (sometimes seen in large breeds, usually not seen unless enlarged)
    Prostate
    Testicles

GI Tract
    Stomach
    Duodenum
    Small and Large intestine

Pancreas
    "Area" of the pancreas—the pancreas itself is not usually visualized, but may be seen in some animals.

Bladder

Lymph Nodes
    Not normally visualized, however the area of the sublumbar, mesenteric, and hepatic nodes should routinely be examined.

Listed below is a suggested way of performing an ultrasound exam. Any order is acceptable as long as you are consistent, thorough, and maintain the proper orientation. The following discussion assumes that you are familiar with abdominal anatomy. Images of "normal" anatomy are given to assist in distinguishing a normal from an abnormal scan. One of the most difficult determination to make in an ultrasound study is whether an organ is normal in size and texture. This determination comes only with experience along with an excellent knowledge of anatomy.

A basic rule to remember in examination of abdominal organs is that of the range of the most echogenic to the least echogenicity within normal organs. That is as follows: spleen > liver > renal cortex > renal medulla.

LIVER

Start with a cross-sectional view of the liver, with the transducer placed near the xyphoid process. Scan to the patients right and back to the left, angling the probe as needed to visualize all of the liver. It may be necessary to apply a fair amount of pressure to displace gas from the stomach and duodenum. Rotate the transducer 90° to yield a longitudinal section. Examine the liver parenchymal "texture" and "echogenicity" (compare the echogenicity of the liver with that of the right kidney), as well as the central vessels, gall bladder, cystic and common bile duct "area", as well as noting any separation of the liver lobes which may indicate free abdominal fluid.

In large breed dogs you may want to scan the liver with a 5MHz transducer to examine as much "texture" and "echogenicity" as possible then switch to a 3.5MHz transducer to evaluate the remainder of the liver.

The liver should be homogeneous, with portal and hepatic veins easily visualized. The portal veins have echogenic walls, while the hepatic veins appear to be without walls. In cats the portal and hepatic veins appear "relatively" larger in relation to the liver than in the dog. The gall bladder is usually anechoic, but may contain echogenic material if the patient has not eaten for several hours. The common bile duct is not normally seen. The borders of the liver should be sharp and not rounded.

During the examination of the liver, remember to examine the diaphragm. It should be smooth and well delineated. Two natural "breaks" appear, these being the post cava and the esophagus passing thru the diaphragm. Do not mistake these for tears when looking for a diaphragmatic hernia.

A partial list of lesions that can be expected from an ultrasound examination of the liver includes:

Mass lesions
    Neoplastic mass lesions
    Abscess/granuloma/hematoma
    Regenerative nodules (nodular hyperplasia)
    Cirrhotic masses
    Focal hepatopathy, (necrosis)

Diffuse parenchymal disease
    Diffuse coarse texture, increase/decrease in echogenicity
    Hepatic fibrosis

Biliary disease
    Obstruction
    Cholangiohepatitis
    Cholecystitis
    Cholelithiasis (stones)
    Biliary neoplasia
    Inspissated bile

Portosystemic shunts

SPLEEN

Use little transducer pressure when examining the spleen as it is a superficial organ. Inspect the parenchymal "texture" and "echogenicity" and compare it to the liver and left kidney. Follow the spleen from tip to tip, noting the size of the splenic veins (usually less than 5mm in diameter).

Splenic texture should be homogeneous, with the splenic veins easily visualized. The spleen can vary greatly in size in normal animals. Splenomegaly has a tendency to be overdiagnosed, especially when sedation has been given.

A partial list of lesions that can be expected from an ultrasound examination of the spleen includes:

Focal lesions
Neoplasia
Hematoma
Infarct/granuloma/abscess

Diffuse parenchymal disease
Neoplasia
Torsion

URINARY TRACT AND ADRENALS

The urinary tract should be scanned beginning with the left kidney. Scan the kidney in transverse as well as longitudinal sections, noting the cortical and medullary "texture" and "echogenicity" as well as the relative thicknesses of each (approximately 2:1—cortex:medulla). There are varying amounts of fat in the renal pelvis which appears very echogenic. While scanning the left kidney look for the left adrenal gland, it should be near the cranial pole and medial to the kidney, and lateroventral to the aorta. Move to the right kidney and repeat the exam, however since the right kidney sits in the renal fossa of the liver, compare the renal cortical echogenicity to that of the liver. Examine the "area" of the right adrenal gland. This gland sits against the caudal borders of the liver and is often times indistinguishable from liver.

The urinary bladder should be imaged next; look for wall thickening, mucosal irregularities, stones, and enlarged sublumbar nodes. Bladder wall thickness is difficult to determine, unless there is free abdominal fluid, which allows the visualization of the exterior bladder wall.

A partial list of lesions that can be expected from an ultrasound examination of the urinary tract includes:

Renal masses
Neoplasia
Abscesses/granuloma/hematoma

Renal fluid collections
Hydronephrosis
Pyelonephritis
Sub-capsular fluid
Peri-renal fluid
Renal cyst(s)

Nephroliths/nephrocalcinosis

Ethylene glycol poisoning

Glomerulonephritis

Tubular Nephrosis

Vasculitis (FIP)

Ureteroliths

Urinary bladder wall masses

Urethral tumors

Cystic calculi and debris

A partial list of lesions that can be expected from an ultrasound examination of the adrenal glands includes adrenal masses or pituitary-dependent hyperadrenocorticism.

PROSTATE OR UTERUS

In male dogs, the prostate should be imaged in both planes, again examining parenchymal "texture" and "echogenicity," as well as the bladder neck region. This organ should be homogeneous and bi-lobed, appearing more echogenic than the spleen or liver. Often times the ureter can be seen running through the center of the prostate.

In the female search the region dorsal to the bladder for the uterine body. The ovaries may sometimes be identified, especially if a follicle is present. It is common not to visualize either the ovaries or the uterus in a normal animal. A nongravid uterus should be less than 1 cm in diameter.

Pregnancy can be easily detected at 20 days of gestation, however earlier pregnancies are easily aborted, often going undetected. A pregnancy exam performed between 28 and 35 days is of the most value. Individual feti can be seen along with a heart beat to determine fetal viability. In general, a gestational sac is seen at about day 14, this continues to grow in size, and about day 21 to 23 a fetus can be seen. At approximately 25 days of gestation a heart beat can be seen. At 35 days internal organs can be seen. At 40 days the bones are dense enough to cast an ultrasound shadow. After about 45 days, pregnancy determination is very easy, but the ability to count the number of feti is greatly reduced due to their size.

A partial list of lesions that can be expected from an ultrasound examination of the prostate and uterus includes:

Prostatic disorders
Focal lesions
Cysts
Abscesses
Neoplasia

Diffuse disease
Hyperplasia
Prostatitis
Neoplasia

Uterine disorders
Infection (metritus, pyometra)

Pregnancy
Normal
Complicated

GASTROINTESTINAL TRACT

The stomach and small intestines should be evaluated for thickness (approximately 4 mm is normal wall thickness). Make several passes through the GI tract in order to avoid missing any abnormalities. You may want to make several passes with very light pressure, and then return with a moderate amount of pressure in order to push some of the gas filled bowel out of the image (Fig. 8-1).

A partial list of lesions that can be expected from an ultrasound examination of the gastrointestinal tract includes:

Obstruction
Foreign bodies
Intussusception
Mural masses (mass lesions with or without obstruction)

PANCREAS

Start in a longitudinal section near the cranial pole of the left kidney, scan across the abdomen (oriented transversely to the pancreas) visualizing the stomach cranially. At the pylorus follow the duodenum, turning the transducer 90° and continue scanning until caudal to the right kidney. Normally the pancreas is not visualized, therefore you must thoroughly evaluate the region of the right and left limbs. Diagnostic hydroperitoneum can be very useful to examine the pancreas, use 60 to 100ml/kg of warm sterile saline, this allows direct visualization of the pancreas. The normal pancreas should be 1 to 2 cm thick, 2 to 3 cm wide, and 5 to 10 cm in length, with an isoechoic granular texture.

A partial list of lesions that can be expected from an ultrasound examination of the pancreas includes neoplasia and pancreatitis.

LYMPH NODES

The sublumbar nodes are dorsal to the urinary bladder at about the bifurcation of the aorta and post-cava into external iliacs arteries and veins. Cecal nodes lie caudomedial to the right kidney. Mesenteric nodes are located in the mid-abdominal region, surrounded by small intestine and mesentery. Hepatic nodes are found lying cranio-dorsal to the body of the stomach. Nodes can range in appearance from almost anechoic to very dense depending on the disease process.

A partial list of lesions that can be expected from an ultrasound examination of the gastrointestinal tract includes lymphadenopathy (hepatic, mesenteric, or sublumbar).

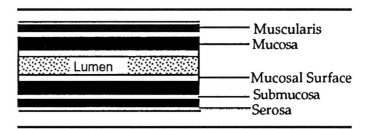

Fig. 8-1
The layers of the stomach and small intestines can be seen on ultrasound and appear as follows:

Muscularis	Thick anechoic layer
Mucosa	Thick anechoic layer
Mucosal Surface	Hyperechoic layer of variable thickness
Serosa	Thin hyperechoic layer
Lamina Propria	Thin hyperechoic line

9. CARDIAC ULTRASONOGRAPHY

As described earlier, a table for cardiac exams is very helpful in obtaining quality images. There are only one to three rib spaces that provide a window for the cardiac exam, usually around the fourth or fifth intercostal space. Shave a small square over the area where the heart can be felt beating with the fingers. Place the cardiac table onto a flat table of standard height, place the patient right side down with the spot you have chosen over the hole in the table. Most ultrasound machines allow the hookup of an ECG while scanning, this can be very useful when evaluating the cardiac cycle while scanning. If contrast is desired, to see a right to left shunt for example, a catheter can be place in a cephalic vein, a syringe of sterile saline shaken vigorously, and then injected. The micro-bubbles that form from being shaken provide excellent contrast.

A partial list of lesions that can be expected from an ultrasound examination of the heart includes cardiomyopathy, aortic stenosis, various masses, and valvular disorders.

With the patient in right lateral recumbency the right side of the heart is used as a window to evaluate the left side of the heart. Again, any order of exam is acceptable as long as you are consistent and thorough.

Right side cross sectional imaging: Start in a cross section at the apex of the heart. Without moving the transducer angle craniodorsal thru the heart. The left ventrical and septum as well as part of the right ventrical can be seen. Continuing craniodorsal, the mitral and tricuspid valves come into view, then the atria and aorta as a circle in the center with a "piece or Mercedes Benz" sign (these are the leaflets of the aortic valve). Passing thru this area, the aortic and pulmonary outflow tract can sometimes be visualized. Make several sweeps to ensure all structures were visualized.

M-Mode sweeps are made in much the same manner. Most measurements are made from M-Mode tracings, it is easier and probably more accurate.

Right side longitudinal imaging: Turn the transducer 90° to obtain a longitudinal image. The left ventricle, septum, part of the right ventricle, mitral and tricuspid valves can be seen in the same slice. Rotate the transducer to bring the aorta and the aortic outflow tract into view. This is a good view for evaluation of aortic stenosis.

Left side imaging: Imaging from the left side provides some additional information. The left side of the heart is used as an offset to evaluate the right side. This only needs to be done if the structures of interest were not adequately visualized from the right side. The view that is obtained only from the left is the four chamber view. With the transducer in a longitudinal orientation, shoot from the apex to the base rotating the transducer until all four chambers, mitral and tricuspid valves come into view (this is easier said than done).

Doppler ultrasound is a useful tool. It is still very expensive to purchase, although used equipment is becoming available and affordable. For the general practitioner it only adds complexity and is of nominal use.

10. BIOPSIES

The two most common techniques for biopsy are freehand and guided. The freehand technique is very useful for large structures that are not highly vascularized, including masses, lymph nodes, and bladder taps. This method of biopsy is not very accurate, especially if you are just learning ultrasound. The guided biopsy consists of the transducer, some sort of fixed guide to keep the needle in the plane of the ultrasound beam. This method is easily mastered and very small lesions (less than 1cm in diameter) can be successfully biopsied. There are several biopsy "guns" on the market, these have the advantage of allowing one person to both scan and biopsy at the same time.

The patient should be sedated for this procedure. Clip and perform a normal ultrasound exam, to ensure nothing is missed. It is always frustrating to examine and biopsy only the liver and totally miss the bladder tumor. Once you have decided what and where to biopsy, prepare the patient by performing a good surgical scrub. Clean the transducer with alcohol or place a sterile sleeve over the transducer, remembering to put gel on the inside of the glove. Attach the sterile guide to the transducer, use sterile gel (KY Gel works fine), and biopsy. If a lesion can be seen, it can be biopsied or aspirated to obtain a diagnosis.

It is highly recommended that a clotting panel be run before a biopsy is performed, and the patient monitored for four to six hours after the biopsy to ensure there are no complications. This should not be considered an outpatient procedure.

11. SUMMARY

EQUIPMENT
- High resolution = High frequency transducer (proper transducer for the exam)
- Proper TGC settings
- Some sort of recording device (hardcopy and/or video tape) When you video tape your exams, it is best to narrate them. Talk your way through the exam, it helps when reviewing the tape at a later date!

PATIENT PREPARATION
- Calm or tranquilized
- Clip hair
- Good transducer coupling—Use plenty of gel to create an airless patient/transducer interface.
- Proper patient and unit positioning

AVOIDANCE OF ARTIFACTS
- Understand their origins
- Proper machine settings (TGC)

SYSTEMATIC PROCEDURE
- Examine and identify all structures, do not stop when one lesion is found
- Scan each structure in two planes
- Avoid pre-conceived ideas of "expected" pathology

KNOWLEDGE
- Knowledge of cross sectional, three dimensional anatomy
- Knowledge of pathologic processes effecting each organ

REFERENCES

BOOKS

Ackerman N. Radiology and Ultrasound of Urogenital Diseases in Dogs and Cats. Iowa State University Press, Ames 1991.

Barr F. Diagnosit Ultrasound in the Dog and Cat. Blackwell Scientific Publications, London 1990.

Bushong SC and Archer BR. Diagnostic Ultrasound: Physics, Biology, and Instrumentation. Mosby-Year Book, Inc., St. Louis 1991.

Feeney DA Fletcher TF and Hardy RM. Atlas of Correlative Imaging Anatomy of the Normal Dog: Ultrasound and Computed Tomography. WB Saunders Co., Philadelphia 1991.

Fleischer AC and James AE. Diagnostic Sonography: Principles and Clinical Applications. WB Saunders Co., Philadelphia 1989.

Kobayashi T and Hayashi M. Clinical Sonographic Atlas. Toshiba, 1981.

Lutz H and Meudt R. Manual of Ultrasound. Springer-Verlag, New York, 1984.

McDicken WN. Diagnostic Ultrasonics: Principles and use of Instruments. Churchill Livingstone, New York 1991.

Metrewel C. Practical Abdominal Ultrasound. William Heinemann Medical Books, Ltd. London, 1978.

Reef VB. Equine Ultrasound. University of Sydney 1992

Taylor KJW. Atlas of Ultrasonography (2nd ed., 2 vol). Churchill Livingstone, New York 1985.

Veterinary Clinics of North America, Diagnostic Ultrasound. Small Animal Practice. Nov. 1985.

Weill Fr. Ultrasonography of Digestive Diseases. CV Mosby Co., St. Louis 1978.

Weill Fr. Renal Ultrasonography. Springer-Verlag, New York, 1981.

PAPERS

Artifacts

Kremkau Fr and Taylor KJW. Artifacts in ultrasound imaging. J Ultrasound Med, 5:227-237, 1986.

Park RD Nyland TG Lattimer JC et al. B-mode gray scale ultrasound: Imaging artifacts and interpretation principles. Vet Radiol 22:31-58, 1980.

General

Kaplan PM. Instrumentation, principles, and pitfalls of ultrasonography. Problems in Veterinary Medicine 3:457-478, 1991.

Nyland TG and Bernard WV. Application of abdominal ultrasound. Calif Vet 2:21-25, 1982.

Nyland TG Park RD Lattimer JC et al. Gray scale ultrasonography of the canine abdomen. Vet Radiol 22:220-227, 1981.

Liver and Spleen

Feeney DA Johnston GR and Hardy RM. Two-dimensional, gray-scale ultrasonography for assessment of hepatic and splenic neoplasia in the dog and cat. J Am Vet Med Assoc 1984:68-81, 1984.

Kantrowitz BM Nyland TG and Fisher PE. Estimation of Portal Blood Flow Using Duplex Real-Time and Pulsed Doppler Ultrasound Imaging in the Dog. Vet Radiol 30:222-226, 1989.

Nyland TG. Hepatic ultrasonography in the dog. Vet Radiol 24:74-84, 1983.

Nyland TG. Hager DA and Herring DS. Sonography of the Liver, Gallbladder, and Spleen. Seminars in Veterinary Medicine and Surgery Vol 4:13-31, 1989.

Nyland TG. Ultrasonic patterns of canine hepatic lymphosarcoma. Vet Radiol 25:167-172, 1984.

Nyland TG and Fisher PE. Evaluation of Experimentally Induced Canine Hepatic Cirrhosis Using Duplex Doppler Ultrasound. Vet Radiol 31:189-194, 1990.

Nyland TG and Gillett NA. Sonographic Evaluation of Experimental Bile Duct Ligation in the Dog. Vet Radiol, 23:252-260, 1982.

Pancreas

Nyland TG et al. Ultrasonic Features of Experimentally Induced, Acute Pancreatitis in the Dog. Vet Radiol 24:260-266, 1983.

Saunders HM. Ultrasonography of the pancreas. Problems in Veterinary Medicine 3:583-603, 1991.

Urogenital and Adrenal

Kantrowitz BM Nyland TG et al. Adrenal Ultrasonography in the dog. Vet Radiol 27:91-96, 1986.

Konde LJ Wrigley RH Park RD and Lebel JL. Ultrasonographic anatomy of the normal canine kidney. Vet Radiol 25: 173-178, 1984.

Nyland TG Kantrowitz BM Olander HJ Fisher PE and Hornof WJ. Ultrasonic Determination of Kidney Volume in the Dog. Vet Radiol 30:174-180, 1989.

Poffenbarger EM and Feeney DA. Use of gray-scale ultrasonography in the diagnosis of reproductive disease in the bitch: 18 cases (1981-1984). J Am Vet Med Assoc 189:90-95, 1986.

Poffenbarger EM Feeney DA and Feeney DW. Gray scale ultrasonography in the diagnosis of adrenal neoplasia: 6 cases (1981-1986). J Am Vet Med Assoc 192, 1988.

Walter PA Feeney DA Johnston GR and O'Leary TP. Ultrasonographic evaluation of renal parenchymal diseases in dogs: 32 cases (1981-1986). J Am Vet Med Assoc 191:999-1007, 1987.

Walter PA Johnston GR Feeney DA and O'Brien TD. Applications of ultrasonography in the diagnosis of parenchymal kidney disease in cats: 24 cases (1981-1986). J Am Vet Med Assoc 192, 1988.

Biopsy

Hager DA Nyland TG and Fisher PE. Ultrasound-guided biopsy of the canine liver, kidney, and prostate. Vet Radiol 23: 82-88, 1985.

Yuan A et al. Ultrasound-guided aspiration biopsy of small peripheral pulmonary nodules. Chest 101:926-930, 1992.

GI Tract

Penninck DG Nyland TG Fisher PE and Kerr LY. Ultrasonography of the Normal Canine Gastrointestinal Tract. Vet Radiol, 30 pp. 272-276, 1989.

Penninck DG Nyland TG Kerr LY and Fisher PE. Ultrasonic Evaluation of Gastrointestinal Diseases in Small Animals. Vet Radiol, 31:134-141, 1990.

Opthalmic

Dziezyc J Hager DA and Millichamp NJ. Two-dimensional real-time ocular ultrasonography in the diagnosis of ocular lesions in the dog. J Am Anim Hosp Assoc 23:501-508, 1987.

Eisenberg HM. Ultrasonography of the eye and orbit. Vet Clin North Am: Sm Anim Prac 15:1263-1274, 1985.

Cardiology

Boon J et al. Echocardiographic Indices in the Normal Dog. Vet Radiol, 24:214-221, 1983.

Pipers FS et al. Echocardiography in the Domestic Cat. Am J of Vet Res, 40:882-886, 1979.

Thomas WA Sisson D et al. Detection of Cardiac Masses in Dogs by Two-Dimentional Echocardiography. Vet Radiol, 25:65-72, 1984.

Thomas WP. Two-Dimensional, Real-Time Echocardiography in the Dog. Vet Radiol, 25:50-64, 1984.

SECTION J

GLOSSARY

Absorbed dose—the amount of energy deposited in tissue by a beam of ionizing radiation—the unit of absorbed dose is the rad or Gray

Absorption—process by which the number of photons is reduced as it passes through matter (see Attenuation, Filtration)

Actual focal spot—area of the focal spot as viewed at right angles to the plane of the target

Added filtration—sheets of aluminum or other material placed in the path of the primary x-ray beam that absorb x-ray photons

Adjustable lead shutter—a type of beam-restricting device that consists of a pair of movable lead shutters

Air gap technique—method of reducing scattered radiation to the film by separating the film and the object being examined

ALARA—an acronym used to express the concept that levels of radiation exposure should be as low as reasonably achievable

Alpha particle—a type of ionizing radiation consisting of 2 protons and 2 neutrons with a charge of +2 (helium nucleus)

Alternating current (AC)—form in which electrical energy is generated with the flow of electrons reversing a specific number of times each second (60 in the U.S.)

Alternating grid—grid that moves during radiographic exposure blurring the grid lines (see Moving grid, Potter-Bucky diaphragm, Potter-Bucky grid, Reciprocating grid)

Aluminum stepwedge—a graduated series of aluminum steps that increase in thickness thus permitting penetration by fewer photons as the thickness increases that is used to help understand the principle of radiographic contrast and film density

Amperage—a term used to describe the flow of electrons through a conductor

Angstrom—unit of length used for measurement of photon wavelength ($1Å = 10^{-8}$ cm)

Anode—the positive electrode in the x-ray tube that contains the target

Aperature diaphragm—a beam-restricting device in the form of a sheet of lead with an opening within the center

Attenuation—reduction in intensity of an x-ray beam as a result of absorption and scattering processes as it passes through matter (see Absorption, Filtration)

Autotransformer—a variable transformer which uses a single coil and is used to select the voltage for the primary of the high-tension transformer

Average Gradient—the slope of the characteristic curve between the end points of the useful range of densities, usually defined as between 0.25 and 2.00 above base plus fog, on an exposed radiograph

Background radiation—radiation received by an entire population primarily due to cosmic radiation, naturally occurring terrestrial radioactive materials, internal isotopes, and diagnostic radiographic examinations

Back-scatter radiation—interaction of photons with the back of the cassette, tabletop, or ground resulting in Compton effect with the scatter photons directed back toward the film where they cause an increase in fogging

Base exposure plus fog—density of the film which has received no exposure through a diagnostic study (also Base density)

Beam restrictor—a device attached to the opening in the x-ray tube housing that regulates the size and shape of the field of exposure (see Collimator)

Beta particle—a high speed electron with kinetic energy and a charge of -1

Binding energy—that energy that must be overcome before an electron can be removed from its orbit

Bremsstrahlung radiation—a method of x-ray generation in which a fast-moving electron comes close to and is deflected by the positively charged nucleus of an atom—the kinetic energy lost is emitted as a photon (see Continuous radiation, General radiation, White radiation)

Bucky—moving grid (named for Dr. Gustave Bucky who invented a stationary grid in 1913)

Bucky factor—required alteration in radiographic technique due to use of a grid

Bucky tray—sliding tray positioned under the radiographic table that holds the grid and cassette

Calcium tungstate—a fluorescent salt used in the manufacture of intensifying screens

Cassette—a light tight film-holding case which positions the x-ray film and intensifying screens in intimate contact (see Film holder)

Cathode—the negative electrode in an x-ray tube that contains the filament from which free electrons are produced by thermionic emission

Cathode beam—the beam of electrons that is accelerated by a high electrical potential and flows from the cathode to the anode in the x-ray tube (see Electron beam)

Caudocranial (CaCr)—a method of describing the direction of the x-ray beam with the entrance caudal and the exit cranial prior to exposure of the x-ray film

Central beam—a term used to describe the imaginary single x-ray photon that is located in the midportion of the primary x-ray beam

Characteristic curve—a curve expressing the relationship between radiation exposure of the film and the resulting film density (see H-D curve)

Characteristic radiation—a method of x-ray generation in which a fast-moving electron removes an electron from a shell in an atom in the target and a photon is released after the vacant space in the shell is filled by another electron (see Line radiation)

Chemical fogging—the generalized graying of the radiograph due to unwanted chemical reactions due to the age or temperature of the developer solution or a change in the developer time

Circuit—a complete path along which electrical current flows —in its simplest form it includes a source of electrons (power source), a load or resistance, and a conductor

Classical scatter—interaction of a photon with an electron in which the photon changes direction but does not lose energy (see Coherent scatter)

Clearing time—time required for the first stage of fixing during which the "milkness" of the radiograph disappears

Coherent scatter—interaction of a photon with an electron in which the photon changes direction but does not lose energy (see Classical scatter)

Collimator—an attachment to the tube-head that restricts the size and shape of the primary beam (see Beam restrictor)

Compton scatter—an attentuation process in which the incident x-ray photon interacts with a loosely-bound electron transferring a portion of the photon's energy to the electron as kinetic energy and the remainder to a newly created scattered photon which travels in a different direction than the incident photon (also Compton effect)

Condenser type unit—x-ray machine that uses a condenser for loading the x-ray tube

Cone—metallic cone-shaped structure that functions as a beam restrictor (see Cylinder)

Constant potential generator—a generator that combines three full-wave rectified circuits slightly out of phase with each other plus other electrical components such that the tube voltage varies between 95% and 100% and never falls to zero

Continuous radiation—a method of x-ray generation in which a fast-moving electron comes close to and is deflected by the positively charged nucleus of an atom—the kinetic energy lost is emitted as a photon (see Bremsstrahlung radiation, General radiation, White radiation)

Contrast—see film contrast, radiographic contrast, subject contrast

Contrast improvement factor—best method of describing the ability of a grid to improve film quality

Convergent line—line along which the lead strips of a linear focused grid would intersect if the strips were extended above the surface of the grid (line is at the focal distance)

Convergent point—the point at which all the lead strips of a crossed focused grid would intersect if the strips were extended above the surface of the grid (point is at the focal distance)

Corpuscular radiation—ionizing radiation consisting of moving particles of matter—usually submolecular such as alpha particles, protons, or electrons (see Particular radiation)

Craniocaudal (CrCa)—a method of describing the direction of the x-ray beam with the entrance cranial and the exit caudal prior to exposure of the x-ray film

Crossover exposure—film darkening and loss of film contrast due to exposure by light from the intensifying screen adjacent to the opposite side of the film

Crossed grid—a grid composed of two linear grids, with the grid lines of one perpendicular to the grid lines of the other (also Crosscut grid, Crosshatch grid)

Curie—a term used to specify the activity of a radionuclide, i.e., the rate at which its atoms disintegrate—one curie equals 3.7×10^{10} disintegrations per second

Cylinder—a metallic tube that functions as a beam restrictor with the feature of possible extension

Definition—feature of film quality in which elements of the patient can be seen on the radiograph—(see Detail, Resolution, Sharpness)

Density—mass per unit volume

Density, radiographic—a measure of the percentage of incident light transmitted through a developed film

Detail—feature of film quality in which elements of the patient can be seen on the radiograph—(see Definition, Resolution, Sharpness)

Development—the chemical reduction of the silver ions to metallic silver in the exposed crystals in the film emulsion

Diaphragm—a beam restrictor consisting basically of a sheet of lead with a hole

Diode—a tube containing a cathode and an anode—an x-ray tube is a special type of diode tube

Direct current (DC)—electrical current whose electron flow is continual in one direction

Direct exposure film—film exposed by the direct action of the x-ray photon (see Non-screen film)

Dorsopalmar (DoPa)—a method of describing the direction of the x-ray beam with the entrance dorsal and the exit on the palmar surface prior to exposure of the x-ray film

Dorsoplantar (DoPl)—a method of describing the direction of the x-ray beam with the entrance dorsal and the exit on the plantar surface prior to exposure of the x-ray film

Dorsoventral (DV)—a method of describing the direction of the x-ray beam with the entrance dorsal and the exit ventral prior to exposure of the x-ray film

Dosimeter—an instrument used to detect and measure an accumulated dosage of radiation

Dual focus tube—an x-ray tube that utilizes two focal spots of different sizes

Duplicating film—single emulsion film that is pre-sensitized and produces a duplication of an existing radiograph upon exposure

Effective focal spot—the area of the focal spot as viewed at right angles to the axis of the x-ray tube as though looking through the window of the x-ray tube (see Projected focal spot)

Electromagnetic radiation—the transmission of ionizing energy through space via photons

Electromagnetic spectrum—grouping of those forms of energy capable of propagating energy through space or matter that have appropriate wave length and energy levels

Electron—one of the smallest fundamental particles of an atom with a negative electrical charge

Electron beam—beam of electrons that is accelerated by a high electrical potential and flows from the cathode to the anode in the x-ray tube (see Cathode beam)

Electron volt (eV)—a unit of energy gained by an electron as it is accelerated through a potential difference of 1 volt

Envelope—that part of the x-ray tube made of glass that provides an evacuated path in which the accelerated electrons can travel (see Glass envelope)

Exposure latitude—variation in machine settings that produces a radiograph that remains technically satisfactory (see Latitude)

Exposure time—that period of predetermined time during which x-rays are produced

Extra-focal radiation—photons that originate within the x-ray tube at other than the focal spot (see Off-focus radiation, Stem radiation)

Filament—part of the cathode from which the electron beam originates

Filament circuit (filament heat control circuit)—low tension circuit that heats the tube filament (see Low tension circuit)

Film badge—a photographic film worn by radiation workers and used as a radiation monitor (see Nuclear emulsion monitor)

Film contrast—a basic feature in film production that influences radiographic contrast

Film density—a measure of the percentage of incident light transmitted through a developed film (see Photographic density, Radiographic density)

Film gradient—a measure of the slope of the characteristic curve at any point

Film graininess—a type of radiographic mottle (loss of detail) caused by the size of the individual silver halide crystals

Film holder—a light-tight film-holding case which positions the x-ray film and intensifying screens in intimate contact (see Cassette)

Film latitude—the range of exposure techniques that produces an acceptable radiographic image

Film marker—devices used in identification of the patient radiographed

Film-screen combination—convenient method of referring to a particular radiographic film when used with a particular type of intensifying screen (also Film-screen system)

Film speed—measure of the exposure necessary to produce a given film density (see Speed)

Filter—material placed in the path of the primary beam that selectively absorbs the lower-energy portion of the x-ray beam

Filtration—action of absorbers in the primary beam to selectively remove lower-energy photons

Fine-line grid—a grid constructed with thin lead strips and interspacers used in a stationary mode (also a Lysholm grid)

Fixation—the removal of undeveloped silver halide crystals after development of the film

Fixing time—time required to fix the film (usually 2X or 3X the clearing time)

Fluorescence—emission of visible light radiation following the absorption of radiation from another source

Fluoroscope—technique whereby observation of a particular fluorescent screen permits visualization of movement of internal organs in the body

Focal distance—the perpendicular distance between the focused grid and the convergent line or point at which the grid functions most correctly

Focal range—the range of distances from the tube to the grid that result in the production of an acceptable amount of grid cut-off (see Focusing range, Grid range)

Focal-film distance (FFD)—distance from the target of the x-ray tube to the plane of the radiographic film (see Target-film distance)

Focal spot—that area of the target (anode) which is bombarded by electrons from the cathode

Focused grid—grid in which the lead strips are slightly angled such that lines drawn through the strips intersect above the midline of the grid

Focusing cup—that part of the cathode in an x-ray tube in which sits the filament

Focusing range—the range of distances from the tube to the grid that result in the production of an acceptable amount of grid cut-off (see Focal range, Grid range)

Fogging—generalized grayness added to radiographs due to exposure to some type of undesired non-information-carrying radiation, also includes chemical fogging

Full-wave rectified current—the flow of electrons across the x-ray tube in which the negative portion of the AC cycle is electronically inverted (also Full-wave rectification)

Gamma—the gradient of the linear portion of the characteristic curve that serves as a measurement of radiographic contrast

Gamma ray—a massless, chargeless packet of energy originating from the nucleus of an atom during radioactive decay—a form of electromagnetic radiation

General radiation—a method of x-ray generation in which a fast-moving electron comes close to and is deflected by the positively charged nucleus of an atom—the kinetic energy lost is emitted as a photon (see Bremsstrahlung radiation, Continuous radiation, White radiation)

Geometric unsharpness—loss of detail due to penumbral effects

Glass envelope—the housing for the cathode and anode of the x-ray tube that permits the creation of a vacuum (see Envelope)

Gray—unit of radiation absorbed equal to 1 joule per kg, equivalent to 100 rads

Grid—a device constructed of alternating strips of lead and a radiotransparent medium which are oriented in such a way that most of the primary radiation passes through the grid while most of the scattered radiation is absorbed

Grid cassette—a cassette permanently fitted with a stationary grid

Grid cutoff—loss of primary radiation that results with use of a grid, especially when the grid is not used correctly—focal spot is not positioned on the convergent line for linear focused grids or at the convergent point for crossed focused grids, central beam is not perpendicular to the surface of the grid, grid is used inverted, or any combination of the above

Grid frequency—the number of lead strips in the grid

Grid holder—a device for supporting the grid alone or the grid and cassette especially used with a horizontally directed x-ray beam

Grid pattern—a description of the orientation of the lead strips within the grid

Grid range—the range of distances from the tube to the grid that result in the production of an acceptable amount of grid cut-off (see Focal range, Focusing range)

Grid-ratio—the ratio of the height of the lead strips to the thickness of interspace material

Half-value layer (HVL)—the thickness of any specified material that attenuates or reduces the intensity of a given photon beam by one half

Half-wave rectified circuit—a circuit through which flows an alternating current in which the negative potential portion of the cycle is eliminated by means of a rectifier, the voltage remaining at zero for that period of the cycle (also Half-wave rectification)

Hard x-ray beam—a subjective term indicating a higher energy, more penetrating x-ray beam

Heat units—the product of kVp x mA x seconds of exposure that produces a method of determining the heat produced at the target during a single x-ray exposure

Hurter and Driefield curve (H-D curve)—a curve expressing the relationship between radiation exposure of the film and the resulting film density (see Characteristic curve)

Heel effect—a consequence of the angle of the target of the tube which results in greater radiation intensities on the cathode side as compared to the anode side of the radiation field

Heterochromatic beam—photon beam containing photons with a spectrum of energies (see Polychromatic beam, Heterogenic beam)

Heterogenic beam—photon beam containing photons with a spectrum of energies (see Polychromatic beam, Heterochromatic beam)

High kVp technique—an arbitrary term commonly applied to diagnostic examinations using upward to 100 kVp that produces a radiograph with a longer scale of contrast

High voltage circuit—the electrical circuit that produces the high potential across the x-ray tube

Incoming line voltage monitor—feature of an x-ray machine that monitors the level of the line voltage supplied to the machine providing the opportunity for adjustment (see Line compensation)

Inherent filtration—the filtration provided by all parts of the x-ray tube and housing through which the beam must pass and includes the glass tube envelope, insulating oil, and x-ray window

Intensification factor—the ratio of the exposure required to produce an image without the aid of intensifying screens to the exposure required to produce an equivalent image using intensifying screens

Intensifying screen—a device for converting the energy of the x-ray photons into light photons, thereby increasing the efficiency of radiographic image formation and reducing the x-ray exposure necessary to produce an image (see Screen)

Intensity—the total energy passing through a unit area per unit time

Inverse square law—a mathematical relationship that describes the decrease in radiation intensity with increasing distance from a point source of radiation

Ionization—process of transferring sufficient energy to an electron of an atom to cause its removal resulting in formation of a pair of subatomic particles

Ionization chamber—a device for measuring radiation exposure by collecting the electrical charge carried by the ions produced in a finite air volume by the incident radiation

Ionizing radiation—high energy electromagnetic or particulate radiation that produces ions as it passes through matter

Isotope—an atom possessing the same number of protons (atomic number) with a variation in the number of neutrons (mass number)

keV—thousand electron volts

Kilovoltage (kV)—the potential difference applied across an x-ray tube to accelerate electrons emitted by the cathode toward the anode

Kilovoltage constant potential—the nearly constant potential difference applied across an x-ray tube by a voltage generator that is designed to decrease the voltage fluctuations to less than 5%

kVp (kilovoltage peak, kilovoltage potential)—the maximum potential difference applied between the anode and cathode by a pulsating voltage generator

Latent image—the information contained by the sensitized "centers" in the film emulsion where some of the silver ions in the silver halide crystal have been converted to neutral silver atoms by the action of the incident radiation

Lateral decentering—an error in grid use resulting from the central beam being positioned lateral to the midline of the grid

Latitude—the range of exposure levels that can be imaged on a film and provide useful optical densities (see Exposure latitude)

Light beam diaphragm—adjustable x-ray beam restricting device consisting of adjustable lead sheets incorporating a light beam to indicate the surface area to be exposed (also Light localizer)

Line compensation—feature of an x-ray machine that monitors the level of the line voltage supplied to the machine providing the opportunity for adjustment (see Incoming line voltage monitor)

Line pair—a unit used to provide a quantitative measure of detectable resolution so that resolution of one line pair per millimeter means that lines 1/2 mm wide and 1/2 mm apart can be detected

Linear grid—either focused or nonfocused grid in which the length of the lead strips are all in the same direction

Line focus—a principle that refers to the apparent decrease in the size of the focal spot by the use of an angled target surface

Line radiation—a method of x-ray generation in which a fast-moving electron removes an electron from a shell in an atom in the target and a photon is released after the vacant space in the shell is filled by another electron (see Characteristic radiation)

Line voltage compensator—a device that permits control of the level of voltage that enters the x-ray machine

Low tension circuit—that part of the circuitry of the x-ray machine that heats the tube filament (see Filament circuit)

Magnification—the exaggeration of image size compared to the actual object size due to: 1) the fact that the image-forming radiation does not emanate from a point source, or 2) increased distance between patient and film

Mammography film—a type of non-screen film originally designed specifically for use in mammography

Mass number—a number equal to the sum of the number of protons and neutrons within an atom

Maximum permissible dose (MPD)—level of radiation exposure above background level that has been established for those working with radiation

Milliamperage (mA)—a measurement of the number of electrons that flow across the x-ray tube during an exposure

Milliampere—measure of current flow equal to one thousandths of an ampere

Milliampere-seconds (mAs)—a combination unit which is the product of the tube current expressed in milliamperes and the exposure time expressed in seconds

Monochromatic radiation—description of a photon beam in which all photons are of a single energy (also Monoenergetic radiation)

Motion unsharpness—the image unsharpness caused by movement of the patient, film, or x-ray tube during the exposure

Moving grid—grid that moves during the radiographic exposure (see Alternating grid, Reciprocating grid, Rotating grid, Potter-Bucky grid)

Neutron—a subatomic particle with no electrical charge

Nonfocused grid—a grid in which the lead strips are all perpendicular to the face of the grid (see Parallel grid)

Non-screen film—an x-ray film designed for exposure by x-ray photons (see Direct exposure film)

Nuclear emulsion monitor—a photographic film worn by radiation workers and used as a radiation monitor (see Film badge)

Object-film distance (OFD)—distance between object being radiographed and the film

Off-focus radiation—photons that originate within the x-ray tube at other than the focal spot (see Extra-focal radiation, Stem radiation)

Off-focus grid—an error in grid usage in which the grid is placed outside the range of usable distances

Optical density—a measure of the percentage of incident light transmitted through a developed film

Orthochromatic film—a type of x-ray film that is sensitive to green light

Palmarodorsal (PaDo)—a method of describing the direction of the x-ray beam with the entrance on the palmar surface and the exit on the dorsal surface prior to exposure of the x-ray film

Plantardorsal (PlDo)—a method of describing the direction of the x-ray beam with the entrance on the plantar surface and the exit on the dorsal surface prior to exposure of the x-ray film

Panchromatic film—a type of x-ray film that is sensitive to the entire light spectrum

Parallel grid—a grid in which the lead strips are all perpendicular to the face of the grid (see Nonfocused grid)

Particulate radiation—radiation which transmits energy from point to point in the form of the kinetic energy of moving particles with mass (see Corpuscular radiation)

Permissible dose—the amount of radiation which may be received by an individual within a specified period of time with the expectation of no harmful result

Phosphor—the substance in the intensifying screens that converts energy carried by the x-ray photon into visible light that results in exposure of the x-ray film

Phosphorescence—the emission of light radiation from a substance after a time delay of greater than 10^{-8} seconds following the absorption of radiation from some other source—(if the time delay is less than 10^{-8} seconds see Fluorescence)

Photoelectric absorption—an x-ray absorption process in which the photon interacts with a tightly-bound inner shell electron of an atom—part of the energy of the photon is used to overcome the forces binding the electron to the atom, and the remainder is expressed as kinetic energy of the emitted electron which is termed a photoelectron (also Photoelectric effect, Photoelectric capture)

Photographic density—the darkness of the radiograph determined by the conversion of silver halide crystals into metallic silver (see Film density, Radiographic density)

Photon—a quantum of electromagnetic energy with a quantity of energy the product of its frequency and Planck's constant (see Gamma ray)

Planck's constant—6.625×10^{-27} erg seconds

Pocket ion chamber—a type of direct-reading personnel radiation monitor

Polychromatic beam—a beam of x-rays containing a spectrum of energies (see Heterochromatic beam, Heterogenic beam)

Potter-Bucky diaphragm—a grid that moves during the radiographic exposure (see Alternating grid, Moving grid, Potter-Bucky grid, Reciprocating grid)

Potter-Bucky grid—a grid that moves during the radiographic exposure (see Alternating grid, Moving grid, Potter-Bucky diaphragm, Reciprocating grid)

Primary radiation—the radiation emitted from the x-ray tube (also Primary beam, Primary x-ray beam)

Projected focal spot—the area of the focal spot as viewed at right angles to the axis of the x-ray tube as though looking through the window of the x-ray tube (see Effective focal spot)

Proton—a subatomic particle with a positive charge

Quality—a term referring to the average energy of the x-ray beam

Quantity—a term referring to the total number of photons in the x-ray beam

Quantum mottle—a type of radiographic mottle (loss of detail) due to the statistical variation in the number of photons incident on any given area of the intensifying screen

RAD—acronym for radiation absorbed dose that corresponds to an energy transfer to the irradiated tissue equal to 100 ergs/gm of tissue (see Radiation Absorbed Dose)

Radiation—a mechanism by which energy is propagated from point to point through space or through matter

Radiation Absorbed Dose—dosage that corresponds to an energy transfer to the irradiated tissue equal to 100 ergs/gm of tissue (see RAD)

Radiation monitor—a device for measuring radiation such as film badge monitor or pocket dosimeter

Radioactivity—process whereby certain nuclides undergo spontaneous disintegration and energy is liberated generally resulting in the formation of new nuclides—accompanied by the emission of one or more types of radiation, such as alpha particles, or gamma radiation (also Radioactive decay)

Radiodense—that characteristic of tissue that permits few of the x-ray photons to pass unaffected and causes a reaction on the radiographic film that enables light to be transmitted through the film (see Radiopaque)

Radiograph—a photographic image produced by a beam of penetrating, ionizing radiation after passing through a patient

Radiographic artifacts—any abnormal appearance on the film which is the result of improper storage, handling, exposure, or processing of the film

Radiographic contrast—the differences in optical densities between different portions of the radiograph which enable image details to be visualized—dependent on subject contrast and film contrast that are independent

Radiographic density—the darkness of the radiograph determined by the conversion of silver halide crystals into metallic silver (see Film density, Photographic density)

Radiographic mottle—the nonuniform density of a uniformly exposed film due to quantum mottle, structure mottle, and film graininess

Radiographic quality—description of the degree the shadows identified on the film clearly depict the anatomical features under investigation

Radiography—technique of producing radiographs

Radioisotope—an element with an unstable nucleus having the same atomic number (Z) but a different mass number (A) with a type of radioactive decay that may be particulate or nonparticulate and with an exponential decay

Radiolucent—that characteristic of tissue that permits most of the x-ray photons to pass unaffected and causes a reaction on the radiographic film that prevents light from being transmitted through the film

Radiopaque—that characteristic of tissue that permits few of the x-ray photons to pass unaffected and causes a reaction on the radiographic film that enable light to be transmitted through the film (see Radiodense)

Rare earth screens—newly constructed intensifying screens that utilize rare earth phosphors

Reciprocating grid—grid that moves during radiographic exposure blurring the grid lines (see Alternating grid, Moving grid, Potter-Bucky diaphragm, Potter-Bucky grid)

Rectification—process of changing the flow of electrical current from alternating current to current moving only in one direction

REM—an acronym for roentgen equivalent man that was devised to allow for the fact that the same absorbed dose in rads delivered by different kinds of radiation does not produce the same degree of biologic effect (see Roentgen equivalent man, Sievert)

Resolution—the ability of an imaging system to define the fine details of an object (see Detail, Definition, Sharpness)

Roentgen—the special unit of exposure defined for the interaction between x or gamma radiation in 0.001293 gram of air (1 cc at standard conditions) that results in ionization equal to one electrostatic unit of charge of either sign

Roentgen, Wilhelm Conrad (1845-1923)—Professor of Experimental Physics at Wurzburg, Germany, who discovered x-rays on November 8, 1895

Roentgen equivalent man—a unit that was devised to allow for the fact that the same absorbed dose in rads delivered by different kinds of radiation does not produce the same degree of biologic effect (see Rem, Sievert)

Rotating anode tube—an x-ray tube design in which the anode is a rotating disk with the actual focal area projected onto an annular region thereby distributing heat over a larger area

Rotating grid—grid that moves during radiographic exposure blurring the grid lines (see Alternating grid, Moving grid, Reciprocating grid)

Scale of contrast—description of the relative densities on the radiograph

Scatter radiation—radiation generated as a result of interaction of the photons within the primary beam with tissue or matter which travels in a different direction and is composed of photons of lower energy than the incident photons which created them (see Secondary radiation)

Screen—a device for converting the energy of the x-ray photons into light photons, thereby increasing the efficiency of radiographic image formation and reducing the x-ray exposure necessary to produce an image (see Intensifying screen)

Screen film—film made with thin emulsions that are specifically sensitive to either the blue or green light of fluorescent screens

Screen-film contact—manner in which the film comes into contact with the intensifying screen

Screen unsharpness—the image unsharpness due to the size of the fluorescent crystals comprising the screens, the thickness of the screens, and the closeness of contract between the film and the screens

Secondary radiation—radiation generated as a result of interaction of the photons within the primary beam with tissue or matter which travels in a different direction and is composed of photons of lower energy than the indicent photons which created them—at the energy used in diagnostic energy it is composed of Compton electrons, characteristic x-rays, and photoelectrons (see Scatter radiation)

Self-rectified circuit—an x-ray tube circuit in which the x-ray tube itself serves as a rectifier and only the positive portion of the alternating current cycle is used—a type of half-wave rectified circuit (also Self-rectification)

Sharpness—feature of film quality in which elements of the patient can be seen on the radiograph—(see Detail, Definition, Resolution)

Sievert (Sv)—a unit of dose equivalence in man or mammals resulting from the absorption of x or gamma radiation—1 Sievert equals 100 rem

Sight development—method of wet-tank film processing where the development time is determined visually

Soft x-ray beam—a subjective term referring to a low energy, low penetrating x-ray beam made at low kVp settings

Solarization—a method of sensitizing x-ray film so that it can be utilized as copy film

Spectral response—a way of classifying screen film by the nature of the visible light to which the films are sensitive

Speed—a measure of the exposure necessary to produce a given film density (see Film speed)

Spinning top—a metal disc with a small hole that rotates and can be used to evaluate the accuracy of the timer and the nature of tube rectification

Static electricity—name given to a common film artifact characterized by increased film density due to exposure of a part of the film to static electricity

Stationary anode tube—an x-ray tube design in which the anode is a single immobile structure

Stationary grid—a grid used in a non-movable mode producing a linear pattern of grid lines (linear grid) or a crossed pattern (crossed grid) on the radiograph

Stem radiation—photons that originate within the x-ray tube at other than the focal spot (see Extra-focal radiation, Off-focus radiation)

Structure mottle—a type of radiographic mottle resulting in a loss of radiographic detail due to variations in the structure of the phosphor in the intensifying screens

Subject contrast—the intensity variations in the x-ray beam emergent from the subject due to the differential attentuation throughout the x-ray field due to tissue densities

Subject density—a measurement of the tissue density affecting the number of x-rays that reach the film that has an inverse relationship with radiographic or film density

Target—area of the surface of the anode of the x-ray tube that contains the focal spot

Target-film distance—distance from the target of the x-ray tube to the plane of the radiographic film (see Focal-film distance)

Technique chart—an organized format to ensure good radiographic quality for each radiographic examination dependent on the measurement of tissue thickness, anatomical part to be radiographed, and the age of the patient

Technique (technic) factors—settings of kVp, mAs, distance, intensifying screen speed, film speed, processing chemistry used to produce a diagnostic radiograph

Thermal overloading—misuse of an x-ray tube causing anode cracking or other injury due to excess heat production

Thermionic emission—the process by which free electrons are produced at the cathode of an x-ray tube when the filament is electrically heated so that the thermal energy imparted to the electrons is sufficient to overcome the atomic forces binding them to the atoms of the filament

Thermoluminescent dosimeter—a form of personnel radiation dosage monitor

Three phase x-ray generator—a generator that combines three full-wave rectified circuits slightly out of phase with each other such that the tube voltage varies between 80% and 100% and never falls to zero

Total filtration—the summation of the effect on the x-ray beam of inherent and added filtration

Transformer—electrical device made of two coils of conductive wire which uses the electromagnetic field that surrounds moving electrons to induce a current in the second coil—the number of turns of wire on each coil determines the level of the induced current and the voltage

Tube rating chart—contains information concerning mA, kVp, and exposure time limits for a single exposure

Tungsten—the metal used to form the filament and the target in an x-ray tube because of the high melting point, thermal conductivity, and high atomic number

Unsharpness—loss of detail in a radiographic image

Valve tube—a thermionic diode that permits the flow of current in one direction only

Ventrodorsal (VD)—a method of describing the direction of the x-ray beam with the entrance ventral and exit dorsal prior to exposure of the x-ray film

Voltage—a term used to describe the energy that can be held by an electron

White radiation—a method of x-ray generation in which a fast-moving electron comes close to and is deflected by the positively charged nucleus of an atom—the kinetic energy lost is emitted as a photon (see Bremsstrahlung radiation, Continuous radiation, General radiation)

Xerography—a dry radiographic process in which the sensitive material consists of a plate carrying an electrical charge on its surface—when light falls on the surface, the charge is released—the plate is dusted with a special powder and an image is formed by the powder being attracted and retained in the charged areas

X-ray—very short wavelength electromagnetic radiation which originates from the extranuclear part of an atom (see Photon)

X-ray spectra—the relative distribution of different photon energies within a photon beam